TEXTBOOK OF
GENERAL AND
ORAL MEDICINE

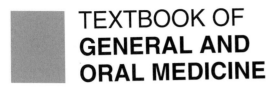

For Churchill Livingstone:

Commissioning Editor: Michael Parkinson
Project Editor: Janice Urquhart
Project Controller: Frances Affleck
Design direction: Erik Bigland
Page make-up: Gerard Heyburn

TEXTBOOK OF GENERAL AND ORAL MEDICINE

David Wray MD BDS MB ChB FDSRCPS FDSRCS(Edin)
Professor of Oral Medicine, University of Glasgow;
Honorary Consultant in Oral Medicine, North Glasgow University Hospitals
NHS Trust, Glasgow, UK

Gordon D. O. Lowe MD FRCP
Professor of Vascular Medicine, University of Glasgow;
Honorary Consultant and Co-Director, West of Scotland Haemophilia Centre,
North Glasgow University Hospitals NHS Trust, Glasgow, UK

John H. Dagg MD FRCP(Glasg) FRCP(Edin)
Honorary Senior Research Fellow, University of Glasgow; Formerly Consultant
Physician, North Glasgow University Hospitals NHS Trust, Glasgow, UK

David H. Felix BDS MB ChB FDSRCS FDSRCPS FDSRCS(Edin)
Consultant in Oral Medicine, North Glasgow University Hospitals NHS Trust;
Honorary Clinical Senior Lecturer, University of Glasgow, Glasgow, UK

Crispian Scully MD PhD MDS FDSRCPS FDSRCS FFDRCSI FDSRCS(Edin) FRCPath FMedSci
Dean and Director of Studies and Research, Eastman Dental Institute for
Oral Health Care Sciences, University of London, UK

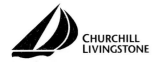

CHURCHILL
LIVINGSTONE

EDINBURGH LONDON NEW YORK PHILADELPHIA ST LOUIS SYDNEY TORONTO 1999

CHURCHILL LIVINGSTONE
An imprint of Harcourt Brace and Company Limited

First published 1999

ISBN 0 443 05189 5

British Library Cataloguing in Publication Data
A catalogue record for this book is available from the British
Library.

Library of Congress Cataloging in Publication Data
A catalog record for this book is available from the Library of
Congress.

Medical knowledge is constantly changing. As new information
becomes available, changes in treatment, procedures,
equipment and the use of drugs become necessary.
The editors, contributors and the publishers have, as far as it
is possible, taken care to ensure that the information given in
this text is accurate and up to date. However, readers are
strongly advised to confirm that the information, especially
with regard to drug usage, complies with current legislation
and standards of practice.

The
publisher's
policy is to use
**paper manufactured
from sustainable forests**

Printed in China

Preface

Health care professionals, regardless of their area of expertise, must have a clear understanding of general medical principles so as to be well placed to provide comprehensive health care. Acquisition of this knowledge must not be overlooked in dentistry which is unique in being taught as an undergraduate medical specialty. A general medical knowledge among the dental profession is also becoming more important because of the increasing numbers of medically compromised patients presenting for treatment. This text, therefore, includes a consideration of general medicine as well as oral medicine and emphasizes the need to integrate an understanding of these two disciplines and highlight areas of overlap.

The first part of this text seeks to educate the student, not only in those aspects of general medicine relevant to oral disease and oral health care, but also in the wide scope of medical disorders which will commonly affect their patients. Thus, this section includes consideration of medical specialties such as dermatology, musculoskeletal disorders and a consideration of reproductive medicine, including pregnancy, and psychological medicine. The general medicine section is designed as a succinct overview of medical problems aimed at clinicians interested in disease processes rather than those directly involved in the treatment of the disorders discussed.

Part two of the text is concerned with the practice of oral medicine. This section is presented in a largely problem-orientated fashion to facilitate differential diagnosis. Because the student will practise oral medicine, this part is necessarily detailed not only in processes of disease but also in management procedures. Oral disease must be treated within the context of general health and so the apposition of information on general and oral medicine is appropriate. The combination of these two subject areas in the one text emphasises the overlap between them and highlights the importance of maintaining a continuum of knowledge throughout the undergraduate curriculum. Students are thus encouraged to read forward to the oral medicine section to gain insight into the relevance of general medicine subjects and to refer back to refresh their memory. The text is also cross-referenced so as to prevent undue repetition.

This textbook is written primarily for undergraduate dental students but is a readable and appropriate source for students of healthcare in any branch of, or those complementary to the medical profession. It will also be useful for postgraduate students studying for exams, especially those working towards the MFDS examination which is designed to test a knowledge of basic sciences integrated with human disease and oral problems. It should also be an invaluable bench book for practitioners engaged in the management of patients with oral soft tissue problems.

The authors hope that the text will be read by all with the enthusiasm and rewards with which it was produced.

Finally the authors would like to record their thanks to Mrs Grace Dobson for typing the manuscript and to Mrs Kay Shepherd and Mrs Gail Drake of the Dental Illustration Department.

D. Wray   Glasgow and London 1999
G. D. O. Lowe
J. H. Dagg
D. H. Felix
C. Scully

Contents

General medicine

Part 1

1 Introduction to general medicine and surgery

Dental students and practising dentists require a knowledge of general medicine and surgery, which should be taught as part of a human disease course in the undergraduate dental curriculum (UK General Dental Council 1997). There are several reasons for this recommendation:

- For effective liaison with other health care professionals:
  - where the patient has coexisting general medical or surgical problems which affect dental practice (e.g. risk of bleeding in patients with bleeding disorders; risk of infective endocarditis in patients with diseased or prosthetic heart valves)
  - where the dentist identifies history or signs of general medical or surgical problems requiring referral (e.g. oral cancer, oral infections suggesting immune deficiency, oral bleeding suggesting bleeding disorders, jaundice, or endocrine disorders such as acromegaly).
- For first aid management of medical emergencies (which may occur in the dental surgery), for example:
  - faints, shock (e.g. anaphylactic shock) or cardiac arrest
  - upper airway obstruction, inhaled foreign body or acute asthma
  - bleeding
  - hypoglycaemia.

- For general knowledge of common diseases and of the principles of disease which one would expect of a health care professional.

The general medicine section of this new textbook replaces *Essentials of Medicine (and Surgery) for Dental Students*, written by teachers of medicine and surgery to dental students at Glasgow University, and published in five editions between 1960 and 1989. It seemed appropriate to the authors and publishers to integrate that part of general medicine and surgery which is relevant to dentists with a textbook on oral medicine, not only to aid cross-referencing but also to emphasize the continuity between general and oral medicine to both undergraduate and postgraduate dentists.

Integration between medicine and surgery progresses in all body systems, and 'general medicine' as covered in this textbook includes mention of surgical aspects of those systemic diseases of which dentists should have some knowledge. Details of surgical procedures are a postgraduate specialty, and are not considered here. Selection of appropriate general medical topics and their presentation in this book has been made with regard to the General Dental Council Guidelines listed above. Following brief chapters on history taking, examination, and the principles of investigation and treatment – the four topics of most importance to dental practice – are considered first. Infections are of dental importance because they often involve the mouth, and because certain infections (e.g. hepatitis B and human immunodeficiency virus (HIV)) may be relevant to the risk of cross-infection in the dental surgery. The cardiovascular system, diseases of the blood and lymph nodes, and the respiratory tract are also considered in some detail because of their dental relevance (General Dental Council 1997). In contrast, chapters on other body systems are relatively short, focusing on common diseases, and include aspects relevant to dental practice (e.g. physical signs which may be observed by the dentist in the clothed patient). Dental students and practitioners seeking more detail on general medical disorders, or on the principles of medicine, are referred to textbooks such as Davidson's *Principles and Practice of Medicine*, also published by Harcourt Brace.

Like medical practice, medical treatments including drugs are constantly changing. In general Part 1 of this book considers only the principles of drug treatment, and quotes commonly used examples of classes of drug. All drug treatments, doses and adverse effects should always be checked in the appropriate national formulary before prescription. In the UK, the *Dental Practitioners'* Formulary is part of the *British National Formulary*, the current version of which should be consulted when prescribing, including prophylaxis of infective endocarditis in dental practice (see Table 6.11).

For management of individual patients, active communication is increasingly important as medical and surgical practice becomes increasingly subspecialized. If there is doubt as to appropriate practice, general dental practitioners are encouraged to seek advice from the patient's general medical practitioner, and/or hospital specialist, or from their local dental hospital.

REFERENCE

General Dental Council 1997. The first five years. The undergraduate dental curriculum. General Dental Council, London

2 Case history taking

History taking is part of the initial communication between any health care professional (dentist, doctor, nurse, therapist, etc.) and his or her patient. Such communication is important for several reasons:

- It is a social and professional introduction.
- It establishes the identities of the professional and his or her patient, and defines his or her roles in the consultation. When a healthy adult patient comes to a general dental practitioner to join the practice, or comes with an acute problem such as toothache, these roles may not be obvious. However, it is appropriate for the dentist to explain his or her role to young children, and to persons with impaired recognition (e.g. those with learning disability, the mentally ill or those confused by acute physical illness or dementia). In clinics, it is important to define who the patient is (when two persons attend together, the person who talks first, or most, is not necessarily the patient!), what his or her problems are, and his or her expectations from the consultation.
- It establishes communication, rapport and trust between the patient and professional, which is important for:
  - elicitation of a full history
  - consent to relevant physical examination, investigations, treatment, and follow-up attendance if required.

Health care professionals learn from their teachers and from their own experiences (positive and negative) a range of professional skills which facilitate communication, rapport and trust. These include:

- An appropriate professional appearance and manner.
- Introducing oneself clearly.
- A considerate approach, appropriate to both the patient's current problem, and to their individual characteristics (e.g. age, intelligence, attitude, mental state such as anxiety, and physical state such as impairment of sight, hearing or mobility).

Current medical problems

Conventionally, medical history taking commences, after preliminary introductions, by identifying the current medical problem(s). This is important, because of the patient's expectation that such problems will be addressed first. It is essential to allow patients to tell their own story, before commencing methodical questioning. 'Leading questions', which suggest the answer, should be avoided: 'open questions', which do not suggest an answer, are preferred.

Having listed these 'presenting symptoms', the practitioner asks further questions which may define both the possible cause of the symptom and its importance to the patient. For example:

- Timing:
  - When did this start?
  - Is it constant, or occasional?
  - If occasional – When does it occur? What makes it worse? What makes it better? (Including self-medications, e.g. analgesics.)
  - Have you had this before? If so, did you attend a doctor/have tests/have treatment?
- Severity, duration and disability – What does it stop you doing? Does it interfere with your work/sleep/family or social life/recreation?
- Questions on pain or discomfort:
  - Site – Where do you feel it most? Can you point to the site?
  - Do you feel it anywhere else? (Radiation.)
  - Character – What does it feel like?

At the end of this part of the history taking, the practitioner should have assessed:

- the patient's current problems
- a differential diagnosis of their causes.

The practitioner then asks a series of relevant questions, often structured by asking in turn about past medical history, family history, social history, drug and allergy history, and a systematic enquiry concerning other symptoms.

Past medical history

This includes:

- previous episodes of similar or related problems, including medical consultations, tests and treatments including hospitalizations and operations
- other previous illnesses, injuries or operations.

Patients may carry warning cards, bracelets or necklets for certain conditions (e.g. allergies, bleeding disorders, endocarditis risk, diabetes or steroid therapy).

Family history

This includes:

- a history of the same problem in blood relatives, which may indicate either a genetic

disorder or predisposition, or common exposure to an environmental factor
- family members, age, cause of death if premature and major illnesses.

Social history

This includes:

- Occupation (current and previous). Specific enquiry concerning occupational exposures (e.g. trauma, fumes or dusts, toxins or noise) and occupational requirements may be relevant.
- Social and family life – partners and relatives.
- Residence. Specific enquiry as to facilities may be appropriate for patients with disabilities.
- Recreations.
- Habits: diet, smoking, alcohol and other recreational drugs.

Drug and allergy history

This includes:

- Current practitioner-prescribed drugs.
- Self-medications.
- Allergies. Details of these should be prominently recorded in the patient's case records, to reduce the risk of prescription. Patients may carry warning cards, bracelets or necklets.

Systematic enquiry

This includes general symptoms (e.g. fever, weight loss), and symptoms related to body systems which have not been considered in the history obtained so far, which may include:

- Infections (see Ch. 5). Hepatitis B and C, HIV and tuberculosis are persistent infections which may be relevant to symptoms in many parts of the body, and which are also capable of cross-infection in clinics and hospitals including the dental surgery.
- Cardiovascular system (see Ch. 6). Congenital heart disease, heart valve disease and

prosthetic heart valves increase the risk of infective endocarditis (including that following certain dental surgical procedures). Chest pain or leg pain on effort, breathlessness and swelling of the legs are common symptoms of cardiovascular disorders.

- Blood disorders (see Ch. 7). Bleeding disorders (e.g. haemophilias), anaemias, leukaemias and lymphomas are of dental relevance. Tiredness, bleeding and swollen glands are common symptoms of blood disorders.
- Respiratory system (see Ch. 8). Asthma, chronic bronchitis and tuberculosis are of dental relevance. Chest pain, breathlessness and cough are common symptoms of chest disorders.
- Nervous system (see Ch. 9). Epilepsy is of dental relevance. Loss of consciousness, headache, disturbance in vision or swallowing, and weakness or sensory disturbance in the limbs are common symptoms of neurological disorders.
- Alimentary tract and liver (see Ch. 10). Liver disease including hepatitis is of relevance. Difficulty in swallowing, vomiting, abdominal pain or swelling, disturbance of bowel habit, and bleeding are common symptoms of alimentary tract disorders.
- Genitourinary system (see Ch. 11). Frequency, difficulty or pain on passing urine, and abnormal discharge or bleeding are common symptoms of genitourinary disease.
- Skin (see Ch. 12). Skin lesions (solitary or rashes), itch or discolorations are common symptoms of skin disease.
- Endocrine and metabolic disorders (see Ch. 13). Symptoms of endocrine and metabolic disorders include changes in weight or temperature, thirst and polyuria (diabetes), and changes in sexual function.
- Musculoskeletal disorders (see Ch. 14). Symptoms of musculoskeletal disorders include pain, joint swelling, and muscle weakness.
- Psychiatric disorders (see Ch. 15). Anxiety and depression are common causes of psychiatric symptoms; hence it is often appropriate to enquire concerning other symptoms suggestive of these diagnoses.

Conclusion

At the end of taking a full history, the practitioner should have refined his or her assessment of the patient's current problems and his or her differential diagnosis; and have assessed their impact on the patient's life in the context of other medical problems, past history, and the family and social context. Examination and investigations can then be performed: these are considered in the following two chapters. However, the importance of the history in diagnosis should be emphasized. For 80% of general medical problems, the diagnosis and management is established by the history; examination alters these in only 10% of patients; and investigations alter these in only the remaining 10%.

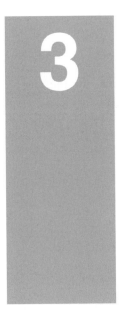

3 Clinical examination

Dentists should be able to observe and interpret physical signs in the clothed patient (General Dental Council – 1997 see Ch. 1). Many such signs give valuable clues to the presence of both organic and functional illness, which may be relevant to both the diagnosis of the patient's presenting complaint, and to the overall management of the patient. Hence, general examination of the patient should be practised by both dentists and doctors as undergraduates; and developed (and never neglected) by postgraduates, however narrow their clinical speciality.

The clinical examination of the patient, whether by doctors or dentists, starts at first encounter. Abnormalities may be noted as soon as outpatients enter the clinic or surgery (e.g. 'illness'; physical disabilities, e.g. walking, sitting, getting on to the dentist's chair, blindness, deafness or speech and language disorder; intoxication; or mental disorders including anxiety, depression, mania, schizophrenia, delirium or learning disability); or become apparent during history-taking, or during dental treatment.

Illness

Assessment of 'illness' in a patient is difficult to define, but develops with clinical experience.

Features may include distress, fever (sweating or warm hands), rapid pulse rate, rapid or difficult breathing, colour change (pallor, jaundice, cyanosis or a grey 'ashen' colour), pain, weakness, obvious weight loss, impaired conscious level or bizarre behaviour. In such patients, the dentist's duties may include:

- A rapid clinical assessment of the patient's medical problem.
- A rapid assessment of their dental problem (if appropriate).
- First aid measures, if required.
- Referral for medical treatment. This may be:
  - an emergency ambulance telephone call (999 in the UK) and/or urgent summoning of medical attention (e.g. a telephone call to the patient's general medical practitioner)
  - a non-urgent contact with the patient's general medical practitioner or hospital specialist (e.g. a letter), with or without postponement of dental treatment as appropriate
  - advice to the patient (or parent/guardian in a child) to attend general medical practitioner.

Physical disabilities

Hemiplegia (weakness of one side of the body) is common and is usually the result of a previous stroke (see Ch. 9); paraplegia (weakness of both legs) is less common and is usually the result of spinal cord injury. Severe arthritis is usually the result of rheumatoid arthritis or osteoarthritis (see Ch. 14). Amputation of the lower limbs usually results from trauma or severe peripheral arterial disease (see Ch. 6), especially in diabetics (see Ch. 13). Such patients may be wheelchair-bound and require assistance with travel to the dentist's surgery or on to the dentist's chair.

Blindness in the UK is usually due to diabetes, glaucoma, macular degeneration, stroke or congenital disease. Such patients may also require assistance in the dental surgery. Deafness in the UK is usually due to old age, middle ear infection, otosclerosis or congenital disease. Such patients may require a hearing aid and loud, clear verbal communication. Speech and language disorders include dysphasia (difficulty in understanding or producing language) and dysarthria (difficulty with forming speech), and are most commonly due to a previous stroke (see Ch. 9). Written communication may be helpful in dysphasia. Intoxication with alcohol may reflect fear of attending the dentist; and is suspected in patients who are garrulous, dysarthric, ataxic and smell of alcohol; however similar features may occur in cerebellar disorders (see Ch. 9) or hypoglycaemia, e.g. diabetics who have taken insulin but have not eaten before visiting the dentist (see Ch. 13). Intoxication with other recreational drugs is increasingly common in Western countries, especially in the young.

Mental disorders (see Ch. 15)

Anxiety is common in patients attending the dentist, and its management is an important part of dental practice.

Depression is common in middle-aged and older patients, and should be suspected in persons with atypical facial pain, a depressed affect (mood), crying or retarded thought and movement. Rapid contact with the patient's general medical practitioner may be appropriate because of the risk of suicide.

Mania presents with pathological hyperactivity and excitement. Urgent summoning of medical

attention is required because of the risks to the patient.

Schizophrenia may present with bizarre behaviour, beliefs and statements; or with a withdrawn, catatonic state. Again, urgent summoning of medical attention is appropriate.

Delirium presents with confusion, disorientation, and clouding of consciousness. Again, urgent summoning of medical attention is appropriate.

Learning disability is usually readily apparent: there may be features of Down's syndrome. The presence of a familiar relative or helper is often useful during dental treatment.

Habitus

Dwarfism may be due to congenital achondroplasia, or growth hormone deficiency (see Ch. 13). Gigantism is due to growth hormone excess before puberty (see Ch. 13). Obesity is common, and often associated with type 2 diabetes mellitus, hypothyroidism, or Cushing's syndrome or corticosteroid drugs (see Ch. 13). Weight loss may be a feature of type 1 diabetes mellitus or hyperthyroidism (see Ch. 13), anorexia nervosa (see Ch. 15), cancer or chronic infections. A humped back may be due to congenital kyphoscoliosis, osteoporosis with vertebral collapse (see Ch. 14), Cushing's syndrome or corticosteroid drugs. Joint deformities may be observed in the gait, or hands, from rheumatoid arthritis, osteoarthritis or gout (see Ch. 14) or haemophilia (see Ch. 7).

Abnormalities in the head and neck

Characteristic facial appearances of endocrine disorders (see Ch. 13) may be associated with acromegaly, hyper- and hypothyroidism, goitre, Cushing's disease and corticosteroid drugs, and Addison's disease (oral pigmentation). Characteristic appearances may also be observed in neurological disorders (see Ch. 9), including facial palsy (resulting from previous Bell's palsy or stroke), oculomotor palsy, and Parkinson's disease. Colour changes include pallor due to anaemia (see Ch. 7), best observed in the conjunctivae; jaundice (Ch. 10), best observed in the sclerae of the eyes; and cyanosis (see Ch. 6), best observed in the lips and tongue. Swellings include parotid swellings (see Ch. 24), cervical lympha-denopathy (see Chs. 7 and 27), and midline neck swellings, e.g. goitre (see Ch. 13).

Skin (see Ch. 12)

Rashes apparent in the face include atopic eczema or measles (see Ch. 8) in children, acne in teenagers, impetigo, erysipelas, urticaria, rosacea, seborrhoeic dermatitis, psoriasis (scalp), drug rashes, and the 'butterfly' rash of systemic lupus erythematosus (see Ch. 14). Skin neoplasms include basal cell and squamous cell carcinomas, and melanomas.

Other manifestations of systemic disease in the head, neck and face

These are considered in the second part of this book.

Other aspects of medical examination

Following general examination as outlined above, medical examination of the patient usually precedes systematically as follows:

- **Cardiovascular system** (see Ch. 6): pulse rate and rhythm, arterial blood pressure, jugular venous pressure, auscultation of the heart with a stethoscope for heart sounds and murmurs,
peripheral arterial pulses, oedema, and signs of peripheral arterial or venous insufficiency.

- **Respiratory system** (see Ch. 8): respiratory rate and effort, palpation of trachea and chest expansion, percussion of the chest to detect dullness (collapse, consolidation, pleural effusion), and auscultation of the chest with a stethoscope for respiratory sounds.

- **Alimentary system** (see Ch. 10) and genitourinary system (see Ch. 11): abdominal and genital inspection (e.g. swelling or scars), palpation (tenderness; organs, e.g. enlarged liver, spleen or kidneys; masses, e.g. tumours, aneurysm, hernia); percussion and auscultation, and rectal and vaginal examination if appropriate. Specific verbal explanation and consent should be obtained by doctors for the latter procedures, due to their intimate nature.

- **Skin** (see Ch. 12): rashes and swellings.

- **Musculoskeletal system** (see Ch. 14): joint deformity, swelling, tenderness and function; bone deformity, swelling and tenderness; and nodules.

- **Nervous system** (see Ch. 9), **and psychiatric examination** (see Ch. 15) if appropriate: conscious level; orientation and cognitive function; memory; cranial nerves; limbs – motor function (tone, power and coordination), sensory function, reflexes.

- **Examination of the eyes, ears, nose and throat:** to include: ophthalmoscopy, otoscopy, rhinoscopy and laryngoscopy if appropriate. Specialist referral to ophthalmologists and ear, nose and throat surgeons is often required in these specialized areas.

- **Examination of the mouth and teeth:** referral to dental surgeons and oral medicine specialists is often required in these specialized areas.

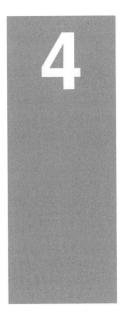

4 Investigations and treatment

Dentists should be aware of the investigations which may be required to establish diagnosis of general medical and surgical problems; and of the principles of treatment, including drug prescription. They should also gain experience of emergency care, and know how to give subcutaneous, intramuscular and intravenous injections (General Dental Council 1997 – see Ch. 1).

Investigations

Following history taking and examination, investigations may be required to confirm or exclude the most likely diagnoses. The general principles are briefly stated here.

Informed consent

While most patients consent to a health care professional taking a history and performing relevant clinical examination, patients may be more concerned about investigations. Routine urine testing is usually accepted as part of medical and insurance examinations. Venepuncture to obtain blood for tests may be complicated by haematomas, infection and even inadvertent arterial puncture; furthermore, the patient may fear the consequences of blood tests (e.g. HIV, hepatitis virus,

cholesterol or genetic tests, which can have implications for their social life or insurance). Hence an explanation of venepuncture and proposed blood tests is required: patients may sometimes refuse consent for such tests. Radiological and other imaging tests often involve radiation exposure, while invasive procedures carry risks of morbidity and even mortality. Hence doctors and dentists should routinely explain the nature of investigations and obtain verbal informed consent (and, for invasive or risky procedures, signed, dated, witnessed, informed consent).

Urine testing

This is routinely performed (with 'dip-sticks') as part of routine medical (including insurance) examinations. It may reveal:

- Glycosuria. This may lead to diagnosis of diabetes mellitus (see Ch. 13), and requires specialist referral.
- Ketonuria. This may be a sign of diabetic ketoacidosis (see Ch. 13), or starvation.
- Bilirubin or urobilinogen. Either of these may indicate hepatobiliary disorders (see Ch. 10) or haemolytic anaemia (see Ch. 7), and require specialist referral.
- Proteinuria or haematuria. Either of these may be due to menstruation, or indicate renal or

urinary tract disease (see Ch. 11), requiring specialist referral.

Urinary culture and microscopy is indicated in persons with proteinuria or haematuria, or with clinical symptoms of urinary tract infection or fever, to exclude urinary tract infection (see Ch. 11).

Blood testing

Blood is routinely obtained by venepuncture from veins in the antecubital fossa, forearm or dorsum of the hand. A tourniquet is applied to distend the veins and render them visible or palpable; and released before the needle is withdrawn. The skin should be cleaned with an alcohol or iodine-soaked swab. A 21G (green hub) or 23G (blue hub) needle is used routinely. Care should be taken to dispose of needles into a sharps box (see section on injections below). Pressure with a swab should be applied to the puncture site for several minutes, to minimize bleeding, and a plaster applied (unless the patient is allergic to these). Blood testing is often required for haematological investigations (see Ch. 7), or biochemical investigations:

- Full blood count. This is one of the laboratory investigations most frequently requested because anaemia and changes in the white blood cell count occur so commonly in a wide variety of diseases. Five millilitres of blood is anticoagulated with dry potassium edetate (EDTA) and should be received in the haematology laboratory within 24 h. Blood cells are usually counted and sized in automatic blood cell counters.
- Blood film. This is prepared from the same sample if indicated by the history, or by the blood count results, for visual inspection of blood cells.
- Erythrocyte sedimentation rate (ESR) or plasma viscosity. These tests can also be performed on the same sample, and are global measurements of non-specific plasma protein changes in disease: principally, increases in the concentration of certain globulins, and a fall in the albumin level. The ESR also increases with anaemia.
- Coagulation screen. This is required to diagnose coagulation disorders. Five millilitres of blood is anticoagulated with liquid sodium citrate and should be received in the haematology laboratory within 4 h (or within 24 h for warfarin control by the prothrombin time).
- Serum iron, transferrin, ferritin, folate and vitamin B_{12} (cobalamin). Levels of these are useful in the diagnosis of anaemias due to deficiencies. Ten millilitres of blood is added to a plain tube, and should be received in the haematology laboratory within 24 h.
- Blood grouping and cross-matching. These are required prior to blood cell transfusion. Ten millilitres of blood is added to a plain tube, and should be received in the haematology laboratory within 4 h.
- Blood glucose. This requires a special tube (sodium fluoride), and is used to diagnose hypoglycaemia or hyperglycaemia, which is often due to diabetes mellitus (see Ch. 13).
- Serum urea, creatinine and electrolytes. These require a plain tube (no anticoagulant), and are used to diagnose renal failure (raised urea and creatinine levels) and electrolyte disturbance (see Ch. 11).
- Serum liver function tests. These require a plain tube and include measurement of bilirubin, alanine aminotransferase, alkaline phosphatase, albumin and globulin, which are useful in the diagnosis of jaundice, liver and biliary tract disorders (see Ch. 10).
- Serum calcium, phosphate and alkaline phosphatase. These require a plain tube, and are useful in the diagnosis of metabolic bone disease (see Ch. 14).
- Serum cardiac enzymes. These require a plain tube, and include measurement of creatine kinase, aspartate aminotransferase and lactate dehydrogenase, which are useful in the diagnosis of acute myocardial infarction (see Ch. 6).
- Serum lipids (cholesterol and triglyceride, lipoproteins). These require a plain tube, and are used to diagnose hyperlipidaemia (see Ch. 6).
- Hormones. These are assayed in the diagnosis of endocrine disorders (see Ch. 13).
- Arterial blood gases (pO_2, pCO_2, H^+ and bicarbonate). These require arterial puncture (usually the radial or brachial artery) and a heparinized syringe. They are used in the diagnosis of respiratory failure (low pO_2, $\pm$ raised pCO_2) (see Ch. 8) and in assessment of acid-base

balance (e.g. diabetic ketoacidosis (see Ch. 13) or renal failure (see Ch. 11).

Immunological investigations

These are performed on serum, and include rheumatoid factor, antinuclear factor and organ-specific autoantibodies.

Microbiological investigations

These include serum antibodies against specific infective agents, and blood cultures in the diagnosis of septicaemia, infective endocarditis and other bacterial infections (see Ch. 5).

Radiological investigations

Pregnancy should always be excluded (risk of fetal irradiation) before performing radiography or other imaging procedures which involve radiation exposure, especially to the abdomen and pelvis.

Plain radiography

This is useful in the diagnosis of fractures, dislocations, bone and tooth disorders, joint disease and foreign bodies. The chest radiograph is valuable in chest disease, heart disease (e.g. heart failure) and in the investigation of general medical problems such as malaise, fever or weight loss (e.g. bronchial carcinoma, tuberculosis and other chest infections). Abdominal radiographs are valuable in diagnosis of gastrointestinal obstruction or perforation, renal stones or gallstones.

Computerized tomography (CT)

CT integrates information from multiple radiographic 'slices' into images of internal organs and tissues, e.g. brain, orbit, sinuses, neck, chest, abdomen and pelvis.

Magnetic resonance imaging (MRI)

MRI also gives sensitive images of the internal organs and tissues, e.g. the brain or spine. It cannot be used in the presence of metal.

Ultrasound scanning

This does not involve radiation exposure, and gives images of internal organs (e.g. heart, abdominal and pelvic organs) and the fetus during pregnancy, as well as imaging blood flow disturbance (e.g. carotid stenosis in the investigation of ischaemic stroke or transient cerebral ischaemic attacks; venous thrombosis or insufficiency in the lower limb; peripheral arterial disease; or aortic aneurysms).

Isotope scanning

This involves intravenous injection of radioactive compounds and visualization of organs with a γ camera. It is most commonly used in the diagnosis of lung disorders (pulmonary embolism) and thyroid disorders (goitre or hyperthyroidism).

Angiography

Angiography is an invasive procedure which requires written, informed consent. It involves injection of radiopaque contrast media into arteries (arteriography, e.g. coronary arteries; aortic arch and carotid and vertebral arteries; lumbar aorta and lower limb arteries; mesenteric or renal arteries) or veins (venography, e.g. diagnosis of deep vein thrombosis in the lower limbs). Arteriography is often combined with angioplasty in the treatment of ischaemic heart disease or peripheral arterial disease (see Ch. 6).

Other contrast studies

These include sialography (see Ch. 24), intravenous urography to image the urinary tract; barium studies of the alimentary tract (barium meals or enemas), and bronchography. The last two are invasive procedures which require written informed consent.

Endoscopy

Endoscopies are invasive procedures which require written informed consent. They are useful investigative and therapeutic tools:

• Flexible endoscopes utilize fibreoptics to visualize internal organs.

• Through separate channels, endoscopes can be used to obtain secretions, washings or biopsies for microbiological, cytological and histological diagnosis of infections, neoplasms and other disorders.

• Per-endoscopic therapeutic procedures can be performed, e.g. haemostasis in gastrointestinal bleeding, and resections of colonic or bladder polyps.

• Example procedures include bronchoscopy, upper gastrointestinal endoscopy (which may include endoscopic retrograde cholangiopancreatography), colonoscopy, cystoscopy (urinary bladder), laparoscopy (peritoneal cavity), and arthroscopy (joints).

Other biopsies

These include biopsies of oral lesions (see part 2 of this book), skin lesions, lymph nodes, lung, pleura, liver, kidney, bone and bone marrow. Written informed consent should be obtained.

Function tests

These include exercise tests for the diagnosis of ischaemic heart disease and peripheral arterial disease, lung function tests, oesophageal function tests, bladder function tests, endocrine tests, and specialized tests of the eye, ear and brain.

Electrophysiological tests

These include electrocardiography (see Ch. 6), electroencephalography (see Ch. 9) and electromyography.

Treatment

Treatment, medical or dental, is more than the prescription of drugs and the performance of surgical procedures. It encompasses professional management of the whole patient, in the context of his or her individual perceptions, general health problems, and social context (as elicited by the history and examination). It includes:

• a professional assessment
• an explanation of identified problems (their nature and possible outcomes) to the patient (and, if appropriate and with the patient's consent, to parents, partners or relatives), in a manner which can be understood easily (avoiding professional jargon)

• an explanation of the proposed management (investigations, treatments and referral to other healthcare professionals), including options for discussion of patient preferences

• advice on what patients themselves can do for their problems, including support from family, partners, friends and other bodies (e.g. obesity, alcohol, smoking or other drug support groups; disease-specific support groups, e.g. local stroke clubs, national societies such as the Haemophilia Society)

• reassurance where appropriate (doctors can make their patients unduly anxious)

• a sympathetic approach: 'to cure sometimes, to help often, to comfort always'.

Principles of drug treatment

Drug prescription is an important part of medical and dental practice. In the UK, a valuable source of information and advice is the *British National Formulary* (BNF), published by the British Medical Association and the Royal Pharmaceutical Society of Great Britain, which is available to all medical and dental practitioners and which includes the *Dental Practitioners' Formulary*. Dental as well as medical undergraduates and postgraduates are well advised to study the general sections of the BNF, and to consult it when prescribing. It is revised twice yearly, to take account of the numerous changes which occur as a result of new information, and the current issue should always be consulted. An electronic version is now available, and development as an intelligent decision-support and prescribing tool is in progress.

The BNF should be consulted for detailed guidance on drug prescription. Some general principles are highlighted here:

• Drug prescriptions must be generic (non-proprietary) if prescribing within the National Health Service, written legibly in English and complete so that the pharmacist can issue the drug to the patient rapidly.

• the prescriber should warn the patient of possible adverse effects. These include:

– Drowsiness. This can occur with carbamazepine (an anticonvulsant, also used in trigeminal neuralgia), chlorpheniramine (an antihistamine), diazepam, nitrazepam and temazepam (benzodiazepine anxiolytics), and dihydrocodeine and pethidine (opiate analgesics). It can affect the performance of skilled tasks (e.g. driving or working with machinery) and the effect is enhanced by alcohol (which should be avoided).

– Allergic reactions, e.g. skin rashes. These often occur with antimicrobials, especially penicillins (e.g. amoxicillin, ampicillin and phenoxymethylpenicillin) and carbamazepine, especially in patients with a history of drug allergy, asthma or hay fever.

– Bone marrow aplasia. This may occur with carbamazepine, and results in anaemia, neutropenia or thrombocytopenia (see Ch. 7). Patients or their carers should be advised to seek immediate medical attention in the event of fever, sore throat, rash, mouth ulcers, bruising or bleeding.

• Drug abuse and dependence are frequent with temazepam (e.g. intravenous injection of the contents of gelatin capsules – 'jellies' – has become epidemic in Glasgow, resulting in a local ban on their prescription), diazepam, nitrazepam, dihydrocodeine and pethidine. Advice on prescribing drugs likely to be misused or raise dependence is given in the BNF, and includes limitation to the lowest dose for the shortest possible time, and care in patients with a history of alcohol or drug abuse or marked personality disorder.

• Care should be taken to avoid certain drugs, or to reduce the dose, in special patient groups:

– children:
  a. guidance on doses is given in the BNF
  b. certain drugs should be avoided, e.g. aspirin should not be given to children under 12 years of age because of the risk of Reye's syndrome
– pregnancy – check the BNF
– the elderly:
  a. the dose may have to be reduced – check the BNF
  b. multiple-drug prescription is common, but should be minimized
  c. clear directions should be given to patients and carers
– bleeding disorders (see Ch. 7) – aspirin and intramuscular injections should be avoided in patients taking anticoagulant drugs, in haemophilia and in thrombocytopenia
– liver disease (see Ch. 10) – doses of drugs which are eliminated by the liver may have to be reduced
– kidney disease (see Ch. 11) doses of drugs which are eliminated by the kidney may have to be reduced.

• Emergency treatment of poisoning, including drug overdose, is summarized in the BNF, which also gives telephone numbers of regional poison information centres that provide 24 h advice. First aid management of the unconscious or semiconscious patient is discussed in Chapter 9.

Injections

Dentists should know how to give subcutaneous, intramuscular and intravenous injections (General Dental Council 1997 – see Ch. 1). Techniques are best learned by practical experience in clinics; however some principles are given here. Dental students gain much practical experience in mucosal injections of local anaesthetics, which is relevant to subcutaneous injection.

• Parenteral administration of drugs by injection is given to achieve a local effect (e.g. subcutaneous injection of local anaesthetic prior to local procedures), to achieve a rapid effect, or to give drugs which cannot be absorbed orally (e.g. insulin or heparin, coagulation factors).

• Sterile, disposable needles and syringes should be used (and not reused), to avoid cross-infection (e.g. with hepatitis B or HIV).

• To avoid infection at the injection site, the skin should be cleaned (e.g. with an alcohol or iodine-soaked swab), infected areas of skin avoided, and the needle should not be touched by the person giving the injection after it is removed from its sterile sheath.

- After injection, great care should be taken to immediately dispose of the needle into an adjacent, secure, leakproof 'sharps container', to avoid the risk of needle-stick injury to the person giving the injection or to others. Sharps containers should be carefully disposed of and not allowed to become full. In particular, resheathing of the needle before its disposal into the sharps container should be avoided as this is a common cause of needle-stick injury. Needle-stick injury can transmit hepatitis B (hence all health care personnel in contact with patients should be vaccinated: see Ch. 5), HIV and other infections. Clear local protocols for management of needle-stick injury should be available in all clinics and situations where injections are given.
- After injections, anaphylactic shock (see Ch. 6) may occur, especially with antimicrobials such as penicillins.

Subcutaneous injection

This is used for local anaesthesia, for injection of insulin or heparin (including self-injection of insulin at home by insulin-dependent diabetics (see Ch. 13)), for emergency self-injection of adrenaline in persons with anaphylactic reactions (e.g. to insect stings (see Ch. 6)), and for injection of opiate analgesics. The last can also be given by continuous subcutaneous infusion in the palliative care of hospital patients with terminal disease. Continuous subcutaneous infusion of fluids for hydration is also given when there is no intravenous access. Subcutaneous injections can be given into a skinfold, pinched up over the anterior abdominal wall or anterior thigh, with vertical insertion of a 25G (orange hub) needle. In diabetics giving themselves regular injections, the sites should be rotated to avoid local fibrosis.

Intramuscular injection

This is used to obtain a more rapid effect than a subcutaneous injection, and where intravenous injection is impractical or carries a greater risk of anaphylactic or cardiac stimulant reaction. A 23G (blue hub) needle is used. Examples include:

- adrenaline in the emergency treatment of anaphylactic shock (see Ch. 6)

- glucagon, in the emergency treatment of hypoglycaemia (see Ch. 13)
- antipsychotics (e.g. chlorpromazine, or haloperidol) in the emergency treatment of acute psychosis (see Ch. 15).
- antimicrobials, e.g. benzathine penicillin in the prophylaxis of rheumatic fever (see Ch. 6).

Adverse effects of intramuscular injections include:

- Pain due to local haematoma formation. Intramuscular injections are contraindicated in patients with coagulation disorders, e.g. haemophilia or induced by anticoagulant therapy (see Ch. 7).
- Nerve damage, which may lead to paralysis, especially in bleeding disorders. This risk is minimized by using either the upper, outer quadrant of the gluteus maximus muscle in the buttock or the deltoid muscle in the upper, outer arm.

Intravenous injection

This is used to achieve a rapid effect in emergencies (e.g. adrenaline in the management of cardiac arrest (see Ch. 6), diazepam in status epilepticus (see Ch. 9), heparin in acute pulmonary embolism (see Ch. 6)). Intravenous infusion through an indwelling catheter is used when administration by other routes is not possible (e.g. blood transfusion (see Ch. 7) or fresh frozen plasma or coagulation factor concentrates (see Ch. 7)). Intravenous infusion is also the route of choice for hydration with intravenous fluids (e.g. saline or dextrose) when oral intake of fluids is not possible (e.g. unconsciousness or semiconsciousness, impaired swallowing (e.g. after stroke), vomiting, or fasting prior to surgery or other procedures). It is also the preferred route for antimicrobial treatment of infective endocarditis (see Ch. 6).

Veins in the antecubital fossa are preferred for intravenous injections; and forearm or dorsal hand veins (which allow joint mobility) for intravenous infusions. Following insertion of the needle (usually 21G (green hub) or 23G (blue hub)) or catheter, intravenous entry should be confirmed by aspiration of blood, and by the absence of local pain or swelling on injection or infusion. Intravenous catheters should be taped in place, and sterile precautions (and rotation of catheter sites) observed to minimize the risk of local thrombosis and sepsis. When prolonged intravenous access is required (e.g. in treatment of endocarditis (see Ch. 6) or malnutrition), a central venous catheter can be inserted (under full sterile conditions) into the internal jugular or subclavian veins. Such central catheters are also useful in monitoring central venous pressure and intravenous fluid replacement in circulatory shock (see Ch. 6).

Principles of surgical treatment

Surgical treatment is increasingly specialized, and has therefore become a postgraduate rather than an undergraduate subject. The General Dental Council (1997 – see Ch. 1) recommends that dental students gain experience in accident and emergency departments of the treatment of acutely ill patients by observing the procedures of triage and resuscitation (see Chs. 6 and 9). Hospital dentists may also be involved in patients with facial fractures as part of multiple injuries, and hence should have knowledge of the surgical management of such patients. These areas are outwith the context of the present book. Dental students and practitioners are referred to text-books such as *Principles and Practice of Surgery*, also published by Harcourt Brace.

5 Infections

Infection is a major cause of disease and death worldwide. A knowledge of the diagnosis and treatment of local and systemic infection is therefore essential. In addition, infections can be transmitted to and by health care workers, making an understanding of cross-infection of paramount importance. Health care workers should also be aware of the possibility of endogenous infections such as endocarditis arising after dental work or infective complications of an inhaled foreign body.

Treatment of infection carries its own risk and health care professionals should be familiar with the adverse effects of antimicrobials which may be severe. Adverse effects and drug reactions are found in the *British National Formulary*.

Many infections are dealt with in the individual chapters dealing with the major organ or system involved. Systemic infections of importance, e.g. HIV, syphilis, are considered here in detail.

Viral infections

Viruses comprise a strand of nucleic acid (either DNA or RNA) enclosed in a protein shell. They grow only within living cells, which they may either destroy, causing acute disease, or transform into neoplastic cells over a longer time period by combining with host cell nucleic acid.

The general symptoms of acute viral infections are well known, due to the universal experience of common virus infections such as upper respiratory tract infections (see Ch. 8):

- fever
- malaise
- muscle pain (myalgia), tenderness and weakness.

The general signs of acute viral infections are:

- slow pulse rate (bradycardia – see Ch. 6)
- low blood pressure (hypotension – see Ch. 6)
- low blood white cell count (leucopenia – see Ch. 7) with relative lymphocytosis.

The diagnosis of a virus infection may be by:

- microscopy, e.g. herpesviruses in skin biopsies, hepatitis B in liver biopsies, viruses in stools, or rabies virus in brain biopsy
- detection of antigen, e.g. hepatitis B or C
- serology – detection of antibody (e.g. HIV or hepatitis A, B or C).

Antiviral drugs interfere with viral nucleic acid or protein synthesis, and include:

- aciclovir, penciclovir and famciclovir – for herpes zoster and herpes simplex infections (see Ch. 22)

- ganciclovir – for cytomegalovirus infection in immunosuppressed patients, e.g. HIV (see below)
- anti-HIV drugs (see below).

RNA viruses

Table 5.1 summarizes the RNA viruses, their clinical features, and the chapters which detail their features and management. HIV infection is considered in detail because of its importance.

Human immunodeficiency virus (HIV) infection and the acquired immune deficiency syndrome (AIDS)

In 1981, cases of a rare neoplasm (Kaposi's sarcoma) and a rare opportunistic infection (*Pneumocystis carinii* pneumonia), both of which had only been reported in patients with severe immunosuppression (due to genetic, neoplastic or drug causes; see Ch. 23), were reported in the USA in previously healthy homosexual men. This epidemic was termed the acquired immune deficiency syndrome (AIDS), which in 1984 was discovered to be due to a new RNA retrovirus, subsequently named the human immunodeficiency virus (HIV). Worldwide, over 20 million people are now thought to be infected with HIV. All countries are involved, but particularly central Africa, South America, the Indian subcontinent and South-East Asia. The high prevalence of this usually disabling and fatal infection in young adults poses major social and economic problems for these countries in the twenty-first

Table 5.1 Diseases due to RNA viruses

Family	Genus or type	Disease
Arenaviruses	Lassa fever	Tropical haemorrhagic fevers (often lethal)
Bunyaviruses	Hantaviruses	
Filoviruses	Marburg/Ebola fever	
Flaviruses	Hepatitis C	Hepatitis (see Ch. 10)
Orthomyxoviruses	Influenza	Respiratory tract infections (see Ch. 8)
Paramyxoviruses	Parainfluenza	
	Mumps	
	Measles	
	Respiratory syncitial virus	
Picornaviruses	Rhinoviruses	
	Enteroviruses	
	Coxsackie viruses	Myocarditis, pericarditis (see Ch. 6)
		Gastroenteritis (see Ch. 10)
	Echoviruses	Pharyngitis (see Ch. 8)
		Meningitis
	Polioviruses	Poliomyelitis (see Ch. 9)
	Hepatitis A	Hepatitis (see Ch. 10)
Retroviruses	Human immunodeficiency virus: HIV-1 and -2	HIV infection/AIDS
	Human T-lymphotropic viruses (HTLV -I and -II)	Leukaemia (see Ch. 7)
Rhabdoviruses	Rabies virus	Rabies (see Ch. 9)
Togaviruses	Rubella virus	Rubella (see Ch. 8)
	Flaviviruses	Yellow fever / Dengue — Tropical fevers
Other	Hepatitis D (incomplete virus)	Hepatitis (see Ch. 10)
	Hepatitis E	

century. Furthermore, HIV-infected persons often develop tuberculosis, which after a brief period of increasing control by antituberculous chemotherapy over the last 40 years has resumed its historical place as the commonest worldwide cause of death (see Ch. 8).

Retroviruses have an RNA genome, and the unique property of transcribing a DNA copy of this genome using the enzyme reverse transcriptase, following penetration of the host cell. The virus principally infects CD4 T-helper lymphocytes, binding to the CD4 receptor using the viral surface membrane glycoprotein 120. The viral DNA may then lie dormant within the cell, or undergo replication of the virus, which buds from the cell surface and is then available to infect other cells. There are two subtypes of HIV: HIV-1 occurs mainly in western Europe, North America and central Africa; while HIV-2 is found mainly in west Africa. The clinical symptoms of these subtypes are similar, and are due to three major effects of HIV infection:

1. Progressive reduction in circulating CD4 lymphocytes (normal blood concentration over 500×10^6/litre), resulting in generalized immunodeficiency, especially cell-mediated immunity (which normally protects against intracellular parasites, e.g. viruses, protozoa and mycobacteria). Failure of antibody responses results in infection with capsulated bacteria. Monitoring of the blood CD4 count allows some prediction of the onset of progressively more severe opportunistic infections or neoplasms (Fig. 5.1; see also Ch. 7) and estimation of survival; and the need for antiretroviral drugs, or antimicrobial prophylaxis of opportunistic infections.

2. Infection of the central nervous system sometimes causes acute viral meningitis or encephalitis at the time of seroconversion, but

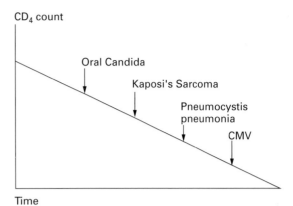

Time

Fig. 5.1 Spectrum of diseases in HIV infection. As the CD4 lymphocyte count in the blood declines, characteristic opportunist infections and neoplasms present clinically.

more commonly chronic infection (encephalopathy, meningitis, myelopathy or peripheral neuro-pathy). This may occur due to migration of HIV-infected monocytes to the brain, where they become microglial cells.

3. Virally-induced tumours.

Transmission of HIV

Transmission of HIV requires exchange of virally infected blood or other body fluids (semen, vaginal secretions or breast milk). Hence the main methods of transmission are sexual intercourse, intravenous drug use with sharing of needles or other equipment, vertical transmission *in utero*, breast feeding, transfusion of infected blood or blood products, and, rarely, organ transplantation. The risk of sexual transmission is higher with anal than with vaginal intercourse, greater for the recipient of penetrative sex (by either route), and is increased by genital trauma or ulceration (such as occurs from other sexually transmitted disorders), as well as by multiple partners. Risk factors for HIV infection are listed in Table 5.2.

Table 5.2 Risk factors for HIV infection	
Sexual transmission	Penetrative (especially for the recipient)
	Anal intercourse
	Genital trauma or ulceration
	Multiple partners
Blood or milk transmission	Intravenous drug use
	Recipient of infected blood, blood products or organs
	Breast feeding by infected mother
Vertical transmission	From infected mother to fetus

The risks from blood or blood products in developed countries have been greatly reduced by screening of blood donors and by viral inactivation of blood products since the 1980s.

Occupational infection of health care workers from HIV-positive patients occurs much less commonly than hepatitis B or C transmission; however, unlike hepatitis B no vaccine is available. Infection is most likely to occur from needle-stick injury (especially when resheathing needles), or prolonged contact of broken skin with contaminated body fluids. Routine precautions against transmission minimize the risk of occupational infection. In the event of occupational exposure to blood or body fluids from a patient with suspected or known HIV infection, health care workers should seek urgent advice from their local occupational health officer, accident and emergency department, or infectious disease unit, according to local protocols. Advice may include risk assessment, counselling and testing for HIV infection, and consideration of a course of prophylactic antiretroviral chemotherapy.

Clinical features of HIV infection

Following a latent period of a few weeks, HIV infection is followed by seroconversion (development of a positive HIV antibody test), which is associated with a short-lived clinical illness in about one-third of patients. Symptoms of such a seroconversion illness include fever, malaise, rash, lymphadenopathy, oral ulceration and, occasionally, encephalitis or meningitis. Patients then become asymptomatic for several years (range 1-15 years or more), although some have persistent generalized lymphadenopathy (PGL). The US Centers for Disease Control (CDC) classification of HIV infection (Table 5.3) classifies patients with these groups of symptoms as Group A.

Group B describes symptoms and signs of progressive HIV infection which are not AIDS-defining, according to the 1987 CDC definition of AIDS. These are listed in Table 5.4, and are sometimes called the AIDS-defining complex.

Group C describes conditions which are AIDS-defining, according to the 1987 CDC definition of the Acquired Immunodeficiency Syndrome. These are listed in Table 5.5. Life expectancy is

Table 5.3 CDC classification of HIV infection

	Clinical group		
Absolute CD4 count ($\times 10^6$/litre)	A	B	C
> 500	A1	B1	C1
200–499	A2	B2	C2
< 200	A3	B3	C3

Group A: acute HIV infection, asymptomatic phase or PGL.
Group B: Symptomatic but not AIDS-defining (see Table 5.4).
Group C: Conditions meeting CDC/World Health Organization case definition for AIDS (see Table 5.5).

Table 5.4 Clinical features of symptomatic HIV disease (group B)

General symptoms	General signs
Fatigue	Lymphadenopathy
Fever	Wasting
Malaise	Oral candidosis ⎫ see Ch. 23
Weight loss	Oral hairy leukoplakia ⎭
Diarrhoea	Herpes zoster (see Ch. 22)
	Immune thrombocytopenia
	Perianal herpes
	Splenomegaly

poor once an AIDS-defining condition is diagnosed (median 18 months); however this is increasing with the use of combination antiretroviral chemotherapy.

In addition to the clinical classification of HIV infection, a decreasing blood CD4 lymphocyte count is associated with an adverse prognosis and is included in the classification (see Table 5.3). Recently, monitoring of blood viral antigenic load has also been used: increasing antigenaemia is associated with an adverse prognosis.

Diagnosis of HIV infection

This is confirmed by demonstrating HIV antibodies in serum, initially by an enzyme-linked immunosorbent assay (ELISA) test, then by confirmation with the more precise Western blot test. The 'window' between infection and seroconversion may be several months, hence repeated testing may have to be performed in patients at risk. HIV antigen levels can also be measured in blood, using the polymerase chain reaction (PCR) test.

Table 5.5 AIDS-defining conditions (group C)

Opportunistic infections
1. Disseminated clinical cytomegalovirus infection (not liver, spleen or lymph nodes)
2. Chronic (> 1 month) mucocutaneous disseminated herpes simplex infection
3. Progressive multifocal leucoencephalopathy (papova (JC) virus)
4. Extrapulmonary tuberculosis or pulmonary tuberculosis with CD4 count < 200×10^6/litre
5. Disseminated *Mycobacterium avium intracellulare* or *Mycobacterium kansasii* infection
6. *Pneumocystis carinii* pneumonia
7. Candidosis of oesophagus, bronchi or lung
8. Chronic (> 1 month) cryptosporidiosis
9. Toxoplasmosis of brain
10. Isosporiasis
11. Disseminated histoplasmosis or coccidioidomycosis
12. Cryptococcosis
13. Extraintestinal strongyloidiasis

Secondary neoplasms
1. Kaposi's sarcoma
2. Primary lymphoma of brain
3. Non-Hodgkin's (immunoblastic) lymphoma

Because of the important medical, psychosocial, financial (life insurance/mortgage) and immigration implications of a positive HIV test, it is important that patients receive adequate pre- and post-test counselling on HIV infection and its possible consequences. Appropriate guidelines for such counselling are available. Practitioners should refer patients with suspected HIV infection and those who request testing to a local counselling and testing clinic. Patients with negative tests should be counselled on risk factor reduction (e.g. safe sex and avoiding sharing needles for intravenous drug use).

Because of the (rare) possibility of transmission of HIV by infected health care workers to their patients, health care workers in direct contact with patients have a duty to seek medical advice if they suspect themselves to be HIV-infected.

Oral manifestations of HIV infection

These are considered in Chapter 23.

Skin manifestations of HIV infection

Skin infections. These are summarized in Table 5.6. Herpes zoster occurs early in HIV infection and often affects more than one dermatome. Chronic herpes simplex infection for more than 1 month is an AIDS-defining diagnosis (see Table 5.5).

Kaposi's sarcoma. This is the commonest opportunistic neoplasm in HIV disease, and is an AIDS-defining condition. Prior to the advent of the HIV epidemic, Kaposi's sarcoma was very uncommon in the USA. However, an endemic form was recognized in parts of Africa, and it also ocurred in Mediterranean Jews. It is common in sexually transmitted HIV infection, but rare in blood-transmitted HIV infection (e.g. in haemophiliacs). This suggests that a sexually-transmitted cofactor is required for its development. A human herpes virus (HHV8) has now been implicated. The sarcoma arises at multiple sites within a short time, usually in the skin (Fig. 5.2), but sometimes in the mouth or hard palate. The nose, penis, limbs (especially lower)

Table 5.6 Skin manifestations of HIV infection

Viral infections	Herpes simplex Herpes zoster } may be disseminated Molluscum contagiosum
Bacterial infections	Staphylococci – folliculitis, impetigo Streptococci – cellulitis Secondary syphilis
Fungal infections	Seborrhoeic dermatitis – *Pityrosporum orbiculare*
Neoplasms	Kaposi's sarcoma Anal carcinoma
Drug rashes	

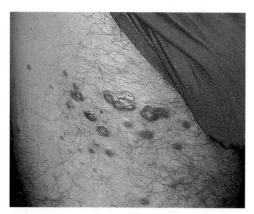

Fig. 5.2 Kaposi's sarcoma affecting the skin of the thigh in an AIDS patient.

and trunk may be involved (see Ch. 23). The lesions are red or violet, well circumscribed, and flat or raised. As the blood CD4 count falls, skin lesions become more aggressive, and lesions occur in the lymph nodes, gut, liver, spleen or lungs.

The diagnosis is confirmed by biopsy: histologically the neoplasm consists of spindle-shaped cells and small, leaky blood vessels. Lesions can be treated by surgery, cryotherapy, local radiotherapy, intralesional chemotherapy or combination cytotoxic therapy.

Anal carcinoma and uterine cervical carcinoma. These are more common in HIV infection, probably due to a higher rate of infection by the human papilloma virus (HPV).

Drug reactions. Drug reactions causing skin rashes are also more common in HIV-infected patients.

Internal manifestations of HIV infection

Many opportunistic infections in AIDS patients are disseminated at clinical presentation, rather than organ-specific. Table 5.5 lists the AIDS-defining disseminated infections, while Table 5.7 lists the common HIV-related problems by organ system.

Table 5.7 Internal manifestations of HIV infection by organ system	

Nervous system	Direct effects of HIV infection
	    Seroconversion illness (encephalitis, meningitis; see Ch. 9)
	    Dementia (see Ch. 15)
	    Myelopathy (see Ch. 9)
	    Peripheral polyneuropathy (see Ch. 9)
	
	Other infections
	    Cytomegalovirus – retinitis, encephalitis
	    Papovavirus (JC virus) – progressive multifocal leucoencephalopathy (PML)
	    Tuberculosis – meningitis, brain abscess
	    Neurosyphilis
	    Cryptococcus neoformans – meningitis
	    Toxoplasma gondii – brain abscess
	
	Tumours – non-Hodgkin's lymphoma (B cell)

Respiratory tract	*Pneumocystis carinii* pneumonia Bacterial pneumonias (pneumococcus) Tuberculosis, *Mycobacterium avium–intracellulare* (MAI) *Candida* spp. Kaposi's sarcoma

Gastrointestinal tract	Oesophagitis – *Candida* spp.
	Intestine – *Cryptosporidium*
	                 Salmonella
	                 Cytomegalovirus

Blood	Immune thrombocytopenia (see Ch. 7)

Cytomegalovirus (CMV). This is a herpesvirus which is a common cause of the glandular fever syndrome (see Ch. 8). Disseminated CMV infection occurs clinically in severe immunosuppresion (CD4 count usually below 50×10^6/litre) and is an AIDS-defining diagnosis (see Table 5.5). In the eye, choroidoretinitis causes haemorrhages and exudates, which can rapidly cause blindness. CMV may also involve the central nervous system, mouth, gut and adrenal glands. Treatment is with intravenous ganciclovir. Pregnant health care workers should avoid contact with HIV positive patients because of the risk of fetal infection with CMV.

Bacterial infections. Bacterial infections, especially with capsulated organisms (pneumococci and salmonellae) are common in HIV infection, and often cause recurrent infection, septicaemia and disseminated infection. Syphilis (see below) and HIV infection commonly coexist.

Tuberculosis. Tuberculosis (see Ch. 8) is common in HIV-infected patients, especially in central Africa and Asia; and is often clinically atypical, and disseminated (outside the lungs). Drug-resistant tuberculosis in HIV-infected patients represents a major problem for both patients and health care workers, who should take appropriate precautions to avoid occupational infection from such patients.

Mycobacterium avium–intracellulare (MAI) and M. kansasii. These are common in severe immunosuppression (CD4 count usually below 50×10^6/litre) and are AIDS-defining diagnoses (see Table 5.5). The usual clinical features are non-specific, and include fever, malaise, night sweats, weight loss, anaemia, lymphadenopathy and hepatomegaly. Diagnosis is by culturing acid-fast bacilli from appropriate specimens. Combination chemotherapy with antimycobacterial drugs is given, as for tuberculosis (see Ch. 8).

Candidosis. Candidosis in the mouth is a common early feature of HIV infection (see Ch. 23). In the later stages of HIV infection, candidal infection often spreads to the oesophagus, bronchi and lung, and then becomes an AIDS-defining diagnosis (see Table 5.5). Oesophageal involvement causes painful difficulty in swallowing, and is diagnosed by endoscopy. Continuous antifungal chemotherapy with an azole drug or amphotericin is required for disseminated infection.

Cryptococcus neoformans. This is the commonest cause of meningitis in AIDS patients, which is often insidious in onset. The fungus is visualized in the cerebrospinal fluid (obtained by lumbar puncture, see Ch. 9) with Indian ink staining. Treatment is with antifungal drugs (an azole drug or amphotericin).

Pneumocystis carinii pneumonia. This is a common, serious protozoal infection in the later stages of HIV infection (CD4 count below 200×10^6/litre or AIDS), and all such patients should be offered primary prophylaxis (e.g. with oral co-trimoxazole). It is an AIDS-defining condition. It usually starts insidiously with a dry cough and breathlessness. Typically, the chest radiography shows diffuse shadowing in both lungs. Diagnosis is by bronchoscopy (see Ch. 8) and bronchoalveolar lavage: *P. carinii* cysts are revealed by silver staining of the lung washings. Treatment is with high-dose co-trimoxazole, given intravenously then orally; followed by secondary prophylaxis.

Toxoplasma gondii. This is a common protozoal infection in humans which, following severe immunosuppression in AIDS patients may cause a brain abscess, that shows as a typical 'ring lesion' on a computerized tomography brain scan (see Ch. 9). Treatment is with pyrimethamine and clindamycin. Prophylaxis of *P. carinii* with co-trimoxazole is also effective in the prophylaxis of toxoplasmosis.

Treatment of HIV infection

This is best managed by an experienced specialist in infectious diseases as part of a multidisciplinary support team (nurse specialists, pharmacists, psychologists, social worker and counsellor), liaising as appropriate with partners, family, friends and patient support groups. Symptomatic care is important in the terminal stages of HIV infection (AIDS), as in terminal cancer.

The principles of treatment are:

- Counselling about HIV infection, lifestyle and infectivity.
- Regular monitoring of clinical and laboratory status (CD4 count and HIV antigen levels).

- Prophylaxis of opportunistic infections at appropriate stages (e.g. co-trimoxazole for *P. carinii* infection and toxoplasmosis).
- Antiretroviral therapy. There are now three groups of antiretroviral drugs for specific chemotherapy of HIV infection (Table 5.8). Treatment is recommended for patients with symptomatic HIV disease; and for asymptomatic patients with falling CD4 counts, especially if accompanied by an increasing viral load. As with chemotherapy of tuberculosis (see Ch. 8), it appears that combination chemotherapy with two or three different types of drug minimizes viral drug resistance and maximizes efficacy.
- Early detection and appropriate treatment of opportunistic infections and neoplasms.

Prevention of HIV cross-infection by health care workers

Transmission of HIV by health care workers is very rare, but may occur through needle-stick injury or reuse of blood contaminated instruments. Because the majority of HIV-infected persons are asymptomatic, and are often unaware of their status, routine precautions against cross-infection are most important. In patients known to be HIV-positive, extra precautions as for hepatitis B appear appropriate (see below).

Viral hepatitis

Viral hepatitis is of major importance because of its potential transmission in the health care setting from carriers of the virus (asymptomatic or symptomatic), through blood and body fluids. Viral hepatitis is the commonest cause of both acute hepatitis and chronic liver disease (see Ch. 10) worldwide, and may be due to several types of virus (A–G). The hepatitis B virus (HBV) (the most important for health care workers) is a DNA virus, and the hepatitis A, C, D and E viruses (HAV, HCV, HDV and HEV, respectively) are RNA viruses.

Viral hepatitis is often asymptomatic, or causes only mild, non-specific symptoms, especially in children. Symptomatic infection occurs in only a minority of cases. After an incubation period of weeks to months, general viral symptoms, often accompanied by nausea and aversion to cigarettes and fatty foods, is followed by jaundice (see Ch. 10). The patient notices yellow discoloration of the skin and sclerae of the eyes, which may be mild or severe. The urine becomes dark and the stools are pale. On examination, there is jaundice, and the liver may be slightly enlarged and tender. About 5% of cases of hepatitis B are complicated by acute glomerulonephritis (see Ch. 11), and about 1% by liver failure (see Ch. 10) with coma and bleeding. Most patients make a clinical recovery within a few weeks, but some may feel generally unwell and depressed for a few months.

The diagnosis is confirmed by abnormal blood liver function tests (raised bilirubin, aminotransferase and alkaline phosphatase levels), and testing for specific virus antigens or antibodies (A–E).

HAV and HEV, which are spread usually by the faecal–oral route, do not cause chronic infection. In contrast, chronic infection (measured by persistence of viral antigen in the blood) is common in hepatitis B (5–10% of cases), C (80% of cases) and D. HBV, HCV and HDV are therefore most commonly transmitted by blood and body fluids (saliva and genital secretions) of carriers, and can also be transmitted vertically from an infected mother to her fetus. Viral carriers are often asymptomatic, but may have symptoms of chronic hepatitis (tiredness or general malaise). Chronic, fluctuating elevated serum transaminases may occur in both asymptomatic and symp-

Table 5.8 Antiretroviral drugs for treatment of HIV infection

Nucleoside analogue reverse transcriptase inhibitors	Zidovudine, didanosine, zalcitabine, lamivudine, stavudine
Non-nucleoside analogue reverse transcriptase inhibitors	Nevirapine, delavardine
Protease inhibitors	Indinavir, ritonavir, saquinavir

.tomatic carriers. Liver biopsy can be performed to assess the histological severity of chronic hepatitis, and to guide treatment with antiviral drugs (α-interferon or ribavirin) which can clear viral antigen from the blood and improve chronic hepatitis in a minority of patients. Progression to hepatic cirrhosis and/or primary hepatoma (see Ch. 10) is common, hence life expectancy is reduced. Patients with chronic hepatitis should be advised against heavy alcohol consumption, which increases the risk of cirrhosis.

Hepatitis A virus

This is endemic in many areas of the world, and travellers to such areas are offered protection with vaccination, or (if time is limited) vaccination combined with an injection of immune serum globulin which contains anti-HAV (passive immunization). HAV is highly infectious and is usually spread by the faecal–oral route; transmission by blood (haemophiliacs) or sexual transmission is rare. No chronic carrier state or progression to chronic hepatitis, cirrhosis or hepatoma occurs.

Hepatitis B virus

Epidemiology. Hepatitis B tests have shown that there are a huge number of asymptomatic carriers, estimated as over 5% of the world's population. HBV infection is one of the World Health Organization's primary targets for eradication of an infectious disease. The prevalence of previous HBV infection (defined as the presence of serum antibody to the viral surface antigen, HBsAb) and of the HBV carrier state (defined as the presence of serum surface antigen, HBsAg) varies markedly worldwide:

- China, South-East Asia, Tropical Africa: 70–95% of the population have antibody and 8–20% are carriers
- eastern Europe, the Mediterranean, former USSR, Central and South America: 20–55% of the population have antibody and 2–7% are carriers
- northern, western and central Europe, North America: 2–6% of the population have antibody, and 0.1–0.5% are carriers.

Even with the low prevalence of carriage in Britain, it is estimated that general dental practitioners could be treating up to 400 undiagnosed carriers of HBV every day. The prevalence of the carrier state is increasing. It is associated with living in towns and with poor socioeconomic conditions.

Groups at increased risk include: immigrants and visitors from high-risk areas; those with learning disabilities living in institutions, especially patients with Down's syndrome and staff in close contact with such patients; persons with multiple sexual partners, including prostitutes, and homosexual or bisexual men; intravenous or percutaneous drug abusers; those living or working in institutions (e.g. prisons and drug and alcohol rehabilitation centres) which have a high prevalence of high-risk persons; and haemophiliacs and other persons who have received regular transfusions of blood or blood products (e.g. renal dialysis, oncology and immunocompromised patients). Health care professionals, especially dentists and clinical dental staff, surgeons, accident and emergency unit personnel, and those working in drug dependency units, renal dialysis units and liver units, and with haemophiliacs or other multitransfused patients, are also at risk, as are laboratory staff, especially those working in blood banks and pathology laboratories.

Partners and close relatives of the above groups, not necessarily with sexual contact, and children of infected mothers are also at increased risk of infection.

Virology. HBV is a DNA virus (hepadnavirus) which differs strikingly from other DNA viruses in that it uses an RNA copy of the genome to integrate itself within the host's chromosomes. It infects hepatocytes, causing acute hepatitis which is often asymptomatic, and which may become chronic, leading to hepatic cirrhosis or hepatocellular carcinoma. The virus is also found in leucocytes in all body secretions (blood, saliva, semen, vaginal and menstrual secretions, breast milk, tears, vomit, faeces, sweat and urine). The concentration of infective virus particles in blood can be very high (up to 10^{12}/ml during acute infection).

Electron microscopy of blood shows several viral forms: intact virus containing the DNA core

(42 nm diameter), and tubular and spherical forms of the surface antigen (22 nm diameter). HBV is a very sturdy virus which can remain viable in the environment for weeks. It is resistant to boiling for less than 30 minutes and to common antiseptics such as chlorhexidine. It can be destroyed only by autoclaving or in hot-air ovens, and by sodium hypochlorite (household bleach), iodine or glutaraldehyde.

Transmission. The high resistance of HBV to inactivation and its high concentration in blood and other body fluids account for its high infectivity by inoculation with blood or body fluids (Table 5.9). Only traces of blood are required, especially if the e antigen (HBeAg) from the virus core is present in serum (see later). Following needle-stick injury from an HBeAg-positive person, the risk of HBV transmission is 40%. Three main routes of transmission are recognized:

1. Transmission from carrier mothers to their babies (vertical transmission) occurs during the perinatal period, especially if the mother has a high titre of HBsAg or contracts acute hepatitis B during or shortly after pregnancy. Most children infected perinatally become chronic carriers of HBV, but this can be reduced by immunization (see later). Vertical transmission is a major factor determining the high prevalence of HBV in eastern and tropical countries.

2. Sexual intercourse, heterosexual or homosexual, especially if unprotected by condoms is also an important method of transmission. Thus, HBV can be a sexually transmitted disease.

3. Inoculation of blood or other body fluids through the skin or mucous membranes may explain cases of non-sexual transmission, and is of most concern to health care workers, especially those involved in invasive procedures. Inoculation can occur in several ways:

a. Transfusion of blood or blood products. This is largely, but not completely, preventable by asking at-risk persons not to donate blood, and by routine testing for HBV. Similar considerations apply to organ transplantation and donation of sperm or breast milk.

b. Dental, surgical and medical procedures, especially:

   (i) injury of health care workers by contaminated needles or other sharp objects (e.g. scalpels, or bone fragments during surgery)

   (ii) contamination of broken skin (e.g. cuts, abrasions, or dermatitis of the hands)

   (iii) inadequate sterilization of dental and surgical instruments prior to reuse, or inappropriate reuse of disposable needles, syringes or other invasive apparatus

   (iv) aerosol spread of infected blood or saliva, e.g. that produced by modern dental equipment, which may infect clinical dental workers through the conjunctivae, mucous membranes or broken skin.

c. Laboratory accidents.

d. Intravenous or percutaneous drug abuse.

e. Tattooing, ear, nose and body piercing, acupuncture, bloodletting, circumcision.

f. Sharing of razors and toothbrushes.

g. Biting and spitting.

h. Theoretically, by bloodsucking insects.

Clinical spectrum and diagnosis.

Acute hepatitis (see Ch. 10). Symptomatic infection occurs in only 20–30% of cases. The incubation period is 6 weeks to 6 months. The diagnosis is established by high serum levels of bilirubin and transaminases (see Ch. 10) and the presence of HBsAg and HBeAg in the serum (Fig. 5.3); core antigen (HBcAg) is only found in the liver. The HBeAg correlates with the number of intact viruses in serum and the infectivity of the blood. These antigens disappear from the serum during convalescence in most persons, but persist in 10–15%, who become chronic carriers. Antibodies to HBcAg, HBeAg and HBsAg appear in that order during convalescence (Fig. 5.3). The presence of HBsAb indicates immunity and lack

---

Table 5.9 Hazards to oral health care staff from hepatitis B

The virus is widespread
Minute traces of body fluids can transmit infection
The virus survives well outside the body
The virus is relatively resistant to disinfection
A chronic infective carrier state is common
Chronic liver disease or cancer may result from infection

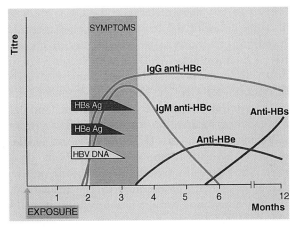

Fig. 5.3 The serological profile in a patient with hepatitis B who recovers normally (Courtesy of Dr J. Bagg, Glasgow Dental School.)

of infectivity. Blood samples from all persons with suspected or known HBV infection should be taken with great care, and sent to laboratories properly packaged to prevent spillage and labelled to indicate high risk of infectivity.

Acute subclinical infection. In most persons acute HBV infection is subclinical, i.e. there are no symptoms or perhaps only non-specific tiredness or malaise. Diagnosis is retrospective by discovery of the presence of HBV antigens or antibodies in serum.

Chronic infection. About 5–10% of healthy heterosexual adults retain the virus for more than 6 months after clinical or subclinical infection: most of these remain seropositive for HBsAg. A higher percentage of the young, old and certain risk groups become carriers. Impaired immune response may partly account for persistent carriage: treatment with α-interferon by injection for several months may produce clearance of the virus.

Diagnosis of carriage may be by follow-up of acute hepatitis, or by discovery when investigating chronic liver disease or performing liver function tests or HBV tests for other reasons. Carriers are usually infectious. The presence of HBeAg (18%) is associated with high infectivity; HBeAb indicates low infectivity in western countries, but not in endemic areas. Liver biopsy may show normal histology, but usually shows chronic hepatitis. Chronic persistent hepatitis has a better prognosis than chronic active hepatitis, which more commonly progresses to hepatic cirrhosis and/or hepatocellular carcinoma (see Ch. 10); 80% of hepatomas are caused by HBV. Most carriers are asymptomatic and unaware of their condition, so their contacts cannot be warned of their infectivity.

Management and prevention of infection. Treatment of acute hepatitis, chronic hepatitis, cirrhosis or hepatoma is symptomatic (see Ch. 10). While recent studies show that interferon (± ribavirin) may clear HBsAg from the serum and improve chronic hepatitis, follow-up studies are required to see if this affects long-term prognosis. Carriers are advised to minimize their alcohol intake, to reduce the risk of progression to cirrhosis.

There are three aspects to prevention of HBV infection.

Active immunization. Effective vaccines are now offered to all persons in the increased risk groups listed above, including dentists and other clinical dental health care workers, as well as dental laboratory staff who are regularly exposed to blood and saliva-contaminated material. A recombinant vaccine containing HBsAg is capable of producing active immunity in up to 95% of healthy persons. It is ineffective in persons already infected by HBV.

Passive immunization. For immediate protection against HBV, anti-HBs immunoglobulin should be given to the following persons at risk:

1. Those who have been acutely exposed to HBsAg-positive blood or other body fluids, especially if highly infective (HBeAg-positive). Examples include inoculation, ingestion, or splashing on mucous membranes, conjunctivae or broken skin, and sexual contacts of acute cases. It will be remembered that following needle-stick injury with an HBeAg-positive blood, the risk of HBV transmission is 40%. Immunoglobulin should be given as soon as possible after exposure, preferably within 24 h, and not more than 7 days after exposure. A second dose is recommended 30 days later.

2. Infants born to HBsAg-positive mothers. The dose of immunoglobulin given does not interfere with the response to active immunization, which should be given simultaneously but at a different site. If HBV infection has already occurred at the time of first immunization, virus

multiplication may not be completely inhibited, but many individuals will be protected from severe illness and from the development of chronic infection.

Prevention of inoculation with infected blood or body fluids. Persons discovered to be carriers of HBV should be counselled and educated concerning their infectivity to others. They should be advised to protect sexual intercourse with a condom, and to limit the number of sexual partners. Sexual partners and spouses should be counselled concerning the risks of infection of themselves and of children, and vaccination offered. Spills of blood and body fluids should be mopped up with disposable tissues and sodium hypochlorite (household bleach) diluted 1:10. Carriers should avoid biting or spitting, sharing razors or toothbrushes, tattooing, body piercing, acupuncture, or blood-letting. They should not inject drugs and never share needles. They and their sexual partners should not donate blood, semen, breast milk, or organs for transplantation. They should be asked to inform any doctor or dentist whom they may attend of their carrier status. Their doctor should inform all health care workers exposed to the patient's blood or body fluids of infectivity, including the patient's dentist: such information is confidential and should not be disclosed to those not directly involved in patient contact. Dentists should take extra precautions against cross-infection in known HBV carriers (see below). However, since most carriers of HBV are asymptomatic, undiagnosed and unaware of their condition, and are already being treated by dentists in large numbers, the only safe policy is to take routine precautions with all patients (see below).

Hepatitis C virus

This RNA flavivirus (which has many genotypes and serotypes) was discovered in 1989. It cannot be cultured, but can infect primates such as chimpanzees. Its prevalence in the UK general population is less than 1%, but is higher in developing countries. Retrospectively, HCV was found (by testing stored serum samples) to be the cause of over 90% of cases of post-transfusion hepatitis before serological tests allowed the routine screening of blood donors for antibody, HCV-Ab

(which commenced in 1991 in the UK). HCV is also the cause of the high prevalence of chronic hepatitis (previously called non-A, non-B hepatitis) in haemophiliacs, treated with factor VIII or factor IX concentrates obtained from thousands of donors (see Ch. 7). The introduction of viral inactivation of such blood products from 1985 (as a precaution against transmission of HIV) greatly reduced the risk of HCV transmission. HCV infection is also common in intravenous drug users. The virus is present in saliva, but sexual, casual or vertical transmission is uncommon. Neither active nor passive immunization is available (Table 5.10).

Hepatitis C infection is usually asymptomatic, but there is a high risk (80%) of chronic carriage of hepatitis C, measured by serum HCV antigen which is detected by PCR. Chronic hepatitis (raised, fluctuating serum transaminase levels, and abnormal liver histology on biopsy) is common in carriers, and there is a high risk of cirrhosis and primary hepatoma after 20 years. Treatment with α-interferon (± ribavirin) may clear the antigen from the blood and reduce chronic hepatitis in a minority of patients, but the long-term benefit is not known. HCV carriers should be counselled to minimize their alcohol intake, and to take care with blood and body fluids, as for HBV carriers. In known carriers, precautions against cross-infection as for HBV appear adequate.

Hepatitis D virus

HDV (previously known as the delta antigen) is an incomplete RNA virus which requires the presence of HBV for its existence. Coinfection with HBV causes a more severe hepatitis in both acute

Table 5.10 Characteristics of hepatitis C, highlighting important differences from B

Less widespread
Less readily transmitted by needle-stick injuries
More vulnerable to antiseptics
Rarely transmitted during dentistry
Acute infection is uncommon and usually mild
No protective vaccine
Infection persists in 80% of individuals
Infection more frequently leads to chronic active hepatitis

and chronic stages, with a high mortality. In the UK, HDV is currently found most often in intravenous drug abusers. HDV infection can be prevented by measures which prevent HBV infection (see above), and is another reason for stressing the importance of such measures.

Hepatitis E virus

Like HAV, the recently discovered HEV is an RNA virus which is spread by the faecal-oral route, and is common in countries with poor sanitation. It can cause epidemics of water-borne hepatitis, and may infect visitors to endemic areas. Neither active nor passive immunization is available. The virus is not transmitted by blood, and chronic infection appears uncommon.

Other causes of viral hepatitis

These include the Epstein–Barr virus (EBV) or cytomegalovirus, often as part of a glandular fever syndrome; and the yellow fever virus in tropical countries.

Routine precautions against cross-infection in the health care environment (Table 5.11)

Health care workers have a duty to ensure the safety of their patients, themselves and their staff, who should be thoroughly trained in precautions, which should be regularly reviewed. Guidelines are issued periodically. Health care workers should be offered HBV vaccination and follow-up for seroconversion tests and booster doses. Health care workers with exudative skin lesions should refrain from direct patient care and from handling equipment in contact with patients until the con-

---

Table 5.11 Basic precautions against transmission of blood-borne infections

All patients should be treated as infectious
Gloves should be worn for all clinical oral health care work
Special care should be taken to avoid needle-stick injuries
Disposable instruments should be used where practical and all others autoclaved
Clinical health care staff should be immunized against hepatitis B

---

dition resolves. Health care workers should inspect their exposed skin every morning and cover any cuts or abrasions with waterproof plasters. They should wear disposable gloves routinely when touching mucous membranes (e.g. examining the mouth) or blood, saliva, other body fluids, or items or surfaces contaminated with blood or body fluids. Between patients, hands should be washed with soap and water or surgical handscrub, and gloves changed. Protective glasses and masks (or chin-length plastic face-shields) should be worn when aerosol spray or splashing of blood or other body fluids is likely. Gowns should be worn if clothing is likely to be soiled with blood or body fluids.

Surfaces which may be contaminated by blood or saliva should be covered with impervious, disposable trays or covers, and changed between patients. Surfaces should be cleaned with disposable absorbent cloths (to remove blood and other organic material) and sodium hypochlorite (household bleach, 1:10 dilution) or glutaraldehyde if metal because hypochlorite corrodes metals.

Needles and other sharp instruments must be handled with great care to avoid accidental injuries. Recapping, bending or breaking needles should be avoided; needles should be disposed into rigid, puncture-resistant containers as close to the area of use as possible, as soon as possible. Disposable equipment should be used wherever possible, and never reused (especially needles or local anaesthetic cartridges). Other solid waste contaminated with blood or body fluids should be placed in stout plastic bags, sealed and incinerated.

Non-disposable equipment should be thoroughly cleaned by scrubbing or ultrasonic cleaners, then sterilized by autoclaving (134°C for at least 3 min) or dry heat (hot air ovens, 160°C for 60 min without interruption). Boiling and cold sterilization are inadequate for HBV: cold sterilization should be considered only for instruments which cannot be exposed to heat (soak for 3 hours in 2% glutaraldehyde). Equipment which cannot be sterilized should be cleaned and disinfected between patients.

Impressions and appliances should be thoroughly cleaned (or sprayed with glutaraldehyde, then sealed in a bag) before sending to the dental laboratory, with which liaison is required regarding cleaning and handling. Biopsy specimens and swabs should be put in secure, leak-proof containers before sending to the pathology laboratory.

Additional precautions for known carriers of HIV, HBV or HCV

Guidelines are issued regularly. Pregnant women should not be involved in treatment. If possible, the appointment should be arranged at the end of the day, with careful cleaning after the procedure. Extraordinary care should be taken to prevent needle-stick injury, or splashing of blood or body fluids into the eye or mouth. If such contamination occurs, the site of contamination should be washed gently but thoroughly, and advice sought immediately from the local hospital (accident and emergency department or infectious diseases department) or dental or medical officer. For

HBV exposure, passive and active immunization may be recommended (see above). For HIV exposure, a course of antiretroviral chemotherapy may be recommended.

DNA viruses

Table 5.12 summarizes the DNA viruses, their clinical features, and the chapters which detail their features and management.

Herpes simplex virus (HSV-1) type 1

This virus is a frequent cause of stomatitis and cold sores in the general population (see Ch. 22), and of finger infections (whitlows). Routine wearing of gloves when examining oral lesions should reduce the risk of occupational whitlows. Herpes simplex encephalitis (see Ch. 9) is a rare complication, which is treated with intravenous aciclovir.

Table 5.12 Diseases due to DNA viruses

Family	Genus or type	Disease
Adenoviruses	Adenoviruses	Upper respiratory tract infections (see Ch. 8)
Hepadnaviruses	Hepatitis B	Hepatitis (see Ch. 10)
Herpesviruses	Herpes simplex virus type 1 (HSV-1)	Stomatitis (see Ch. 22) Finger infections (whitlows) Encephalitis
	Herpes simplex type 2 (HSV-1) Varicella–zoster (VZV)	Genital infections Chickenpox Shingles
	Epstein-Barr virus (EBV)	Glandular fever (see Ch. 8) Burkitt's lymphoma (see Ch. 7) Hairy leukoplakia (HIV) (see Ch. 23) Nasopharyngeal carcinoma
	Cytomegalovirus (CMV)	Glandular fever Congenital Disseminated (HIV)
	Human herpesvirus 6 (HHV6) Human herpesvirus 8 (HHV8)	Exanthem subitum Kaposi's sarcoma (see Ch. 23)
Papovaviruses	Human papillomavirus (HPV) JC virus	Warts, squamous carcinoma Leucoencephalopathy (HIV)
Parvoviruses	B19	Anaemia
Poxviruses	Variola Vaccinia Molluscum contagiosum Orf	Smallpox Cowpox Water warts Sheep warts

Varicella–zoster virus (VZV)

This virus is the cause of chickenpox (varicella), a common and highly infectious disease usually affecting children under the age of 10 years. It is spread by droplets from the upper respiratory tract, or by contact with ruptured skin lesions on patients with chickenpox or shingles. General symptoms are usually mild in children, but can be severe in adults. On the second day of infection, a characteristic rash appears on the trunk, spreading to the face and then the limbs. The rash progresses from macular (flat red lesions) to papular (raised red lesions), vesicular (clear fluid-filled blisters) then pustular (pus-filled lesions). The itchy rash is often scratched, leading to secondary bacterial infection. The pustules dry up in a few days to form scabs; residual scars may occur. Complications include encephalitis (see Ch. 9), septicaemia and pneumonia (especially in adults and immunosuppressed patients). Treatment is symptomatic. Immunosuppressed patients are given aciclovir. Secondary infection is treated with local antiseptics (e.g. chlorhexidine) and antibiotics (e.g. flucloxacillin). Immunosuppressed persons in contact with VZV-infected patients should receive human anti-varicella immunoglobulin.

Shingles is due to reactivation of the VZV within a posterior nerve root ganglion, causing pain, followed after 3–4 days by a vesicular rash in the relevant dermatome. It is common in divisions of the fifth (trigeminal) cranial nerve (see Ch. 22), and may cause inflammation and blindness if the eye is affected. It is also a common cause of lateral chest pain (see Ch. 8) when it involves the intercostal nerves. Treatment is with systemic aciclovir (especially in the immunosuppressed and those with ophthalmic infection), and management of secondary infection is as for chickenpox. Aciclovir is most effective when started early. Postherpetic neuralgia is common in older persons.

Human herpesvirus 6 (HHV6)

This herpesvirus is a recently discovered virus causing a mild febrile rash in children (exanthem subitum).

Parvovirus B19

This virus may cause acute anaemia. It may be transmitted by blood and blood products, and is resistant to viral inactivation of the latter.

CHLAMYDIAE AND RICKETTSIAE

Table 5.13 summarizes diseases due to these microbes, which like viruses are intracellular pathogens, but which unlike viruses have both RNA and DNA. Treatment is with certain antimicrobials, e.g. erythromycin or tetracycline (Table 5.14).

BACTERIAL INFECTIONS

The general symptoms of acute severe bacterial infections are:

- fever – often high and swinging, with sweats
- malaise
- rigors – attacks of shivering.

Table 5.13 Diseases due to chlamydiae and rickettsiae

Chlamydia trachomatis	Keratoconjunctivitis (trachoma) (commonest cause of blindness in tropical countries) Non-gonococcal urethritis, pelvic inflammatory disease
Chlamydia psittaci	Psittacosis (borne by birds) (see Ch. 8)
Chlamydia pneumonia	Atypical pneumonia (see Ch. 8)
Rickettsiae	Typhus fevers (borne by lice, fleas, ticks, mice)
Coxiella burnetii	Q fever (borne by ticks) Infective endocarditis

The general signs of acute bacterial infections are:

- rapid pulse rate (tachycardia – see Ch. 6)
- low blood pressure (hypotension – see Ch. 6)
- high blood white cell count, due to increased neutrophils (neutrophilia – see Ch. 7)
- septicaemic shock (see Ch. 6), due to massive bacteraemia and endotoxaemia, causing multiple organ damage and with a high mortality; treatment is with intensive care unit support and high-dose intravenous antimicrobials.

Diagnosis of bacterial infection may be by:

- microscopy, for example:
  - staphylococci in pus smear
  - pneumococci in purulent sputum
  - acid-fast bacilli (e.g. *Mycobacterium tuberculosis*) in sputum or in urine
  - *Corynebacterium diphtheriae* in throat swab
- culture, for example:
  - from blood – infective endocarditis or septicaemia
  - from urine – urinary tract infections
  - from throat swab – upper respiratory tract infections
  - from sputum – lower respiratory tract infections
  - from faeces – gut infections
  - from pus
- detection of antigen, e.g. meningococcus or pneumococcus (from blood, sputum or cerebrospinal fluid)
- serology – detection of antibodies (e.g. syphilis, typhoid or brucellosis).

Table 5.14 summarises some commonly-used antibacterial drugs.

Tables 5.15 and 5.16 summarise the common bacterial infections, their clinical features, and the chapters which detail their features and management. Syphilis is considered in detail because of its importance.

Syphilis

Like HIV infection, syphilis is a chronic, systemic infectious disease which is usually transmitted by sexual intercourse (it may also be transmitted from mother to fetus, or by blood contact or blood transfusion); and which may present with clinical features in many body systems after a latent period of months to years. Unlike HIV infection, it can be cured by early detection and treatment with penicillin. A high index of suspicion is required for early detection, especially in the following high risk groups of men and women:

- young, sexually active (aged 16–34 years)
- frequent overseas travellers, e.g. military personnel and airline and shipping personnel
- prostitutes and homosexuals
- persons with sexually acquired HIV infection (see above).

The cause is the spirochaete *Treponema pallidum*, which can penetrate intact skin or mucosae; hence, skin and mucosal lesions are highly infectious. Classically, syphilis presents clinically in four stages:

1. *Primary.* After an incubation period (usually 2–4 weeks), a primary lesion (chancre) develops at the site of infection. This is usually on the genital organs, but may be in the mouth (oral intercourse) or anus or rectum (rectal intercourse). The lesion starts as a small, flat pink spot (macule), which then becomes raised (papule) and ulcerates. The regional lymph nodes become enlarged: they are painless, non-tender, mobile, discrete and rubbery. Primary syphilis should be considered in the differential diagnosis of oral, genital or anorectal ulcers, especially in high-risk groups.

2. *Secondary.* The second stage usually starts 6–8 weeks after the primary chancre. It is due to systemic spread of the treponemal infection, and causes lesions which (like the primary chancre) are highly infectious: hence disposable gloves should be routinely worn when examining lesions in high-risk patients. The clinical features include:

- Skin. A rash occurs in 75% of patients. It usually starts on the trunk and becomes generalized, affecting the palms and soles. It consists of copper-coloured macules or dull red papules, which do not itch and which turn scaly. Condylomata lata are flat papules in moist areas (e.g. mouth, anus).
- Lymphadenopathy. This occurs in 50% of patients, and is usually generalized,

however, the nodes have the characteristics of the regionally enlarged lymph nodes of primary syphilis.

- Mucosal ulcers. These occur in 30% of patients, and affect the mouth (see Ch. 19), pharynx, larynx and genitals. Superficial early lesions may form 'snail tracks': they develop a white base with a red margin. Like the primary chancre, these lesions are highly infectious, and disposable gloves should be worn routinely.

3. *Tertiary.* The third stage is now rare, and occurs after an asymptomatic 'latent' stage of at least 2 years. This classic lesion is a granuloma (gumma) which affects skin, mucosa and bones,

including the palate and nasal septa. It is a hard, painless lump which may ulcerate.

4. *Quaternary.* The fourth stage is now also rare, and occurs after a latent stage of several (up to 30) years. It involves the cardiovascular system (usually causing thoracic aortic aneurysms or aortic valve incompetence, see Ch. 6) and the central nervous system (usually causing Argyll Robertson pupils, dementia or spinal cord disease, see Ch. 9).

Congenital syphilis

Fetal infection, acquired from a mother with early acquired syphilis, may cause intrauterine death,

Table 5.14 Some antibacterial drugs

Drug	Route of administration	Indications
Penicillins		
Phenoxymethylpenicillin	Oral	Mild streptococcal infections, e.g. dental infections, sore throat
Benzylpenicillin	Injection	Streptococcal (including endocarditis)
Procaine penicillin	Injection	and meningococcal infections, diphtheria, syphilis, gonorrhoea, anthrax, actinomycosis
Ampicillin	Oral/injection	Dental infections, endocarditis
Amoxycillin	Oral/injection	prophylaxis, streptococcal, *Haemophilus influenzae*, *Salmonella* and *Shigella* infections
Flucloxacillin	Oral/injection	*Staphylococcus* infections
Ticarcillin	Injection	*Pseudomonas* infections
Cephalosporins		
Cefuroxime	Oral/injection	Empirical therapy of undiagnosed
Cefotaxime	Injection	infections (e.g. septicaemia, pneumonia, meningitis, urinary tract infection, sore throat, *H. influenzae* epiglottitis
Others		
Gentamycin	Injection	Endocarditis prophylaxis and treatment, serious Gram-negative infections
	Eyedrops	Purulent conjunctivitis
Streptomycin	Injection	Tuberculosis (combination therapy)
Erythromycin	Oral/injection	As for penicillin (use in penicillin allergy), *Legionella* pneumonia, *Campylobacter* enteritis, *Mycoplasma* and *Chlamydia* infections
Tetracyclines	Oral	Chronic destructive periodontal disease, syphilis (if penicillin allergy), *Mycoplasma* and *Chlamydia* infections
Clindamycin	Oral/injection	Acne, rosacea, endocarditis prophylaxis, *Staphylococcus* infections
Vancomycin	Injection	Endocarditis prophylaxis
Teicoplanin	Injection	and treatment
Co-trimoxazole	Oral/injection	Prophylaxis and treatment of *Pneumocystis* infection
Trimethoprim	Oral/injection	Urinary tract infections, exacerbations of chronic bronchitis
Fusidic acid	Oral/injection	*Staphylococcus* infections (bone, joint)
Ciprofloxacin	Oral/injection	Serious Gram-negative infections
Metronidazole	Oral/injection	Anaerobic bacterial infections (including dental infections, peritonitis), protozoal infections

Table 5.15 Diseases due to bacteria: streptococci and staphylococci

Streptococci

Strep. pyogenes	Sore throat (tonsillitis, see Ch. 8)
	Skin and soft tissue infections/rashes,
	e.g. erysipelas, cellulitis, scarlet fever (see Ch. 12)
	Bone and joint infections (see Ch. 14)
	Rheumatic fever (see Ch. 6)
	Glomerulonephritis (see Ch. 11)
Strep. faecalis (enterococcus)	Urinary tract infection
	Endocarditis (see Ch. 6)
Viridans streptococci	Endocarditis (see Ch. 6)
Strep. pneumoniae (pneumococcus)	Pneumonia (see Ch. 8), meningitis (see Ch. 9)
Anaerobic streptococci	Dental infections, peritonitis

Staphylococci

Staph. aureus	Skin infections, e.g. boils, styes, carbuncles, abscesses, wound infections (see Ch. 12)
	Endocarditis (intravenous drug users) (see Ch. 6)
	Bone and joint infections (see Ch. 14)
	Chest infections, e.g. pneumonia, lung abscess, empyema (see Ch. 8)
	Central nervous system infections, e.g. brain abscess (see Ch. 9)
	Enterocolitis
Staph. epidermidis	Endocarditis (see Ch. 6)

Table 5.16 Diseases due to other bacteria

Haemophilus influenzae	Exacerbations of chronic bronchitis, pneumonia, epiglottitis (see Ch. 8)
Neisseria meningitidis (meningococcus)	Meningitis (see Ch. 9)
Neisseria gonorrhoeae (gonococcus)	Gonorrhoea
Corynebacterium diphtheriae	Diphtheria (see Ch. 8)
Bacillus anthracis	Anthrax
Bordetella pertussis	Whooping cough (see Ch. 8)
Salmonella spp.	Typhoid and paratyphoid fever, gastroenteritis
Campylobacter jejeni	Gastroenteritis
Shigella spp.	Bacillary dysentery
Vibrio cholerae	Cholera
Brucella abortus	Brucellosis
Yersinia pestis	Plague
Mycobacterium tuberculosis	Tuberculosis (see Ch. 8)
Mycobacterium avium–intracellulare (MAI)	Disseminated infection in HIV infection (this chapter)
Mycobacterium leprae	Leprosy
Leptospira spp.	Leptospirosis
Borrelia spp.	Lyme disease
	Relapsing fevers (tick, lice)
Treponemal infections	Syphilis (this chapter) yaws, pinta, bejel

or characteristic features in the baby, which include:

- nasal inflammation (snuffles), leading to destruction of the nasal cartilages and a saddle-nose deformity
- moist papules at the angles of the mouth, which heal to leave fine, radiating scars (rhagades).

In later childhood, other lesions include lesions of the permanent teeth:

- incisors – widely spaced, tapering and notched (Hutchinson's teeth)
- first molars – round or domed (Moon's molars).

Congenital infection is now rare in countries which routinely perform serological screening at antenatal clinics, because treatment during pregnancy usually eradicates the infection in the mother and fetus.

Diagnosis

All suspected cases should be referred to a genitourinary medicine clinic, for assessment, diagnosis, treatment and counselling. Tracing of potentially infected partners for confidential counselling, diagnosis and treatment is equally important.

T. pallidum may be identified (by dark ground microscopy) in scrapings from genital, oral or anal ulcers in the primary or secondary stages of infection. Because the microbe is readily killed by antiseptics, these should not be applied to the lesion before the sample is taken.

Serological tests for syphilis are positive from the fourth week of acquired infection, and at birth in congenital infection. Non-specific screening tests (which identify a lipoidal antigen) such as the Venereal Disease Research Laboratory (VDRL) test may be falsely positive, e.g. in connective tissue disorders such as rheumatoid arthritis (see Ch. 14). Hence, positive screening tests should be followed by specific tests for treponemal infection, such as the *T. pallidum* haemagglutination assay.

Treatment

Syphilis is cured by antibacterial therapy with daily intramuscular procaine penicillin, or in penicillin-allergic patients with tetracycline or erythromycin. The duration of treatment varies from two weeks (in the first three stages) to four weeks (for quaternary syphilis).

All patients with syphilis should be counselled and screened for other sexually transmitted diseases (Table 5.17) at the genitourinary medicine clinic, because they commonly coexist. The incidence of all sexually transmitted diseases can be reduced by public health advice on safe sex.

Fungal infections (mycoses)

Candida species

Candida species, especially *C. albicans*, are a cause of mucosal infections, often with a thick, white discharge (thrush). They are discussed fully as a cause of oral infection in Chapter 22. *Candida* also infects the vagina (Table 5.17), nails and skin (intertrigo, see Ch. 12), and causes disseminated infection in immunosuppressed (e.g. HIV-infected) persons (e.g. pharyngitis and oesophagitis; see above). Treatment is with topical nystatin, or systemic (oral or intravenous) imidazole (ketoconazole) or triazole (fluconazole or itraconazole) antimicrobials.

Tinea infections

These infections of the skin (ringworm) are due to dermatophyte fungi, which invade skin keratin (see also Ch. 12). They include:

- *T. pedis* (athlete's foot)

Table 5.17 Sexually transmitted diseases

Viral	HIV infection (this chapter) Hepatitis B, especially homosexuals (rarely hepatitis C) Anogenital herpes simplex virus type 2 (HSV-2) Genital warts, cervical cancer (human papillomavirus, HPV) Molluscum contagiosum
Bacterial	Syphilis (this chapter) Gonorrhoea (*Neisseria gonorrhoeae*) – urethritis, orchitis, pelvic inflammatory disease, arthritis
Chlamydial	*Chlamydia trachomatis* (cause in about 50% of non-gonococcal urethritis) Lymphogranuloma venereum (in tropics)
Fungal (Yeast)	*Candida* species – vaginitis
Protozoal	*Trichomonas vaginalis* – vaginitis, urethritis

- *T. unguium* (nails)
- *T. manum* (hands)
- *T. cruris* (groin)
- *T. corporis* (trunk)
- *T. capitis* (scalp).

Diagnosis is by skin microscopy. Treatment is with local ointments, or systemic griseofulvin or terbinafine.

Systemic fungal infections

Infections such as aspergillosis, blastomycosis, coccidioidomycosis, cryptococcosis and histoplasmosis are common in immunosuppressed (e.g. HIV-infected) patients, and are treated with systemic amphotericin or azole antifungals.

Protozoal infections

Apart from *Trichomonas vaginalis* vaginitis (Table 5.17), in developed countries these are usually encountered in:

- immunosuppressed (e.g. HIV-infected) patients (pneumocystis and toxoplasmosis)

- visitors from, or travellers returning from, tropical countries.

Tropical protozoal infections are summarized in Table 5.18.

Helminth infections

These are also common in tropical countries, and are summarized in Table 5.19.

Arthropods and infection

Scabies (mites), lice and tick infestations are common causes of skin disorders (see Ch. 12). Arthropods (including flies and fleas) may also act as vectors of microbial infections, especially in tropical countries (Table 5.20).

Prion infections

Prions are recently discovered proteins which are infectious in the absence of an associated nucleic

Table 5.18 Protozoal infections

Malaria	*Plasmodium falciparum, vivax, ovale or malariae*; transmitted by anopheline mosquitoes infect blood cells and liver Annual infection rate 100 million; mortality 1% Causes periodic fever, sweats, anaemia, enlarged liver and spleen *Falciparum* causes severe infection with coma, intravascular haemolysis, shock and acute renal failure Diagnosis – blood films show parasites Treatment – chloroquine (or other drugs if resistant) Prophylaxis – chloroquine, proguanil or mefloquine
Trypanosomiasis	Africa – sleeping sickness (*Trypanosoma brucei* or *rhodesiense*); transmitted by the tsetse fly South and Central America – Chagas' disease (*T. cruzi*); transmitted by a winged bug Treatment – suramin, pentamidine (Africa), nifurtimox (America)
Leishmaniasis	*Leishmania* species; transmitted by sandflies infects liver, spleen (visceral, kala-azar) and skin (cutaneous) Diagnosis – smears or culture of bone marrow, lymph node or liver Treatment – pentavalent antimicrobials
Giardiasis	*Giardia lamblia;* infection through contaminated water causes diarrhoea, abdominal pain, nausea and vomiting; may become chronic Diagnosis – stool examination for cysts Treatment – metronidazole or tinidazole
Toxoplasmosis	See HIV infection (this chapter)

Table 5.19 Helminth infections

Trematodes (flukes)	Blood: *Schistosoma* ssp. (blood flukes) – schistosomiasis Lungs: *Paragonimus westermani* (lung fluke) Hepatobiliary system: *Fasciola hepatica* (sheep liver fluke)
Cestodes (tapeworms)	Intestine: *Taenia saginata* (beef tapeworm) or *solium* (pork tapeworm) Tissue: *Taenia solium* – cysticercosis *Echinococcus granulosus* (dog tapeworm) – hydatid disease of liver, lung or brain
Nematodes (roundworms)	Intestine: *Enterobius vermicularis* (threadworm of anus), *Ascaris lumbricoides* (roundworm), *Necator americanus* (hookworm), *Ancylostoma duodenale* (hookworm) Tissue: *Wuchereria bancrofti* – filariasis, *Dracunculus medinensis* (Guinea worm)

Table 5.20 Arthropod infections

Infestations of skin (see Ch. 12)

Mites	Scabies
Lice	Pediculosis
Fleas	

Infections transmitted by arthropods

Mosquitoes	Malaria
	Yellow fever, dengue, other arboviruses
	Filariasis
Tsetse fly	African trypanosomiasis
Ticks	Lyme disease, relapsing fever
Winged bug	American trypanosomiasis
Mites	Scrub typhus fever
Lice	Epidemic typhus fever, relapsing fever
Fleas	Plague, endemic typhus fever

acid, in contrast to viruses. Creutzfeldt–Jakob disease (CJD) is an uncommon cause of rapidly progressive dementia (see Ch. 9), which is transmissible in the laboratory to chimpanzees, and rarely from person to person, e.g. by human growth hormone for treatment of growth hormone deficiency (see Ch. 13), which was historically extracted from human pituitary glands at postmortem examinations. Recently, a new variant of CJD has been described, which to date has been described mostly in young persons in the UK, and which may be the human equivalent of bovine spongiform encephalopathy, transmitted by eating beef contaminated by brain or spinal cord tissue. Because of the hypothetical possibility of transmission of the prion by blood or blood products, blood from UK donors has been treated by leucodepletion (removal of white blood cells) from 1998, and multiple-donor blood products from UK donors phased out. Whether or not prion infections can be transmitted in the health care environment is unknown. There is no known treatment and prions are resistant to sterilization.

Vaccination

Routine vaccination against selected infectious diseases is an important part of public health medicine and infection control. The current UK schedule is given in Table 5.21. Additionally, hepatitis B vaccination is recommended for all health care workers in close contact with patients, starting in the student years. Visitors to other parts of the world may be advised to have vaccinations against certain endemic infections: current advice can be obtained from travel clinics.

Table 5.21 Schedule of vaccinations in the UK

Age	Visits	Vaccine	Intervals
3-12 months	3	Three administrations of diphtheria, tetanus and pertussis triple vaccine (DTP), oral poliomyelitis, and *Haemophilus influenzae* type B	6–8 weeks 4–6 months
12-24 months	1	Measles, mumps and rubella (MMR)	
1st year at school	1	Booster diphtheria and tetanus (DT), oral poliomyelitis	
10-13 years	1	BCG (Bacille Calmette–Guérin; see Ch. 8) for tuberculin-negative individuals.	
Girls: 11-13 years	1	Rubella	
15-19 years or on leaving school	1	Booster diphtheria (low dose) and tetanus (toxoid), oral poliomyelitis	

6 Disorders of the cardiovascular system

Introduction

Cardiovascular disorders, especially coronary heart disease and stroke, are the commonest cause of death (including premature death) in developed countries. Symptoms of cardiovascular disease such as pain in the chest or legs, or breathlessness, are also common causes of morbidity, and cardiovascular disease may complicate the management of patients with concomitant illnesses.

Assessment of the cardiovascular system

Symptoms and signs pertaining particularly to the cardiovascular system will be discussed in the first instance, along with consideration of the special investigations which are helpful in assessing cardiovascular disorders.

Cardiovascular symptoms

Important symptoms of cardiovascular disease are shown in Table 6.1. To assess cardiovascular status, several questions are pertinent in eliciting relevant information; a simple scheme is shown in Table 6.2.

Table 6.1 Symptoms of cardiovascular disease
Chest pain or discomfort
Lower limb pain or discomfort
Shortness of breath
Palpitations
Oedema of the legs

Chest pain or discomfort

Chest pain may be the presenting manifestation of several pathological conditions. These are listed in Table 6.3.

Chest pain is the commonest clinical presentation of ischaemic (coronary) heart disease. When the coronary arteries are narrowed by coronary atherosclerosis, transient chest pain or discomfort (angina pectoris) may occur as a result of local myocardial ischaemia when the demands of the heart are increased by exercise or emotion. It is usually felt behind the sternum, and radiates across the chest and down the arms; it may also radiate to the back or to the mandible. In stable angina, the pain or discomfort is typically brought on by exertion or emotion, and is relieved by a few minutes' rest. Recovery is accelerated by sublingual nitrates.

Pain of a similar type, and site, is experienced when the coronary arteries are acutely occluded by

Table 6.2 Cardiovascular history taking

Heart valve problems	Have you ever had heart murmurs, heart tests or heart surgery? Has a doctor ever told you about telling your dentist about heart problems? Do you carry a card about this? Have you ever been given antibiotics for tooth extractions?
Anticoagulant (blood-thinning) drugs	Do you take these drugs? Do you carry a card about this? Do you attend an anticoagulant clinic? Why do you take them? (Heart valve problems, irregular heart or pulse, blood clots)
High blood pressure	Have you ever had this? Are you on treatment for this? Which drugs? (Ask patient/doctor about nifedipine if gum hyperplasia is present)
Chest pain or discomfort	Do you ever get this? If so, where and when? Do you also get this in your arms or jaw? Are you on treatment for this? Which drugs? (ask patient/doctor about nifedipine if gum hyperplasia is present)
Shortness of breath	Do you ever get this? If so, is it at rest, or only on exercise? How much exercise can you do?
Swelling of the legs	Do you ever get this? Are you on treatment for this, e.g. water tablets (diuretics)?

Table 6.3 Causes of central chest pain or discomfort

Ischaemic heart disease
  Stable angina
  Unstable angina
  Myocardial infarction

Pulmonary embolism

Pericarditis

Dissecting aortic aneurysm

Acute tracheitis (see Ch. 8)

Reflux oesophagitis/
oesophageal spasm (see Ch. 10)

coronary artery thrombosis. However, in contrast to stable angina, the pain is spontaneous; it is not brought on by exertion or emotion, it is not relieved by rest, or by sublingual nitrates, it lasts longer than a few minutes, it is often more severe and it may be accompanied by cardiac arrest, pallor, sweating, nausea, fainting or shock, shortness of breath, and a pulse which may be fast, slow or irregular.

Other cardiovascular causes of central chest pain include massive pulmonary embolism, pericarditis and dissecting aortic aneurysm. Non-cardiovascular causes include acute tracheitis (see Ch. 8) and reflux oesophagitis or oesophageal spasm (see Ch. 10).

Lower limb pain or discomfort

A tight or cramping pain in the lower limb muscles on exercise (intermittent claudication) is the commonest clinical presentation of peripheral arterial disease, which causes narrowing by atherosclerosis of the arteries supplying the lower limb. Like stable angina, the pain is relieved by rest, and lasts only a few minutes.

Shortness of breath

The main causes are shown in Table 6.4.

Normal persons are unaware of their breathing unless under stressful conditions (e.g. unaccustomed exercise or acute anxiety). Shortness of breath (dyspnoea) is commonly due to heart diseases which impair the ability of the heart to

Table 6.4 Causes of shortness of breath

Heart failure

Any severe lung disease (see Ch. 8), especially asthma or chronic bronchitis

Anaemia (see Ch. 7)

Abdominal swelling
    Ascites (see Ch. 10)
    Late pregnancy
    Tumours

pump blood through the lungs from the right ventricle to the left atrium, i.e. heart failure. The resulting pulmonary venous congestion reduces gas exchange across the alveolar membrane, resulting in hypoxaemia and compensatory hyperventilation. The congested lungs also become more resistant to expansion during ventilation, resulting in increased ventilatory effort.

In chronic progressive heart failure, breathlessness is initially experienced only on effort (e.g. climbing hills or stairs, or running) and is relieved by rest. The degree of effort required to provoke shortness of breath decreases with time, and eventually progresses to breathlessness at rest. Patients with breathlessness due to heart failure often experience breathlessness on lying flat (orthopnoea), which is relieved by sitting up or using extra pillows in bed: this reduces pulmonary venous congestion.

In acute left-sided heart failure, severe breathlessness occurs due to acute pulmonary oedema. Patients often wake at night with a feeling of choking or suffocation; they have rapid and difficult breathing, cough up frothy sputum which may be pink due to traces of blood, and have central cyanosis (see below). This picture may result from acute myocardial infarction or as an intercurrent event in patients with chronic left ventricular dysfunction, e.g. due to coronary heart disease and/or hypertension.

Shortness of breath may also result from lung diseases (see Ch. 8), anaemia (see Ch. 7), or abdominal swelling (e.g. ascites – see Ch. 10), late pregnancy, or abdominal tumours such as ovarian cysts) (Table 6.4). These causes frequently coexist; for example, heavy smokers may have shortness of breath as a result of both heart failure

from coronary heart disease, and also chronic bronchitis and emphysema (see Ch. 8).

Palpitation

This can be defined as an awareness of the action of the heart, and is very common in anxious or introspective individuals. It can, however, have its basis in organic cardiac disease, and is occasioned by unduly forceful heart beats, or by disturbances of rhythm.

Oedema of the legs

Bilateral leg swelling due to oedema is a common and important feature of chronic heart failure, but can occur in other systemic diseases, or in chronic venous insufficiency affecting both legs. Unilateral oedema usually has local causes.

Cardiovascular examination

Signs of cardiovascular disease detectable by simple observation are listed in Table 6.5.

Difficulty in breathing

Patients with severe heart failure (acute or chronic) may show evidence of respiratory distress, including rapid laboured breathing (over 20/minute), and the use of accessory muscles of respiration, e.g. neck muscles.

Cyanosis

Cyanosis is defined as a blue colour of the skin and mucous membranes, and is due to the

Table 6.5 Signs of cardiovascular disease

Difficulty in breathing

Cyanosis
    Peripheral
    Central

Finger clubbing

Swollen legs – oedema

Distended neck veins

Arterial pulse – fast, slow or irregular

presence of an excessive amount of de-oxygenated haemoglobin in these tissues.

Central cyanosis. This reflects impaired oxygenation of blood in the lungs, resulting in the systemic circulation of deoxygenated blood: all visible tissues are affected, including the lips, tongue and hands, which are warm. The common causes are severe heart failure (see below), cyanotic congenital heart disease with right heart to left heart shunts (see below), severe respiratory failure (see Ch. 8) and abnormal blood pigments (e.g. sulph-haemoglobin or met-haemoglobin, which are usually adverse drug effects).

Peripheral cyanosis. This is due to slow flow through the peripheral circulation and hence stagnation of circulating blood allowing exaggerated deoxygenation. It is best seen in the hands and feet, which are cold. Since oxygenation of blood in the lungs is normal, sites such as the tongue and lips are unaffected. Causes of peripheral cyanosis include all types of peripheral vasoconstriction, e.g. Raynaud's syndrome, shock, and chronic heart disease with pump failure. Local venous obstruction may lead to impaired perfusion by back pressure through the capillary bed.

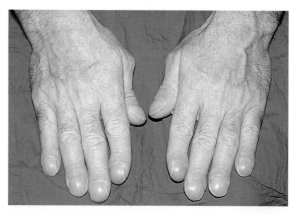

Fig. 6.1 Finger clubbing.

Finger clubbing

This describes filling in of the angle of the nailbed and a round expansion of the fingernails (Fig. 6.1). This can be a feature of two cardiac disorders (congenital cyanotic heart disease and infective endocarditis); two chest disorders (bronchial carcinoma and lung sepsis; see Ch. 8) and two alimentary disorders (cirrhosis of the liver and inflammatory bowel disease; see Ch. 10). It can also be congenital.

Swelling of the legs due to peripheral oedema

As noted above, bilateral swelling of the legs due to peripheral oedema may be due to chronic heart failure. Oedema (excess tissue fluid) is detectable by fingertip pressure over the tibial bone for about 30 s; a 'pit' due to physical displacement of excessive tissue fluid is observed (Fig. 6.2).

Distended neck veins

Systemic fluid retention and the inability of the right heart to pump blood into the lungs may be

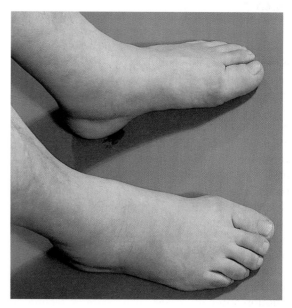

Fig. 6.2 Pitting oedema of the ankles.

reflected in distension of the neck veins, which act as a 'manometer' of systemic venous pressure (Fig. 6.3). When patients are reclining at about 45° to the horizontal the blood level in the jugular veins is normally below the level of the clavicle. In heart failure, this level rises, and may be visible pulsating above the clavicle.

Arterial pulses

Heart rate and rhythm are usually assessed by palpating the radial artery pulse and timing it over 15 s. The resting rate in adults averages about

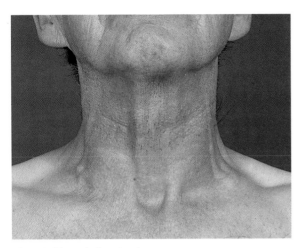

Fig. 6.3 Distended neck veins.

72 beats per minute (18 beats per 15 s), but varies widely between 60 and 90 beats per minute. Children and pregnant women have faster pulse rates.

The internal carotid pulse in the neck should be palpated in patients with acute collapse, to distinguish patients with cardiac arrest (absent carotid pulsation) from those with faints or shock (carotid pulsations are present, but there is reduced peripheral perfusion pressure which may cause the radial pulse to be impalpable).

Lower limb pulses (femoral, popliteal, dorsalis pedis and posterior tibial) assess the presence and site of peripheral arterial disease.

Tachycardia (pulse rate over 100 beats per minute) is a physiological response to exercise, emotion and pain. It also occurs as a normal reaction to injury (including haemorrhage and shock) or infection. Other diseases causing tachycardia include myocardial infarction, heart failure and hyperthyroidism (see Ch. 13). Drugs which increase the heart rate include adrenaline (given to treat anaphylactic shock) and adrenaline analogues such as salbutamol (given to treat acute asthma, see Ch. 8).

Bradycardia (pulse rate under 60 beats per minute) is commonly seen in physically trained persons such as athletes, or as a result of increased vagal tone. Acute bradycardia occurs during simple faints (vasovagal syncope), and in acute heart block, e.g. complicating acute myocardial infarction. Chronic bradycardia may be due to β-adrenergic blocker drugs (e.g. atenolol) used for treatment of angina or hypertension, digoxin therapy, heartblock or hypothyroidism (see Ch. 13).

Arterial blood pressures are routinely examined using a sphygmomanometer in recumbent patients. After inflation of the pneumatic cuff around the upper arm to occlude the brachial artery (as shown by disappearance of the radial pulse), the cuff is slowly deflated while the examiner listens with a stethoscope over the brachial artery in the antecubital fossa and observes the mercury column. The systolic arm blood pressure is recorded as soon as the pulse beat can be detected audibly (Korotkoff sounds). The diastolic blood pressure is recorded at the point when these sounds disappear. The systolic and diastolic blood pressures are expressed in millimetres of mercury read on the column, e.g. 120/80 mmHg.

Clinical examination of the heart itself is outside the scope of this chapter. Important information about chamber size and function can be obtained by palpation. Auscultation will provide additional data on cardiac rate and rhythm, and detection of murmurs is vital in the diagnosis of valvular and congenital heart disease.

Cardiovascular investigations

The cardiovascular investigations which are available are shown in Table 6.6 along with their use in diagnosing cardiovascular disorders.

Cardiovascular disorders

A wide range of disorders can affect the heart and vascular system. These will be considered under the headings 'Dysrhythmias' 'Collapse', 'Cardiac disorders characterized by anatomical derangements of the heart' and 'Blood vessel disorders'.

Dysrhythmias

Dysrhythmias (disorders of heart rhythm) may be suspected clinically by a history of palpitations, and by examining the arterial pulse. Electrocardiography (Fig 6.4) confirms the diagnosis. If intermittent dysrhythmias are suspected, patients can be fitted with an ambulatory (Holter)

Table 6.6 Cardiovascular investigations and their uses

Investigation	Usefulness
Electrocardiography (Fig. 6.4)	Heart rate, rhythm, ischaemia, pericarditis, ventricular hypertrophy
Exercise electrocardiography	Ischaemia
Chest radiography (Fig. 6.5)	Heart size, pulmonary venous congestion, pulmonary oedema, pulmonary effusion, heart failure, valvular disease, congenital heart disease
Cardiac enzymes	Acute myocardial infarction (creatinine kinase, transaminases, lactate dehydrogenase)
Cardiac ultrasound scanning (echocardiography)	Valve disease, ventricular dysfunction, pericardial effusion, dissecting aortic aneurysm, major pulmonary embolism
Isotope scanning (thallium or technetium)	Ischaemia (especially after exercise)
Cardiac catheterization	Valve disease
Coronary angiography	Coronary artery disease
Peripheral ultrasonography	Peripheral vascular disease, carotid artery disease
Peripheral angiography	Peripheral arterial disease, carotid artery disease
Peripheral venography	Deep venous thrombosis
Pulmonary isotope scanning	Pulmonary embolism
Pulmonary angiography	Pulmonary embolism

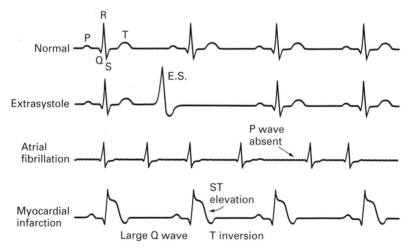

Fig. 6.4 Electrocardiograms (ECGs) showing the normal pattern, an extrasystole, atrial fibrillation, and acute myocardial infarction. Sinus rhythm describes the normal pattern of electrical coordination of the cardiac cycle. Electrical activity starts in the sinoatrial node, passes across the atria (detected as the P wave on the ECG), then travels across the atrioventricular node before causing ventricular depolarization (detected as the QRS complex on the ECG) and ventricular repolarization (detected as the T wave on the ECG).

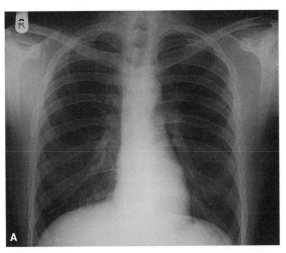
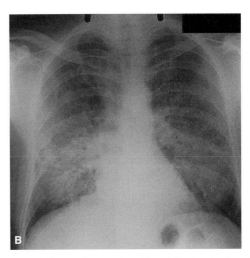

Fig. 6.5 Chest X-rays. **A** Normal appearance. **B** Heart failure: note the enlarged heart, the prominent lung hilar due to chronic pulmonary congestion, and opacification over both lower lung fields indicating pulmonary oedema.

monitor, which records the electrocardiogram (ECG) over a 24 h period, during which patients make a timed record of their symptoms.

The causes of sinus tachycardia and sinus bradycardia have been considered above. Sinus arrhythmia is a physiological finding in young persons: it consists of an increased heart rate during inspiration followed by a decreased heart rate during expiration, resulting from altered tone in the vagus nerve.

Extrasystoles are additional heart beats initiated in some focus of excitation outside the sinoatrial node (ectopic focus). The ECG shows whether this focus is supraventricular (atrial, or from the atrioventricular node) or ventricular (Fig. 6.4). The patient may experience palpitations, and the arterial pulse is irregular. Causes include increased adrenergic activity (anxiety, smoking, coffee, tea or unaccustomed exercise), drugs (adrenaline, adrenaline analogues (e.g. salbutamol used for treatment of asthma) or digoxin), and underlying heart disease. Treatment includes avoiding precipitating factors, and sometimes β-adrenergic blockers (e.g. atenolol).

Paroxysmal tachycardias are rapid runs of extra heart beats arising from an ectopic focus; the ECG shows whether this focus is supraventricular or ventricular. The patient is often aware of a sudden onset of sustained, rapid palpitations, and the arterial pulse is rapid and regular. The causes are

as for extrasystoles. The tachycardia may precipitate heart failure if there is underlying heart disease. Treatment is monitored by the ECG, and includes physical vagal stimulation (e.g. unilateral carotid sinus massage) or drugs (e.g. intravenous adenosine, verapamil, amiodarone, or β-adrenergic blockers). Hospital admission may be required if the tachycardia does not resolve in the hospital emergency department.

Atrial fibrillation is the commonest chronic dysrhythmia, and may be paroxysmal or sustained. It is unusual before the age of 50 years, but the incidence rises with age thereafter, reaching a prevalence of about 10% in people aged over 80 years. Patients may be aware of palpitations. The arterial pulse is totally irregular, and may be rapid. The ECG shows uncoordinated atrial activity (an irregular, wavy baseline), and in the absence of normal atrial contraction, P waves are not seen; the ventricular response is rapid and unpredictable (Fig. 6.4). Causes include chest infection, hyperthyroidism (see Ch. 13), ischaemic heart disease, alcoholic cardiomyopathy and rheumatic heart disease (especially mitral stenosis).

Like paroxysmal tachycardias, atrial fibrillation reduces cardiac output, and may precipitate heart failure. In addition, thrombi form in the non-contracting left atrium, and may cause systemic thromboembolism: such emboli usually occlude either cerebral vessels, causing cerebral infarction and stroke (see Ch. 9), or limb vessels, causing limb ischaemia or gangrene.

Treatment of atrial fibrillation includes electrical defibrillation (cardioversion) performed under a short-acting general anaesthetic, control of rapid ventricular rate by digoxin and/or β-adrenergic blockers, and anticoagulation with warfarin to reduce the risk of thromboembolism. Aspirin is less effective than warfarin in long-term prophylaxis, but is given when the bleeding risk of warfarin outweighs the benefit.

Atrial flutter has similar causes and treatment to atrial fibrillation. However, the rapid atrial rhythm is regular (appearing as a 'saw-tooth' pattern on the ECG). The atrioventricular node transmits every second, third or fourth atrial impulse to the ventricles.

'Heart block' implies impaired electrical conduction within the heart (usually within the atrioventricular node). Causes include degenerative changes with age, ischaemic heart disease including acute myocardial infarction, and digoxin therapy. First-degree heart block consists of delayed conduction through the bundle of His, and is only detectable by the ECG. Second-degree heart block results in irregular impulses passing down the bundle, and thus an irregular ventricular response, and pulse. In third-degree (complete) heart block, no atrial impulses reach the ventricles, which then adopt their own intrinsic capacity to contract at about 32 beats per minute (idioventricular rhythm). When third-degree heart block occurs suddenly, it may take several seconds before an idioventricular rhythm occurs, hence there is a transient cardiac arrest (Stokes–Adams attack) with loss of consciousness, pallor, cyanosis and absent pulse; followed by recovery. Treatment is with a battery-operated pacemaker. For temporary use (e.g. in acute myocardial infarction) the pacer wire is passed from an external pacemaker through a central vein into the right ventricle; permanent pacemakers are implanted under the skin of the chest wall.

Collapse

Collapse may arise for a number of cardiovascular reasons and these are shown in Table 6.7.

Table 6.7 Cardiovascular causes of collapse

Cardiac arrest
Fainting
Circulatory shock
Anaphylactic shock
Haemorrhagic shock

Cardiac arrest

Cardiac arrest is cessation of spontaneous cardiac output, which is detected by sudden loss of consciousness; pallor, followed by cyanosis; absent large arterial pulses (feel the carotid pulse in the neck – Fig. 6.6a); and cessation of respiration within a few seconds or minutes (cardiorespiratory arrest). Breathing may be noisy, irregular or intermittent before ceasing. Brain death occurs unless effective life support is initiated promptly; this is characterized by fixed dilated pupils. Delayed resuscitation may result in recovery of heartbeat and breathing, but persistent coma due to irreversible hypoxic brain damage.

Cardiac arrest is due to one of three mechanisms which can be distinguished on the emergency ECG:

- *Ventricular fibrillation.* The normal QRS complex is absent, and replaced by chaotic activity on the ECG. This is most commonly due to acute myocardial infarction (when it may be preceded by a typical history of acute, severe central chest pain), but may be due to any type of heart disease, pulmonary embolism, anaphylactic shock, electrocution, drowning or asphyxiation. In many cases, emergency life support and electrical defibrillation restore sinus rhythm and an effective heartbeat.
- *Ventricular asystole.* The ECG tracing is flat. Asystole is more common than fibrillation in patients with severe terminal disease (e.g. heart failure). In this situation, asystole can be converted to ventricular fibrillation by intravenous adrenaline or atropine, and, if so, electrical defibrillation may subsequently restore sinus rhythm and an effective heartbeat.
- *Electrical–mechanical dissociation.* The ECG is normal, hence there is a lack of mechanical pumping action of the heart despite normal electrical conduction. This may be due to

hypovolaemic shock, pulmonary embolism, cardiac tamponade from a large pericardial effusion, tension pneumothorax (see Ch. 8), drug overdose, hypothermia or electrolyte imbalance.

If cardiac arrest occurs, cardiopulmonary resuscitation should be initiated immediately (Fig. 6.6), and a cardiac arrest team summoned if the incident occurs in hospital or a cardiac ambulance if the arrest occurs elsewhere.

Fainting (syncope)

A faint is transient loss of consciousness, due to a fall in systemic arterial blood pressure which reduces the blood supply to the brain. It is manifested by loss of consciousness, which is usually less sudden than in cardiac arrest, and is preceded by feeling and looking unwell for seconds or minutes. The patient also has features of cerebral hypoperfusion, and feels light-headed, giddy and nauseated. Breathing is shallow. There are signs of compensatory adrenergic activity, which attempts to maintain blood pressure: the skin is pale and cold (due to vasoconstriction) with profuse sweating. The radial pulse is weak or impalpable (however the carotid pulse is present), and may be slow in a vasovagal attack or heart block, or rapid due to compensatory adrenergic activation. The arterial blood pressure is low.

Causes of faints include:

- *Vasovagal attacks (simple faints)*. The fall in blood pressure is due to the combined effects of increased vagal tone (which slows the heart) and widespread vasodilatation. Simple faints are common in healthy young persons, including trained sportsmen and athletes who have a slower heart rate and lower blood pressure than the general population. Precipitating factors include pain, fear, seeing needles or blood; hearing bad news or witnessing an accident; and prolonged standing, especially in hot weather, which promotes vasodilatation; and drugs causing hypotension, e.g. those used for treatment of hypertension or angina.
- *Dysrhythmias*, e.g. paroxysmal tachycardia, atrial fibrillation, and complete heart block (Stokes–Adams attack).
- *Heart disease*, e.g. acute myocardial infarction and aortic valve stenosis.

Management of faints. Cardiac arrest should first be excluded by ensuring that there is an arterial pulse (feel the carotid pulse in the neck, because the radial pulse may be impalpable due to low blood pressure; Fig 6.6) and that respiration is maintained. Patients should be laid flat and their legs raised to 45°. These procedures increase cerebral blood flow, especially if blood is pooled in the legs due to systemic vasodilatation. The

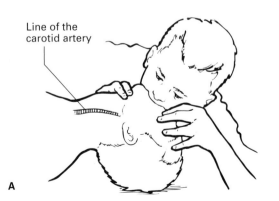

Line of the
carotid artery

A

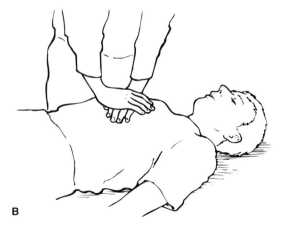

B

Fig. 6.6 **A** Life support in cardiac arrest: mouth-to-mouth breathing, and line of the carotid artery for detection of an arterial pulse. **B** Life support in cardiac arrest: external cardiac compression.

following are also important: loosen any tight clothing around the neck (e.g. collars and ties); clear any hazards around the patient who has fainted on the ground (e.g. motor traffic in the street, fires in the house); and observe the patient carefully until recovery occurs. Emergency medical attention should be sought if the patient does not make a full and rapid recovery. One should avoid giving alcohol, which is a vasodilator drug.

Shock (circulatory collapse)

This is a medical emergency, characterized by a prolonged fall in systemic arterial blood pressure and reduced perfusion of vital organs, including the brain, kidney, liver and lungs. The clinical features are similar to those of faints (see above) but do not recover rapidly. Prolonged hypoperfusion of vital organs results in secondary changes, which may be fatal even if the primary cause of shock is treated ('irreversible' shock):

- kidney – acute tubular necrosis, causing acute renal failure (see Ch. 11)
- liver and gut – acute liver failure and enterotoxaemia
- lungs – acute respiratory distress syndrome, comprising alveolar damage, pulmonary oedema and consolidation, and respiratory failure with severe hypoxia.

Disseminated intravascular coagulation, is an additional complication, resulting in consumption of plasma fibrinogen and other coagulation factors with generalized bleeding (see Ch. 7).

It is therefore important that shock is recognized and treated early, before these complications occur.

Causes of shock include:

- *Anaphylaxis.* A severe allergic reaction to drugs (especially if injected), foods, bee or wasp stings etc. This is discussed below.
- *Cardiogenic shock*, e.g. acute myocardial infarction or massive pulmonary embolism.
- *Major bleeding*, e.g. trauma, surgery, gastrointestinal bleeding (see Ch. 10), or obstetric accidents.
- *Septicaemia.* This is especially likely with Gram negative organisms such as *Escherichia coli.*

- *Loss of plasma*, e.g. severe skin burns.
- *Loss of salt and water*, e.g. severe vomiting, diarrhoea, diabetic coma (see Ch. 13), hypoadrenalism (see Ch. 13) or heat stroke.

Management of the severely shocked patient requires the monitoring and therapeutic resources of a hospital intensive care unit. Transfer should thus be arranged urgently, using a specialized ambulance team if available. Other than first-aid treatment of the primary cause, e.g. adrenaline in anaphylactic shock, any delay should be avoided.

Anaphylactic shock. This is a severe allergic emergency, which may be encountered following drug administration, especially if injected (e.g. antibiotics or aspirin or other non-steroidal anti-inflammatory drugs (NSAIDs)). Other causes include blood products and vaccines; wasp and bee stings and insect bites; foods, e.g. eggs, fish, nuts including peanuts and cow's milk protein; and food additives, e.g. peanut oil (arachis oil).

Atopic persons (those with a history of asthma, hay fever or atopic eczema) are at increased risk. It is important always to ask about known allergies before prescribing drugs, especially antibiotics or aspirin.

Symptoms of anaphylaxis usually occur within minutes of exposure to the allergen, which reacts with the host IgE antibody to release histamine and other vasoactive substances. As a result there is hypotension and shock, due to intense dilatation and leakage of small blood vessels. There is also bronchospasm (acute wheeze and breathlessness), due to increased permeability and constriction of bronchioles (as in asthma, see Ch. 8) and stridor (gasping for breath through a narrowed larynx) due to laryngeal oedema (angioedema) from increased vascular permeability.

Emergency treatment includes ensuring an adequate airway; lying the patient flat and raising the legs to restore blood pressure; summoning a cardiac ambulance; and emergency medical treatment which includes oxygen and adrenaline by intramuscular injection (0.5–1 mg, i.e. 0.5–1 ml of a 1:1000 adrenaline injection). Patients with previous anaphylactic reactions may be trained to carry and to self-administer 0.3 mg (i.e. 0.3 ml of a 1:1000 adrenaline injection). The dose can be repeated every 10 min until improvement occurs.

Other measures include antihistamine, e.g. chlorpheniramine 10–20 mg by slow intravenous injection; corticosteroid, e.g. hydrocortisone 100–300 mg by slow intravenous injection; and tracheal intubation or tracheostomy, which may be required for severe laryngeal oedema.

Haemorrhagic shock. Removal of 0.5 litre of blood from healthy persons (e.g. blood donors) is usually well-tolerated; however, after loss of 1 litre or more, hypovolaemia develops, with an increase in pulse rate, fall in blood pressure, and other clinical features of syncope or hypovolaemic shock. Because both blood cells and plasma are lost from the circulation, the blood haematocrit and haemoglobin concentration are normal for several hours, falling only after expansion of the plasma volume (by endogenous retention of salt and water, or by therapeutic infusion of plasma expanders). Signs of hypovolaemia (e.g. pulse rate over 100 beats per minute, systolic blood pressure under 100 mmHg, low central venous pressure or shock) indicate the need for blood transfusion.

Management of haemorrhagic shock includes general management of shock (see above). In addition, the patient requires rapid infusion of plasma expanders (e.g. dextran, gelatin, starch, albumin or plasma protein solution) to restore blood volume while blood is cross-matched for transfusion.

Direct control of bleeding points is of immediate importance. Temporary control may be obtained by local pressure, including local pressure on a spurting artery or application of a limb tourniquet as first aid in trauma. Surgical control is obtained by clamping, ligation or undersewing of arteries, or by suturing, packing or electrocoagulation of smaller vessels. Endoscopy or open surgery may be required for access in internal bleeding to allow these procedures to be performed.

Cardiac disorders characterized by anatomical derangements of the heart

Several cardiac lesions result in disruption of the blood flow through the heart, and these are shown in Table 6.8.

Congenital heart disease

Congenital heart disease may be a consequence of genetic disorders such as Down's syndrome, or

Table 6.8 Conditions causing disruption of cardiac blood flow

Congenital heart disease
Rheumatic fever
Chronic rheumatic heart disease
Other valvular diseases
Infective endocarditis

infections in early pregnancy such as rubella (see Ch. 5). The incidence in the newborn is about 1% of live births. In addition, minor defects can present in later life (e.g. a further 1% of the population have bicuspid aortic valves). Table 6.9 lists the common defects detected at birth.

Although clinical features of congenital heart disease may be apparent at birth, some patients may not present till later in life (e.g. at routine medical examinations). Features include heart murmurs, heart failure due to abnormal haemodynamics, and central cyanosis if the lesion causes shunting of deoxygenated blood from the right heart to the left heart (e.g. in Fallot's tetralogy, Table 6.9). Such patients may also develop finger clubbing and secondary polycythaemia (see Ch. 7).

There is often a risk of infective endocarditis, which may follow dental procedures. All such

Table 6.9 Common congenital heart defects

Defect	Congenital heart disease detected at birth (%)
Ventricular septal defect (VSD)	32
Persistent ductus arteriosus (PDA)	10
Pulmonary stenosis (PS)	8
Atrial septal defect (ASD)	7
Coarctation of the aorta	6
Fallot's tetralogy (VSD, PS, right ventricular hypertrophy, overriding aorta)	5
Aortic stenosis (AS)	4
Transposition of the great arteries (TGA)	4
Others	23

patients should be given an endocarditis risk card, and their dentists informed of the need for antimicrobial prophylaxis.

Diagnosis of congenital heart disease is usually confirmed by cardiac ultrasound ± catheterization.

Treatment of congenital heart disease includes correction (usually surgical) of the defect – either at open-heart surgery (see below), at cardiac catheterization or even occasionally by medical treatment, thus, for example, patent ductus arteriosus between the aorta and the pulmonary trunk can be closed by medical treatment with a prostaglandin synthesis inhibitor (indomethacin).

Rheumatic fever

Rheumatic fever is an abnormal immune reaction in certain persons to an acute infection with certain strains of *Streptococcus pyogenes* (group A), usually streptococcal sore throats (see Ch. 8), occurring in school-age children (5–15 years).

In developed countries, the incidence of rheumatic fever (and subsequently of rheumatic heart disease) has declined markedly since the 1940s, due partly to changes in the bacterium, partly to improved social conditions (less poverty and overcrowding) and partly to the introduction of effective antimicrobial therapy for streptococcal infections (e.g. penicillins). However, both rheumatic fever and rheumatic heart disease remain major health problems in developing countries.

The clinical features of acute rheumatic fever are shown in Table 6.10. Treatment of acute rheumatic fever includes bed rest, anti-inflammatory drugs (aspirin ± corticosteroids) and antimicrobials (penicillin, or erythromycin in patients with penicillin allergy). These are given both as treatment of the primary infection, and as secondary prophylaxis to prevent further attacks of rheumatic fever and development of rheumatic heart disease.

Chronic rheumatic heart disease

About 70% of patients with rheumatic fever develop chronic rheumatic heart disease. The fibrous tissue reaction to the endocardial inflammation may produce either narrowing of the affected valve (stenosis) which reduces blood flow

Table 6.10 Features of acute rheumatic fever

Preceding history of streptococcal infection
Pyrexia
Migrating acute polyarthritis of large joints
Pancarditis
   Endocarditis, especially of valves
   Myocarditis
   Pericarditis
Skin rashes
Chorea (involuntary jerky movements) – basal ganglia of brain affected

through the valve, or incompetent closure (incompetence) with regurgitation of blood flow; the valves exposed to high pressures (mitral and/or aortic) are most likely to be involved. Patients are usually young or middle-aged adults. Clinical features in women often worsen in pregnancy, due to increased circulatory demands.

Clinical features of chronic rheumatic heart disease include a history of rheumatic fever or chorea (only obtained in 50% of cases); heart murmurs (these may be found at routine medical examinations, e.g. antenatal clinics during pregnancy); and superimposed infective endocarditis, which can occur at any time and which may follow dental procedures. All patients should be given an endocarditis risk card, and their dentist informed of the need for antimicrobial prophylaxis. Patients may also develop heart failure and atrial fibrillation (especially in mitral stenosis), which carries a high risk of thromboembolism, and requires longterm prophylactic oral anticoagulants.

Diagnosis of individual valvular lesions is made clinically, and confirmed by cardiac ultrasound and catheterization.

Treatment of rheumatic heart disease includes antimicrobial prophylaxis of infective endocarditis, including for some dental procedures; anticoagulant prophylaxis, especially in the presence of atrial fibrillation; treatment of heart failure; and surgical correction of the defect. Most procedures (usually heart valve replacement) require open-heart surgery, during which the heart and lungs are temporarily bypassed with an extracorporeal circulation including an artificial pump and oxygenation device. Full anticoagulation with heparin is required to prevent thrombosis within this circuit. After the circuit is established, ventricular fibrillation is induced to stop the pumping action of the heart and allow surgery to be performed. After completion of surgery, normal cardiac rhythm is re-established by electrical defibrillation, and the artificial circulation is removed.

Prosthetic heart valves may be either mechanical or biological (porcine tissue valves). Mechanical prostheses have a longer life expectancy, but are more thrombogenic and often require long-term oral anticoagulant prophylaxis. Bioprostheses have a shorter life-expectancy, but are less thrombogenic, and often require only short-term oral anticoagulant prophylaxis followed by long-term oral antiplatelet prophylaxis (e.g. aspirin). Both types of prostheses are susceptible to infective endocarditis (which may develop during their insertion), hence all patients should be given an endocarditis risk card, and their dentists informed of the need for antimicrobial prophylaxis.

Other causes of heart valve disease

Syphilis (see Ch. 5) may involve the aortic valve, causing destruction and aortic regurgitation. Degenerative aortic stenosis is common in older patients, and usually results from progressive calcification of congenitally bicuspid aortic valves (which occur in 1% of the general population).

Infective endocarditis

Infective endocarditis is infection of the heart valves or endocardium by bloodborne microbes. These are usually bacteria (streptococci or staphylococci), but sometimes yeasts (*Candida albicans*), rickettsiae, mycoplasmas or chlamydiae. The heart valves may be normal, especially if the microbe is virulent (e.g. *Staphylococcus aureus*). However, there is an increased risk if the heart valves or endocardium are abnormal, e.g. congenital heart disease (valve disease, septal defects or patent ductus arteriosus), rheumatic heart valve disease; degenerative or syphilitic heart valve disease, or prosthetic heart valves.

Sources of infection include:

- *Oral sepsis (gingivitis, periodontitis).* Bacteraemia (e.g. *Streptococcus mutans* or *sanguis*)

is common during normal chewing or oral hygiene procedures, and its severity and magnitude correlate with the severity of gingival inflammation. Good oral health reduces the likelihood of endocarditis in at-risk patients, and should therefore be encouraged in all such patients.

- *Invasive dental procedures.* Procedures which induce gingival bleeding (e.g. dental extractions, periodontal scaling and other surgery involving gingival tissues) also induce bacteraemia. Hence, antimicrobial prophylaxis is recommended in at-risk patients for such procedures. Table 6.11 summarizes the recommendations in the *British National Formulary* (September 1998) for patients in the UK, which reflect the recommendations of the Working Party of the British Society for Antimicrobial Chemotherapy (Simmonds 1993). Such recommendations are updated regularly: current recommendations should be consulted. In the USA, the American Heart Association (Dajani et al 1997) recommends prophylaxis for all dental procedures that induce gingival bleeding.

Although fewer than 5% of endocarditis cases can be related to recent dental treatment, a high level of awareness is necessary among all professionals carrying out invasive medical or surgical procedures, to prevent this serious illness.

Infective endocarditis, usually occurring on the tricuspid valve, is an increasing problem in intravenous drug users who use non-sterile equipment.

The clinical features of infective endocarditis are very variable and their severity is often dependent on the infecting organism. For example, *Staph. aureus* endocarditis is highly destructive to the valve involved, and results in a rapidly progressive illness if not treated; less virulent organisms such as *Strep. viridans* present more insidiously (subacute bacterial endocarditis).

The principal manifestations consist of (1) septic emboli from friable vegetations on the affected valve, (2) deteriorating valve function and resulting cardiac failure, and (3) the general effects of debilitating infection such as fever, malaise, anorexia and anaemia.

Diagnosis is established by repeated blood cultures to identify the causal microbe (which is not identified in about one-third of patients), and by cardiac ultrasound, which may show abnormal heart valves or vegetations.

Table 6.11 Prevention of endocarditis in patients with a heart-valve lesion, septal defect, patent ductus or prosthetic valve[1]

Dental procedures[a] under local or no anaesthesia

Patients who have not received more than a single dose of a penicillin in the previous month, including those with a prosthetic valve (but not those who have had endocarditis), oral amoxycillin 3 g 1 h before a procedure; Child under 5 years, quarter adult dose; 5–10 years, half adult dose

Patients who are penicillin-allergic or have received more than a single dose of penicillin in the previous month, oral clindamycin[b] 600 mg 1 h before a procedure; child under 5 years, quarter adult dose; 5–10 years, half adult dose

Patients who have had endocarditis, amoxycillin + gentamicin, as under general anaesthesia

Dental procedures[a] under general anaesthesia

No special risk (including patients who have not received more than a single dose of a penicillin in the previous month): IV amoxycillin 1 g at induction, then oral amoxycillin 500 mg 6 h later; Child under 5 years quarter adult dose; 5–10 years half adult dose
or oral amoxycillin 3 g 4 h before induction then oral amoxycillin 3 g as soon as possible after procedure; Child under 5 years, quarter adult dose; 5–10 years, half adult dose
or oral amoxycillin 3 g + oral probenecid 1 g 4 h before procedure

Special risk (patients with prosthetic valve or who have had endocarditis), IV amoxycillin 1 g + IV gentamicin 120 mg at induction, then oral amoxycillin 500 mg 6 h later; Child under 5 years, amoxycillin quarter adult dose, gentamicin 2 mg/kg; 5–10 years amoxycillin, half adult dose, gentamicin 2 mg/kg

Patients who are penicillin-allergic or who have received more than a single dose of a penicillin in the previous month:

either IV vancomycin 1 g over at least 100 min then IV gentamicin 120 mg at induction or 15 min before procedure; Child under 10 years, vancomycin 20 mg/kg, gentamicin 2 mg/kg

or IV teicoplanin 400 mg + gentamicin 120 mg at induction or 15 min before procedure; Child under 14 years teicoplanin 6 mg/kg, gentamicin 2 mg/kg

or IV clindamycin[b] 300 mg over at least 10 min at induction or 15 min before procedure then oral or IV clindamycin 150 mg 6 h later; Child under 5 years, quarter adult dose; 5–10 years, half adult dose

---

1   Reproduced from the *British National Formulary* (September 1998), with the permission of the British Medical Association and Royal Pharmaceutical Society of Great Britain.
   IM, intramuscular; IV, intravenous.
a   Dental procedures that require antibiotic prophylaxis are extractions, scaling, and surgery involving gingival tissues. Antibiotic prophylaxis for dental procedures may be supplemented with chlorhexidine gluconate gel 1% or chlorhexidine gluconate mouthwash 0.2%, used 5 min before the procedure.
b   If clindamycin is used, periodontal or other multistage procedures should not be repeated at intervals of less than 2 weeks.

Treatment is with antimicrobials, selected according to the known (or suspected) microbe and its drug sensitivity. Antimicrobials should be bactericidal (often given in combination to prevent drug resistance), and therapy for several weeks may be necessary. Patients should be monitored clinically, and with repeated C-reactive protein assays (as a measure of ongoing infection) and cardiac ultrasound (to detect vegetations and valve damage). Heart valve replacement of damaged valves may be required, as will local treatment of dental sepsis (including extractions if required) during or after therapy.

Blood vessel disorders

Several disorders are considered here such as hypertension, atheroma, peripheral arterial diseases and venous and lymphatic diseases. Chronic heart failure is also considered here because it is usually due to atheroma or hypertension.

Heart failure

Chronic heart failure is defined as the symptom complex arising from both the inability of the heart to maintain cardiac output and the resulting venous congestion in the pulmonary and/or systemic circulations (congestive heart failure). Symptoms and signs include features of a low cardiac output: tiredness, low exercise tolerance, low pulse volume and blood pressure, and cold cyanosed peripheries. There are also features of cardiomegaly, pulmonary venous congestion and oedema (see Fig. 6.5), progressive breathlessness, orthopnoea and attacks of acute pulmonary oedema. Central cyanosis may occur due to hypoxia. Features of systemic venous congestion include swelling of the legs due to pitting oedema (see Fig. 6.2), distended neck veins (see Fig. 6.3) and an enlarged, tender liver.

Causes of heart failure and precipitating factors are summarized in Table 6.12. In the UK, most patients with heart failure are aged over 65 years, and ischaemic heart disease is the commonest cause.

Management of heart failure includes hospitalization and bed rest if there are severe, disabling symptoms. While mobility is restricted, prevention of venous thromboembolism by subcutaneous heparin is important in patients who are not already receiving anticoagulants. Treatment of causal and precipitating factors is also required. Oxygen should be administered as required for breathlessness. Diuretic drugs (e.g. frusemide or bendrofluazide) should be given as they increase renal excretion of salt and water, relieving features of pulmonary and systemic congestion. Vasodilator drugs, especially angiotensin-converting enzyme (ACE) inhibitors (e.g. captopril), are also useful as these improve cardiac output, effort tolerance and mortality.

Heart transplantation has an established place but due to limited availability of human donor hearts is usually reserved for younger patients with severe symptoms. Complications include rejection, infection and accelerated atherosclerosis.

Hypertension (high blood pressure)

Hypertension is defined as a systemic arterial blood pressure which is consistently higher than average, and which requires treatment to reduce the risk of complications. These complications arise from mechanical effects on the blood vessels and the heart, and include ischaemic heart disease, stroke, heart failure and renal failure (Table 6.13). Screening of adults for hypertension, and its treatment, are an important part of preventive medicine.

In younger adults, resting systolic blood pressure is usually less than 140 mmHg and diastolic blood pressure usually less than 90 mmHg. Blood pressure rises with age, and in those aged over 60 years the corresponding levels are 160 and 95 mmHg. Persons found to have either systolic or diastolic blood pressure readings above these levels for their age should have their resting blood pressure levels monitored over a period of time. Persistent elevations require patient–doctor discussions about treatment to prevent complications, and investigations to exclude an underlying cause.

In 95% of patients, no single underlying disease is identified, and the term 'primary hypertension' is used. The increased blood pressure arises from a sustained increase in arteriolar tone, which increases peripheral resistance. The cause is unknown, but is probably due to an interaction of multiple genetic and racial factors with environmental stresses and metabolic factors. A family

Table 6.12 Causes of heart failure and precipitating factors	
Causes	*Precipitating factors*
Ischaemic heart disease	Atrial fibrillation
Hypertension	Infections (e.g. chest)
Chronic lung disease (e.g. chronic bronchitis)	Anaemia (see Ch. 7)
Alcoholic cardiomyopathy	Thyroid overactivity or underactivity (see Ch. 13)

Heart valve disease
    Congenital
    Rheumatic
    Degenerative
	Drugs – β-adrenergic blockers, corticosteroids, non-steroidal anti-inflammatory drugs (NSAIDs)
	
	Pulmonary embolism
	
	Pregnancy

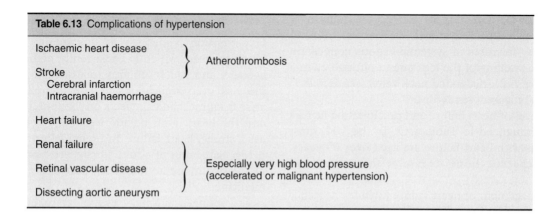

Table 6.13 Complications of hypertension

Ischaemic heart disease	} Atherothrombosis

Stroke
    Cerebral infarction
    Intracranial haemorrhage	

Heart failure	
Renal failure	} Especially very high blood pressure (accelerated or malignant hypertension)
Retinal vascular disease	
Dissecting aortic aneurysm	

history of hypertension is common, probably reflecting the contributions of many genes. Persons of African and Asian descent have an increased risk of hypertension under the conditions of Western lifestyle. Such lifestyle changes include certain stresses, and the development of obesity which is also associated with increasing blood pressure. Central obesity in particular is associated with insulin resistance, which may be clinically manifest as non-insulin-dependent diabetes mellitus (see Ch. 13). Drugs including tobacco, alcohol, oral contraceptives, corticosteroids, and potent NSAIDs (e.g. indomethacin) also increase blood pressure. Hypertension may also appear in pregnancy, when it may cause the additional complication of cerebral oedema and epileptic seizures (eclampsia).

In about 5% of cases, the hypertension is secondary to underlying renal or renovascular disease (renal arterial disease rendering one or both kidneys ischaemic) or endocrine diseases (see Ch. 13). These disorders elevate blood pressure through hormonal effects (Table 6.14). They are identified by routine clinical examination; testing of urine for protein and blood to detect renal disease; testing of blood urea, creatinine and electrolytes to detect renal disease or aldosterone excess; and hormone tests if endocrine disease is suspected.

Management of hypertension is summarised in Table 6.15.

Because the major complications of hypertension (ischaemic heart disease and stroke due to cerebral infarction) are due to atherothrombosis,

Table 6.14 Causes of hypertension

Primary (idiopathic or essential) – 95% of cases	Genetic factors
	Racial factors (Africans, Asians)
	Obesity (especially central), insulin resistance and
	    non-insulin dependent diabetes mellitus
	Stress
	Drugs – tobacco, alcohol, oral contraceptives,
	    corticosteroids, potent NSAIDs
	Pregnancy

Secondary – (5% of cases)	Renal or renovascular disease (excess renin/angiotensin) Endocrine diseases (see Ch. 13) Phaeochromocytoma (excess catecholamines) Cushing's syndrome (excess cortisol) Conn's syndrome (excess aldosterone) Acromegaly (excess growth hormone) Coarctation of the aorta.

Table 6.15 Management of hypertension

Assess and treat other risk factors for complications (smoking, cholesterol, diabetes mellitus)

Assess complications/target organ damage (ischaemic heart disease, stroke, heart failure, retinal vascular disease, renal impairment, left ventricular hypertrophy on ECG)

Identify and treat causes of secondary hypertension (see Table 6.14)

Lifestyle advice – reduce weight, smoking, alcohol, relevant drugs, stress, and dietary salt

If blood pressure remains elevated, antihypertensive drugs are indicated:

Thiazide diuretics, e.g. bendrofluazide
β-adrenergic blockers e.g. atenolol
ACE inhibitors, e.g. captopril
Calcium antagonists, e.g. amlodipine or nifedipine
α-adrenergic blockers, e.g. doxazosin.

it is important to modify any coexisting risk factors such as smoking, high blood cholesterol and diabetes mellitus. Evidence of complications or target organ damage also increases the case for active treatment. Causes of secondary hypertension should be identified and treated and appropriate lifestyle advice and support given.

If hypertension persists despite these measures, antihypertensive drugs should be prescribed, and blood pressure monitored regularly. The long-term aim of treatment is to reduce the risk of cardiovascular events by maintaining blood pressure levels of 140/90 mmHg or less. Many antihypertensive drugs are available: examples are given in Table 6.15. More than one drug may be needed for adequate blood pressure control. Long-term compliance is often poor, hence treatment should be as simple as possible (as few drugs as possible, given once or twice daily if possible) and free of adverse effects. The choice of drug(s) in the individual depends on patient preferences, and on the presence of other disorders including diabetes, gout, obstructive airways disease, angina, heart failure or renal failure, each of which may contraindicate (or indicate) certain types of drug.

Ischaemic heart disease and atherothrombosis

Ischaemic heart disease (coronary artery disease or coronary heart disease) is the major cause of death in developed countries, and is due to atherothrombosis of the coronary arteries. This is a systemic arterial disease which progresses throughout life and affects not only the coronary arteries but also the aorta, the lower limb arteries (peripheral arterial disease) and the carotid, vertebral and cerebral arteries (cerebrovascular disease).

Atherothrombosis comprises atherosclerosis and arterial thrombosis. Atherosclerosis is the development of raised fibro-fatty lesions (plaques) at sites of blood flow disturbance (bends and bifurcations) in the arterial tree. Such lesions may grow large enough to cause stenosis, reducing blood flow on exercise to the heart (angina) or lower limb muscles (claudication). However, the most serious complications of atherothrombosis (myocardial infarction, sudden cardiac death, stroke, and critical limb ischaemia/infarction) result from arterial thrombosis. This usually occurs following rupture of an atherosclerotic plaque, which exposes flowing arterial blood to the plaque contents including lipids and collagen: this stimulates formation of a 'haemostatic plug' of platelets and fibrin (see Ch. 7). An occlusive thrombus will then cause myocardial, cerebral or limb infarction.

Risk factors for ischaemic heart disease are listed in Table 6.16.

Primary prevention of ischaemic heart disease is an important part of preventive medicine. It has two complementary strategies. First, health education of the whole population with lifestyle

Table 6.16 Risk factors for ischaemic heart disease

Non-modifiable	Modifiable
Age	Smoking
Male sex	Cholesterol (total/high-density lipoprotein ratio)
Family history	Blood pressure
Race	Diabetes mellitus
Area	Obesity, lack of exercise
Social deprivation	Fibrinogen
	Periodontal disease
	Menopause

Table 6.17 Primary prevention of ischaemic heart disease: lifestyle advice on health education of whole western populations

Stop smoking
Take regular exercise – e.g. 30 min walking three times per week
Lose weight if obese – ideal body mass index (weight/height^2) is under 25 kg/m^2
Diet
  Eat fruit or vegetables at each meal
  Eat fish twice a week
  Restrict:
    animal fat
    salt (<100 mmol/day)
    alcohol (<28 units/week in men; <21 units/week in women)

Table 6.18 Primary and secondary prevention of ischaemic heart disease in 'high-risk persons' (persons who have multiple risk factors, or clinical evidence of ischaemic heart disease, peripheral arterial disease or cerebrovascular disease)

Lifestyle advice (see Table 6.17)
Treat high blood pressure
Treat high blood lipids – increased total: high-density lipoprotein cholesterol ± increased triglycerides
Treat diabetes
Consider aspirin (75–300 mg/day) unless contraindicated (e.g. allergy, peptic ulcer, bleeding disorder)

advice (Table 6.17); second, screening to identify 'high-risk' persons who, in addition to lifestyle advice, may merit drug treatments (antihypertensives, lipid-lowering drugs, antidiabetics, or antithrombotic drugs (e.g. aspirin)). (Table 6.18).

Secondary prevention of ischaemic heart disease in persons with clinical evidence (e.g. angina or myocardial infarction) is equally important, because persons with clinical evidence of arterial disease have the highest risk of a further arterial thrombotic event (e.g. myocardial infarction or stroke) – on average, about 5% per year. The measures in Table 6.18 are also appropriate for such patients.

Angina pectoris is the commonest clinical presentation of ischaemic heart disease. It is infrequent before the age of 40 years, but increasingly common thereafter (prevalence about 5% of the population aged over 40 years). Angina and its precipitants have already been described (see page 43).

Diagnosis of stable angina is usually made from a typical history, since there are few relevant clinical signs. Evidence of myocardial ischaemia may be evident on a resting ECG (ST segment depression; T wave flattening or inversion); if not, exercise ECG testing can be considered in an attempt to elicit these changes. Cardiac catheterization and coronary angiography may be indicated if the diagnosis remains unclear, or if coronary angioplasty or bypass surgery are being considered.

Treatment of stable angina is summarized in Table 6.19. All patients should initially be treated

medically, with risk factor reduction and antianginal drugs. For treatment of acute anginal attacks, patients are given short-acting glyceryl trinitrate, which acts rapidly by causing vasodilatation both peripherally (reducing cardiac work) and in the coronary arteries. It is given orally as sublingual, buccal or spray preparations, which are rapidly absorbed and effective within seconds or minutes. Adverse effects include headache and faints.

For prevention of attacks, long-acting nitrates (oral, or skin patches), β-adrenergic blockers or calcium antagonists are effective (Table 6.19). These drugs reduce cardiac workload, and the last two types of drug are also effective in treating associated hypertension. As with hypertension, more than one drug may be needed for adequate control of anginal attacks, and the choice of drugs in the individual depends on patient preferences and on the presence of other disorders (hyperten-

Table 6.19 Treatment of stable angina

Risk factor reduction (see Tables 6.17, 6.18)
Treatment of attacks: short-acting nitrates (glyceryl trinitrate)
Prevention of attacks
    Long-acting nitrates (e.g. isosorbide)
    β-adrenergic blockers (e.g. atenolol)
    Calcium antagonists (e.g. amlodipine, nifedipine)
If inadequate control by medical therapy
    Percutaneous transluminal coronary angioplasty
      (PTCA)
    Coronary artery bypass grafting (CABG)

sion, diabetes, obstructive airways disease or heart failure), each of which may contraindicate (or indicate) certain types of drug. If anginal attacks are not adequately controlled by medical treatment, percutaneous transluminal coronary angioplasty (PTCA) or coronary artery bypass grafting (CABG) can be considered.

In coronary angioplasty, the coronary narrowing is defined by angiography, then a deflated balloon is passed across the narrowed area (using a guidewire) and inflated. Dilation of the balloon enlarges the arterial lumen by stretching the vessel wall and by forcing the atherosclerotic plaque into the medial layer. Restenosis occurs in about 40% of patients: this can be prevented in some patients by inserting a metal stent (expandable wire cage).

Coronary artery bypass grafting may be indicated when angiography shows stenosis of the left main coronary artery or the first part of its anterior descending branch, disease of both branches of the left coronary artery as well as the right coronary artery (triple-vessel disease), or poor ventricular function; and if the patient is fit for open-heart surgery. In such patients, survival is improved as well as anginal symptoms. Coronary stenoses are bypassed either by using the saphenous vein (from the patient's leg) or the left internal mammary artery. The mortality from this operation is about 3% in the UK.

Myocardial infarction and unstable angina. As noted above, these usually result from rupture of a coronary artery plaque (which is usually non-stenotic) and formation of a platelet–fibrin arterial thrombus, often with local, reactive coronary artery spasm. If the artery is totally occluded, myocardial necrosis (infarction) results;

partial occlusion results in a similar clinical picture but without evidence of myocardial infarction on serial ECGs and plasma cardiac enzyme tests (unstable angina).

Myocardial infarction may be clinically silent and discovered incidentally when an ECG is performed at a later date. More commonly, it presents as acute myocardial ischaemic pain, of similar character and site as stable angina pectoris, but usually is more severe; more prolonged (over 20 min); accompanied by nausea, vomiting, breathlessness, abnormal heart rate or rhythm, low blood pressure, fainting or circulatory shock, and is not relieved by rest or by nitrate drugs.

The diagnosis is confirmed by serial changes on the ECG (abnormal Q waves, ST segment elevation, and T wave inversion; see Fig. 6.4) and by elevation in plasma cardiac enzyme levels (creatine kinase, transaminases and lactate dehydrogenase). Infarction usually occurs spontaneously, but may be precipitated by unaccustomed vigorous exercise, major surgery, or infections (it is commoner in the winter months). There may or may not be a previous history of angina or infarction. Complications of infarction are listed in Table 6.20. The most important is sudden death due to ventricular fibrillation, which occurs in 50% of heart attack patients before they can be admitted to hospital. Many hospital deaths result from large infarcts, and infarct size and hospital mortality can be reduced by prompt thrombolytic therapy. For these reasons, all patients with acute central chest pain, 'collapse' or shock require urgent first aid, a cardiac ambulance team, and rapid admission to a hospital cardiac care unit.

First aid management of acute chest pain is summarized in Table 6.21; and hospital diagnosis and management in Table 6.22. Hospital mortality is about 15% overall, and is poorer in older patients. After recovery, rehabilitation and secondary prevention (Table 6.18) are coordinated initially by hospital-based coronary nurses and subsequently in primary care. Exercise ECG and/or myocardial perfusion isotope scanning are usually performed also, to identify patients whose prognosis may be improved by PTCA or CABG procedures. Other types of surgery should be deferred for several months if possible, because general anaesthesia may cause dysrhythmias and hypotension.

Table 6.20 Complications of acute myocardial infarction

Cardiac arrest/sudden death (ventricular fibrillation or asystole)
Other dysrhythmias – paroxysmal tachycardia, atrial fibrillation, heart block
Cardiogenic shock
Acute left heart failure, chronic heart failure
Acute pericarditis
Mural ventricular thrombus and systemic embolism leading to brain or limb infarction

Table 6.21 Management of acute chest pain in the dental surgery

Stop dental treatment
Clear airway
Check consciousness, respiration and arterial pulse
If patient is known to have angina and glyceryl trinitrate, encourage its use
If pain does not settle within 5 min, call a cardiac ambulance (via a 999 call) and the general practitioner
Monitor patient for cardiac arrest; institute life support immediately (see Fig. 6.6)
If patient is not taking regular aspirin, give 300 mg orally (soluble or chewable tablet)

Table 6.22 Management of acute chest pain in ambulance and hospital

Monitor ECG; defibrillate if ventricular fibrillation and institute other measures for cardiac arrest
Give high-flow oxygen
Insert intravenous catheter; give intravenous opiate analgesic (e.g. morphine or diamorphine) and antiemetic
Give oral aspirin (see Table 6.18)
If ECG shows ST elevation, give thrombolytic therapy
Monitor cardiac enzymes (intravenous streptokinase or alteplase)
Detect and treat complications early

Unstable angina may present with a similar clinical picture to acute myocardial infarction, but there is no evidence of myocardial necrosis on serial ECGs or plasma cardiac enzyme measurements, and a lower risk of complications. Thrombolysis is not beneficial. The risk of myocardial infarction is increased in the subsequent few months, due to further coronary artery thrombosis: this risk is reduced by aspirin and anticoagulation for a few days with intravenous or subcutaneous heparin. Intravenous nitrates are usually effective in relieving recurrent chest pain.

Patients with persisting chest pain may require urgent coronary angiography, PTCA or CABG.

Other causes of acute central chest pain are summarized in Table 6.3.

Acute pericarditis may result from virus infections (e.g. Coxsackie B) or recent myocardial infarction: the ECG shows ST elevation without T wave flattening, and cardiac ultrasound may show a pericardial effusion, which may cause heart failure and require drainage.

Dissecting aortic aneurysm usually occurs in hypertensive patients, and causes severe 'tearing' chest pain. Diagnosis is by cardiac ultrasound or angiography; management includes control of hypertension and sometimes urgent surgical repair.

Peripheral arterial disease

As noted in the previous section, peripheral arterial disease is another common manifestation of atherothrombosis: it affects the lower limbs much more often than the upper. The risk factors are generally similar to those for ischaemic heart disease (Table 6.15); smoking and diabetes are particularly strong risk factors for peripheral arterial disease.

Intermittent claudication. This is the commonest clinical presentation of peripheral arterial disease, particularly in those aged over 50 years. Like stable angina, claudication is intermittent, occurring predictably after exercise. The symptoms arise from transient lower limb muscle ischaemia when exercise (particularly, walking up hills or stairs) increases muscle work, and local blood flow becomes inadequate to meet these demands because of atherosclerotic arterial narrowing. On examination, the peripheral arterial pulses palpated at the ankle (posterior tibial, dorsalis pedis) may be weak or absent. The skin of the leg and foot may be cold and hairless.

Chronic critical limb ischaemia. In a minority of patients (especially smokers and diabetics), atherothrombotic disease of the lower limb arteries progresses to a critical stage where limb viability is threatened and there is a major risk of limb infarction (gangrene) requiring amputation. Clinical features include rest pain, which is usually felt in the foot and at night when the lower limb is elevated. Patients often put their feet on the floor, which raises perfusion pressure through gravity. Skin changes also occur, which include cold, cyanosed feet and infarction (gangrene) of the toes. Additional problems include superimposed infection, and ulceration: these complications are particularly likely in diabetic patients.

A diagnosis can usually be made clinically, although arteriography can define the extent of arterial lesions in patients in whom angioplasty or bypass grafting are contemplated.

Management of peripheral arterial disease includes the important factors shown in Table 6.23.

Acute peripheral arterial occlusion. This is a surgical emergency presenting with sudden onset of pain, pallor and coldness, pulselessness and paralysis in the affected limb as a result of distant embolism from the heart (e.g. atrial fibrillation, heart valve disease or prosthesis, or acute myocardial infarction) or more locally from a major lower limb arterial thrombus arising on an ulcerated plaque. It may be possible to save the limb by emergency angiography to visualize the thrombus, followed by catheter embolectomy, and/or thrombolysis by local infusion of streptokinase. Reconstructive surgery for underlying stenosis can also be considered. If such measures are unsuccessful, gangrene will occur, requiring amputation.

Aortic aneurysms. Atherosclerosis of the aorta can weaken the wall, leading to focal expansion into an aneurysm. Thrombus often forms within the aneurysm, which may embolize, causing distal ischaemia. The commonest site is the bifurcation of the abdominal aorta. Clinical features include pain in the abdomen and back, and a pulsatile swelling in the abdomen. Rupture presents with severe pain and haemorrhagic shock, and is usually rapidly fatal. Diagnosis is by ultrasound, computerized tomography scanning or arteriography. Treatment is surgical, bypassing the aneurysm with a synthetic graft.

Dissection of a thoracic aortic aneurysm. This has already been discussed as a cause of acute chest pain. Thoracic aneurysms may be due to syphilis as well as atherosclerosis.

Raynaud's disease (peripheral vasospasm). This is a common disorder which usually affects premenopausal women and may have a hormonal cause. A family history is often present. Attacks may be precipitated by cold exposure. There is paroxysmal vasoconstriction of the digital arteries, causing the fingers and toes to become white and cold. Stagnation of blood in the skin capillaries results in peripheral cyanosis. Reactive vasodilatation causes the fingers finally to become red, tingling and throbbing.

The history is usually diagnostic. People working with vibrating tools may develop Raynaud's disease as an occupational disorder, and should stop such work. Underlying rheumatic disorders (e.g. scleroderma or systemic lupus erythematosus, see Ch. 14) should be excluded. Treatment includes avoiding cold, wearing gloves, stopping smoking, and using the vasodilator drug nifedipine.

Venous disease

Varicose veins. These are very common in the lower limbs, and result from incompetence of the venous valves. Risk factors include a family history, obesity, prolonged standing, and a past history of deep vein thrombosis (DVT) which blocks deep veins and damages venous valves. In some patients, cosmetic surgery is performed (injection of sclerosants, ligation or stripping): this is inappropriate in post-thrombotic cases because the distended superficial veins are the only route for venous blood to return to the heart.

Venous insufficiency. This may occur in patients with primary varicose veins, but is commoner in varicose veins secondary to DVT (post-thrombotic leg syndrome). Heaviness of the legs is followed by local oedema, brown pigmentation (deposition of haemosiderin from small haemorrhages), skin fibrosis, and ulceration which becomes infected. The skin over the medial malleolus is usually affected. Management includes

Table 6.23 Management of peripheral arterial disease
Risk factor reduction
Care of feet and nails
Regular exercise
Angioplasty or bypass surgery in selected cases

weight reduction in the obese, oedema reduction by compression bandages and keeping the legs elevated while sitting, and regular dressing of the ulcers until healing occurs (which is often slow).

Superficial thrombophlebitis. Attacks of local, sterile inflammation with secondary thrombosis are common in superficial veins, especially if varicose. The vein becomes red, hot, firm and tender. Treatment is with NSAIDs, e.g. ibuprofen. Recurrent thrombophlebitis may be due to congenital thrombophilias (see below) or underlying malignant disease.

Venous thromboembolism. DVT is a common complication of bedrest following trauma, surgery or medical illnesses (e.g. myocardial infarction, heart failure, stroke, severe infections, or cancer). Stasis of blood in the deep veins of the leg, combined with systemic activation of blood coagulation, are the major mechanisms involved. Many thrombi remain confined to the calf veins and asymptomatic; others extend to the popliteal, femoral and iliac veins and cause symptoms:

- Acute symptomatic DVT. Occlusion of the major veins causes pain, tenderness, unilateral leg swelling with pitting oedema, blue discoloration and distended superficial veins.
- Chronic post-thrombotic leg syndrome (see above).
- Acute pulmonary embolism (PE). This feared complication often results from a non-occlusive, asymptomatic DVT. The features are dependent on size, and whether the embolism lodges in the main pulmonary vessels or can be carried more peripherally into the lung. The condition may thus present as massive PE, characterized by acute central chest pain, breathlessness and shock, which is often rapidly fatal, or submassive PE which is characterized by breathlessness, lateral pleuritic chest pain (see Ch. 8) from lung infarction, and haemoptysis.

Suspected DVT is confirmed by ultrasound or venography of leg veins. PE can be confirmed by isotope lung scanning or by pulmonary angiography through a catheter placed in the right heart.

In DVT, oedema is treated acutely by leg elevation, followed by elastic compression stockings. Management with anticoagulants reduces further extension and embolization of thrombi; a typical regime consists of intravenous or subcutaneous heparin for 3–5 days followed by oral warfarin for 3 months. Oxygen and analgesics are given in PE; in massive PE thrombolysis or embolectomy is considered if shock continues. Prophylaxis of DVT and PE during immobilization is important in high-risk hospital patients by the use of low-dose subcutaneous heparin, or mechanical prophylaxis with elastic compression stockings, intermittent compression, or foot-moving devices. DVT and PE may be the presenting feature of cancer, polycythaemias (see Ch. 7) or thrombophilias (see below).

Thrombophilias. Just as congenital deficiencies of blood coagulation factors (haemophilias, see Ch. 7) cause excessive spontaneous, post-traumatic or postoperative bleeding; congenital deficiencies of blood coagulation inhibitors cause an increased risk of venous thromboembolism – spontaneous, or following trauma or surgery. These deficiencies include antithrombin, protein C and protein S deficiency; and activated protein C resistance, which is due to a mutation in coagulation factor V. These disorders are autosomal dominant, and there is often a family history. Patients in whom thrombophilias are identified require counselling for prophylaxis in at-risk situations (trauma, surgery, bed rest, pregnancy and puerperium), and for risks of oestrogen-containing oral contraceptives or hormone replacement therapy. They also should be counselled regarding family screening and require longer duration warfarin after DVT or PE.

Lymphatic disease

Lymphoedema. Lymphatic obstruction causes unilateral limb oedema which is often chronic, and hence fibrous and non-pitting. It may be congenital (Milroy's disease), result from filariasis (see Ch. 5) in tropical countries, or result from lymphatic invasion by cancer (e.g. breast cancer for the upper limb or pelvic cancers for the lower limb).

Lymphadenopathy. Enlargement of lymph glands is considered in Chapter 7.

REFERENCES

Dajani AS, Taubert KA, Wilson W et al 1997. Prevention of bacterial endocarditis. Recommendations by the American Heart Association. Journal of the American Medical Association. 277: 1794–1801

Simmonds NA 1993. Recommendations for endocarditis prophylaxis. The Endocarditis Working Party for Antimicrobial Chemotherapy. Journal of Antimicrobial Chemotherapy. 31: 437–438

7 Disorders of the blood and lymphatic system

Introduction

The circulating blood consists of a suspension of cellular elements in a fluid plasma medium (about 45 and 55% by volume respectively). Much haematological work is concerned with abnormalities of the blood cells, but normal haemostasis is dependent on coagulation factors present in the plasma. Blood viscosity is dependent largely on the concentrations of cells in the plasma, but is also influenced by rises in certain plasma proteins, such as globulins or fibrinogen. In anticoagulated blood samples, the erythrocytes will sediment on standing. The erythrocyte sedimentation rate (ESR) rises in certain inflammatory conditions associated with increased concentrations of acute phase proteins, and can be a useful pointer to underlying organic disease and its response to therapy.

In normal individuals, cell numbers are maintained homeostatically within quite close limits.

Abnormalities of cell numbers are thus an important sign of haematological disease; some commonly used terms are shown in Table 7.1. In the case of white cells, it is possible to apply more precise terminology to indicate which subtype may be affected, for example agranulocytosis, neutropenia, lymphocytosis, monocytosis, etc. Increased numbers of leucocytes may be reactive to infection or inflammation (physiological) or malignant (leukaemia).

A full blood count is therefore the essential investigation. Blood cells are usually counted and sized in an automatic cell counter. In addition, the haemoglobin concentration is measured chemically. Table 7.2 lists generally accepted values for blood counts and sizes; however, the reference ranges of the local laboratory should be used for interpreting results. Visual inspection of blood cells for morphological changes is also needed in all cases where numerical screening is abnormal; a

Table 7.1 Commonly used terms describing haematological disorders

	Erythrocytes	Leucocytes	Platelets
Increased numbers	Polycythaemia	Leucocytosis	Thrombocytosis or thrombocythaemia
Reduced numbers	Anaemia	Leucopenia	Thrombocytopenia

Table 7.2 Full blood count – adult reference range

Haemoglobin (Hb)	Male: 13–18 g/dl Female: 11.5–16.5 g/dl
Haematocrit (Hct) (packed cell volume, PCV)	Male: 0.40–0.54 Female: 0.37–0.50
Red cell count (RCC)	Male: 4.5–$6.5 \times 10^{12}/l$ Female: 3.8–$5.8 \times 10^{12}/l$
Mean red cell volume (MCV)	76–96 l
White cell count (WCC)	4.0–$11.0 \times 10^9/l$
Neutrophil count	2.0–$7.5 \times 10^9/l$
Lymphocyte count	1.5–$4.0 \times 10^9/l$
Platelet count	150-$400 \times 10^9/l$

stained blood film is therefore prepared from the same sample and examined microscopically.

Other investigations include levels of the haematinics – iron, folic acid and vitamin B_{12} – as discussed later, and, occasionally, bone marrow or lymph node biopsy. Bone marrow is usually obtained by aspiration from the iliac crest or sternum following infiltration with a local anaesthetic, and films are prepared on a glass slide. Sometimes a bone marrow biopsy is required using a trephine needle to obtain a core of marrow which is fixed, sectioned and stained. If lymph node histology is required, fine needle aspiration or preferably, excision biopsy can be performed under local anaesthesia.

Anaemias

Anaemia is characterized by a reduction in haemoglobin concentration, usually accompanied by a reduction in red cell numbers, and is the commonest haematological disease presentation. All cases merit precise diagnosis and appropriate management.

The symptoms of anaemia are listed in Table 7.3. Most symptoms are consequences of reduced oxygen carriage by the blood (hypoxaemia) due to the low haemoglobin level, which in turn causes tissue hypoxia. Tiredness and breathlessness are the most common complaints. The haemoglobin level at which symptoms of anaemia develop varies widely from person to person. Symptoms occur at a higher haemoglobin level if the anaemia develops rapidly (e.g. due to bleeding), and in older persons with cardiovascular disease; thus

anaemia can precipitate or worsen angina, claudication or mental confusion in the elderly.

There are two compensatory processes which act to reduce tissue hypoxia in anaemia. First, the concentration of 2,3-diphosphoglycerate increases in the red blood cells: this shifts the haemoglobin–oxygen dissociation curve, such that more oxygen is liberated to tissues from circulating haemoglobin at any given tissue oxygen level. Second, the circulation becomes hyperdynamic, resulting in increased blood flow to tissues (and thus an increased rate of oxygen delivery). The heart rate and stroke volume both increase, resulting in increased cardiac output. There is also a generalized vasodilatation. As a result of these circulatory changes, anaemic patients may become aware of a rapid, stronger heart beat (palpitations) and may develop headaches (due to dilatation of cranial blood vessels). These increased demands, and hypoxia of the cardiac muscle itself, may lead to heart failure.

The signs of anaemia are also listed in Table 7.3. Pallor of the skin and mucous membranes may be apparent, but is more reliably assessed in the conjunctivae than the mouth. In deficiency anaemias, other tissue signs may be present; those result from the direct effects of the deficiency itself, and not from anaemia per se. Thus, koilonychia, a spoon-shaped depression of

Table 7.3 Symptoms and signs of anaemia

Symptoms	Tiredness (initially on effort) Breathlessness (initially on effort) Weakness Palpitations Dizziness Fainting Tinnitus Angina Calf claudication Confusion Throbbing headache
Signs	Pallor Rapid, high volume arterial pulse Leg oedema (heart failure) Oral signs (see Ch. 26) (iron, folate or B_{12} deficiency) Jaundice (haemolytic anaemias) Koilonychia (iron deficiency) Splenomegaly

the nails (Fig 7.1), may be a confirmatory sign in iron deficiency anaemia, and oral signs (see Ch. 26) may occur in deficiencies of iron, vitamin B_{12} and folic acid. Mild jaundice (see Ch. 10) may be present in haemolytic anaemias: it is most reliably assessed in the sclera of the eye and, in combination with the pallor of anaemia, may cause a lemon-yellow skin colour. Splenomegaly is a feature of many haematological disorders, and does not necessarily imply malignancy.

Red cell morphology is very helpful in the diagnosis of anaemias. Attention is given to the size of the red cells, their shape, and their degree of haemoglobinization, and these visual impressions confirm the measurements given in Table 7.2. For example, poorly haemoglobinized microcytes are characteristic of haemoglobin deficiency as occurs in impaired haem synthesis (usually due to iron deficiency), or in impaired globin chain production (thalassaemias and haemoglobinopathy diseases). On the other hand, circulating macrocytes usually reflect disturbed maturation of red cells during their development in the bone marrow. These observations allow the simple classification of anaemia illustrated in Table 7.4.

An alternative way of classifying anaemia is according to mechanism, and such a classification is shown in Table 7.5.

Following diagnosis, appropriate therapy should be possible. Red cell transfusion is usually reserved for anaemic patients who are either actively bleeding, or who have symptomatic, severe anaemia (e.g. blood haemoglobin under 8 g/dl) for which specific treatment is either not available or will not increase the haemoglobin level within an acceptable time. Synthetic oxygen-carrying fluids (haemoglobin substitutes) are currently undergoing clinical trials.

Table 7.4 Classification of anaemia according to red cell morphology

Type of anaemia	Mean cell volume
Normochromic,[a] normocytic[b]	Normal
Hypochromic,[a] microcytic[b]	Low
Normochromic,[a] macrocytic[b]	High

[a] Applies to degree of haemoglobinization.
[b] Applies to cell size.

Microcytic anaemias

As indicated above, this group of diseases is characterized by impaired haemoglobin synthesis. Since iron is a prerequisite for haem manufacture, the usual cause is iron deficiency, but they may also arise due to altered iron metabolism (Table 7.6): in a secondary anaemia accompanying chronic infection and inflammation there is a block of release of iron from macrophages and in sideroblastic anaemia, a rare disorder, iron enters the normoblast but cannot be utilised. Thalassaemias may also be microcytic, but are considered with the other haemolytic anaemias later.

Iron is essential for synthesis of the haem component of haemoglobin; it is also required by enzymes in epithelial cells. Iron is continuously lost from the body in epithelial cells shed from the

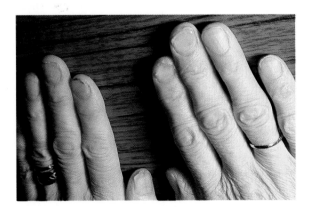

Fig. 7.1 Koilonychia in a patient with iron deficiency.

Table 7.5 Classification of anaemia according to mechanism

Excessive loss or destruction of red cells
  Haemorrhage – posthaemorrhagic anaemia
  Excessive destruction – haemolytic anaemia

Failure of production of red cells
  Diminished production with marrow aplasia (aplastic anaemia) or replacement
  Diminished production with marrow hyperplasia – dyshaemopoietic anaemia (e.g. iron deficiency, megaloblastic anaemia)

skin and gut; and also in chronic blood loss (e.g. from the uterus in menstruating women). Iron deficiency arises when dietary intake of iron is insufficient to replace such losses.

Iron deficiency is the commonest cause of anaemia. It may occur at any age, and is most commonly due to chronic blood loss (Table 7.6). In the UK and other developed countries, increased menstrual bleeding (menorrhagia) in women is the commonest cause. This is usually primary, but sometimes may be due to uterine diseases (see Ch. 16) or to the congenital bleeding disorder, von Willebrand's disease (see below). Severe menorrhagia can be treated with oral tranexamic acid, which reduces uterine blood loss by inhibiting the fibrinolytic system (see below).

If uterine blood loss is not obviously the cause of iron deficiency, other causes of chronic blood loss must be sought. These include recurrent urinary bleeding (haematuria, e.g. from carcinoma of the bladder) and recurrent nosebleeds (epistaxes). However, chronic gastrointestinal bleeding is the commonest cause of iron deficiency in men, and in non-menstruating women. This is often occult, that is, it is not visible as vomiting of blood (haematemesis) or the passage of altered blood in the stools (melaena). Occult blood in the stools can be detected by a simple chemical test strip, to which a small amount of faeces is applied. In many developing countries, the commonest cause of iron deficiency anaemia due to occult gastrointestinal blood loss, is hookworm infestation of the intestine. For a full consideration of gastrointestinal blood loss see Ch. 10 (Fig. 10.5).

Iron deficiency may also be due to increased demands, for example during pregnancy to supply iron to the fetus, and during lactation. Prophylactic iron supplements are therefore given during pregnancy, combined with folic acid supplements (see below). Dietary deficiency of iron-containing foods (meat, fish and vegetables) may also cause iron deficiency, for example in poverty and in widowers. Iron deficiency may also be due to malabsorption, such as after gastrectomy or in coeliac disease.

Clinical features of iron deficiency include the general symptoms and signs of anaemia and signs of epithelial deficiency of iron-containing enzymes such as oral changes (see Ch. 26) and koilonychia. Rarely, iron deficiency causes a postcricoid

Table 7.6 Causes of microcytic anaemia
Iron deficiency
Chronic blood loss, e.g.:
uterus (menorrhagia)
urinary tract (bladder cancer)
nosebleeds
gastrointestinal (see Ch. 10)
Increased demands (pregnancy, lactation)
Dietary deficiency
Malabsorption
Anaemia of chronic infection or inflammation
Siderobastic anaemia
Thalassaemias

pharyngeal web. This is a rare cause of difficulty in swallowing (dysphagia – see Ch. 10): the Paterson–Brown–Kelly syndrome. It can be visualized by endoscopy or barium swallow.

Laboratory findings of iron deficiency include low levels of haemoglobin, red cell count and mean red cell volume (MCV). Inspection of the blood film confirms that the red cells are smaller than normal (microcytosis) and stain poorly (hypochromia), due to their low haemoglobin content (Fig. 7.2a). The white cell count and platelet count are usually normal. The serum iron concentration is low, and the serum transferrin and iron-binding capacity are increased. The most useful test, however, is serum ferritin, which when reduced is indicative of iron deficiency. Bone marrow examination is not routinely indicated, but if performed shows absent stainable iron and small red cell precursor cells (microblasts).

Treatment of iron deficiency is usually with oral iron salts (e.g. ferrous sulphate 200 mg three times daily). Patients should be advised to take their tablets with meals (to minimize gastric adverse effects such as nausea), and also that iron may colour the stools grey-black. Occasionally, intramuscular iron injections or red cell transfusion are required. Causes of chronic blood loss should be identified and treated (e.g. avoidance of aspirin and other non-steroidal anti-inflammatory drugs if these have caused gastritis or gastric erosions).

Macrocytic anaemias

Deficiencies of either vitamin B_{12} (cobalamin) or folic acid are the commonest causes of anaemia

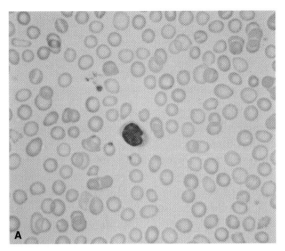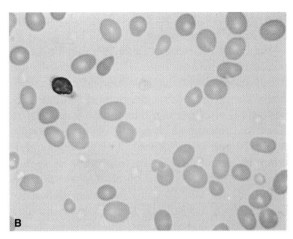

Fig. 7.2 A Blood film in iron deficiency anaemia (microcytic, hypochromic). **B** Blood film in megaloblastic anaemia (macrocytic, normochromic).

with macrocytosis (large red blood cells; MCV over 96 f1) (Table 7.7). These vitamins are required for synthesis of white blood cells and platelets as well as red cells; marrow examination shows abnormally large red cell precursors (megaloblasts) with impaired nuclear maturation but normal haemoglobin synthesis. Folic acid and vitamin B$_{12}$ are also required for normal epithelial and neurological function

Macrocytosis may sometimes occur in the presence of a normal haemoglobin concentration: the commonest cause of this is a heavy alcohol intake.

The commonest cause of vitamin B$_{12}$ deficiency is autoimmune gastritis: antibodies to gastric parietal cells or intrinsic factor are often detectable in the serum, and atrophy of these cells results in failure to secrete gastric acid, and also intrinsic factor, which normally binds to dietary vitamin B$_{12}$ in the

stomach and small intestine. As a result, normal absorption of the vitamin B$_{12}$–intrinsic factor complex in the terminal part of the ileum fails to occur, and when liver stores of vitamin B$_{12}$ are exhausted, deficiency arises. This cause of permanent failure to absorb oral vitamin B$_{12}$ was originally called pernicious anaemia because it was progressive and untreatable prior to the introduction of parenteral vitamin B$_{12}$ therapy, which is required lifelong. The onset is usually in the second half of life. There is often a family history of this condition, and a familial association with auto-immune thyroid disease (see Ch. 13). Because of its slow onset, which allows compensatory adaptions for anaemia to occur (see above), the haemoglobin level may be very low (under 6 g/dl) before symptoms occur.

Rarer causes of vitamin B$_{12}$ deficiency include other causes of malabsorption (e.g. gastrectomy,

Table 7.7 Causes of macrocytic anaemia	
Vitamin B$_{12}$ (cobalamin) deficiency	Autoimmune gastritis (pernicious anaemia) Malabsorption (gastrectomy, Crohn's ileitis) Dietary deficiency (e.g. in vegetarians)
Folate deficiency	Increased demands pregnancy haemolysis Malabsorption (coeliac disease) Dietary deficiency (alcoholics and the elderly) Antifolate drugs (phenytoin, methotrexate)

involvement of the terminal ileum by Crohn's disease or tuberculosis (see Ch. 10), and dietary deficiency (e.g. in vegetarians).

Folic acid deficiency (Table 7.7) may be due to increased demands, especially in pregnancy (as noted above, prophylactic folate and iron supplements are given during pregnancy). Folate prophylaxis is also given in haemolytic anaemias, to meet the increased demand of compensatory increased red cell synthesis. Folate deficiency is common in malabsorption (especially in coeliac disease, which affects the jejunum where folate is absorbed, see Ch. 10) and in dietary deficiency (especially in alcoholics). Drugs which interfere with folate metabolism include anticonvulsants (e.g. phenytoin) and cytotoxic drugs (e.g. methotrexate).

Clinical features of vitamin B_{12} or folate deficiency include general features of anaemia and oral changes (see Ch. 26). Neurological disorders are associated with vitamin B_{12} deficiency (see Ch. 9), usually peripheral neuropathy (tingling, numbness and weakness of the feet and hands), and, rarely, spinal cord degeneration (severe leg weakness and postural disturbance).

Laboratory features of vitamin B_{12} or folate deficiency include low levels of haemoglobin and a low red cell count, with an increased MCV. Inspection of the blood film confirms that the red cells are large (macrocytosis), well filled with haemoglobin, and vary in size and shape (Fig 7.2b). The white cell and platelet counts are low. Bone marrow examination is important to confirm the diagnosis, especially in autoimmune gastritis, for which lifelong vitamin B_{12} therapy is required. Since the blood and marrow appearances in vitamin B_{12} and folic acid deficiency are identical, these disorders can only be distinguished by estimation of blood levels of each vitamin. Serum antibodies to parietal cells or intrinsic factor may be present in autoimmune gastritis, and decreased intestinal absorption of radiolabelled vitamin B_{12} in this disorder can be demonstrated by the Schilling test.

Vitamin B_{12} is given as hydroxocobalamin by intramuscular injection (1 mg daily for 5 days, then every 3 months for life). Folic acid is given orally (5 mg daily). Deficiency of the appropriate vitamin is confirmed by an increase in the reticu-locyte count within a few days of treatment, followed by normalization of the low haemoglobin concentration.

Normocytic anaemias

There are many possible causes of normocytic anaemias (Table 7.8). These will be briefly discussed in turn.

Anaemias associated with systemic diseases. Many systemic diseases are associated with a normocytic anaemia. Normal red cell synthesis requires not only iron, vitamin B_{12} and folate but also vitamin C, thyroxine and erythropoietin. Normocytic anaemia is therefore part of the clinical picture of scurvy (see below), hypothyroidism or myxoedema (see Ch. 13), and renal failure (see Ch. 11). Treatment with vitamin C, thyroxine or erythropoietin, respectively, is usually effective.

The blood haemoglobin level usually falls as part of the body's response to tissue injury (e.g. trauma, surgery, infection and other causes of inflammation). The mechanisms are poorly defined, but may involve cytokines such as interferon (treatment of viral hepatitis with recombinant interferon can also cause anaemia), and impaired utilization of iron by red cell precursors. A persistent normocytic anaemia, (sometimes called the 'anaemia of chronic disease') is often seen in chronic infections (e.g. endocarditis, tuberculosis, HIV infection), chronic immunological diseases (e.g. rheumatoid arthritis) and malignant diseases.

Management includes the exclusion of other causes of anaemia, treatment of the disease process if possible and in some cases erythropoietin or red cell transfusion.

Anaemias associated with marrow aplasia or hypoplasia. Marrow aplasia or hypoplasia is diagnosed by bone marrow histology. It may be primary, or secondary to viruses, radiation, toxins (e.g. carbon tetrachloride) or drugs. Drug-induced aplasia may be predictable (e.g. cytotoxic drugs) or idiosyncratic. It may affect only the red cell precursors or also the white cell and platelet precursors. In this case blood neutrophil and platelet counts are also low (pancytopenia) and clinical features of these may be

Table 7.8 Causes of normocytic anaemias

General cause	Specific cause
Systemic diseases	Infections (e.g. endocarditis, tuberculosis, HIV infection) Immune diseases (e.g. rheumatoid arthritis) Renal failure (erythropoietin deficiency) Malignancy Thyroid deficiency (myxoedema) Vitamin C deficiency (scurvy)
Marrow aplasia/hypoplasia	Primary Drugs (e.g. cytotoxics), toxins, viruses Radiation exposure (e.g. radiotherapy)
Marrow neoplasia (leucoerythroblastic anaemias)	Leukaemias Lymphomas Myeloproliferative disorders Metastatic carcinoma (e.g. breast, bronchus)

Haemolytic anaemias	Congenital
	    Haemoglobin defects (sickle cell disease, thalassaemias)
	    Membrane defects (e.g. spherocytosis)
	    Enzyme defects (e.g. glucose-6-phosphate dehydrogenase deficiency)
	Acquired (e.g. autoimmune, malaria)

Acute haemorrhage	

apparent in addition to anaemia. Serious haematological reactions to drug administration are now a major problem, and it is good practice to question the necessity for any drug before prescribing it.

Management includes removal of exposure to any potential causal factor (e.g. drugs); transfusion of red cells, platelets and granulocytes as required; and treatment of infections. Corticosteroids or anabolic steroids sometimes increase marrow cell function. Stem cell transplantation may be considered in severe, persistent cases (see below).

Anaemias associated with marrow neoplasia. Marrow neoplasia is diagnosed by bone marrow histology, which may reveal leukaemias, lymphomas or myeloproliferative disorders (see below), or secondary carcinomatous deposits (commonly from breast or bronchial carcinoma). In some cases, neoplastic replacement of red cell and white cell precursors stimulates the latter to appear in the circulation (leucoerythroblastic anaemia).

Management includes treatment of the underlying neoplasm, and transfusion of red cells as required.

Haemolytic anaemias

These anaemias are characterized by accelerated red cell destruction, which may be intravascular, or more commonly extravascular, especially in the spleen. This can be the result of many disorders, either congenital (where faults in the red cell itself are usually responsible, and where there is often a positive family history) or acquired (where the red cells themselves are normal but where their environment has become hostile). Congenital disorders include haemoglobin defects, which are widespread throughout the world (e.g. sickle cell disease in persons of African origin, or thalassaemias in persons of Mediterranean or Asian origin); membrane defects (e.g. spherocytosis), and enzyme defects (e.g. glucose-6-phosphate dehydrogenase deficiency). Acquired disorders include autoimmune haemolytic anaemias in which antibodies to red cells are detectable, and infections (e.g. malaria).

Clinical features of haemolytic anaemia include all the symptoms affecting any anaemic patient. In haemolytic disease, jaundice is characteristic, due to increased bilirubin formation from excess haemoglobin breakdown, and splenomegaly is often present. In chronic haemolytic states, there is enormous compensatory hypertrophy of the marrow, and in children this may alter the skeleton, including the facial bones (see Ch. 26). In sickle cell disease, the red cells take up a crescentic shape during episodes of hypoxia, infection or dehydration when the abnormal HbS precipitates: these cells are rigid and tend to sludge in small blood vessels. This causes a wide variety of painful vaso-occlusive events, especially in bones, abdominal viscera and the brain; infarcts of the spleen are frequent, leading to atrophy rather than enlargement.

Laboratory features of haemolytic anaemias include a low haemoglobin, low red cell count, increased reticulocyte count, increased serum bilirubin level, abnormal red cell appearance on the blood film, e.g. spherocytes or sickle cells (after acidification in a 'sickle cell preparation') and abnormal haemoglobin electrophoresis in haemoglobinopathies, abnormal red cell enzymes in enzyme defects, and antibodies to red cells, causing lysis (Coombs' test) in autoimmune haemolytic anaemias.

Management of haemolytic anaemias includes red cell transfusions for haemolytic crises, folic acid prophylaxis to meet increased demands, and specific treatments (e.g. corticosteroids for autoimmune haemolytic anaemias; antimicrobials for infections causing haemolysis such as malaria; splenectomy, in patients with recurrent anaemia due to splenic destruction, and symptomatic treatment of vaso-occlusive crises in sickle cell disease with analgesics and hydration).

Anaemia due to acute haemorrhage. An acute normocytic anaemia occurs following major haemorrhage, e.g. after trauma or surgery, gastrointestinal bleeding, or uterine bleeding from complications of pregnancy and labour. The fall in the haemoglobin concentration takes several hours to develop, and follows dilution of the residual circulating red cell mass by a compensatory increase in plasma volume, caused by endogenous retention of salt and water (and also treatment with intravenous fluids). In acute haemorrhage the need for blood transfusion should be based on clinical features of hypovolaemia (e.g. increased pulse rate and low blood pressure) rather than a fall in the haematocrit.

Polycythaemias

Polycythaemia is defined as an increased concentration of haemoglobin (over 18 g/dl), associated with an increased concentration of red blood cells and an increased haematocrit (over 0.50). The polycythaemias are less common than the anaemias, but are important to diagnose because the increased haematocrit results in increased blood viscosity which slows blood flow and increases the risk of ischaemia and thrombosis, especially in the brain (stroke), eye, and leg veins.

Increased haemoglobin and haematocrit levels may be due to an increased red cell mass (absolute polycythaemias) or to a decreased plasma volume (relative polycythaemias). These can be differentiated by isotope studies.

Primary polycythaemia is one of the malignant disorders of the bone marrow termed myeloproliferative disorders (see below). There is an increase in red cell mass, due to excessive production of red blood cells by their precursor cells in the bone marrow. There is often also excessive marrow production of granulocytes and platelets. Clinical features include increased redness of the skin and mucous membranes, enlargement of the spleen, and itching. In addition to the increased risk of thrombosis, myeloid leukaemia may develop. The prognosis is relatively good provided the raised red cell mass can be controlled, initially by venesection and thereafter by marrow suppression using chemotherapy (oral hydroxyurea) or irradiation of the bone marrow with radioactive phosphorus (^{32}P).

Secondary polycythaemias are absolute polycythaemias in which the increased red cell mass is an apparent compensation for chronic hypoxia. It occurs in high-altitude dwellers (e.g. in the Andes), in congenital cyanotic heart disease (see Ch. 6), in chronic lung diseases (e.g. chronic bronchitis, see Ch. 8), and in heavy smokers. Treatment includes treatment of the cause of hypoxia, and sometimes venesection.

Relative polycythaemia is due to a low plasma volume. This occurs acutely in dehydration or in major burns (due to loss of plasma); and chronically in cigarette smokers and in hypertension. Treatment is that of the underlying condition.

Disorders of white blood cells

Leucocytosis and leucopenia are common findings on a full blood count and a differential diagnosis of these conditions is considered in turn.

Leucocytosis

Table 7.9 summarizes the commoner causes of a raised white cell count (leucocytosis). Neutrophil leucocytosis is usually due to bacterial infection, tissue death following infarction (e.g. myocardial infarction or stroke), or major trauma, burns or surgery. Lymphocytosis is usually due to viral infections. Marked leucocytosis is characteristic of the leukaemias, but also occurs in certain infections (leukaemoid reactions). In glandular fever (see Ch. 5), the combination of marked leucocytosis, atypical mononuclear cells on the blood film, cervical lymphadenopathy, sore throat and fever may mimic acute leukaemia.

Leucopenia

Table 7.10 summarizes the commoner causes of a low white cell count (leucopenia).

Neutropenia

Neutropenia is commonly due to virus infections (including HIV infection), bone marrow neoplasia, or treatment of haematological or other neoplasms with cytotoxic drugs or radiotherapy. Occasionally it may result from an idiosyncratic drug reaction (e.g. with carbimazole): any possibly causal drugs should be stopped immediately. Bone marrow aspiration may be required to establish the diagnosis. Extreme neutropenia is also called agranulocytosis, and may coexist with aplastic anaemia (see above).

Neutropenia increases the risk of bacterial infections, often with commensal organisms, especially affecting the mouth and throat (necrotic ulcers), respiratory tract and skin; septicaemia can occur through any of these portals of entry, and through the gut. Care should be taken to minimize these risks in patients with severe neutropenia in hospital (e.g. isolation, reverse-barrier

Table 7.10 Causes of leucopenia

Drugs
    Cytotoxic drugs
    Antirheumatic drugs (e.g. gold)
    Antithyroid drugs (e.g. carbimazole)

Infections, e.g. viral hepatitis

Malignancy, e.g. marrow invasion

Splenomegaly

Systemic lupus erythematosus

Megaloblastic anaemia

Table 7.9 Causes of leucocytosis

Neutrophilia	Bacterial infection
	Sterile inflammation
	Trauma and surgery
	Haemorrhage
	Infarction (e.g. myocardial, cerebral)
	Gout
	Malignancy
	Cancer
	Myeloproliferative disorders
Lymphocytosis	Viral infections e.g. Epstein–Barr virus, cytomegalovirus, herpes simplex virus
	Protozoal infections, e.g. toxoplasma
	Malignancy
	Lymphatic leukaemias
	Lymphomas

nursing, laminar air flow, and sterile food). Infections should be detected early and treated with high doses of bactericidal chemotherapy. Transfusions of granulocytes, or injections of granulocyte colony-stimulating factor (G-CSF) are given in selected cases.

Lymphopenia

Lymphopenia is characteristic of HIV infection (see Ch. 5), which selectively destroys T-helper (CD4) lymphocytes.

Neoplastic disorders of white blood cells

Neoplastic disorders of white blood cells can usually be considered under the headings shown in Table 7.11. Among the myeloproliferative disorders is included primary polycythaemia, which is a purposeless red cell proliferation, and is considered in this chapter under the section on red cell disorders. In addition, myeloid leukaemia is a myeloproliferative disease, whilst lymphatic leukaemia is a haematogenous form of lymphoid neoplasm. Both are considered together here because of their shared clinical features.

Lymphoreticular malignancies

These are malignant proliferations of lymphoid cells, usually involving the lymph glands, spleen and liver; spread to skin and bone marrow may occur. As with other haematological neoplasms, the cause is usually unknown. Epstein–Barr virus infection is a causal factor in Burkitt's lymphoma, which occurs mainly in tropical Africa and is implicated in some other lymphomas.

Hodgkin's disease (Hodgkin's lymphoma). This is the commonest type of lymphoma, and usually occurs in young adults: it is commoner in men. It usually presents with persistent enlarged superficial lymph nodes, most commonly in the neck. The enlarged glands are not usually painful, although pain may occur on drinking alcohol. On examination, the glands are discrete, firm and 'rubbery' in texture, and not tender or associated with local inflammation (in contrast to 'reactive' lymphadenopathy). Enlargement of deep lymph nodes also occurs:

enlarged mediastinal glands can cause bronchial compression and lung collapse, or vena caval compression (see Ch. 8). Enlargement of the spleen and liver may occur, while bone marrow replacement may cause anaemia, neutropenia and thrombocytopenia. Fever may occur due to Hodgkin's disease itself, as well as due to infection secondary to neutropenia.

The blood count and film are usually normal at presentation, although eosinophilia can occur. The diagnosis is usually made by lymph gland biopsy. Histology shows replacement of normal structure by a mixed proliferation of lymphocytes, large reticulum cells, which may be multinucleate (Reed–Sternberg giant cells), eosinophils, plasma cells, and fibrous tissue; depending on the proportions of these elements, several subtypes can be recognized which correlate with the prognosis.

Since successful eradication of the disease depends on treating all involved areas, following biopsy diagnosis, patients undergo extensive imaging investigations of the chest, abdomen, pelvis and skeleton, and further biopsy of tissues likely to be affected, especially bone marrow and liver. Occasionally, laparotomy and operative biopsies may be required. Localized disease is treated by radiotherapy, whereas chemotherapy with multiple cytotoxic drugs is given for more extensive disease. Of patients presenting with early localized disease 80–90% can be cured; but the 5-year survival is about 60% in patients with generalized disease.

Non-Hodgkin's lymphoma (NHL). NHLs are commoner than Hodgkin's disease, and their frequency increases with advancing years. They are extremely heterogeneous, and classification of

Table 7.11 Neoplastic disorders of white blood cells
Lymphoreticular malignancy
Hodgkin's disease
Non-Hodgkin's lymphoma
Myeloproliferative diseases
Primary polycythaemia
Leukaemia
Thrombocytosis
Myelofibrosis
Plasma cell tumours
Multiple myeloma
Waldenström's macroglobulinaemia

the histology has been contentious for many years; numerous subtypes are recognized, and only a simplified outline is given in Table 7.12. In general, low-grade lymphomas are less aggressive, more often widespread before diagnosis, and, although difficult or impossible to eradicate, usually have a better prognosis. Chronic lymphocytic leukaemia is best regarded as a low-grade NHL with cells exfoliating into the blood. High-grade lymphomas include some very aggressive tumours, and often appear to begin in one anatomical site, with spread following subsequently; paradoxically, cures with intensive chemotherapy are possible in this group, although for the majority of patients the outlook is poor. The clinical features are similar to those of Hodgkin's disease.

Low-grade lymphomas, not immediately life-threatening, are usually only treated when symptomatic, using intermittent suppressive oral chemotherapeutic agents such as chlorambucil and prednisolone; a good quality of life is possible for many years. Management of high-grade lymphomas requires radical multiagent chemotherapy, and the supportive resources of a specialized hospital unit.

Myeloproliferative disorders

This is a group of diseases characterized by malignant proliferation of precursor cells in the bone marrow. In pure form, only a single cell line is involved, thus producing the myeloid (granulocyte) leukaemias, primary proliferative polycythaemia, myelofibrosis or primary thrombocytosis. Each myeloproliferative disorder may exist in an acute aggressive form, or in a chronic relatively well-differentiated form. It is possible, however, for some of the features of these conditions to overlap at the time of diagnosis, or for one to evolve later into another. Their causes are largely unknown.

Leukaemias. This is a group of diseases characterized by a malignant, clonal proliferation of white blood cell precursors, which can lead to death in a few weeks or months (acute leukaemias) or a few years (chronic leukaemias). The causes are not well-defined, but include chromosomal abnormalities e.g. the 9:22 reciprocal chromosomal translocation in chronic myeloid leukaemia, and radiation exposure which can cause chromosomal damage especially in the fetus (for this reason, care is taken to minimize radiological studies during pregnancy, especially of the pelvis and abdomen).

Clinical features of leukaemias include anaemia. This is usually due to replacement by proliferating cells of normal red cell precursors in the bone marrow, but may also be due to bleeding (thrombocytopenia), infection, folate deficiency (cytotoxics) or autoimmune haemolysis (especially in chronic lymphatic leukaemia).

Neutropenia also occurs (due to replacement of normal neutrophil granulocyte precursors in the bone marrow) and/or lymphocyte dysfunction (especially in lymphatic leukaemias). Signs and symptoms include oral and throat ulceration and opportunistic infections such as candidosis (see Ch. 22), respiratory and urinary tract infections, and septicaemia from any of these sites of infection.

Tissue infiltration by proliferating cells is also seen. Symptoms and signs include gingival swelling and bleeding. This is typical of acute myelomonocytic leukaemia (see Ch. 26, Fig. 26.3). Lymph node enlargement (cervical, axillary and inguinal) occurs, especially in lymphatic leukaemias. Cervical lymph node enlargement may also reflect associated oral or throat infections. Enlargement of spleen and liver is seen, especially in myeloid leukaemias, and brain infiltration may cause cerebral haemorrhage.

If leukaemia is suspected from any of the above clinical features, it is important to ensure early

Table 7.12 Classification of non-Hodgkin's lymphomas	
Low grade	Small, mature lymphocytes (well differentiated) Nodular structure in affected tissues Low mitotic rate Best prognosis
High grade	Large, immature lymphoid cells (poorly differentiated) Diffuse structure in affected tissues High mitotic rate Worst prognosis

diagnosis and treatment. Diagnosis relies on the following investigation: a full blood count may show anaemia, thrombocytopenia and often a raised white cell count (although this may be normal or low in acute leukaemias). The blood film usually shows white cell precursors (blasts) in acute leukaemias, or an increased number of (usually) mature white cells in chronic leukaemias. Bone marrow histology (supplemented by immunological and chromosomal studies) usually confirms the diagnosis, showing increased clonal proliferation of a white cell precursor, and allows classification of the type of leukaemia (Table 7.13).

Acute leukaemias can occur at any age, but particularly in children in whom it is usually lymphatic in origin (acute lymphoblastic leukaemia, ALL). In adults, acute leukaemia is usually myeloid in origin (acute myeloid leukaemia, (AML) or myelomonocytic leukaemia), and may develop from pre-existing chronic leukaemia. Symptoms develop rapidly, and enlargement of the lymph nodes, spleen and liver is usually not marked. The blood film usually shows primitive blast cells, marked anaemia and thrombocytopenia.

Patients should be transferred at once to a specialized leukaemia unit. The anaemia is corrected with red cell transfusions, and bleeding with platelet transfusions; and infection treated with antibiotics, which should be bactericidal and given intravenously, and sometimes with granulocyte transfusion or injections of granulocyte colony-stimulating factor. Oral problems may dominate the clinical picture, as discussed fully in Chapter 26. Courses of cytotoxic drugs in combination are then given to kill the leukaemia cells.

In childhood ALL, 90% of patients achieve a remission. Relapses are common, especially in the central nervous system, hence prophylactic cranial irradiation and intrathecal cytotoxic drugs are given. After 5 years, 40% are still in remission, and many of these are probably 'cured'.

In adult AML the remission rate is 70%, but relapses usually occur within a few months or years. The prognosis has been improved by bone marrow (stem cell) transplantation. The patient is given 'lethal' doses of radiation and cytotoxic drugs to kill all leukaemic cells and also all normal bone marrow cells. Bone marrow, usually from a sibling, is then infused, and stem cells 'seed' in the marrow cavities to restore normal marrow.

Chronic myeloid leukaemia (CML) has its maximum incidence in the middle years of life, while chronic lymphatic leukaemia (CLL) tends to occur rather later.

The onset is insidious, and the patient usually presents with a complaint of tiredness, a dragging sensation in the upper left abdomen due to splenic enlargement, or enlargement of lymph nodes. The splenic enlargement is often so marked in CML that the spleen may come to fill the left side of the abdomen; it is less of a feature in CLL. Lymph node enlargement is usually prominent in CLL and relatively slight in CML. The white cell count is characteristically very high (e.g. $100–200 \times 10^9$/litre). Examination of the stained blood film shows that the great majority of white cells present are either granulocytes (CML) or lymphocytes (CLL). Most are mature. A moderate degree of anaemia is usually present while the platelet count may be normal, increased or decreased (due to removal by the large spleen).

In most cases life can be maintained for some 2–5 years after the diagnosis of CML has been made, and often considerably longer in the lymphatic form. Towards the end of the illness, CML may become acute, with severe anaemia, thrombocytopenia, and the appearance of blast cells in the blood film.

Conventional therapy for the chronic leukaemias is by oral alkylating agents (e.g. hydroxyurea or

Table 7.13 Classification of leukaemias	
Acute lymphoblastic (ALL)	Usually pre-B cell Sometimes T cell/B cell/undifferentiated
Acute myeloid (AML)	Several subtypes recognizable on morphological grounds carrying a different prognosis
Chronic lymphatic	Usually B cell, rarely T cell
Chronic myeloid	Philadelphia chromosome-positive Philadelphia chromosome-negative Eosinophilic

busulphan for CML and chlorambucil for CLL) if the patient is symptomatic. Cure is not achieved in the chronic leukaemias, although radical eradicative chemotherapy followed by bone marrow transplantation is under investigation in CML. Radiotherapy has only a limited role in these conditions. Autoimmune haemolytic anaemia and thrombocytopenia are common in CLL, and may respond to treatment with corticosteroids.

Thrombocythaemia. In essential thrombocythaemia, proliferation of bone marrow megakaryocytes results in a very high blood platelet count (often 1000×10^9/l). Bone marrow histology is required to distinguish this disorder from reactive thrombocytosis, in which the high blood platelet count is a reaction to infections or inflammatory disorders (e.g. rheumatoid arthritis or inflammatory bowel disease). Clinical features include thrombosis, and also bleeding (due to dysfunctional platelets).

Myelofibrosis. In myelofibrosis, the bone marrow is replaced by cells which produce fibrous tissue: this often causes a 'dry tap' on marrow aspiration. Patients develop anaemia, neutropenia and thrombocytopenia; and the spleen and liver become markedly enlarged due to compensatory extramedullary haemopoiesis (production of blood cells outside the bone marrow). Treatment is symptomatic, with red cell transfusions, platelet transfusions, and treatment of infections as required. Survival is usually a few years.

Plasma cell tumours

Plasma cell tumours are derived from B lymphocytes, which are normally responsible for the synthesis and secretion of antibodies. Tumours of these cells, therefore, commonly produce large amounts of immunoglobulin, which may be detected in the plasma or urine. The most frequent tumour type is myeloma, but others include Waldenström's macroglobulinaemia and heavy chain disease, both of which are very rare.

Myeloma. This a malignant proliferation of plasma cells largely confined to the bone marrow, which may be local (plasmacytoma) or generalized (multiple myeloma or myelomatosis). The main clinical features (Table 7.14) are bone pains

Table 7.14 Important features of multiple myeloma

Skeleton	Musculoskeletal pain Pathological fractures Hypercalcaemia Diffuse osteoporosis
Bone marrow replacement	Anaemia Neutropenia Thrombocytopenia

Serum and urine paraprotein	High plasma viscosity
	Chronic renal failure
	Low normal plasma
	   immunoglobulin levels
	Interference with blood
	   coagulation

(especially in the spine), pathological bone fractures, recurrent infections, anaemia and renal failure. The ESR and plasma viscosity are very high, due to production of an abnormal monoclonal immunoglobulin (IgG or IgA), which can be detected by plasma protein electrophoresis. The high blood viscosity may cause neurological symptoms and breathlessness. The urine may contain immunoglobulin fragments (Bence–Jones protein). Bone radiographs show 'punched-out' lytic areas, particularly in the skull, ribs and spine. Hypercalcaemia may occur due to bone lysis (see Ch. 14). Bone marrow histology shows increased plasma cells. Despite treatment with radiotherapy for bone lesions, corticosteroids and the cytotoxic drug melphalan, survival is usually only a few years. Stem cell transplantation is sometimes performed, and treatment of hypercalcaemia or hyperviscosity (with plasmapheresis to remove the immunoglobulin) may be required (see also Ch. 26).

Waldenström's macroglobulinaemia. In Waldenström's macroglobulinaemia, the proliferating cells produce large amounts of monoclonal immunoglobulin (IgM), which (as in myeloma) greatly increases the ESR and plasma viscosity and may cause a clinical hyperviscosity syndrome requiring treatment with plasmapheresis.

The porphyrias

The porphyrias are rare inherited disorders involving the biosynthetic pathway of the porphyrin haem, ocurring mostly in the liver (hepatic por-phyrias) but also less commonly in the bone mar-row (erythropoietic porphyrias). Single-enzyme deficiencies determine the particular variants of porphyria; biochemically these lead to accumula-tion and increased excretion of precursor prod-ucts up to the level of the block in biosynthesis.

Acute intermittent porphyria is characterized by increased production and urinary excretion of the porphyria precursors, δ-aminolevulinic acid and porphobilinogen. Clinically it causes severe peripheral neuropathy, which can include respira-tory paralysis, and neurovisceral attacks charac-terized by abdominal pain. The metabolic defect is exacerbated by a variety of drugs, catastrophi-cally so in the case of barbiturates or barbiturate-based anaesthetics, and specialized anaesthetic care is mandatory in such patients.

Porphyria cutanea tarda (cutaneous hepatic porphyria) leads to overproduction and accum-mulation of formed tetrapyrrole porphyria mole-cules. This causes a bullous dermatosis on the basis of photosensitivity, pigmentation and facial hirsutism. Overt hepatic disease, especially from alcohol, worsens the biochemical and clinical abnormalities.

Congenital (erythropoietic) porphyria is extremely rare, but historically was the first por-phyria disease to be described. It also causes pho-tosensitivity, and accumulation of porphyrins in the teeth (erythrodontia), which leads to a brown-red discoloration (see Ch. 26).

Bleeding disorders

Haemostasis

Following tissue injury which ruptures smaller blood vessels (including injections, surgical inci-sions and dental extractions), a series of interac-tions between the vessel wall and the blood normally occurs, which results in cessation of blood loss within a few minutes (haemostasis). Haemostasis results from effective sealing of the severed vessels by a haemostatic plug. This is ini-tially formed of blood platelets, which are also called thrombocytes (primary haemostasis), and is subsequently stabilized by fibrin, which is formed locally as a result of the interaction of plasma clot-

ting factors (secondary haemostasis). Over the next few days, the haemostatic plug is gradually digested by the fibrinolytic system, in parallel with tissue repair processes.

Generalized bleeding disorders can arise due to a defect in any one of the four interactive compo-nents of haemostasis:

- the vessel wall
- the platelets – low number (thrombocytopenia) or platelet dysfunction
- the coagulation system
- the fibrinolytic system.

These bleeding disorders are considered in turn.

Vessel wall disorders

Congenital vessel wall disorders

Congenital vessel wall disorders include heredi-tary haemorrhagic telangiectasia and the Ehlers–Danlos syndrome.

Hereditary haemorrhagic telangiectasia. This is a group of disorders whose inheritance is autosomal dominant, hence men and women are affected equally, and the risk of siblings and off-spring also being affected is 50%. Telangiectasia describes the formation of dilated, thin-walled, small blood vessels which do not contract nor-mally after trauma, resulting in prolonged bleed-ing. These lesions develop during early adult life, and are visible as purple vascular malformations a few millimetres in diameter on the face, lips, tongue and hands (Fig. 7.3). They do not occur in tooth sockets, hence do not cause excessive postextraction bleeding; however, oral lesions can bleed excessively following trauma, includ-ing accidental trauma in the dental surgery. The main clinical problem is recurrent nosebleeds and gastrointestinal bleeding from lesions in the nose and gastrointestinal tract, which cause iron deficiency anaemia in most patients and require oral iron. Acute bleeding may require treatment with endoscopy and local coagulation proce-dures at the bleeding site. The fibrinolytic inhibitor tranexamic acid may reduce the risk of bleeding.

Ehlers–Danlos syndrome. This is a heterogeneous group of disorders whose inheritance may be dominant, recessive or, occasionally,

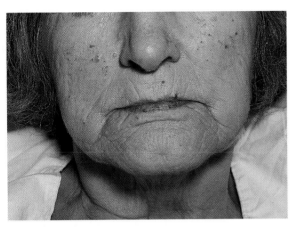

Fig. 7.3 Hereditary haemorrhagic telangiectasia.

x-linked. They result in defective formation of collagen, which supports small blood vessels, and hence in excessive bleeding, both after surgery and spontaneously. Hyperextensible joints also occur in such patients. Treatment is symptomatic.

Acquired vessel wall disorders

Acquired vessel wall disorders usually cause only bleeding into the superficial layers of the skin (purpura), and are sometimes termed the vascular purpuras to distinguish them from purpura due to thrombocytopenia (see below). The common disorders all begin with the letter 'S', which may help the reader to remember them.

Scurvy. Vitamin C deficiency due to dietary lack of fruit and vegetables – scurvy – which impairs collagen synthesis, is an exception to the 'purpura-only' rule because it also causes internal bleeding, especially from the gums. This only occurs in the presence of teeth, and is aggravated by poor dental hygiene. In developed countries, scurvy is usually seen in alcoholics, widowers and the elderly, and occasionally in young people with unusual diets. Associated clinical features include normocytic anaemia (see above), impaired wound healing, bone tenderness (from subperiosteal haemorrhage), and features of associated nutritional deficiencies. Treatment is with oral vitamin C (initially 1 g/day then 50 mg/day).

Steroid-induced purpura. Excess of adrenal corticosteroids may be endogenous (overproduction in Cushing's syndrome, see Ch. 13), but is more commonly exogenous from high doses of corticosteroid drugs (e.g. prednisolone) given to suppress immunological diseases such as rheumatoid disorders, asthma, or certain blood or skin disorders. Their catabolic effects include breakdown of skin collagen, resulting in thinning of the skin, easy bruising due to rupture of small blood vessels (Figure 7.4), and bruising after venepuncture. This is usually seen in the arms, and is only of cosmetic significance.

Senile purpura. This is commonly seen in older people (who are not necessarily senile!). Like steroid-induced purpura, it is due to breakdown of skin collagen, resulting in thin skin, easy bruising, and bruising after venepuncture. It is usually seen only in the arms and hands (Fig. 7.5), and may reflect the combined effects of age and light exposure. It is only of cosmetic significance.

Septicaemia. This disorder, due to certain bacteria, can present with fever and acute purpura, due to direct bacterial toxic effects on small blood vessel walls. This is classically seen in acute meningococcal septicaemia (Fig. 7.6), which may occur with or without clinical features of meningitis (see Ch. 9). This is a medical emergency, requiring immediate injection of penicillin, because death can occur rapidly. A similar picture may be seen in postoperative septicaemia due to Gram-negative bacteria. Disseminated intravascular coagulation (see below) may also be present in septicaemia, and cause purpura and other types

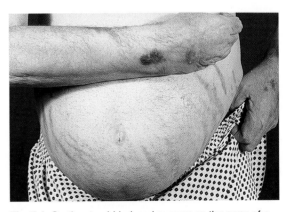

Fig. 7.4 Corticosteroid-induced purpura on the arms of a patient with Cushing's syndrome. Note also truncal obesity and abdominal striae.

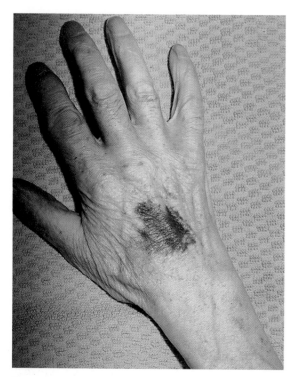

Fig. 7.5 Senile purpura.

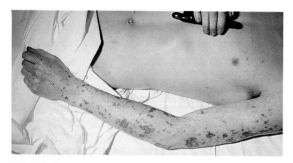

Fig. 7.6 Acute spreading purpura in meningococcal septicaemia.

of bleeding. Haemorrhagic skin rashes can also be seen in viral or rickettsial haemorrhagic fevers, which are uncommon in the UK.

Schönlein–Henoch purpura. This is the commonest clinical syndrome of acute vasculitis: a sterile inflammation of small blood vessels. This initially causes a raised, red papular rash (due to inflammation and oedema) which becomes haemorrhagic after a day or two due to leakage of blood from damaged blood vessels. Unlike other forms of purpura, which are 'flat', vasculitic skin lesions

are raised due to the presence of inflammation as well as bleeding ('palpable purpura'). Schönlein–Henoch purpura usually occurs in children, often about 10 days after an upper respiratory tract infection, which triggers formation of immune complexes that are deposited in small blood vessels. The rash occurs on the buttocks and extensor aspects of the limbs. Vasculitis may also occur in the joints (joint pains), gut (abdominal pains) and kidney (glomerulonephritis with haematuria and proteinuria, see Ch. 11). Corticosteroids are given in severe cases.

Platelet disorders

Platelets participate in haemostasis by adhering to the damaged vessel wall and to each other (aggregation), forming the primary haemostatic plug which initially stops bleeding within a few minutes of injury. Platelet function can be tested by the skin bleeding time, in which a standardized incision is made on cleaned forearm skin with a sterile device, the bleeding wound touched gently with filter paper every 30 s, and the time to cessation of bleeding recorded. The normal range is 2–10 minutes. As may be expected, the bleeding time increases with decrease in the blood platelet count. The bleeding time test is usually used to assess suspected platelet dysfunction in patients with normal platelet counts, e.g. in suspected von Willebrand's disease.

Like vascular bleeding disorders, platelet disorders usually present as purpura: bleeding into the superficial layers of the skin, which usually appears as a 'rash' of red spots (Fig. 7.7). A purpuric rash can be distinguished from other red rashes in that the red spots do not disappear on pressure, because the blood is extravascular. In red rashes due to local vasodilatation (e.g. drug-induced rashes or viral infections such as measles) the blood remains intravascular, so the red spots disappear on pressure. Unlike most vascular purpuras, platelet disorders frequently cause internal bleeding: oral bleeding from characteristic 'blood blisters' (Fig. 7.8), nosebleeds (epistaxis), heavy uterine bleeding (menorrhagia), gastrointestinal bleeding (haematemesis and melaena), and intracranial bleeding. The last two types of bleeding may be fatal.

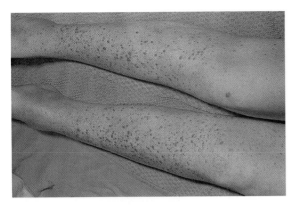

Fig. 7.7 Purpura in thrombocytopenia.

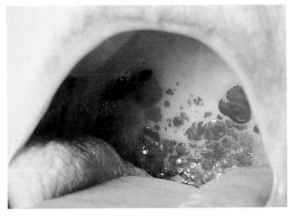

Fig. 7.8 Palatal blood blisters in a patient with thrombocytopenia.

Platelet defects also cause excessive bleeding after venepuncture, hence it is important to compress the venepuncture site for at least 15 min in order to conserve veins. Platelet defects also cause excessive bleeding after trauma or surgery, including dental extractions, so preoperative correction of the defect is required.

Thrombocytopenia

The normal blood platelet count is 150–400 × 10^9/l. Purpura and other types of bleeding are often evident when the platelet count falls to 50–100 × 10^9/l. Haemostatic cover with platelet transfusions for surgery (including dental extractions) or invasive procedures should be discussed with the haematologist in patients with platelet counts below 80 × 10^9/l. Platelet transfusion may also be required to treat internal bleeding in thrombocytopenia.

Table 7.15 includes the commoner causes of a low blood platelet count. A bone marrow aspiration is often performed to distinguish two main groups: conditions in which bone marrow histology is abnormal and platelet production is reduced, and conditions in which bone marrow histology is normal and thrombocytopenia results from increased removal of platelets from circulating blood. The former group includes several disorders previously considered in this chapter, including marrow aplasia, neoplasia, and megaloblastic anaemia (in which the platelet count is rarely low enough to cause bleeding). Treatment of thrombocytopenia in these disorders is that of the underlying disorder, with platelet transfusion as required.

There are three main groups of disorders causing increased platelet removal from circulating blood. In immune thrombocytopenic purpura (ITP), antiplatelet antibodies develop and result in increased removal of platelets from the blood by the reticuloendothelial system (especially the spleen). This most commonly presents as purpura about 10 days after an upper respiratory tract infection in children, and is usually transient; this clinical picture is similar to Schönlein–Henoch purpura (see above), from which it is distinguished by the low platelet count and by the absence of clinical features of vasculitis. ITP also occurs in adults, again often due to infections (especially HIV infection) or to neoplasms. Platelet transfusion is often ineffective in ITP because the antiplatelet antibodies result in very short survival of the infused platelets. Treatment options include intravenous infusion of purified human immunoglobulin, corticosteroids, or splenectomy if the condition persists.

Splenomegaly from any cause can result in thrombocytopenia due to sequestration/destruction of platelets in the enlarged spleen. Common causes include cirrhosis of the liver and rheumatoid arthritis (see Ch. 14).

Disseminated intravascular coagulation (DIC) can cause acute platelet consumption. It is discussed in the next section.

Table 7.15 Bleeding disorders

Vessel wall disorders

Congenital	Hereditary haemorrhagic telangiectasia
	Ehlers–Danlos syndrome
Acquired	Scurvy
	Steroid purpura (Cushing's syndrome, drugs)
	Senile purpura
	Septicaemia (e.g. meningococcal)
	Schönlein–Henoch purpura

Platelet disorders

Thrombocytopenia
Acquired

Decreased formation (abnormal bone marrow)	Marrow aplasia
	Marrow neoplasia
	Megaloblastic anaemias
Increased destruction (normal bone marrow)	Immune thrombocytopenic purpura (ITP)
	Splenomegaly
	Disseminated intravascular coagulation (DIC)

Platelet function disorders

Congenital	Von Willebrand's disease
Acquired	Aspirin
	Renal failure (see Ch. 11)

Coagulation disorders

Prolonged activated partial thromboplastin time (APTT) (intrinsic defects)

Congenital	Haemophilia A (factor VIII deficiency)
	Haemophilia B (factor IX deficiency)
Acquired	Heparin therapy

Prolonged prothrombin time (PT) (extrinsic defects)

Acquired	Liver disease
	Vitamin K deficiency, malabsorption, obstructive jaundice
	Oral anticoagulant therapy (e.g. warfarin, vitamin K antagonists)

Prolonged thrombin time (TT) (fibrinogen defects)

Acquired	Disseminated intravascular coagulation (DIC)

Fibrinolytic disorders

	Thrombolytic therapy (streptokinase, alteplase)
	Primary pathological fibrinolysis (e.g. tumours)

Platelet function disorders

These disorders cause a 'platelet-type' clinical pattern of excessive bleeding and a prolonged skin bleeding time, in the presence of a normal platelet count.

Von Willebrand's disease. This is a group of congenital bleeding disorders which are common (affecting at least 1 in 1000 persons) but usually mild, and therefore often not diagnosed. The inheritance is usually autosomal dominant, hence men and women are equally affected, and the risk of siblings and offspring also being affected is 50%. The clinical features are easy bruising, nose-bleeds, oral bleeding, menorrhagia in women, gastrointestinal bleeding, and excessive bleeding following trauma or surgery, including dental extractions.

The excessive bleeding is due to low plasma levels of von Willebrand factor, which is released from endothelial cells and platelets, and which plays an important role in platelet adhesion to the damaged vessel wall, and in the subsequent process of platelet aggregation to form the primary haemostatic plug. The von Willebrand factor also carries coagulation factor VIII (anti-haemophilic factor) in the circulation, and delivers it to sites of injury, facilitating coagulation and formation of the secondary, fibrin haemostatic plug. Plasma levels of coagulation factor VIII are therefore often moderately reduced in von Willebrand's disease, reflecting the low plasma level of its carrier protein, von Willebrand factor. Low levels of von Willebrand factor and factor VIII confirm the diagnosis of von Willebrand's disease, as does defective platelet aggregation in response to the antibiotic ristocetin. Patients with von Willebrand's disease commonly present with prolonged bleeding after dental extraction, which can be treated by raising the low plasma level of von Willebrand factor (and factor VIII) to normal. This is usually done by intravenous infusion of desmopressin, a synthetic analogue of vasopressin or antidiuretic factor (see Ch. 11), which releases von Willebrand factor from vascular endothelium into the plasma. Intravenous infusion of human plasma von Willebrand factor/factor VIII concentrates (e.g. Hemate P) may be required in severe cases of von Willebrand's disease in whom desmopressin is ineffective.

Patients with suspected von Willebrand's disease should be referred to regional haemophilia centres for diagnosis, registration, issue of a bleeding disorders card (to show to any doctors and dentists), and counselling and education (of both the patient and other affected family members). They should avoid aspirin, which aggravates the platelet function defect (see below). Dental extractions and other operations or invasive procedures should be arranged in advance with the haemophilia centre. Intravenous desmo-pressin is usually given just prior to surgery, then every 12–24 h for 2–3 days (after which it usually loses its effect due to exhaustion of endothelial stores of von Willebrand factor). Intravenous infusion of plasma von Willebrand factor/factor VIII concentrate may be required as haemostatic cover in severe cases of von Willebrand's disease in whom desmopressin is ineffective. Oral tranexamic acid (1 g thrice daily) is also given prior to dental extractions and continued for 7 days. It inhibits oral fibrinolytic enzymes which break down the fibrin haemostatic plug in the tooth socket, reducing the risk of delayed bleeding.

Aspirin therapy. Aspirin induces a mild platelet function defect, due to inhibition of platelet prostaglandins. This effect is shown by prolongation of the skin bleeding time (e.g. from 5 to 10 min), occurs within an hour, and lasts for about 7 days until most circulating platelets are replaced by new platelets released from the bone marrow. In persons with normal haemostasis, this effect of aspirin has little effect on postoperative bleeding, and it is not necessary to stop aspirin prior to dental extraction or most other types of surgery. However, aspirin should be avoided in persons with bleeding disorders (e.g. thrombocytopenia, von Willebrand's disease or coagulation disorders) because it increases their risk of bleeding. Because of its antiplatelet effect, aspirin is used as an antithrombotic drug (see Ch. 6).

Renal failure. Acute or chronic renal failure also causes a platelet function defect (see Ch. 11). This is partly due to retention of platelet inhibitory toxins, which are normally excreted by the kidney (this is reversed by dialysis treatment), and partly due to anaemia (this is reversed by erythropoietin treatment in chronic renal failure). Prior to dental extraction or other types of surgery, patients should be adequately dialysed to minimize the risk of excessive bleeding.

Coagulation disorders

These are the bleeding disorders of most importance to the dentist, not only because they are the commonest but also because they are the most likely to cause prolonged bleeding following dental extraction, nerve block injections or other invasive procedures.

The clinical pattern of bleeding in coagulation disorders differs from that in platelet disorders. Instead of purpuric spots in the superficial skin, bleeding into the skin occurs at a deeper level, and results in large, spreading bruises. Nosebleeds, oral bleeding and menorrhagia are less common than in platelet disorders; however, haematuria (blood in the urine), bleeding into muscles and joints (haemarthrosis) is common in severe haemophilia. As with platelet defects, gastrointestinal bleeding and intracranial bleeding can occur, and can be fatal.

Coagulation defects do not cause excessive bleeding after venepuncture, but do cause excessive bleeding after intramuscular injections (which should therefore be avoided in such patients; intravenous or subcutaneous injections should be used instead). Excessive bleeding is common after surgery, dental extractions and nerve block injections (Figs 7.9 and 7.10). Whereas postoperative bleeding usually occurs immediately in platelet disorders (due to defective formation of the primary, platelet haemostatic plug), in coagulation disorders bleeding after surgery is often delayed for several hours or days (due to initial haemostasis by a normal primary, platelet haemostatic plug, which is later washed away, and bleeding recurs because of defective formation of the secondary, fibrin haemostatic plug).

The coagulation system is outlined in Fig. 7.11. Following vessel wall injury, blood is exposed to tissue factor in the subendothelium, which initiates blood coagulation by sequential activation of plasma protein clotting factors, which are enzymes denoted by roman numerals. Tissue factor initiates the extrinsic pathway of blood coagulation (so called because tissue factor is normally extrinsic to circulating blood). This extrinsic pathway is screened in the haematology laboratory by the prothrombin time, in which tissue factor is added to citrated plasma and the clotting time recorded (normal range 10–15 s). Coagulation factors in this pathway include factor VII, which activates factor X in the presence of its cofactor, factor V. In turn, factor II (prothrombin) is activated to thrombin, which converts soluble fibrinogen (factor I) to insoluble fibrin. This last stage of the coagulation pathway

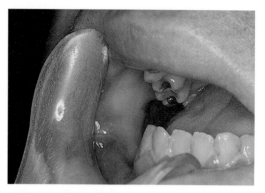

Fig. 7.9 Intraoral bruising and clotting after molar extraction in a haemophiliac.

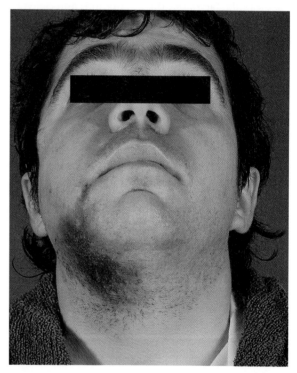

Fig. 7.10 Bleeding in the soft tissues of the neck after molar extraction in a haemophiliac.

is screened in the haematology laboratory by the thrombin time, in which thrombin is added to plasma and the clotting time recorded (normal range 10–15 s).

While the extrinsic pathway is important in initiating blood coagulation, maintenance of thrombin and fibrin formation depends on the intrinsic pathway (so called because all factors are intrinsic

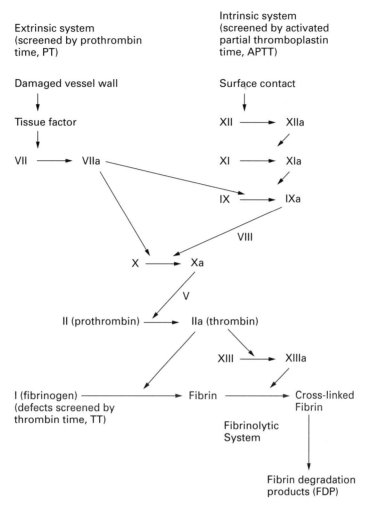

Fig. 7.11 The coagulation cascade showing the numbered factors (a, activated form). The factors involved in the intrinsic system, beginning with the activation of factor XII and ending with the activation of factor X, are all present in the circulating plasma: the extrinsic system consists of tissue thromboplastin and includes factor VII, not involved in the intrinsic system. Activated factor X, along with factor V, initiates the final steps, culminating in the conversion of fibrinogen to fibrin by thrombin.

to circulating blood). This pathway is screened by the activated partial thromboplastin time (APTT), in which citrated plasma is exposed to a standard surface (kaolin suspension). The normal range of the APTT is 30–50 s. Surface contact activates in turn factors XII, XI and IX (Christmas factor), which in the presence of its cofactor, factor VIII (antihaemophilic factor), activates factor X (Fig. 7.11). While surface contact is a useful stimulant of the intrinsic pathway in the laboratory, the relevance of this part of the pathway is questionable because patients with factor XII deficiency

and many patients with factor XI deficiency do not bleed excessively. Activation of factor IX in the intrinsic system may largely be due to its activation by factor VII (Fig. 7.11).

In a suspected coagulation disorder, a screen of these three clotting times is performed, which in combination with the clinical features usually provides an initial diagnosis. Specific assays of individual clotting factors can then be performed, if required, to provide a specific diagnosis. Three main groups of coagulation disorders can be distinguished by the coagulation screen:

- Intrinsic defects (prolonged APTT):
  - congenital deficiencies of factor VIII or IX (haemophilias)
  - anticoagulant therapy with heparin (see Ch. 6).

- Extrinsic defects (prolonged prothrombin time) usually due to acquired deficiencies of factors II, VII and X, which are synthesized in the liver in the presence of vitamin K:
  - liver disease (see Ch. 10)
  - vitamin K deficiency (e.g. malabsorption, obstructive jaundice, see Ch. 10)
  - oral anticoagulant therapy with warfarin (a competitive antagonist of vitamin K, see Ch. 6).

- Fibrinogen defects (prolonged thrombin time), usually due to acquired consumption of fibrinogen in DIC.

Haemophilias

The haemophilias are congenital coagulation disorders, due to genetic deficiencies of either factor VIII (classic haemophilia or haemophilia A; 80% of families) or factor IX (Christmas disease or haemophilia B; 20% of families). The prevalence of haemophilia is about 1 in 10 000; hence, there are about 6 000 haemophiliacs in the UK. The clinical features of factor VIII deficiency and factor IX deficiency are identical.

Both types of haemophilia are X-linked recessive disorders. The genes controlling synthesis of factor VIII and factor IX are on the X chromosome. In affected males, the abnormal X chromosome cannot synthesize the relevant clotting factor, resulting in low plasma levels and an increased bleeding tendency (haemophilia). Affected males pass their Y chromosome to their sons and not their abnormal X chromosome, hence the sons of haemophiliacs and their descendants are unaffected. In contrast, all the daughters of affected males receive their father's abnormal X chromosome, hence they are carriers (usually asymptomatic) of haemophilia, whose sons have a 50:50 chance of being haemophiliacs, and whose daughters have a 50:50 chance of being carriers (Fig. 7.12). All female relatives of haemophiliacs

should be offered genetic counselling concerning the possibility of sons with haemophilia: some opt for prenatal diagnosis and termination of pregnancy in the event of an affected male with severe haemophilia.

The severity of the bleeding disorder in haemophilia generally reflects the plasma level of factor VIII (or factor IX). The normal range of plasma factor VIII (or factor IX) is about 50–200% of the mean normal level (defined as 100%). In about half of families with haemophilia, the plasma level of the relevant factor is slightly reduced (10–50% of normal), and the disorder is termed 'mild': excessive bleeding occurs infrequently, usually only after trauma or surgery (including dental surgery). In the other half of families, the disorder is 'moderate' (factor level 2–10% of normal), with bleeding occurring more frequently, often after minor trauma or surgery, or 'severe' (factor level 0–2% of normal) with frequent bleeding, often occurring 'spontaneously' after minimal trauma or surgery.

In families with severe or moderate haemophilia, affected males usually have bleeding episodes in childhood. Bleeding into joints (haemarthosis) is characteristic of severe haemophilia. It usually occurs in the knees, ankles, elbows or wrists. The joint becomes acutely painful, warm and swollen, with greatly

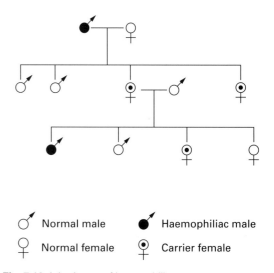

Fig. 7.12 Inheritance of haemophilia.

reduced movement. Recurrent joint bleeds cause chronic arthritis (see Ch. 14) with chronic pain, swelling, restricted movement and disability. Bleeding into muscles is also common, and often follows minor trauma, including intramuscular injections which should never be given to haemophiliacs (intravenous and subcutaneous injections can be given instead). Muscle bleeds cause large, painful, warm swellings which impair movement. Other bleeding episodes which are common in severe or moderate haemophilia include large, spreading skin bruises; bleeding into the urine (haematuria) or gastrointestinal tract (haematemesis, melaena); intracranial bleeding; and excessive bleeding following surgery, including dental surgery.

In families with mild haemophilia, bleeding into joints or muscles is less common, and excessive bleeding may not be recognized until adult life. Such excessive bleeding often occurs following the first episode of significant trauma: this may be an accidental injury, or a surgical operation, which is often the first extraction of an adult tooth (deciduous teeth are usually lost with little trauma). Excessive bleeding after dental extractions (or other dental surgical procedures) should always raise the suspicion of haemophilia in a male, even if there is no past history or family history of excessive bleeding. In about one-third of newly-presenting haemophiliacs, there is no family history. This may occur (1) because of a new genetic mutation in that patient, (2) because of a lack of affected males in recent generations – the disorder can 'skip' generations because of its recessive inheritance (Fig. 7.12), or (3) because the family history is not recalled, or not given.

The diagnosis of haemophilia is confirmed by a haematologist or haemophilia centre from a typical personal and family history, the APTT, which is usually prolonged (in contrast to the prothrombin time and thrombin time, which are usually normal), and by low plasma levels of either factor VIII (haemophilia A) or factor IX (haemophilia B). In patients with low factor VIII levels, it is important to exclude von Willebrand's disease by also measuring plasma levels of von Willebrand factor (see above).

Management of haemophilia as well as von Willebrand's disease is best organized by regional haemophilia centres, staffed by haematologists, physicians, nurses, physiotherapists, social workers and dentists who have experience with the many complications of this uncommon but important disease. Comprehensive haemophilia care includes:

• Accurate diagnosis (type and severity of disorder).
• Registration of affected patients, who are given a bleeding disorders card (Figure 7.13) which records the type and severity of the disorder, blood group, and the name and telephone number of the haemophilia centre. Patients are asked to show this card to any doctor or dentist whom they attend. Haemophilia centres can be contacted at any time for consultation and advice, including cover of emergency dental or other surgical treatment.
• Education and counselling of patients and families, including genetic counselling of patients and their female relatives who may be carriers, and advice to avoid aspirin, intramuscular injections, and traumatic activities.

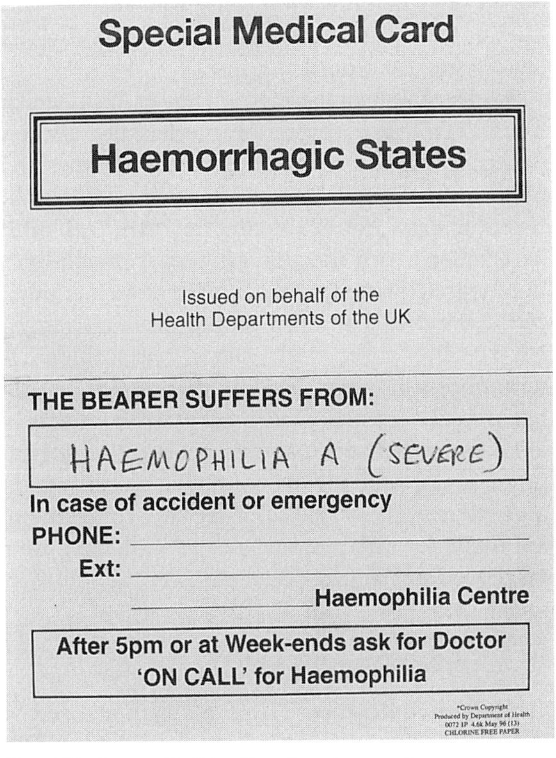

Special Medical Card

Haemorrhagic States

Issued on behalf of the
Health Departments of the UK

THE BEARER SUFFERS FROM:

HAEMOPHILIA A (SEVERE)

In case of accident or emergency
PHONE: _____
Ext: _____
_____**Haemophilia Centre**

**After 5pm or at Week-ends ask for Doctor
'ON CALL' for Haemophilia**

*Crown Copyright
Produced by Department of Health
0072 1P 4.6k May 98 (13)
CHLORINE FREE PAPER

Fig. 7.13 Congenital bleeding disorders card.

- Regular review (at least annually).
- Provision of treatment (hospital or home treatment) including desmopressin and coagulation factor concentrates. Severe haemophiliacs, especially children, often receive prophylaxis with regular concentrate infusions (2–3 times weekly) to prevent haemarthoses.
- Vaccination against hepatitis B and hepatitis A, which may occasionally be transmitted by plasma-derived coagulation factor concentrates. No vaccine is currently available against hepatitis C or HIV. Unfortunately, many haemophiliacs treated with plasma-derived coagulation factor concentrates before 1985 became carriers of hepatitis C, HIV, and/or hepatitis B. Full precautions against cross-infection should be observed in such patients, including during dental surgery (see Ch. 5). The introduction of blood donor screening and of antiviral treatment of concentrates (e.g. heat treatment) in 1985 has greatly reduced the risk of haemophiliacs acquiring such infections. Since 1995, haemophiliacs have been increasingly being transferred to recombinant coagulation factor concentrates, which are produced by mammalian cells transfected with human factor VIII or factor IX genes, and which appear free from human viruses.
- Dental management. This is outlined in Table 7.16. For severe or moderately affected patients, the haemophilia centre dental specialist often provides all dental treatment. For mild haemophiliacs, routine dental treatment can often be arranged with the general dental practitioner, but invasive procedures (e.g. extractions, regional block injections or deep scaling), which require haemostatic cover with factor replacement or desmopressin, are usually performed at the haemophilia centre. The important principle is close liaison between patients, their general dental practitioner, and the haemophilia centre dentist and other staff, so that appropriate arrangements are made for safe performance of individual dental procedures in individual patients.

Acquired coagulation disorders

Extrinsic defects. These are characterized by a prolonged prothrombin time, and are usually due to acquired deficiencies of factors II, VII or X (the prothrombin complex) which are synthesized in the liver in the presence of vitamin K:

- Liver disease (see Ch. 10), including acute hepatic failure (e.g. caused by paracetamol overdose or viral hepatitis) and chronic liver failure (cirrhosis). Treatment of bleeding (or prophylaxis of bleeding prior to surgery, including dental surgery) is with fresh frozen plasma to normalize the prothrombin time. Vitamin K is ineffective.
- Vitamin K deficiency (see Ch. 10), including malabsorption and obstructive jaundice. Treatment or prophylaxis of bleeding is with vitamin K injections to normalize the prothrombin time.
- Induced by oral anticoagulant therapy with warfarin, which is a competitive antagonist of vitamin K (see Ch. 6). Patients receiving warfarin should be given an oral anticoagulant booklet (Fig. 7.14), which records their general medical practitioner, hospital specialist, current warfarin dose and intensity of anticoagulant effect. This is measured by the ratio of the patient's prothrombin time to the normal prothrombin time, using laboratory reagents which are internationally standardized. This ratio is the international normalized ratio (INR) of the prothrombin time, e.g.

$$INR = \frac{\text{patient's prothrombin time (30 s)}}{\text{normal prothrombin time (15 s)}} = 2.0$$

The target therapeutic range of the INR is usually 2.0–3.0, except for patients with mechanical

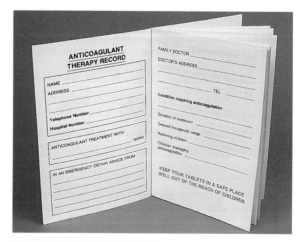

Fig. 7.14 Anticoagulant booklet.

Table 7.16 Dental management in haemophiliacs

Prophylaxis	All diagnosed patients to be reviewed regularly by haemophilia centre dental specialist and dental hygienist
	Appropriate cross-infection precautions in patients known to be carriers of hepatitis B, hepatitis C or HIV (or whose status is unknown)
Invasive procedures	Always check with haemophilia centre, who will establish: type and severity of haemophilia presence or absence of inhibitors/viral infections past history of bleeding after invasive procedures Agree joint individual management plan with dental practitioner, patient and relatives.

Type of procedure	General guidelines
Low risk Supragingival or subgingival scaling Simple restoration Local anaesthetic injection in well-defined areas over bone Restoration with subgingival preparation	No haemostatic cover usually required, unless previous bleeding with such procedures
Moderate risk Regional injection of local anaesthetic Simple extraction of single tooth	Raise plasma level of deficient factor to 100% shortly before procedure by intravenous infusion of factor/ desmopressin as appropriate at haemophilia centre. Repeat dose next day, then for rebleeding if required. Give oral tranexamic acid (adult dose 1 g three times a day) starting before procedure and continuing for 7 days
High risk Extensive surgery (e.g. multiple extractions)	As for moderate risk above, but (1) admit to haemophilia centre hospital overnight after procedure and (2) give additional intravenous infusion of factor/ desmopressin on evening after procedure (or earlier if excessive bleeding)

All patients should be given clear, written instructions prior to leaving hospital to attend the haemophilia centre in the event of bleeding after the procedure, for haematological and dental assessment and hospital admission if appropriate.

heart valve prostheses, who require a higher target range (3.0–4.0) to prevent valve thrombosis (see Ch. 6). There is a wide variation between patients in the daily dose of warfarin required to achieve their target INR (1–15 mg). The daily required dose in an individual patient also varies with time, due to variations in dietary intake of vitamin K-containing foods and of alcohol, and to interactions with other drugs. It is therefore important that the INR be regularly monitored (by the general medical practitioner, or by a hospital anticoagulant clinic), at least every 6–8 weeks, and the dose adjusted to maintain the target INR.

In the event of bleeding, the INR should be checked as an emergency, and the anticoagulant effect reduced by either intravenous vitamin K, or by fresh frozen plasma.

The anticoagulant effect may also have to be reduced prior to surgery, including dental surgery (e.g. extractions). As with haemophilia, it is important that the general dental practitioner liaises with the patient's general medical practitioner and/or hospital specialists to agree a management plan for the individual procedure in the individual patient. General guidelines are summarized in Table 7.17.

Fibrinogen defects. These are characterized by a prolonged thrombin time. The usual cause is acquired consumption of fibrinogen in DIC. This is due to excessive thrombin generation, which converts plasma fibrinogen into microthrombi throughout the body, leading eventually to low plasma fibrinogen and bleeding. The platelet count may also be low, due to consumption of platelets in the microthrombi. DIC can be a complication of circulatory shock (e.g. trauma, septicaemia, or complications of pregnancy such as uterine bleeding) or of disseminated malignant disease. Treatment is usually with fresh frozen plasma, and platelet transfusion if required.

Disorders of fibrinolysis

The body's fibrinolytic system has a physiological role in the digestion of fibrin. If it did not exist, unopposed blood coagulation would cause excessive fibrin formation and thrombosis (see Ch. 6). Fibrin formation stimulates vascular endothelial cells to produce tissue plasminogen activator (t-PA), which activates circulating plasma plasminogen to plasmin, an enzyme which digests fibrin to soluble fibrin degradation products.

Excessive bleeding due to excessive fibrinolysis (Table 7.15) may occur during thrombolytic therapy for acute myocardial infarction with streptokinase or alteplase (recombinant t-PA) (see Ch. 6), or, rarely, due to excessive production of endogenous t-PA by tumours (primary pathological fibrinolysis). Treatment is with the fibrinolytic inhibitor drug tranexamic acid.

Blood transfusion

Blood transfusion is usually given as red cell concentrates, plasma being fractionated for specific use as plasma protein solution, albumin, coagulation factor concentrates, etc. Prior to transfusion of red cells, patient serum is sent to the blood bank for cross-matching, to prevent transfusion of donor-incompatible blood, agglutination and haemolysis, which can be fatal. The ABO blood groups, defined by the presence of antigens on red cells and the presence of antibodies in serum, are shown in Table 7.18.

Table 7.17 Dental management of patients receiving oral anticoagulant therapy

Type of procedure	General guidelines (Always check with patient's haematologist)
Low risk Supragingival or subgingival scaling Simple restoration Local anaesthetic injection in well-defined areas over bone Restoration with subgingival preparation Regional injection of local anaesthetic	Treat as normal
Moderate risk Simple extraction of single tooth	Adjust INR to lower end of therapeutic range (about 2.0 for normal-intensity anticoagulation; about 2.5 for high-intensity anticoagulation)
High risk Extensive surgery (e.g. multiple extractions)	Adjust INR to lower end of therapeutic range ± local management of sockets. Admit to hospital overnight after procedure

Table 7.18 ABO blood groups, cellular antigens and serum antibodies

Group	Cell antigens	Serum antibodies
O	–	Anti-A, anti-B
A	A	Anti-B
B	B	Anti-A
AB	A, B	–

Table 7.19 Complications of blood transfusion

Incompatible blood reactions
Febrile reactions
Infection with blood-borne viruses

In addition, donor blood is tested for the rhesus blood group (Rh). Rh-negative patients should receive only Rh-negative blood where possible.

Complications of blood transfusion are shown in Table 7.19.

Incompatible blood reactions should be prevented by cross-matching (see above). Agglutination and haemolysis occur, causing loin pain, shock, rigors, breathlessness, renal failure and jaundice. Transfusion should be stopped, and samples of patient and donor blood saved for investigation. When febrile reactions occur, transfusion should be stopped. Infection with blood-borne viruses (e.g. hepatitis B or C, HIV, syphilis or malaria) is now very rare due to screening of blood donors.

8 Diseases of the respiratory system

Introduction

Diseases of the respiratory system are important for several reasons: upper respiratory tract infections are major causes of morbidity and sickness absence; inhaled foreign bodies (including extracted teeth, portions of teeth and dental instruments) can cause bronchial obstruction, lung collapse and serious complications; acute asthma is common and may require first aid treatment; chronic lung diseases (e.g. chronic bronchitis) are major causes of disability and death, and increase the risks of major surgery and general anaesthesia or sedation; and lung cancer and pulmonary tuberculosis are major causes of death world-wide, and are major concerns in preventive medicine and public health.

Specific aspects concerning the history, examination and investigation of respiratory disease will be followed by consideration of the individual disorders.

History

Table 8.1 summarizes the important parts of history taking for diseases of the respiratory system. Cigarette smoking, occupation (exposure to irritants), and weight loss (indicating lung cancer,

tuberculosis or chronic lung sepsis) are also relevant.

Cough

Coughing is a normal defensive reflex initiated by irritation of the mucosa lining the respiratory tract. It protects against entry of foreign material, and expels mucous secretions. Increasing coughing is a common symptom of respiratory disease. Acute cough is a common symptom of acute upper and lower respiratory tract infections and allergies: it may be 'dry', produce clear (mucoid) sputum, or produce yellow-green (purulent) sputum if there is bacterial infection (e.g. acute tracheobronchitis or pneumonia). Chronic cough

---

Table 8.1 History taking and the respiratory system

Upper respiratory tract
  Sneezing, nasal discharge, nosebleeds
  Facial pain (sinusitis)
  Ear pain or discharge
  Deafness
  Sore throat, hoarseness
Lower respiratory tract
  Cough
  Sputum
  Haemoptysis
  Breathlessness (see Table 6.1)
  Chest pain (see Table 6.2)

is the typical symptom of chronic bronchitis, but may also be due to tuberculosis or lung cancer.

Haemoptysis

This is the coughing up of blood from the respiratory tract. It may be due to acute pulmonary oedema (heart failure, see Ch. 6), pulmonary embolism (see Ch. 6), or lung diseases including pneumonia, lung cancer, tuberculosis or chronic lung sepsis.

Breathlessness

This may be due to heart failure (see Ch. 6), anaemia (see Ch. 7), abdominal swelling, or to any lung disease which is extensive enough to cause impaired oxygenation of blood passing through the lungs. Common lung causes include chronic bronchitis, asthma, pneumonia, lung collapse, pneumothorax and pleural effusion.

Chest pain

Chest pain due to respiratory disease may be centrally sited in acute tracheitis: the patient describes a raw, sharp pain under the sternum on coughing. Lateral chest pain is usually due to pleurisy: a sharp, stabbing pain due to involvement of the pain-sensitive parietal pleural membrane by lung or chest wall disease. This pain is often well localized by the patient, and is characteristically increased by deep breathing, coughing or moving. Common causes include pulmonary embolism (infarction), pneumonia, pneumothorax, rib fracture, infections, with Coxsackie virus and herpes zoster (shingles) virus.

Examination

Table 8.2 summarizes the signs of respiratory disease which may be observed.

Central cyanosis

Central cyanosis (see Ch. 6) can be a sign of severe respiratory failure, which may result from

Table 8.2 Examination of the respiratory system

Sneezing, nasal discharge, nasal polyps
Difficulty in breathing (increased rate or effort)
Cyanosis (see Ch. 6)
Finger clubbing (see Ch. 6)
Barrel-shaped chest

any severe lung disease, most commonly a severe infective exacerbation of chronic bronchitis.

Finger clubbing

Finger clubbing (see Ch. 6, Fig. 6.1) may be a sign of bronchial carcinoma or chronic lung sepsis.

Barrel-shaped chest

A barrel-shaped chest results from hyperinflation due to obstructive airways disease (asthma or chronic bronchitis). Increased respiratory effort in such patients often involves the accessory respiratory muscles such as the sternomastoid.

The chest can also be examined by palpation, percussion and by auscultation (using a stethoscope) for other signs of chest disease.

Investigations

Examination of the upper respiratory tract often requires referral to an ear, nose and throat surgeon and includes examination of the ears (otoscopy); nose (rhinoscopy) from the front and from the back using a pharyngeal mirror; and the larynx, which can also be examined by mirror. These structures can also be examined and biopsied by direct endoscopy. Radiographs of the nasal bones and sinuses are useful in diagnosis of fractures, sinusitis and tumours.

Investigations of the lower respiratory tract are listed in Table 8.3.

Upper respiratory tract infections

Colds, coughs, sore throats and their complications are very common, especially in the winter months, and are a major cause of absence from

Table 8.3 Investigation of the lower respiratory tract

Chest radiography
Isotope lung scanning
Computerized tomography
Lung function tests
Skin tests for allergy
Sputum – microscopy, culture, cytology
Bronchoscopy, bronchial biopsy
Aspiration of pleural effusion, pleural biopsy
Lung biopsy

Table 8.4 Complications of upper respiratory tract infections

Complication	Symptom
Sinusitis	Facial pain and tenderness, discharge
Oropharyngitis	Sore throat
Laryngitis	Hoarse voice, pain on talking
Epiglottitis	Laryngeal obstruction (infants)
Otitis media	Ear pain and discharge
Tracheobronchitis	Central chest pain, cough and sputum
Bronchopneumonia	Breathlessness, chest pain, cyanosis

school or work. The great majority are viral infections, usually with rhinoviruses, which have high infectivity and are spread from person to person in droplet sprays: 'coughs and sneezes spread diseases'. Rhinoviruses have many strains, and immunity is thus unlikely to protect against recurrent attacks. The incubation period is usually short (2–3 days).

Common cold (coryza)

The clinical features of the common cold are known to all. A mild to moderate toxaemia is followed by symptoms of rhinitis and nasopharyngitis: nasal irritation, sneezing, and production of a watery mucous exudate from the nasal passages and sinuses (catarrh). Nasal congestion arises from mucosal oedema. Conjunctivitis frequently occurs, with red, watery eyes. Symptoms usually settle in a few days, unless complications occur. There is no specific antiviral treatment. Management includes staying off school or work in the acute stage to minimize spread to other persons and advice to rest, to keep warm and avoid cold, and to take symptomatic measures: hot drinks, aspirin (adults) or paracetamol, and steam inhalations or decongestants for nasal congestion.

Complications of the common cold (Table 8.4) are frequent, and are often due to secondary bacterial infection (e.g. by staphylococci, streptococci, pneumococci or *Haemophilus influenzae*), which causes increasing malaise, fever, a raised blood neutrophil count, and local symptoms.

Acute sinusitis

This causes aching pain and tenderness over the frontal or maxillary sinuses, sometimes with a purulent nasal discharge which can be cultured. Sinusitis is included in the differential diagnosis of facial pain (see Ch. 25). Radiographs may show opacification and fluid levels within the sinuses. Treatment is with oral amoxycillin or ampicillin (or erythromycin in persons with penicillin allergy), and should be given for 2 weeks. Occasionally sinus aspiration or irrigation by an ear, nose and throat surgeon may also be required. Patients with persistent sinus symptoms should be referred to an ear, nose and throat surgeon for investigation for chronic sinusitis or tumour.

Acute oropharyngitis

Several viruses (rhinoviruses, adenoviruses, Coxsackie viruses) cause a sore throat, often with discomfort on swallowing. On examination, oropharyngeal redness, swelling and exudate (which may involve the tonsils) can be observed. The cervical lymph nodes may be enlarged and tender. In adenovirus infection, there is often associated conjunctivitis, causing red, swollen, watery eyes: this infection is highly contagious and cross-infection may occur. A throat swab should be taken to exclude bacterial causes of pharyngitis (*Streptococcus pyogenes*, *Corynebacterium diphtheriae*: see below), and blood count and serial serum samples taken for detection of antibodies to Epstein–Barr virus (EBV), cytomegalovirus (CMV) and toxoplasma if glandular fever is suspected (see below). Treatment of viral pharyngitis is symptomatic, with drinks, pastilles or syrups, and aspirin (adults) or paracetamol. Antimicrobials are only indicated if bacterial pharyngitis is confirmed by a throat swab (see below). The role of tonsillectomy in the prevention of recurrent attacks is controversial.

Acute laryngitis

This is often associated with acute rhinitis/oropharyngitis, and causes a hoarse or absent voice and pain on talking. Treatment is as for acute rhinitis/oropharyngitis, with additional advice to rest the voice. Patients with persistent hoarseness should be referred to an ear, nose and throat surgeon for investigation to exclude cancer (e.g. of the larynx, or bronchus with involvement of the recurrent laryngeal nerve), tuberculosis or syphilis.

Acute epiglottitis

This is a specific infection by *H. influenzae* in infants, which causes laryngeal obstruction and stridor, and can be fatal. It requires urgent admission to a paediatric intensive care unit and intravenous cefotaxime or chloramphenicol.

Acute otitis media

This is a common infection in children, and is associated with adenoid hypertrophy and nasal obstruction. Spread of bacterial infection (e.g. *Streptococcus pneumoniae* or *H. influenzae*), characteristically following a viral infection such as measles, ascends from the nasopharynx up the eustachian tube to the middle ear, causing a stuffed feeling in the ear followed by severe pain which often causes the child to cry all night. Examination of the eardrum at otoscopy shows redness and bulging of the tympanic membrane, sometimes with rupture and discharge of mucoid or purulent material. Antimicrobial treatment is with oral amoxycillin or ampicillin (or erythromycin in persons with penicillin allergy), and should be given for 10–14 days; in severe infections, initial parenteral benzylpenicillin can be given. Nasal decongestants and paracetamol can also be given for symptomatic relief, and incision of the tympanic membrane (myringotomy) should be considered if there is severe pain and a bulging tympanic membrane. Complications include mastoiditis, facial nerve paralysis, meningitis, and brain abscess (see Ch. 9). Patients with persistent symptoms should be referred to an ear, nose and throat surgeon, to exclude chronic exudation ('glue ear', which requires drainage by grommets) or chronic infection of the mastoid sinus (which often required mastoidectomy before antimicrobial use became widespread). The role of adenoidectomy in prevention of recurrent attacks is controversial.

Acute tracheobronchitis

This causes a cough productive of mucoid sputum, which becomes purulent if there is secondary bacterial infection, and a 'raw' central chest pain which is increased by coughing. The former is common in patients with chronic bronchitis (acute infective exacerbations; see below), and requires urgent treatment (which can be issued to patients to initiate) with amoxycillin or ampicillin (or trimethoprim or tetracycline in persons with penicillin allergy). Symptomatic treatment is as described for coryza.

Specific upper respiratory tract infections

These include influenza, measles, rubella, mumps and whooping cough (see also Ch. 5).

Influenza

Influenza viruses tend to cause epidemics of infection about every 10 years, due to an antigenic change in the virus, which then spreads through the non-immune population. Worldwide spread can occur (pandemics): that which occurred in 1918–1919 killed 20 million people (more than the First World War of 1914–1918). Like the common cold, influenza is spread by droplet spray and has a short incubation period of a few days. Unlike the common cold, the clinical features of rhinitis are relatively mild, whereas symptoms of toxaemia are severe: these include intense malaise, fatigue, generalized pains; including headache, limb and trunk pains; fever, sweating and vomiting. Patients often have little choice but to collapse into bed. General medical practitioners rapidly become familiar with the clinical features of local influenza epidemics. Treatment is with bed rest and symptomatic treatment as for the common cold. Most patients recover within a few days. In some, secondary bacterial infection with acute tracheobronchitis and bronchopneumonia (which may be staphylococcal) occurs: this can be rapidly fatal. Antimicrobials should be given to those with features of secondary bacterial infection, which is commonest in the old or frail, infants, and persons with chronic lung or heart disease. Influenza virus vaccines should be given annually (usually in October), and at times of epidemics.

Measles

The measles virus usually affects children, is spread by droplet infection, and initially presents as an upper respiratory tract infection. Its incubation period is 10 days to onset of symptoms, and 14 days to onset of the characteristic rash. Its distinguishing features from the common cold are as follows: the child is febrile, irritable, restless and red eyed (conjunctivitis). There is a characteristic buccal mucosal rash (Koplik's spots). These are small, grey-white spots which resemble grains of salt and are set on a red base. They are most often seen along the occlusal line. The characteristic skin rash appears 3–4 days after the onset of symptoms, usually behind the ears and spreading to the face and trunk. It is blotchy and red, and usually lasts a few days, resolving together with the fever.

Measles is important because of the high risk of bacterial complications, including otitis media and bronchopneumonia, which may result in bronchiectasis. Viral encephalitis is unusual but may cause permanent brain damage (see Ch. 9). Management is as for upper respiratory tract infections, but with more intensive observation for complications and their treatment (often in a hospital infectious disease unit). Prevention of measles by vaccination with an attenuated virus is an important part of preventive medicine: in the UK it is offered to children aged 1–2 years, combined in the measles, mumps and rubella vaccine (MMR vaccine). Measles immunoglobulin (derived from plasma of persons with previous measles) can also be used to give passive immunity to exposed, immunodeficient persons (e.g. those with HIV infection).

Rubella (German measles)

The rubella virus is spread by droplet infection and has an incubation period of 2–3 weeks. It causes a mild febrile illness with rhinitis, tender enlargement of cervical lymph nodes, and a transient rash behind the ears. Its only importance is that if infection occurs in women during the first 4 months of pregnancy, there is a high risk of congenital defects including congenital heart disease (see Ch. 6). Hence, in the UK, immunization is offered to children aged 1–2 years (as part of the MMR vaccine; see above); to non-immunized girls aged 11–13 years; and also to pregnant women found to be non-immune (after delivery) to protect the fetus in further pregnancies.

Mumps

The mumps virus is also spread by droplet infection and has an incubation period of 2–3 weeks. It affects glandular organs, usually the parotid salivary glands (see Ch. 24), causing bilateral tender swelling with inflammation of the parotid duct orifice. The other salivary glands may also be involved. Complications include encephalitis and meningitis (see Ch. 9), and pancreatitis (see Ch. 10) or orchitis, which are commoner in adults. Treatment is symptomatic, e.g. oral hygiene and a fluid diet for acute parotitis. Vaccination with an attenuated virus is offered to children aged 1–2 years in the UK (as part of the MMR vaccine; see above).

Whooping cough (pertussis)

Unlike other primary respiratory tract infections, this is caused by a bacterium (*Bordetella pertussis*), which is spread by droplet infection and has an incubation period of 1–3 weeks. It usually affects children under 5 years old. It presents as a severe upper respiratory tract infection (often with conjunctivitis), and the diagnosis becomes apparent when the child develops paroxysms of severe cough, followed by an inspiratory 'whoop' caused by spasm of the glottis. Complications include vomiting, ulceration of the frenum of the tongue, and bronchopneumonia, which may result in bronchiectasis. Treatment is with antimicrobials and oxygen. Vaccination in the first year of life (together with diphtheria and tetanus) is valuable in prevention; encephalitis is a very rare complication of the procedure, but over-concern about it has reduced parental acceptance of vaccination, resulting in increased incidence and fatality of this preventable disease.

Specific causes of acute sore throat

As noted previously, specific bacterial causes of acute oropharyngitis include *Strep. pyogenes* and *C. diphtheriae*. The glandular fever syndrome may be due to EBV, CMV, HIV or toxoplasmosis.

Streptococcal sore throat

The commonest infection caused by *Strep. pyogenes* (β-haemolytic streptococci) is an acute oropharyngitis. Other streptococcal infections include otitis media and skin infections (erysipelas and cellulitis, see Ch. 12) and wound infections. Spread is by droplet infection or skin contact, and infectivity is high: cross-infection may occur from patients. The incubation period is short. Infection is most common in school-age children and young adults: small epidemics may occur, especially in the winter months.

The clinical features are those of acute oropharyngitis (see above). Compared to the (much commoner) viral oropharyngitis, bacterial oropharyngitis is more likely to cause a purulent (yellow) tonsillar exudate; fever, malaise and leucocytosis; or a skin rash (e.g. scarlet fever). However, it is often impossible to distinguish between streptococcal and viral oropharyngitis on clinical grounds: hence the importance of a throat swab to establish whether or not streptococcal infection is present. This can also be demonstrated retrospectively by a rising blood antistreptolysin O titre.

The importance of a throat swab to confirm or exclude streptococcal infection is twofold.

First, streptococcal infection should be treated with antimicrobials. *Strep. pyogenes* is usually sensitive to penicillin (oral phenoxymethylpenicillin, amoxycillin or ampicillin; or parenteral benzylpenicillin in severe cases). Erythromycin or a cephalosporin should be given to persons allergic to penicillin. Amoxycillin or ampicillin should not be given if glandular fever is suspected, because of a very high risk of allergic skin rash. Antimicrobials reduce the risk of complications of streptococcal sore throat, which include otitis media (see above); peritonsillar abscess (quinsy), which may require surgical drainage; rheumatic fever and rheumatic heart disease; chorea (see Ch. 6); and acute post-streptococcal glomerulonephritis (see Ch. 11).

Secondly, viral infections should not be treated with antimicrobials. Antimicrobials are ineffective against viral sore throat, and their inappropriate use increases bacterial resistance and exposes patients to adverse reactions (e.g. allergic reactions, especially in glandular fever) and wastes money.

Diphtheria

Following the widespread adoption of immunization with a toxoid in the first year of life (together with whooping cough and tetanus), this previously common, life-threatening illness of young children is now rare. The causative bacterium, *C. diphtheriae*, is spread by droplet infection and has an incubation period of 2–7 days. The initial clinical features are of an oropharyngitis; however, two major complications occur: an adherent grey-yellow membrane can extend from the oropharynx to obstruct the larynx, causing stridor and asphyxiation which requires emergency tracheostomy; and production of a toxin which causes severe toxaemia, myocarditis and paralysis (e.g. paralysis of the soft palate).

Treatment includes admission to a hospital intensive care unit, parenteral penicillin and diphtheria antitoxin, and tracheostomy and ventilation if required.

Glandular fever

This clinical syndrome is commonest in adolescents and young adults. It may be due to one of three possible agents, each of which usually causes a subclinical illness in young children. Chronic latent infection may result, which may be reactivated or transmitted to others, usually by close contact (e.g. kissing). Patients with immuno-suppression (e.g. HIV infection, see Ch. 5) can develop severe, generalized infections. In pregnant women, two of the three agents can infect the fetus. Clinical features include fever and malaise; sore throat, often with white tonsillar exudate and palatal purpura; lymphadenopathy (especially in the neck); splenomegaly; skin rashes; viral hepatitis; and, lastly, atypical, large lymphocytes on the blood film (mononucleosis).

Epstein–Barr virus

This herpesvirus is the commonest cause of glandular fever. The illness (infectious mononucleosis) is usually mild but can be prostrating. Diagnosis is made by the Paul–Bunnell or monospot tests, in which a characteristic heterophile antibody in the patient's serum agglutinates red blood cells of other species. An increase in EBV antibodies also occurs. Treatment is symptomatic. If antimicrobials are given for suspected strepto-coccal pharyngitis, amoxycillin and ampicillin should be avoided because of the high risk of skin rash. A short course of corticosteroids may be given if the illness is severe. Fetal infection does not occur.

Cytomegalovirus

This is another herpesvirus, and can cause a similar glandular fever illness to EBV. The Paul–Bunnell and monospot tests are negative; an increase in serum CMV antibodies is diagnostic. Treatment is symptomatic.

Acquired toxoplasmosis

This causes a similar illness, and is due to an intracellular protozoon (*Toxoplasma gondii*) which occurs in all mammals. Infection can occur by eating undercooked meat, or by contact with cat faeces, either directly or from contaminated soil. The Paul–Bunnell and monospot tests are negative; an increase in serum toxoplasma antibodies is diagnostic. In immunosuppressed HIV patients, cerebral lesions occur (see Ch. 5). Treatment is with

antimicrobials (spiramycin or cotrimoxazole) for severe illness.

Glandular fever and pregnancy

In pregnant women, CMV and *T. gondii* can cause fetal infection and abnormalities. No pregnant women should be exposed to patients with glandular fever illness, hepatitis, or HIV infection (in which generalized clinical or subclinical infection is common). This rule applies to health care professionals, including dentists and their clinical assistants.

Candidosis

This common oral infection may also involve the throat. It is considered in Chapter 22.

Allergic rhinitis

This is a common allergy, which may be seasonal or perennial.

Seasonal rhinitis (hay fever)

This is a type 1 allergic reaction to inhaled grass pollen, which is common in the early summer months especially in the young. The symptoms comprise rhinitis (sneezing, profuse watery nasal discharge, conjunctival irritation and lacrimation, and nasal congestion). Treatment includes avoiding grassy places when air pollen counts are high; nasal decongestants and oral antihistamines, e.g. chlorpheniramine. Drowsiness is a common adverse effect of these drugs, and can affect driving and other skilled tasks. Alcohol increases the drowsiness, and should be avoided. Non-sedative antihistamines are now available, however. Other treatments are nasal sprays of cromoglycate, which blocks release of histamine from mast cells, and nasal sprays of corticosteroids.

Perennial rhinitis (vasomotor rhinitis)

This is a year-round allergic reaction to viruses, bacteria, house dust mites or nasally applied drugs. Symptoms and treatment are similar to seasonal rhinitis.

Nasal polyps

These are reactive outgrowths of nasal mucosa due to chronic allergic rhinitis. They can cause obstruction, and may require surgical removal.

Carcinoma of the nasopharynx or nasal sinuses

Carcinoma of the maxillary antrum is of dental importance because it may erode into the oral cavity. It may also present as pain, halitosis, persistent sinusitis, anaesthesia or unilateral facial swelling. The diagnosis is confirmed by imaging techniques, endoscopy and biopsy. Treatment is by surgery (maxillectomy) and radiotherapy.

Carcinoma of the larynx

This is usually squamous cell carcinoma, and may arise from areas of premalignant change (leukoplakia). It is strongly associated with cigarette smoking, and also alcohol. Clinical symptoms include persistent hoarseness (when the vocal cords are affected); throat pain on swallowing (which can be referred to the ear); metastatic enlargement of cervical lymph nodes; and laryngeal obstruction. The diagnosis is confirmed by laryngoscopy and biopsy. Radiotherapy is the treatment of choice in early laryngeal tumours.

Acute upper airway obstruction

Laryngeal obstruction can be caused mechanically by the inhalation of a foreign body, e.g. a lump of meat, peanuts, or toys in children, or by trauma – physical or chemical (e.g. swallowed corrosives). Angioedema is usually caused by an acute allergic reaction, which may occur as part of anaphylactic shock (see Ch. 6), or with an acute skin rash (urticaria), and leads to severe swelling of the face, lips, and oropharyngeal mucosa. Parenteral adrenaline is a specific treatment (see Ch. 6).

Laryngeal obstruction may also be caused by infections, e.g. whooping cough, *H. influenzae*

epiglottitis, diphtheria (see above) or tumour, e.g. carcinoma of the larynx (see above).

The clinical features of acute upper airway obstruction are respiratory distress, with stridor (a whistling noise caused by airflow in the narrowed larynx), and central cyanosis if hypoxia occurs. Urgent tracheostomy may be required to bypass the obstructed airway. In an emergency, a wide-bore needle can be inserted through the cricothyroid membrane, and oxygen, if available, connected to the needle.

Inhalation of a foreign body causing acute laryngeal obstruction is a common emergency requiring urgent first aid. An adult may have been chewing food (especially lumps of meat); a child may have been playing with small toys, coins or nuts. The patient becomes distressed, turns blue and cannot talk (but may indicate with signs what has happened). Small children can be swung upside down and thumped on the back to dislodge the foreign body. Adults can also be thumped on the back, or the Heimlich manoeuvre applied. In this manoeuvre, the adult first-aider stands behind the erect patient, with fists clenched together; a sudden pull of their fists towards them acutely raises intra-abdominal and intra-thoracic pressures, which may dislodge the foreign body. If these attempts to dislodge the foreign body fail, emergency ambulance and medical attention should be called, and a wide-bore needle tracheostomy performed, if possible by a skilled attendant.

Nosebleeds (epistaxis)

These are common, especially in children, and usually occur from erosion of the vascular plexus in the anterior nasal septal mucosa (Little's area); they cause much alarm, but are rarely severe. Bleeding may be due to trauma (e.g. picking the nose or insertion of a foreign body by the child) or upper respiratory tract infections. Recurrent nosebleeds are common in hypertension (see Ch. 6), and in bleeding disorders, especially hereditary haemorrhagic telangiectasia, thrombocytopenia or von Willebrand's disease (see Ch. 7).

First aid management of nosebleeds includes reassuring the patient, who should sit with the head forward, applying gentle but firm, sustained pressure to the affected side of the nose, compressing it against the bleeding nasal septum for several minutes. The first-aider can apply the pressure in the case of younger children. Patients should breathe through the mouth. Gloves should be worn if available (and can be supplied to teachers) to avoid blood contact with any cuts or sores. If bleeding persists despite first aid, the patient should be sent to the nearest accident and emergency department or doctor's surgery. Persistent bleeding is treated either by electrical or chemical cautery of the bleeding point, or by nasal packing with gauze soaked in lubricant jelly, either from the front of the nose or from the back. Rarely blood loss is severe, requiring blood transfusion and sometimes surgery.

Halitosis

Halitosis may be caused by smoking, drinking and foods (e.g. onions or garlic); oral and upper respiratory tract infections; and lung sepsis, e.g. lung abscess and bronchiectasis. Like oral sepsis, anaerobic bacteria are responsible for the foul odour. Patients may give a history of purulent sputum, and finger clubbing may be observed. Other causes of halitosis include: vomiting, diabetic ketoacidosis, where the breath smells of ketones; renal failure, where the breath smells of ammonia; or liver failure, where the breath smells of mice.

Halitosis is considered in further detail in Chapter 27.

Bronchial asthma

Asthma is a respiratory disorder characterized by recurrent, reversible attacks of acute breathlessness, wheeze and cough due to bronchial obstruction. The three elements contributing to bronchial obstruction are bronchoconstriction due to spasm of the circular smooth muscle surrounding the bronchi; swelling of the bronchial mucosa, due to inflammatory oedema; and mucous exudate, which may be coughed up as bronchial 'plugs'.

In early onset (childhood) asthma, hypersensitivity to inhaled allergens can be frequently demonstrated; such allergens include inhaled pollens, feathers (in pillows), animal dander (e.g. from cats or dogs) or house dust mites; ingested foods (e.g. eggs or shellfish); and drugs, (e.g. aspirin or penicillin). Such persons often have a family history, and often have more generalized type 1 allergies (atopy), e.g. hay fever, infantile eczema of the face, and skin flexures (see Ch. 12). Common allergens can be identified by skin prick or patch tests, applied to the forearm skin. In late-onset asthma, which starts in middle age, allergies occur less often.

Other precipitants of asthma include emotion; exercise; inhalation of cold air; respiratory tract infections; β-adrenergic blocking drugs (e.g. atenolol), which are used for treatment of angina and hypertension (see Ch. 6); and atmospheric pollution, e.g. from road traffic. This last cause may be responsible for the recent major increase in childhood asthma in the UK and other developed countries. It should be remembered that if a drug has recently been administered, an acute attack of bronchospasm may be part of an anaphylactic reaction, accompanied by circulatory shock (see Ch. 6).

Diagnosis of asthma is established from the history, and by wheezing expirations on auscultation of the chest; it is confirmed by lung function tests which demonstrate airways obstruction, reversible by administration of a bronchodilator drug.

Acute asthma develops suddenly over a few minutes. Treatment of an acute asthmatic attack in a dental patient is as follows: stop the procedure; check that the airway is patent, and that a foreign body has not been inhaled; allow the patient to sit up; and loosen any tight clothing around the neck. Many patients with asthma carry an inhaler containing a bronchodilator drug (β_2-adrenergic agonist, e.g. salbutamol or terbutaline) in metered doses. If so, the patient should be encouraged to use the inhaler, which often aborts an attack. The patient should sit, under supervision, in a quiet room until the attack settles. The current procedure should be postponed until the patient has fully recovered. Urgent ambulance and medical attention should be sought if there are features of anaphylactic shock (see Ch. 6), the attack does not settle rapidly, or there is a suspicion of an inhaled foreign body (see below).

Further treatment of acute asthma includes high-dose oxygen (40–60%); nebulized bronchodilators (e.g. salbutamol or terbutaline); monitoring of arterial blood gases and the peak flow rate; systemic steroids (e.g. oral prednisolone 30–60 mg or intravenous hydrocortisone 200 mg); intravenous aminophylline (another bronchodilator); antimicrobials, if infection is suspected; and artificial ventilation in an intensive care unit, which may be required for status asthmaticus.

Prophylaxis of asthmatic attacks includes: avoidance of allergens (e.g. using hypoallergenic pillows) and other precipitating factors; inhaled bronchodilators (e.g. salbutamol or terbutaline) as required; and regular inhaled corticosteroid (e.g. beclomethasone), 2–4 times daily. Inhaled corticosteroids have fewer systemic effects than systemic corticosteroids (see Ch. 13), but can cause oral candidosis (see Ch. 22). Regular inhaled cromoglycate reduces the histamine secretion from mast cells during allergic reactions; it is more effective in children and in the prevention of exercise-induced asthma.

Chronic bronchitis and emphysema

These two disorders frequently coexist, and are often referred to jointly as chronic obstructive airways disease (COAD) or chronic obstructive pulmonary disease. They are the commonest causes of chronic cough and breathlessness in adults in the UK and in other industrialized countries. Causal factors are listed in Table 8.5, and often coexist.

Chronic bronchitis

This is defined as a productive cough, for at least 3 months of the year, for at least 2 years. The typical history is that of a cigarette smoker living in an industrial city who has a persistent 'smoker's cough' productive of mucoid sputum. The pathological basis for these symptoms is chronic overproduction of bronchial mucus by increased goblet cells, in response to inhaled pollutants, which also reduce mucus clearance by ciliated columnar cells. Superinfection of retained tracheobronchial mucus by *Strep. pneumoniae* and *H. influenzae* from the upper respiratory tract occurs readily in acute upper respiratory tract infections (especially in the winter months), and from chronic sinusitis. Bacterial superinfection results in infective exacerbations of chronic bronchitis, in which the patient develops fever, malaise, worsening dyspnoea, purulent sputum, and central chest pain from acute tracheobronchitis. Each of these infections causes further pathology and deterioration in lung function. Acute infections may also cause asthma ('wheezy bronchitis'), which is partly reversible by bronchodilator drugs. Clinical examination may reveal nicotine-stained fingers, cough, and wheeziness on auscultation of the chest (sounds due to narrowed, mucus-containing airways). The chest radiograph is usually normal. Lung function tests show airway obstruction which is usually poorly reversible (unlike asthma).

Emphysema

This is a common sequel of chronic bronchitis, but may also develop as a result of chronic asthma or pneumoconioses. Prolonged overdistension of alveoli, and weakening of their walls by chronic

Table 8.5 Causal factors in chronic bronchitis and emphysema

Smoking	Active and passive
Smog	Atmospheric pollution (traffic, industry, mines, foundries) combined with a damp, foggy climate
Sex	Males rather than females
Social class	Lower socio-economic groups rather than higher
Susceptibility	Family history common
Superinfection	*Strep. pneumoniae*, *H. influenzae*
Sinusitis	Chronic sinusitis predisposes to bronchitis

infection, leads to alveolar destruction and rupture, with the formation of larger air-containing spaces (bullae). The lungs become hyperinflated, and the patient develops a 'barrel chest'. Reduction in the alveolar surface available for gas exchange results in hypoxia and retention of carbon dioxide. Resistance to blood flow through the lungs (pulmonary hypertension) leads to right ventricular hypertrophy and heart failure (cor pulmonale).

The patient with advanced chronic bronchitis and emphysema lives a precarious and often miserable existence; in population terms the cigarette-induced cumulative morbidity of this condition is arguably greater than that of bronchial carcinoma. The main complications are summarized in Table 8.6.

Prevention of COAD includes public and personal health education against smoking, along with other government measures to reduce tobacco consumption and atmospheric pollution. Prompt antimicrobial therapy for acute infective exacerbations, (e.g. amoxycillin or ampicillin), is important, and patients may be given a starter pack to take as soon as an exacerbation starts. Annual influenza vaccination, usually in October, may help to reduce exacerbations. Drug therapy includes bronchodilators, if reversible airway obstruction is demonstrated, treatment of heart failure (see Ch. 6); and domiciliary oxygen for the management of severe chronic hypoxia in selected patients who stop smoking. Acute respiratory failure requires hospital admission.

Prior to major surgery, patients require careful assessment by a skilled anaesthetist: in many cases, local or spinal anaesthesia can be used rather than general anaesthesia; such patients should be encouraged to stop smoking and should receive chest physiotherapy. After surgery, intensive physiotherapy and antimicrobials are given to reduce the risks of postoperative lung collapse and pneumonia.

Lung diseases due to dusts (pneumoconioses)

These are usually due to industrial exposure, and have become less common in the UK and other developed countries due to control measures, e.g. dust limitation, wearing of masks or respirators, and monitoring. Financial compensation is available for prescribed industrial diseases.

Silicosis

This is due to inhalation of silica dust by miners, stonemasons and sandblasters. Progressive lung fibrosis occurs over several years, causing increasing breathlessness and disability. The chest radiograph may show diffuse shadows. Complications include heart failure and pulmonary tuberculosis. Treatment is by removal from dust exposure.

Asbestosis

This results from inhalation of asbestos dust (previously used for insulation). It causes lung fibrosis, bronchial carcinoma and pleural malignancy (mesothelioma).

Cystic fibrosis

This is a genetic disorder with autosomal recessive inheritance. Viscid mucous secretions cause chronic pulmonary infection and fibrosis from childhood, requiring intensive physiotherapy and antimicrobials for survival into adult life. Pancreatic fibrosis also occurs, causing malabsorption (see Ch. 10).

Table 8.6 Complications of advanced COAD

Respiratory failure (hypoxia, carbon dioxide retention)

Right heart failure

Recurrent infective exacerbations

Pneumonia from mucus retention, e.g. after surgery

Poor toleration of surgery and anaesthesia

Polycythaemia secondary to chronic hypoxia

Pneumothorax – rupture of surface emphysematous bulla

Severe restriction of physical activity, social life and employment

Bronchial obstruction and its consequences

Bronchial obstruction has several serious consequences, including collapse of a lung segment, bronchopneumonia, and chronic lung sepsis (lung abscess or bronchiectasis) (Fig. 8.1).

Bronchial obstruction

Causes of bronchial obstruction include:

• *Inhalation of a foreign body.* This is of major dental importance, because extracted teeth, portions of teeth, dental instruments or blood clot can be aspirated by the patient during dental surgery, especially if the patient is sedated or anaes-

thetised. Other foreign bodies which may be inhaled include coins or small toys (by children) or nuts (e.g. trying to catch a peanut, tossed into the air, in the mouth).

• *Inhalation of vomit.* Aspiration is a major risk in semiconscious or unconscious persons (e.g. due to alcohol intoxication, self-poisoning, head injury, stroke, diabetic coma or general anaesthesia). It can be prevented by placing such persons in the 'coma position' (on the left side, head downwards, knees flexed) and inserting an oral airway if available.

• *Mucus plug.* Retention of mucus occurs most commonly after general anaesthesia, particularly in patients with chronic bronchitis, and can be prevented by intensive chest physiotherapy before and after surgery.

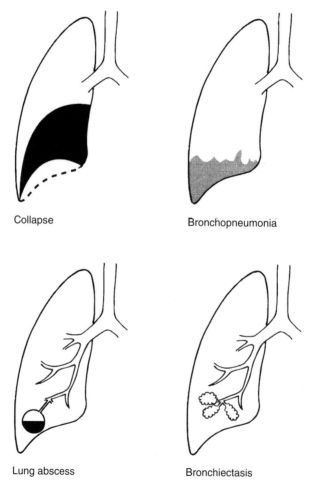

Collapse   Bronchopneumonia

Lung abscess   Bronchiectasis

Fig. 8.1 The complications that may follow inhalation of foreign material into the respiratory passages.

- *Bronchial carcinoma.* Chronic progressive bronchial obstruction is a common clinical presentation of lung cancer.
- *External compression.* Enlarged mediastinal lymph nodes, e.g. metastatic bronchial carcinoma, lymphoma or tuberculosis, can cause compression resulting in bronchial obstruction.

Clinical features of acute bronchial obstruction include sudden breathlessness, with cyanosis if there is major lung involvement. Distal to bronchial obstruction, air is absorbed into the bloodstream, and the lung or lung segment collapses. Signs may be found on chest examination but the chest radiograph is much more sensitive in demonstrating lung collapse, which appears as a triangular area of opacification, sometimes accompanied by a raised hemidiaphragm, and deviation of the trachea to the affected side (Fig. 8.1). A foreign body may also be visualized if it is radio-opaque (e.g. a tooth or metal instrument). The chest radiograph can also show evidence of bronchial carcinoma or enlarged lymph nodes. Inhalation of diffuse material (e.g. blood clot or vomit) is more likely to appear as diffuse, patchy opacities of bronchopneumonia on the chest radiograph, rather than as a single area of lung collapse (Fig 8.1). Spreading infection in the lung causes fever, malaise, chest pain, breathlessness, cyanosis, a rapid pulse and neutrophil leucocytosis.

Great care must be taken to avoid inhalation of foreign bodies during dental treatment. In suspected cases, lean the patient forward and encourage coughing, combined with a thump on the back, to encourage dislodgement of the foreign body. Seek medical advice urgently, and transfer the patient to hospital for chest radiography and consideration of bronchoscopy to identify and remove foreign bodies. A full record of events should be made in case of future litigation.

Lung abscess

A lung abscess (Fig. 8.1) may arise as a consequence of bronchial obstruction, or without obstruction as a consequence of severe cavitating pneumonia (especially due to *Staphylococcus aureus*). Clinical features include: sepsis, a high swinging fever, neutrophil leucocytosis, halitosis and purulent sputum. Finger clubbing and weight loss may develop after several weeks; and brain abscess (metastatic infection) is a feared complication.

The diagnosis is confirmed by chest radiography or computerized (CT) scanning, which shows a thick-walled abscess, often containing a fluid level. Treatment is with antimicrobials and physiotherapy; surgical drainage of the abscess or lobectomy may also be required.

Bronchiectasis

In this condition there is dilatation and chronic sepsis of the terminal bronchioles, especially in the lower lobes of the lung (Fig. 8.1). It usually results from bronchial obstruction, either by a foreign body, or by tenacious mucus plugs as in cystic fibrosis, measles or whooping cough (see above). The clinical features are similar to those of lung abscess, but due to communication with the bronchial tree, halitosis and copious purulent sputum are more common. The diagnosis cannot be confirmed by chest radiography, and requires CT scanning or bronchography (instillation of radiopaque material into the bronchial tree). Treatment is with antimicrobials and physiotherapy; surgical lobectomy may also be required.

Pneumonia

Pneumonia is a severe lung infection, in which the alveoli are filled by fluid and cells (consolidation), causing impaired gas exchange, and often respiratory failure, especially in those with pre-existing impaired lung function. It is a common cause of death, especially in the very young, the very old, those with severe chronic disease, and in developing countries.

Three patterns of pneumonia can be distinguished by their clinical and radiological features: bronchopneumonia, lobar pneumonias and diffuse pneumonias. The causes are listed in Table 8.7.

Bronchopneumonia

This follows the descent of pathogenic organisms from the upper respiratory tract to the lower; and

Table 8.7 Causes of pneumonia

Bronchopneumonia	Upper respiratory tract bacteria (staphylococci, streptococci, *H. influenzae*)
Lobar pneumonias	*Strep. pneumoniae* (pneumococcus) *Legionella pneumophila* *Staph. aureus* *H. influenzae* *Mycoplasma pneumoniae* *Chlamydia psittaci* *Coxiella burnetii*
Diffuse pneumonias	*Pneumocystis carinii* (immunosuppression, e.g. HIV infection) Influenza Tuberculosis

usually involves staphylococci, streptococci (including *Strep. pneumoniae*) and *H. influenzae*. Bronchopneumonia may also follow bronchial obstruction (see above), and aspiration of food or fluids, and may complicate oesophageal obstruction (see Ch. 10) or neurological disorders such as stroke (see Ch. 9).

Bronchopneumonia may also arise from acute infective exacerbations of chronic bronchitis (see above); severe upper respiratory tract infections, e.g. influenza, measles or whooping cough (see above); or terminal illness, e.g. cancer, heart failure, respiratory failure, stroke or dementia – in this context, it has been called the 'old man's friend'.

Lobar pneumonias

In contrast to bronchopneumonias, these usually occur in healthy persons. *Strep. pneumoniae* (pneumococcus) remains the commonest cause of lobar pneumonia. In recent years, *Legionella pneumophila* (causing legionnaires' disease) has been increasingly recognized. This organism lives in stagnant water, causing epidemic spread in ventilation systems involving humidifiers, and in showers (e.g. in hotels and hospitals: it was first described in a hotel convention of legionnaires, hence the name). *Staph. aureus* is an increasingly common cause of lobar pneumonia, often with cavitation and lung abscess formation; it is often a complication of tricuspid valve endocarditis in intravenous drug users (see Ch. 6). Mycoplasmas, chlamydiae, and rickettsiae can also cause lobar pneumonia (Table 8.7).

Diffuse pneumonias

Diffuse pneumonias may occur in some persons with influenza, often combined with staphylococcal superinfection. The immunosuppression of HIV infection (see Ch. 5) is frequently complicated by *Pneumocystis carinii* pneumonia, a protozoal infection which is a major cause of death in AIDS patients. Prophylaxis is described in Chapter 5.

Clinical features

Clinical features of pneumonia include fever, malaise, rapid arterial pulse, and leucocytosis (in bacterial pneumonias); breathlessness and central cyanosis; cough and purulent sputum, often tinged with blood (in lobar pneumonias); pleuritic chest pain (especially pneumococcal pneumonia); herpes simplex infection of the lips (herpes labialis); and signs of lung consolidation on examining the chest.

Diagnosis is by chest radiography (which shows opacities due to areas of consolidation); and bacteriological cultures of blood and sputum. Bronchoscopic aspiration of secretions is particularly important in detecting *P. carinii* in immunosuppressed patients. Serum antibodies are also useful in retrospective diagnosis of legionella, myoplasma, chlamydia, rickettsia and viral infections. Pneumococcal antigen can be detected in urine.

Treatment includes appropriate antimicrobials, usually amoxycillin, ampicillin, or (in persons allergic to penicillin) erythromycin or cotrimoxazole. Flucloxacillin is given for staphyloccal infection; erythromycin and rifampicin for legionella pneumonia; and tetracycline for mycoplasma or chlamydia pneumonia. Oxygen for hypoxia is also required, as are analgesics for pleuritic chest pain and physiotherapy.

Complications of pneumonia include pleural effusion, empyema, lung collapse, lung abscess, and venous thromboembolism from prolonged bedrest. Because of modern effective antibiotic therapy these are less commonly seen than hitherto.

Tuberculosis

Historically, tuberculosis has been the commonest infective cause of death worldwide. When effective antituberculous drugs were introduced in the 1950s, temporary control was achieved in many countries in western Europe and North America. However, with the worldwide epidemic of HIV infection during the 1980s and 1990s, tuberculosis has regained its position as the world's pre-eminent fatal disease. Furthermore, drug-resistant strains of *Mycobacterium tuberculosis* are increasingly prevalent. Persons at increased risk of tuberculosis are listed in Table 8.8, and include dentists and their assistants, who are exposed to droplet spray from their patients.

Primary tuberculous infection in the lung usually results from inhaled droplet spray, but sometimes occurs in the tonsils or ileum when infection is acquired from infected milk (bovine tuberculosis). Caseous lesions form in the regional lymph nodes (mediastinal, cervical or mesenteric, respectively). Many primary infections heal by natural immunity, without declaring themselves clinically; both primary and node lesions calcify.

Occasionally, healing does not occur, and haematogenous spread occurs to the lungs, bones, joints, kidneys or meninges; local spread to adjacent structures is also possible, e.g. from lung to pleura or pericardium.

The commonest clinical manifestation of pulmonary tuberculosis arises from reactivation of previous infection (postprimary tuberculosis), and may form a cavity in the upper lobes of the lungs. Clinical features of active tuberculosis are summarized in Table 8.9. The diagnosis should be suspected if any of these occur in at-risk persons (Table 8.8).

Active tuberculosis is suggested by the presence of upper lobe opacities and cavities on the chest radiograph, and by a strongly positive tuberculin test. The diagnosis is confirmed by demonstration of *M. tuberculosis* in sputum, which appears as acid- and alcohol-fast bacilli using the Ziehl–Neelsen stain. Culture of bacilli is important to identify drug sensitivity.

Patients with active tuberculosis should be closely supervised by a specialist physician. In the UK, combinations of rifampicin, isoniazid, pyrizinamide and ethambutol are usually used, to reduce the development of drug resistance. Treatment is usually initiated in hospital; thereafter, supervised outpatient treatment should be given for 12 months. Isolation is rarely required if effective antimicrobial therapy is given. Following diagnosis, close contacts (including dentists and other clinical staff) should be screened for active tuberculosis.

Sarcoidosis

This is a granulomatous multisystem disease; the lesions resemble those of tuberculosis but do not

---

Table 8.8 Persons at increased risk of tuberculosis

Children and young adults
Contacts of patients with active disease
Immunosuppressed patients (HIV, immunosuppressive drugs)
Health workers in close contact with many patients
Socially disadvantaged persons living in crowded conditions
Persons with alcoholism, diabetes mellitus or silicosis

Table 8.9 Clinical features of pulmonary tuberculosis

Loss of appetite and weight
Tiredness
Fever and sweating, often at night
Cough, sputum and haemoptysis
Breathlessness due to pleural effusion, pneumothorax or lung collapse

caseate. The cause is not known. The lungs, skin, eyes and lymph nodes may be involved. Corticosteroids may be indicated for treatment in some cases (see also Ch. 26).

Bronchial carcinoma

In the UK (as in many other western countries), this is the commonest cause of death from malignant disease in men (8% of all deaths), and the second commonest in women after breast cancer (4% of all deaths). At least 90% of cases are directly due to personal cigarette smoking, which causes squamous metaplasia and malignant change in bronchial epithelium. Passive smoking may account for another 5% of lung cancer deaths. Such evidence justifies public education against tobacco, and the progressive restriction of smoking in public places in developed countries. Asbestos exposure also accounts for a significant percentage of cases. The incidence is increasing in developing countries, following their adoption of cigarette smoking.

Clinical features of lung cancer are summarized in Table 8.10. There are few early symptoms, and unfortunately spread has often occurred before the condition declares itself. The tumour may extend within the thoracic cavity, producing many effects by invasion or pressure; it can also spread by lymphatics to the lymph nodes in the neck and axillae, or disseminate widely by the bloodstream to liver, bones, brain and other tissues. Non-metastatic neurological and endocrine features can also occur, due to secretion of hormones (e.g. adrenocorticotrophic hormone or antidiuretic hormone).

A diagnosis of lung cancer is often suggested by the presence of suspicious opacities on the chest radiograph (or CT scan) in a cigarette-smoker, and can be confirmed histologically by sputum cytology; bronchoscopy and endobronchial biopsy; or by biopsy of peripheral lung tumours, lymph nodes, pleura, liver or skin nodules. There are four main histological varieties: squamous cell in 50%; small cell in 25%; adenocarcinoma in 15%; and large cell in 10%. Bone involvement is detected by isotope bone scanning and bone marrow biopsy; liver involvement by ultrasound scanning; and brain involvement by CT scanning.

Management is difficult, because curative treatment by surgical resection is rarely possible due to distant spread prior to clinical presentation. The 5 year survival after diagnosis is less than 10%. Radiotherapy is used for symptomatic treatment of superior vena caval obstruction, recurrent haemoptysis, and bone nerve pain. Small cell carcinoma is often initially responsive to chemotherapy. Palliative care is important in most patients.

Table 8.10 Clinical features of bronchial carcinoma	
General	Anorexia, weight loss, fever
Local bronchial involvement	Cough, sputum, haemoptysis Lobar or lung collapse Pneumonia Lung abscess
Local spread within the thorax	Pleural effusion Dysphagia Diaphragmatic paralysis (phrenic nerve) Hoarseness (recurrent laryngeal nerve) Superior vena caval obstruction
Spread outside the thorax	Lymph nodes Liver Skeleton – pathological fractures Brain
Non-metastatic or humoral/ hormonal effects	Finger clubbing Cushing's syndrome and other endocrinopathies Peripheral neuropathy Cerebellar degeneration

Other lung tumours

Bronchial adenoma is much less common than bronchial carcinoma. It usually presents as cough and haemoptysis, and is cured by surgical resection.

Secondary carcinoma is common, and usually arises from the breast, thyroid, prostate, kidney, stomach, colon or bone. The chest radiograph often shows multiple, round 'cannonball' deposits.

Pleural effusion

Bilateral accumulation of fluid in the pleural cavity most commonly results from congestive heart failure (see Ch. 6). Unilateral effusions may result from pulmonary embolism, lobar pneumonia, bronchial carcinoma or tuberculosis. The clinical presentation is usually breathlessness, sometimes with pleural pain. Chest radiography shows dense opacification of the hemithorax with a near-horizontal fluid level. Pleural aspiration is performed under local anaesthesia both to relieve breathlessness and for diagnosis of the underlying cause; pleural biopsy can also be performed at the time of aspiration. The fluid may be bloodstained in pulmonary embolism or bronchial carcinoma: in the latter case, carcinoma cells may be visualised at cytology or in the pleural biopsy. Tuberculous effusions are straw-coloured, contain lymphocytes and may grow tubercle bacilli after guinea-pig inoculation. Postpneumonic effusions contain neutrophils; sometimes pus is aspirated (empyema). Empyema may be associated with clinical features of chronic lung sepsis (as in lung abscess or bronchiectasis), and may require surgical drainage as well as antimicrobial therapy.

Pneumothorax

Air in the pleural cavity may result from a penetrating wound of the chest wall (often accompa-

nied by blood: haemopneumothorax), or may occur spontaneously due to rupture of the visceral pleura over the lung surface. The latter may occur in emphysema or tuberculosis, but usually results from a congenital defect in young, healthy men – sometimes after exercise. Significant entry of air into the pleural space is always associated with some degree of collapse of the underlying lung; spontaneous absorption or therapeutic removal of this air allows re-expansion. A tension pneumothorax arises when the leak on the lung surface behaves like a valve and allows more air out than can be reabsorbed; the resulting progressive rise of pressure in the pleural cavity then causes not only complete collapse of the lung on the affected side but also displaces the mediastinum to the opposite side, with potential collapse of the healthy lung.

Clinical features include pleuritic chest pain, breathlessness, and central cyanosis if there is major collapse of the underlying lung. Chest radiography confirms air in the pleural cavity and collapse of the lung. If the pneumothorax is small, simple aspiration of air under local anaesthesia may be sufficient treatment. Larger pneumothoraces require insertion of a chest drain under local anaesthesia, which is connected to an underwater drainage system to allow air to escape from the pleural cavity on expiration, without admitting air on inspiration. The lung usually re-expands over a few days. If it does not, thoracotomy may be required to seal the lung leak. Tension pneumothorax is a medical emergency requiring immediate insertion of a needle on the affected side, as soon as this condition is known with certainty, even before tube drainage is instituted. Recurrent pneumothorax is treated by surgical or chemical pleuradesis, which seals the parietal and visceral pleura together.

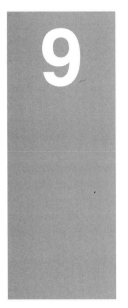

9 Disorders of the nervous system

Introduction

Neurological disorders are extremely common: vascular disease in particular is an important cause of stroke, which is the third commonest cause of death after cardiovascular disease and cancer. Its prevention and treatment form a major part of preventive medicine and of hospital and community care. Cerebrovascular disease is considered here along with other important neurological disorders including impaired consciousness. Cardiovascular causes of impaired consciousness (faints and cardiac arrest) are considered in Chapter 6. Pain is a common presenting symptom of many disease processes, and is not considered separately here. A detailed consideration of pain is found in Chapter 25.

History

Table 9.1 summarizes some important parts of history taking for diseases of the nervous system. Alcohol, drug and tobacco consumption, occupation, and evidence of systemic disease are also relevant.

Examination

Table 9.2 summarizes examination of the nervous system. Detailed assessment of conscious level, orientation, cognitive ability and limb function is important in medical examination of patients with nervous system impairment. Examination of the cranial nerves (Fig. 9.1) will be described in order.

First nerve

The olfactory nerve transmits smell sense from the nose to the brain. It is of little clinical impor-

Table 9.1 History taking and the nervous system
Past or family history of epilepsy (fits)
Loss of consciousness (blackouts)
Intellectual impairment and personality change
Headache
Difficulty with sight hearing swallowing
Weakness of face, arms or legs
Sensory disturbance in face, arms or legs loss of sensation (numbness, anaesthesia) disturbance of sensation (pins and needles, 'shooting' pains along the nerve)
Difficulty with passing urine or faeces (retention or incontinence)

Table 9.2 Examination of the nervous system

In patients with impaired conscious level, orientation or cognitive function
  Conscious level
    Response to questions?
    If none, response to stimulation (e.g. moving limbs, pressure on tips of fingers or toes)
  Orientation
    Place
    Time (year, month, day)
    Person (who am I?)
  Cognitive function
    Tests of memory and recognition

In all patients
  Physical disabilities
    Hemiparesis (e.g. due to stroke)
    Paraparesis (e.g. due to spinal cord injury)
    Blindness
    Deafness
    Tremor (e.g. Parkinson's or cerebellar disease)
  Speech and language disorders
    Dysphasia (difficulty in understanding or producing language)
    Dysarthria (difficulty in forming speech)
  Facial appearance
    Parkinson's disease (immobile, drooling)
    Ptosis (drooping eyelid(s))
    Oculomotor weakness (squint)
    Facial weakness
  Cranial nerves (see text)
  Limbs
    Motor function (tone, power, coordination)
    Sensory function
    Reflexes

tance. Loss of smell (anosmia) is most commonly associated with local conditions of the nose (e.g. the common cold). Anosmia may also result from skull fractures of the anterior cranial fossa involving the cribriform plate.

Second nerve

The main steps on the visual pathway are the optic nerves, the optic chiasma, which is closely related to the pituitary gland, the optic tracts, the optic radiation, which passes through the internal capsule, and the visual area of the cerebral cortex in the occipital lobe. The fibres from the medial side of the retina cross in the optic chiasma, and those fibres are relayed to the opposite occipital lobe. Fibres from the lateral side of the retina remain uncrossed, and therefore pass back to the ipsilateral visual area.

Visual acuity

Visual acuity is examined by asking the patient to count fingers, read print, or to read standardized print on a chart (Snellen's types).

Visual fields

Visual fields are compared to the examiner's, or examined formally by perimetry. A stroke commonly causes loss of the contralateral half of each visual field (homonymous hemianopia). A pituitary tumour (see Ch. 13) may press on the optic chiasma, resulting in loss of vision in the lateral half of each visual field (bitemporal hemianopia).

The retina

The retina is examined by ophthalmoscopy, taking account of the optic nerve head (disc), the blood vessels, and the background appearances. A healthy disc has a distinct margin and a centrally depressed portion, or cup. Optic atrophy results in a pale disc. The term 'papilloedema' describes the swollen appearance of the optic disc which develops if the intracranial pressure is increased, e.g. in cerebral tumour, intracranial bleeding or severe hypertension (see Ch. 6).

Third, fourth and sixth nerves

The oculomotor, trochlear and abducens nerves are collectively responsible for the nerve supply to the extrinsic ocular muscles. The nuclei lie in the brainstem, and the nerves pass through the cavernous sinus on their way to the eye muscles. The fourth nerve supplies the superior oblique muscle, the sixth nerve the lateral rectus muscle, while the third nerve supplies the four remaining extrinsic muscles, i.e. the inferior rectus, superior rectus, medial rectus, and inferior oblique. The third nerve also supplies the voluntary part of the levator palpebrae superioris and the parasympathetic fibres to the muscles of accommodation, stimulation of which causes constriction of the pupil.

An isolated lesion of the fourth or sixth nerve on one side causes paralysis of one extrinsic muscle, and this results in a squint (strabismus)

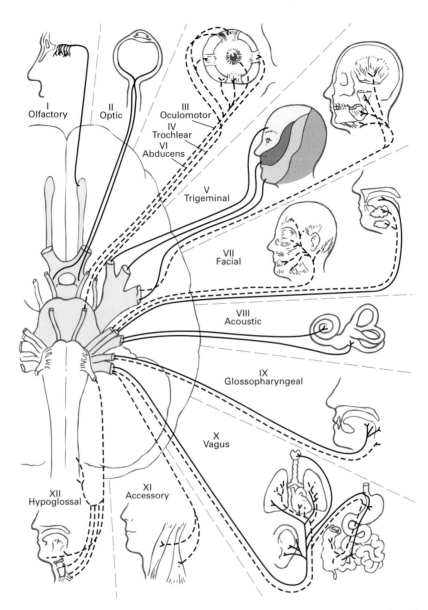

Fig. 9.1 The cranial nerves. An interrupted line (- - - -) indicates a motor pathway and a continuous line (——) a sensory pathway. (After F. H. Netter, The Ciba Collection of Medical Illustrations.)

and double vision (diplopia). A third nerve palsy also causes a squint and diplopia, and in addition drooping of the upper eyelid (ptosis), and a dilated pupil which does not react to light or convergence (Fig. 9.2). Other causes of a dilated pupil (mydriasis) are brain damage (e.g. acute rise in intracranial pressure due to an intracranial haematoma; or brain death due to hypoxia), or anticholinergic (e.g. atropine) or sympath-

omimetic drugs (e.g. adrenaline or cocaine). The Holmes–Adie pupil is a benign condition in which one pupil is dilated and reacts only slowly to light or convergence.

Causes of a constricted pupil include a lesion of the cervical sympathetic nerve fibres (Horner's syndrome), central lesions (Argyll-Robertson pupil), cholinergic drugs (e.g. neostigmine) and opiate drugs.

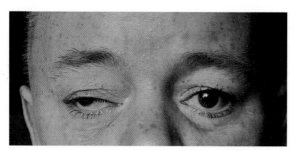

Fig. 9.2 Unilateral third nerve palsy, causing ptosis, a squint and a dilated pupil on the patient's right side.

Horner's syndrome comprises unilateral:

- ptosis (drooping of the upper eyelid)
- miosis (constricted pupil)
- hypohydrosis (loss of sweating of the ipsilateral face).

It is most commonly due to cancer at the apex of the lung (see Ch. 8), which can infiltrate the superior cervical sympathetic ganglion, or to neck trauma.

Argyll-Robertson pupils are small, irregular and unequal; they fail to react to light but still react to convergence. The condition may result from neurosyphilis, diabetes mellitus or multiple sclerosis.

Fifth nerve

The motor component is responsible for the muscles of mastication, and the sensory component carries sensation from the side of the face and head, including the cornea, from the teeth and mucosa, and from the anterior two-thirds of the tongue.

The principal disorders of the trigeminal nerve are trigeminal neuralgia (see Ch. 25) and herpes zoster (see Ch. 22).

Seventh nerve

The facial nerve supplies the muscles of facial expression and also the taste fibres to the anterior two-thirds of the tongue. The nucleus is in the pons close to that of the sixth nerve, and receives fibres from the opposite motor cortex. The nerve passes across the posterior fossa of the skull in close proximity to the eighth nerve, traverses the bony facial canal in the petrous portion of the temporal bone, where it is related to the middle ear and the mastoid air cells, emerges from the skull through the stylomastoid canal and foramen, and passes forward through the parotid gland before dividing up into branches for distribution to the various facial muscles and to taste buds in the tongue. Pathology of the facial nerve is discussed in Chapter 25.

Eighth nerve

The eighth nerve has an auditory component and a vestibular component. The principal symptoms that may follow lesions of the eighth nerve are vertigo, tinnitus (a ringing noise in the ears) and deafness.

Patients with vertigo have an illusion of movement or of visible objects moving about them, and may stagger or fall. There is often associated vomiting. Vertigo is caused by disordered function of the labyrinthine mechanism responsible for normal equilibrium. Ménière's disease is a degenerative form of paroxysmal vertigo, associated with tinnitus and deafness. Viral labyrinthitis is common, and may occur in small outbreaks.

Deafness may be due to an eighth nerve lesion (e.g. an acoustic neuroma), but is more commonly due to wax, chronic suppurative middle ear disease, fusion of the bones of the middle ear (otosclerosis), or from primary nerve degeneration associated with advancing age or noise exposure.

Ninth, 10th, 11th and 12th nerves

Isolated lesions of these nerves are rare. Glossopharyngeal neuralgia is considered in Chapter 25. Unilateral hypoglossal (12th nerve) lesions cause weakness and atrophy of the ipsilateral tongue muscles. The tongue deviates towards the weak side on protrusion (Fig. 9.3).

Combined bilateral lesions of these nerves are more common. Bulbar palsy is characterized by lower motor neurone weakness, usually due to motor neuron disease, which is an idiopathic degeneration of the nuclei in the medulla. Symptoms include difficulty in eating, swallowing (dysphagia) and articulating speech (dysarthria). The tongue is small, atrophic, shows quivering

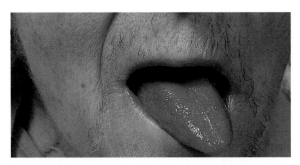

Fig. 9.3 Unilateral 12th nerve palsy, causing weakness (deviation to the weak side on protrusion) and atrophy of the ipsilateral tongue muscles.

muscle fibres (fasciculation) and cannot be protruded.

Pseudobulbar palsy involves upper motor neuron weakness, usually due to bilateral strokes. The symptoms and signs are similar; however, there is no atrophy or fasciculation of the tongue.

Examination of the limbs

A resting tremor may be observed in basal ganglia disorders (e.g. Parkinson's disease), and may be accompanied by muscle rigidity. Tremor on movement (intention tremor) is observed in cerebellar disorders (e.g. alcohol toxicity), and may be seen in the eyes (nystagmus), arms (past-pointing when the patient is asked to touch his or her nose or the examiner's finger) or legs (unsteady walking –

ataxia). Other causes of tremor include anxiety, hyperthyroidism (see Ch. 13) and adrenergic drugs (e.g. salbutamol inhalers for treatment of asthma).

Weakness (paresis) of the limbs may be mild or severe. The term 'hemiparesis' is applied when loss of power affects both an arm and a leg on the same side; paralysis of both legs is termed paraparesis (paraplegia). The clinical features of upper and lower motor neuron lesions are summarized in Table 9.3. Muscle tone is tested by gently moving the limbs after asking the patient to relax. Tendon reflexes are elicited by tapping muscle tendons with a tendon hammer, e.g. the knee jerk (Fig. 9.4). The plantar reflex is performed by gently stroking the outer plantar surface of the foot; normally this causes flexion of the toes, but

Table 9.3 Comparison of the clinical features of weakness due to upper and lower motor neuron lesions

Feature	Upper	Lower
Muscle wasting	Absent	Present
Fasciculation	Absent	Sometimes present
Muscle tone	Increased (spastic)	Decreased (flaccid)
Tendon reflexes	Increased	Decreased
Plantar reflex	Extensor	Flexor

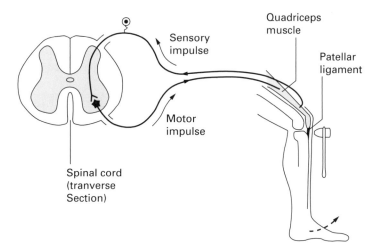

Fig. 9.4 The reflex arc of the knee jerk.

in upper motor neuron lesions (e.g. strokes) the response is extensor.

Sensory testing includes light touch (cotton wool), vibration (tuning-fork), pain (a sharp point), temperature, and position sense (proprioception).

Investigations

Specialized investigations of the cranial nerves can be performed by ophthalmologists and ear, nose and throat specialists; and of the peripheral nerves by the neurophysiology laboratory, which also performs electroencephalography in investigation of epilepsy.

Skull radiography is useful in the diagnosis of skull fractures, and pituitary tumours may cause enlargement of the pituitary fossa. Causes of spinal cord or nerve root compression may be shown on spinal radiographs (e.g. trauma, pathological fractures or tumours). Chest radiography may show bronchial carcinoma, which is a common cause of brain metastases, nerve root compression or peripheral neuropathy.

Computerized tomography (CT) or magnetic resonance imaging (MRI) scans are valuable in identifying lesions of the brain, spinal cord, nerve roots, and pituitary. Cerebral angiography is used to demonstrate aneurysms (e.g. after subarachnoid haemorrhage) or vascular malformations (angiomas). Carotid arteriography is used to demonstrate carotid artery stenosis in patients with carotid territory strokes or transient ischaemic attacks, but is increasingly replaced by Doppler ultrasound imaging, which is non-invasive.

Lumbar spinal puncture is performed under local anaesthesia to obtain cerebrospinal fluid for laboratory examination in suspected:

- meningitis (white blood cells or microbes)
- subarachnoid haemorrhage (blood cells or their pigment)
- tumours
- multiple sclerosis (immunoglobulins).

Epilepsy

Epilepsy is defined as recurrent seizures (fits), which are paroxysms of uncontrolled electrical activity in the brain (general or focal) with associated clinical features. The condition is common, the prevalence being about 1 in 200 persons. In most cases, the cause is unknown (idiopathic epilepsy) although a family history is common, suggesting genetic predispositions. There may be a history of previous brain damage, e.g. trauma or hypoxia (including birth injury and brain surgery), infection (e.g. meningitis) or tumour; it is important also to consider metabolic causes of fits.

Investigations for an underlying cause include brain scanning to exclude intracranial tumour (especially in adults), blood glucose (hypoglycaemia) and serum calcium (hypercalcaemia). Many persons have only one seizure, which is often precipitated by an obvious cause such as:

- fever (especially in infants – 'febrile convulsions')
- prolonged faints (see Ch. 6)
- withdrawal of alcohol or addictive drugs.

The common clinical types of epilepsy are summarized in Table 9.4. It is particularly important to obtain a description of attacks from witnesses of patients with fits.

In major (grand mal) epilepsy the individual has recurrent convulsions. Sometimes there is a brief warning (aura), but more frequently the seizure occurs without warning. Consciousness is suddenly lost, and the patient may fall heavily to the ground, suffering injury. For a few moments the limbs and trunk muscles are rigid and tense (the tonic phase); this includes the respiratory muscles and cyanosis is characteristic. This is quickly followed by violent uncontrolled move-

Table 9.4 Major clinical types of epilepsy

General
Grand mal
   Convulsive
     Non-convulsive
Petit mal

Focal
Jacksonian
   Motor cortex
     Sensory cortex
Temporal lobe

ments of the limbs (clonic phase). Frothing at the mouth is common, and the tongue may be bitten. Incontinence of urine often occurs. Each attack may last from a few moments up to many hours; the term 'status epilepticus' is used when seizures follow each other without remission. After the attack the patient is often drowsy and confused and may sleep deeply or be semiconscious for several hours. In major non-convulsive seizures, consciousness is lost but there is no motor activity. The electroencephalogram (EEG) is often generally abnormal in major epilepsy.

Petit mal epilepsy is characterized by a transient mental blank, but there is no convulsion. This form of epilepsy occurs mostly in children. The attacks occur without warning and last for a few seconds to a minute or so. The child is unresponsive during the attack, and may be scolded by teachers or parents for inattention before the diagnosis is made. The EEG shows a characteristic 'spike and wave' abnormality.

In temporal lobe epilepsy, the patient does not lose consciousness but experiences peculiar complex sensory disturbances and may exhibit inappropriate, complex behaviour attacks of which they have no recollection. In Jacksonian epilepsy, the focus is in the motor or sensory cortex, causing unilateral convulsions or sensory disturbance, often without loss of consciousness.

Management

The most important step during a convulsive seizure is to prevent self-injury. Patients should be removed from anything dangerous such as a fire, machinery (e.g. dental equipment) or a cooking stove. They should be laid on their side when convulsions cease, and a clear airway maintained. Patients should be kept under supervision until consciousness has returned to normal. Depending on the circumstances and duration of the attack, this may necessitate hospital admission. This is urgently required for status epilepticus to avoid hypoxic brain damage; intravenous anticonvulsants (e.g. diazepam) and/or general anaesthesia may be required.

Management of the patient between seizures is very important. In the UK, patients should not drive unless free from seizures for 1 year, and cannot hold public service or heavy goods vehicle licences. They should avoid working at heights or with machinery. For epileptic children, a suitable occupation should be chosen so that if seizures occur while at work the chance of injury to the patient and others is minimal.

The principal drugs employed to reduce frequency and severity of seizures are phenytoin, sodium valproate, carbamazepine, lamotrigine and vigabatrin. These are preferably employed singly but can be combined. In petit mal epilepsy, ethosuximide is also used.

If dental treatment is required in a known epileptic patient, a local rather than a general anaesthetic is preferred, because transient cerebral anoxia may occur with the latter and precipitate an attack. The anaesthetist should be aware of the patient's epilepsy and treatment.

The incidence of febrile convulsions can be reduced in children by the use of antipyretics such as paracetamol to control fever.

Vascular disease

A stroke is an acute focal disturbance in the brain, almost always due to cerebral infarction or cerebral haemorrhage; a small number of strokes are due to cerebral tumours, some arising acutely because of haemorrhage into the tumour. Stroke is the third most common cause of death (after myocardial infarction and cancer), and is the most common cause of hospital bed occupancy and of disability in the community. The incidence increases with age, and hypertension is the most important risk factor. Smoking, diabetes and hyperlipidaemia are also risk factors for cerebral infarction.

Cerebral ischaemia and infarction

Cerebral infarction is the cause of 80% of strokes. The usual cause of infarction is thrombosis occurring on a ruptured atherosclerotic plaque, commonly at the carotid bifurcation in the neck. The thrombus may fragment, causing embolism in the distal cerebral arteries. Thromboembolism may also occur from the heart, e.g. from atrial fibrillation, especially in the presence of rheumatic valve disease, artificial heart valves, infective endocarditis, or mural thrombus after acute myocardial infarction (see Ch. 6). Lacunar infarction is due to thrombosis of small, penetrating arteries in the base of the brain.

Small thrombi or emboli may cause transient cerebral ischaemic attacks with a duration of less than 24 h, or minor strokes, the duration of which is greater than 24 h but from which patients recover with little or no disability. Such patients should be treated with aspirin (75–300 mg daily), which reduces the risk of subsequent major strokes due to larger thromboemboli. Hypertension, smoking, diabetes and hyperlipidaemia in such patients should also be treated, and anticoagulants considered in patients with a suspected cardiac source of embolism (e.g. atrial fibrillation).

The symptoms and signs of transient ischaemic attacks and strokes due to cerebral infarction depend on the site of arterial occlusion. Occlusion of an internal carotid artery or its branches (the ophthalmic artery and anterior and middle cerebral arteries) is most common, and may result in ipsilateral monocular blindness (ophthalmic artery occlusion); contralateral hemianopia (visual tracts); contralateral hemiparesis (weakness of arm and leg) or monoparesis (weakness of only arm or leg) from motor cortex involvement; or contralateral hemi-anaesthesia (sensory cortex).

Involvement of the speech centres in the dominant hemisphere causes dysphasia – disability in understanding or using language (spoken or written). In right-handed people the left cerebral hemisphere is dominant, whereas in left-handed people either hemisphere may be dominant. Dysphasia must be distinguished from dysarthria, which is difficulty in speaking due to dysfunction of the ninth to 12th cranial nerves (this may occur after stroke, e.g. pseudobulbar palsy), and which may be associated with difficulty in eating and swallowing.

Occlusion of the vertebral or basilar arteries or their branches may cause transient loss of consciousness, vertigo or ataxia (infarction of the brainstem or cerebellum) or cortical blindness (infarction of the occipital lobe, supplied by the posterior cerebral arteries).

Intracranial haemorrhage

Intracranial haemorrhage, which is usually spontaneous, is the cause of 20% of strokes. A significant proportion of these are due to intracerebral haemorrhage from small congenital aneurysms in the internal capsule, cerebellum or brainstem; this is especially common in hypertension. In all patients with intracranial bleeding, it is important to detect and treat any generalized bleeding disorders, e.g. anticoagulant drug-induced, haemophilias or thrombocytopenia (see Ch. 7).

Bleeding from aneurysms of the circle of Willis at the base of the brain results in subarachnoid haemorrhage. Such aneurysms are again associated with hypertension; prior to rupture they may press on adjacent cranial nerves (second to sixth), causing cranial nerve symptoms and signs. Subarachnoid haemorrhage causes the abrupt onset of severe occipital headache, neck stiffness due to meningeal irritation by blood, and frequently transient or permanent loss of consciousness. Focal signs may be present, often due to associated cerebral arterial spasm. Suspected subarachnoid haemorrhage should be confirmed by CT scanning; blood-stained cerebrospinal fluid is also seen at lumbar puncture, but this should not be performed routinely due to the risk of 'coning' of the brainstem through the foramen magnum, causing cardiorespiratory arrest and death. Cerebral angiography may show aneurysms, which can be ligated by a neurosurgeon to reduce the risk of subsequent bleeding, which is high in the next few weeks and frequently fatal.

Progress and management of strokes

Strokes are usually sudden in onset; slowly progressive focal symptoms and signs are more suggestive of subdural haemorrhage following head injury, tumours or degenerative diseases. In major strokes, consciousness is often impaired or lost, with incontinence of urine and faeces. Loss of consciousness, headache and vomiting due to raised intracranial pressure are common at the onset in intracranial haemorrhage, and occur after a day or two in major cerebral infarction due to cerebral oedema. Focal symptoms and signs depend on the site of the lesion. Contralateral hemiparesis (with or without hemianopia, hemi-anaesthesia or dysphasia) is the most common presentation of major strokes.

An accurate diagnosis of the underlying cause cannot be made clinically, and requires CT scanning. Occasionally CT scanning reveals causes that are potentially treatable by a neurosurgeon (subarachnoid haemorrhage or subdural haemorrhage, tumour), but usually it shows untreatable pathology (intracerebral haemorrhage or cerebral infarction). Coagulation defects (e.g. anticoagulant therapy, haemophilia or thrombocytopenia) should be reversed urgently in patients with intracranial bleeding. Aspirin is given as secondary prevention in patients with cerebral infarction.

About one-third of patients with major stroke die, either in the acute stage from a large brain lesion, or in subsequent weeks or months from infection (bronchopneumonia, urinary tract infection or bedsores) or pulmonary thromboembolism. One-third recover but are dependent on others for their care. One-third recover to an independent existence but have an increased risk of subsequent cardiac or cerebral vascular events.

Treatment of major strokes is largely symptomatic, with nursing care and physiotherapy. Patients must be turned every 2 h to prevent bedsores and pneumonia, and may require bladder catheterization. Care of the skin and mouth is important to prevent infection, and fluids are given by intravenous or nasogastric tubes to prevent dehydration, since oral fluid intake is often poor because of impaired consciousness or swallowing. If swallowing difficulty persists, patients should be fed through a nasogastric tube, or sometimes through a tube inserted through the abdominal and stomach wall at endoscopy.

Physiotherapy to the paralysed limbs initially involves passive movement to prevent contractures and maintain posture, and subsequently help to regain active movements and the ability to walk. The affected limbs are often stiff, with extension of the leg and flexion of the arm. The stiff leg can aid return of walking, but arm function is often permanently lost. Dysphasia and dysarthria can be helped by speech therapy. Occupational therapists play an important role in adapting home circumstances to suit disability.

Medical treatment includes treatment of infections with antibiotics, and identification of the small number of patients who may benefit from neurosurgery.

After recovery from stroke, preventive measures against further strokes should be considered as for transient ischaemic attacks and minor strokes, i.e. aspirin in cerebral infarction, anticoagulants in cerebral infarction due to embolism from proven cardiac lesions, and hypotensive drugs for persistent hypertension. In patients with transient ischaemic attacks and/or minor cerebral infarction, ulcerated atherosclerotic plaques at the carotid bifurcation can be visualized by ultrasound scanning and arteriography, and may be removed surgically (carotid endarterectomy) if there is stenosis greater than 75% of the lumen.

Along with Alzheimer's disease, repeated minor strokes account for the majority of patients with progressive dementia.

Multiple sclerosis

This is another common and serious disease affecting the central nervous system. The cause is unknown. Pathologically the disorder is characterized by areas of demyelination (plaques) scattered throughout the spinal cord, the cerebral hemispheres and the cerebellum. The clinical picture depends on the site of these lesions and their progression.

Multiple sclerosis usually starts in early adult life. The first expression of the disease is most often a transient weakness or sensory disturbance affecting a limb, cranial nerve (see Ch. 25) or disturbed vision (optic neuritis or diplopia). Characteristically these early symptoms remit after only short duration, but later the individual develops more areas of demyelination throughout the nervous system, and although there may be some temporary improvement after each episode there is often progressive disability.

In the fully developed case there is usually evidence of pyramidal tract involvement shown by weakness of the legs with increased tendon jerks and extensor plantar responses, loss of bladder control, slurring of the speech, and tremor. Incoordination resulting both from cerebellar disease and from proprioceptive dysfunction is often pronounced.

No curative treatment is known for multiple sclerosis. Physiotherapy and occupational therapy are helpful. The duration and severity of acute episodes may be reduced by a course of corticosteroids or adrenocorticotrophic hormone. Recently, interferon has been shown to benefit some people. The disorder may be aggravated by anaesthetics or operations, and this fact may influence the nature and extent of dental procedures in these patients.

Parkinson's disease (parkinsonism)

This is a common disorder of unknown aetiology occurring in middle or later life; there is often a positive family history. The basal ganglia are depleted of dopamine, leading to unbalanced cholinergic activity. A similar clinical picture can arise from the use of neuroleptic drugs such as phenothiazines, from toxic damage to the basal ganglia, and as part of other diffuse brain diseases; it also arose as an aftermath of the worldwide epidemic of viral encephalitis lethargica seen in 1918–1930.

The clinical picture of Parkinson's disease is characteristic:

- slowness and poverty of movements, including facial movements and blinking (the expression is 'mask-like')
- rigidity of limbs, due to increased muscle tone
- coarse tremor of the arms, head and jaw, present at rest
- a flexed posture of the trunk
- a shuffling gait
- dysarthria
- drooling of saliva, due to retarded swallowing.

The administration of levodopa (usually in combination with carbidopa, which inhibits enzymes which metabolize it) benefits many patients with parkinsonism, at least in the short term; it is converted into dopamine in the brain.

Other degenerative disorders of the nervous system

Syringomyelia

In this disorder, cystic cavities develop within the spinal cord, usually at the cervical level. They cause progressive pressure damage to both motor and sensory pathways within the cord. The sensory loss is often 'dissociated', in that pain and temperature sensation is lost while deep sensation is not affected. It is now postulated that the condition is due to blockage of the exit foramina of the fourth ventricle leading secondarily to distension of the vestigial central canal of the cord. Surgical decompression may be helpful.

Cervical spondylosis (see Ch. 14)

Pressure damage to the cervical part of the spinal cord and the posterior nerve roots can result from degenerative changes in the cervical intervertebral discs. Clinical features include pain in the back of the neck, shoulders and arms; or weakness and sensory disturbances in the legs. The latter may require surgery in selected cases.

Motor neuron disease

This is an uncommon disorder of older persons, of unknown aetiology, characterized by progressive degenerative changes in the anterior horn cells, the cranial nerve nuclei, and the pyramidal pathway. It progresses to severe disability and death. Bulbar or pseudobulbar palsy results from involvement of the lower cranial nerves. There is no specific treatment.

Huntington's chorea

This rare form of chorea may be distinguished from chorea of rheumatic origin (see Ch. 6) by a family history of the disorder, and progressive dementia. The onset is in middle age. The involuntary movements are often extremely marked. The recent development of gene probes may allow antenatal diagnosis and selective termination of affected pregnancies.

Subacute combined degeneration of the cord

This is a serious disorder of the nervous system caused by deficiency of vitamin B_{12} (see Ch. 7). Degenerative changes in the pyramidal tract and the posterior sensory columns result in leg weakness and sensory loss. Peripheral polyneuropathy is usually associated. Urgent vitamin B_{12} therapy is required.

Intracranial tumours

Primary tumours

Most primary neoplasms of the brain are malignant, but they have the peculiarity that they never metastasize to other tissues. Tumours, benign and malignant, also arise from other structures within the skull. Important examples include:

- pituitary tumours (see Ch. 13)
- acoustic (eighth nerve) neuromas
- meningiomas
- gliomas.

Clinical features include:

- increased intracranial pressure – headache, vomiting usually without nausea, visual upset due to papilloedema, and bradycardia
- focal damage – muscle weakness, sensory defects, personality changes, etc., depending on the site of the tumour.

Tumours can be localized by CT or MRI and their nature determined by brain biopsy. Treatment may be by radiotherapy or surgery. The prognosis is poor in the majority of cases. Symptoms of raised intracranial pressure are often helped by corticosteroids (e.g. dexamethasone), which reduce cerebral oedema.

Secondary tumours

The brain is a common site for secondary neoplasia, often metastasizing from the lung, breast, kidney or thyroid. Treatment is symptomatic.

Intracranial abscess

Abscesses may occur in the extradural or subdural spaces. The commonest sources of brain abscess involve spread of chronic infection from the middle ear; or the facial sinuses; it follows that most abscesses are found in the frontal or temporal lobes, or in the cerebellum. Metastatic infection from the chest (lung abscess or empyema) is less likely (see Ch. 8). The clinical features may be similar to those of a cerebral tumour, though the course of the illness is usually more acute, with fever and leucocytosis. Precise diagnosis by CT scanning allows the surgeon to perform drainage, which may be curative in combination with antibiotics.

Meningitis

Infection of the meninges which cover the brain and spinal cord is most commonly due to viral infections; but may also be due to bacteria, tuberculosis, fungi or tumours (Table 9.5). The clinical features include:

- headache, which is often acute, severe and global
- neck stiffness, due to reactive muscle spasm, and detectable when the patient's neck is flexed
- fever
- drowsiness, irritability and photophobia (discomfort on looking at the light)

Table 9.5 Causes of meningitis

Viral	Herpes simplex Mumps Enteroviruses (echo, Coxsackie, polio) Influenza HIV Lymphocytic choriomeningitis (arenovirus) Rabies
Bacterial	*Neisseria meningitidis* (meningococcus) *Streptococcus pneumoniae* (pneumococcus) *Haemophilus influenzae* *Streptococcus pyogenes* Gram-negative bacilli
Tuberculous	*Mycobacterium tuberculosis*
Fungal	Cryptococcal (in immunosuppressed patients, e.g. HIV infection)
Malignant	Carcinoma Leukaemia, lymphoma

- an acute purpuric rash (see Ch. 7) – this is characteristic of meningococcal meningitis, and is due to direct vascular damage and disseminated intravascular coagulation from meningococcal septicaemia.

The diagnosis is confirmed by urgent examination of the cerebrospinal fluid obtained by lumbar spinal puncture under local anaesthesia (Table 9.6). Blood cultures may also be positive in bacterial meningitis.

Viral meningitis

Viral meningitis is usually a benign, self-limiting illness which requires no specific treatment. Occasionally there is an associated encephalitis, clinically evident as impairment of consciousness with focal neurological signs. Suspected viral encephalitis should be treated with intravenous aciclovir, because it may be effective in encephalitis due to herpes simplex.

Bacterial meningitis

Bacterial meningitis is a more serious illness, which may be rapidly fatal or cause permanent brain damage, and which requires urgent treatment with intravenous antimicrobial chemotherapy. For *Neisseria meningitidis* (the meningococcus), the commonest cause in children and young adults, benzylpenicillin is the drug of choice; chloramphenicol or cefotaxime is an alternative in patients allergic to penicillin. Pneumococcal infection is common in older patients and in patients without a functioning spleen (see Ch. 7), and is treated with

cefotaxime or chloramphenicol. *Haemophilus influenzae* infection is common in young children, and is treated with chloramphenicol or cefotaxime. Household and other close contacts of patients with meningococcal infections should be given prophylactic rifampicin for 2 days. Treatment of tuberculous infection is considered in Chapter 8.

Other infections of the nervous system

Herpes zoster

Herpes zoster infection of the trigeminal nerve (shingles) is considered in Chapter 25. Infection of non-cranial peripheral nerve roots is commonest in the intercostal nerves, causing chest pain followed by a local rash (see Ch. 8). Disseminated infection may occur in the immunocompromised, e.g. due to HIV infection.

Poliomyelitis

Poliomyelitis is due to an enterovirus infection, which may be asymptomatic, cause a viral meningitis or encephalitis, or progress to damage the spinal cord anterior horn cells, causing muscle weakness. This may result in respiratory failure, requiring artificial ventilation, or permanent lower motor neuron weakness and wasting, usually of the leg muscles. Routine immunization has greatly reduced the frequency of poliomyelitis.

Myalgic encephalitis (ME)

ME is also known as the postviral syndrome or chronic fatigue syndrome. It may follow glandular fever (see Ch. 7) in young adults, and possibly other viral infections (e.g. enteroviruses). Symptoms include malaise, fatigue, headaches and muscle pains. There are no abnormal physical signs or confirmatory tests, although serology may show evidence of previous Epstein–Barr virus or Coxsackie B virus infection. Treatment is supportive; antidepressants may be effective. Some patients become chronically disabled.

Table 9.6 Cerebrospinal fluid findings in meningitis

Cause	Cells	Microbes	Glucose	Protein
Viral	Lymphocytes	-	Normal	Normal
Bacterial	Polymorphs	+	Low	High
Tuberculous	Mixed	±	Low	High
Fungal	Lymphocytes	±	Low	High
Malignant	Lymphocytes	-	Low	High

HIV and syphilis infections of the nervous system are considered in Chapter 5.

Head and spinal injuries

Common causes of head or spinal injury in developed countries include road traffic accidents, violence, and intoxication with alcohol or other drugs.

First aid measures in patients with suspected head or spinal injuries include:

- Assessment and maintenance of airway, breathing and circulation. Cardiopulmonary resuscitation is described in Chapter 6, and is essential to minimize hypoxic brain damage, which is additive to traumatic brain damage.
- Avoidance of further spinal cord injury. Flexion of the spine should be avoided, and an appropriate cervical spinal splint or stretcher fitted by the emergency medical/paramedical team.
- Assessment and management of other injuries, e.g. chest, abdominal, pelvic or limb fractures and their complications (e.g. bleeding, pneumothorax or haemothorax, see Ch. 8).
- Urgent transfer to an accident and emergency centre for further management.

Hospital management includes:

- Monitoring of conscious level and neurological signs. Conscious level is accurately monitored by the Glasgow Coma Scale (Table 9.7). Neurological signs are monitored to detect progressing brain damage due to intracranial bleeding (subarachnoid, extradural, subdural or intracerebral), or progressing spinal cord damage in spinal injuries.
- Assessment of cerebrospinal fluid leakage from the nose or ear, which carries a risk of infection (meningitis or brain abscess), and which requires antimicrobial prophylaxis and surgical repair of persistent leaks.
- Radiographs of the skull and spine to detect fractures and guide surgical management. Compound skull fractures or penetrating wounds require urgent surgery.
- CT scans of the head, to identify the presence and site of intracranial bleeding, which may require surgical decompression.

Table 9.7 Glasgow Coma Scale

Assessment	Score
Eye-opening (E)	
Spontaneous	4
To speech	3
To pain	2
Nil	1
Best motor response (M)	
Obeys	6
Localizes	5
Withdraws	4
Abnormal flexion	3
Extensor response	2
Nil	1
Verbal response (V)	
Orientated	5
Confused conversation	4
Inappropriate words	3
Incomprehensible sounds	2
Nil	1
Coma score = E + M + V	
Minimum	3
Maximum	15

- Haematological monitoring, to detect and treat bleeding disorders (e.g. anticoagulant drug-induced, haemophilia, thrombocytopenia or disseminated intravascular coagulation secondary to circulatory shock; see Ch. 6), anaemia due to blood loss, or infection.
- Biochemical monitoring, to detect and treat fluid, electrolyte or glucose imbalance.

Intracranial haemorrhage

Intracranial haemorrhage following head injury may occur at four sites:

- *Extradural.* This is usually due to laceration of a branch of the middle meningeal artery. Classically, the patient regains consciousness after a head injury, only to relapse into a coma due to lateral compression of the brain by an enlarging haematoma. The ipsilateral pupil dilates (due to stretching of the third cranial nerve), with contralateral hemiparesis and an extensor plantar response. Urgent surgical decompression through a burr hole on the side of the dilating pupil is indicated.
- *Subdural.* This is usually due to tearing of a small vein after relatively mild head injury,

especially in infants, the elderly, alcoholics, and patients with coagulation defects (e.g. anticoagulant drug-induced, haemophilia or liver disease). Symptoms and signs usually develop more gradually than with extradural haemorrhage (over days or weeks rather than hours), and the minor head injury may have been forgotten. Gradually progressive headache, confusion or personality change is the usual presentation, sometimes with the focal neurological signs of lateral brain compression (dilating ipsilateral pupil, contralateral hemiparesis and extensor plantar response). The diagnosis is confirmed by CT or isotopic brain scanning. Treatment is usually by surgical decompression.

• *Subarachnoid and intracerebral.* These haemorrhages are commonly found on CT brain scanning after head injury. Surgical decompression may be required for accessible progressing intracranial haematomas.

Cerebral oedema is also common after head injury, and may respond to intravenous infusion of hyperosmolar solutions (e.g. mannitol).

Paraplegia (paralysis and anaesthesia below the waist level) is a common complication of thoracic spinal cord injury. Complications include retention or incontinence of urine and faeces, urinary infection, pressure sores, which may become infected, deep vein thrombosis and pulmonary embolism, leg muscle spasms and contractures, psychosocial and sexual problems, and depression. Management and rehabilitation is optimally conducted in specialized spinal injury units. Quadriplegia (paralysis and anaesthesia below the neck level) is a common complication of cervical spinal cord injury, and may result in death from respiratory failure, or require permanent nursing care.

Coma

Assessment and management of the unconscious or semiconscious patient is an important part of medical care. Table 9.8 lists the common causes of coma. A history from witnesses, friends or relatives of the mode of onset of coma, precipitating events (head injuries, drugs or alcohol) and previous medical history (epilepsy, diabetes, thyroid or adrenal disease, liver or kidney disease, chest or

Table 9.8 Causes of coma

Metabolic	Drug or alcohol overdose
	Diabetes mellitus (see Ch. 13)
	Hypoglycaemia
	Hyperglycaemia
	Hyponatraemia (see Ch. 11)
	Renal failure (see Ch. 11)
	Liver failure (see Ch. 10)
	Respiratory failure (see Ch. 8)
	Hypothermia
Trauma	Intracranial bleeding, cerebral oedema
Stroke	Subarachnoid haemorrhage
	Intracerebral haemorrhage
	Major cerebral infarction
	Brainstem infarction or haemorrhage
Infections	Meningitis
	Encephalitis
	Cerebral abscess
	Septicaemia
	Malaria
Others	Epilepsy
	Intracranial tumour
	Hysteria

heart disease) is critical to establishing the cause. Further management includes:

• Assessment and maintenance of the airway, breathing and circulation.

• Neurological examination, especially for head injury, meningism (meningitis or subarachnoid haemorrhage), papilloedema (raised intracranial pressure), and focal neurological signs indicating a focal neurological lesion (e.g. brain haemorrhage, infarct, tumour or abscess).

• Assessment and management of any head and other injuries.

• Biochemical screening, especially glucose, alcohol, drugs, blood gases and pH, urea, electrolytes and drugs.

• Haematological screening (infection or bleeding disorders).

• Skull radiography, CT brain scanning (skull fractures or intracranial lesions).

• Consideration of lumbar spinal puncture (meningitis or subarachnoid haemorrhage).

SPINAL CORD DISORDERS

Spinal injury has been considered above.

Spinal cord compression may arise from lesions in the vertebral column, the spinal meninges, or the spinal cord. The common causes are listed in Table 9.9. Symptoms may be acute or chronic, and include:

- pain – in the spine or nerve root distribution
- paraesthesia or numbness – usually in the lower limbs
- weakness – usually in the lower limbs
- difficulty in passing urine, leading to retention.

Investigations to establish the cause include spine and chest radiography, spinal scanning (CT or MRI), and sometimes myelography. Treatment depends on the cause, and may include surgical decompression.

Multiple sclerosis, poliomyelitis and subacute degeneration of the spinal cord are considered elsewhere in this chapter.

Nerve root disorders

The causes of nerve root compression include prolapsed intervertebral disc, spondylosis due to osteoarthritis of the cervical or lumbar spine (see Ch. 14), trauma, and infiltration by tumour.

Prolapsed intervertebral disc

This is most common in the lower lumbar spine, and in young adults. It may follow sudden muscular exertion such as lifting a heavy object. The patient experiences severe pain in the lower back, buttock and down the back of the leg. The pain is increased by attempting to raise the straight leg. It results from compression of the nerve roots which form the sciatic nerve (sciatica; Fig. 9.5). The prolapsed disc may be visualized by MRI.

The majority of cases respond to initial rest on a firm mattress, analgesics, and active mobilization with exercises. A plaster cast to hold the spine extended is rarely required. In refractory cases, surgical removal of the prolapsed disc (laminectomy) may be helpful.

Tumour

A few cases of sciatica are secondary to pressure from tumour deposits in the spine, which are visualized by MRI or radioisotope scanning.

Peripheral polyneuropathy

Generalized disorder of the peripheral nerves may be due to many toxic or metabolic disorders (Table 9.10); because of the diffuse nature of the pathogenesis, the manifestations are usually symmetrical. Some acute cases are apparently due to a hypersensitivity reaction following virus or other infection (Guillain–Barré syndrome); plasma exchange is beneficial in the treatment of this condition, and ventilation is occasionally required for respiratory paralysis.

The clinical features reflect motor or sensory function, or a mixture of both; there is thus lower motor neuron weakness, with wasting of peripheral muscles, loss of reflexes, paraesthesia and sensory loss of all types over the distal parts of the limbs, and tenderness of the calves. Treatment is of the underlying cause.

Damage to individual peripheral nerves

Direct damage to peripheral nerves may occur as a result of trauma, or involvement by tumour. There is lower motor neuron weakness in the affected group of muscles, with wasting, loss of

Table 9.9 Causes of spinal cord compression	
Vertebral (80% of cases)	Trauma Osteoporosis and crush fracture Prolapsed intervertebral disc Secondary carcinoma (e.g. lung) Myeloma Tuberculosis
Meninges (15% of cases)	Meningioma Neurofibroma Ependymoma Secondary carcinoma Leukaemia, lymphoma Abscess
Spinal cord (5% of cases)	Glioma Ependymoma Secondary carcinoma

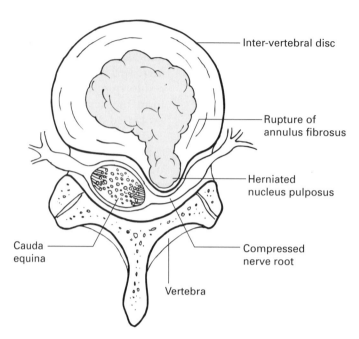

Fig. 9.5 Prolapse of a lumbar intervertebral disc, compressing a nerve root to cause sciatica.

reflexes and, in sensory nerves, associated sensory loss. After trauma, excision of the damaged nerve ends and accurate repair can be followed by a degree of recovery. Common examples of damage to peripheral nerves include trauma to the inferior dental nerve during extraction of teeth, or to the lingual nerve during the removal of impacted lower molar teeth. The infraorbital nerve or the inferior dental nerve may be damaged in fractures of the facial skeleton.

Muscle disorders

Muscular dystrophies

This is a group of genetic disorders of voluntary muscle which occur mainly in children and adolescents. A family history is often present. The affected muscles show progressive weakness and wasting. There are several different clinical varieties, named according to the muscle groups involved. The facioscapulohumeral type is often recognizable by the fact that the masticatory muscles are usually more markedly affected than the other facial muscles, leading to weakness of retraction of the angles of the mouth and a characteristic 'transverse smile'. Treatment is symptomatic.

Myasthenia gravis

This is a disease in which the muscles show an abnormal fatiguability on exercise, reversible after

Table 9.10 Causes of peripheral polyneuropathy	
Genetic	Charcot–Marie–Tooth disease
Metabolic	Diabetes mellitus Renal failure Porphyria
Toxic	Alcohol Heavy metals, e.g. mercury or lead Solvents Drugs, e.g. phenytoin
Deficiencies	Vitamins B_2, B_6, and B_{12}, folate
Infections	Diphtheria HIV Leprosy
Malignancies	Lung
Connective tissue disorders	Rheumatoid arthritis Polyarteritis nodosa Systemic lupus erythematosus

rest. Cranial nerve involvement causes double vision (diplopia), ptosis, and difficulty in chewing, swallowing or speaking. The symptoms are usually more prominent at the end of the day. The disease shows a tendency to remission and relapse. It usually affects younger women. It is due to an autoimmune disorder of conduction at the myoneural junction with antibodies to acetylcholine receptors, which may be relieved by cholinergic drugs, e.g. neostigmine or pyridostigmine.

Polymyositis (see Ch. 12)

This is a connective tissue disease which affects older adults, causing weakness and wasting of muscles, often with a skin rash (dermatomyositis). Treatment is with corticosteroids. An underlying tumour may be causal.

Metabolic myopathies

Muscle weakness may result from hyperthyroidism, corticosteroid therapy, Cushing's syndrome, hypercalcaemia, hypokalaemia, or glycogen storage diseases.

10 Disorders of the gastrointestinal tract

Introduction

The alimentary tract runs from the mouth to the anus, and includes the oesophagus, stomach, small intestine, colon and rectum. A brief description of the anatomy and physiology of these organs will be followed by a description of the important disorders which affect them. There is then a general consideration of gastrointestinal bleeding.

The chapter concludes with disorders of the liver, biliary tract, and pancreas.

Disorders of the oesophagus

Anatomy and physiology

The oesophagus is a hollow tube 25 cm in length stretching from the cricoid cartilage (C6) to the cardiac orifice (T11); the distance from the incisor teeth to the gastric entry is normally 40 cm. The oesophagus runs posteriorly on the vertebral column through the mediastinum, initially in relation to the larynx, trachea and thyroid, and lower down to the aortic arch and left main bronchus. During swallowing it is closed at the upper end by the cricopharyngeus to prevent aspiration. At the lower end, reflux is prevented by the lower oesophageal sphincter, by the diaphragm, and,

during increased intra-abdominal pressure, by a reflex rise in the tone of the sphincter. It takes 5 s for a swallowed bolus to travel from the pharynx to the stomach.

Investigations

Techniques for visualizing the oesophagus include plain chest radiography, which may show widening, tortuosity, or an external lesion exerting pressure; direct fluoroscopy during barium swallow, which is especially good for demonstrating strictures and motility problems; and endoscopy, which allows inspection of the mucosa itself, and biopsy. Motility disorders may also be studied using manometry to obtain pressure readings.

Dysphagia

The two main complaints arising from oesophageal disease are pain in the back or chest, often widely referred, and difficulty swallowing (dysphagia). Physical signs are few. It is important first to distinguish those patients with difficult swallowing due to painful or neurological oropharyngeal conditions, and this can normally be done by careful history taking. It is usually not safe to diagnose psychogenic or anxiety-associated dysphagia (*globus hystericus*) without adequate investigation. Patients with long-standing or severe obstruction may develop profound nutritional and hydration problems; weight loss is thus the rule in organic obstruction.

Dysphagia from extrinsic pressure

Pressure from organs in close relationship with the oesophagus may obstruct swallowing. Examples include mediastinal lymph nodes (tuberculosis, malignant lymphoma or metastatic carcinoma), bronchial carcinoma, thyroid enlargements and aneurysm of the aorta. Pharyngeal diverticula may exert extrinsic pressure on the oesophagus when they fill with food or fluid.

Intrinsic oesophageal lesions

Carcinoma of the oesophagus. Although formerly there was a great preponderance of squamous carcinomas, adenocarcinoma has become equally common. There are strong geographical links with the condition even within a single country, pointing to environmental factors such as nutritional deficiencies, ingested carcinogens and infection. In temperate countries there is a strong link with tobacco and alcohol excess; non-malignant abnormalities such as the Paterson–Brown–Kelly syndrome (Plummer–Vinson syndrome), simple strictures or Barrett's oesophagus also predispose (see later). Squamous carcinoma is commoner in blacks, and adenocarcinoma in whites, and men are more likely to be affected than women.

The prognosis is still dismal, with most patients surviving only 6 months after diagnosis; the cure rate is less than 10%. Surgical resection, radiation and chemotherapy are all used; palliation may be achieved by the insertion of indwelling tubes or stents, and by laser irradiation of intraluminal tumour.

Simple strictures and peptic oesophagitis. Fibrous strictures may result from ingestion of corrosive substances or foreign bodies. Much the commonest cause of stricture, however, is gastro-oesophageal reflux disease (Table 10.1), in which acid, pepsin or even bile, regurgitate freely into the lower oesophagus. Heartburn is thus the classic symptom. The condition results in reflux oesophagitis, ulceration with or without bleeding, stricture, or metaplasia of the epithelium (Barrett's oesophagus). High reflux of acid may result in dental erosion. Patients with occult gastrointestinal bleeding may present with iron deficiency anaemia (see Ch. 7).

Drug therapy for peptic oesophagitis includes simple antacids and layering agents, H_2 receptor blockers such as cimetidine or ranitidine, which inhibit gastric acid secretion, and prokinetic agents such as cisapride or metoclopramide to increase tone in the lower oesophageal sphincter. Proton pump inhibitors such as omeprazole, which inhibit acid production, produce a dramatic alleviation in symptoms, and corresponding gratitude from patients, but the long-term effects are still under investigation. Surgery has a limited role, mainly for failures in medical therapy, for organic strictures, and for those with recurrent aspiration pneumonia. Established strictures may also be palliated by the regular use of a heavy bougie to dilate the stricture.

Other disorders. The Paterson–Brown–Kelly syndrome (Plummer–Vinson syndrome) (see Ch. 7) is associated with chronic iron deficiency states, and may cause dysphagia associated with the presence of a crescentic web in the upper oesophagus, demonstrable on barium swallow (see Ch. 26). Other signs of iron deficiency such as koilonychia, atrophic glossitis, oral ulcers and angular cheilitis may also be present.

Neuromuscular and motility disorders

Neuromuscular disorders. Dysphagia is a common and distressing result of diseases affect-

Table 10.1 Factors favouring gastro-oesophageal reflux[a]
Increased intra-abdominal pressure – pregnancy, obesity
Hiatus hernia
Recumbent posture
Non-steroidal anti-inflammatory drugs
Factors reducing lower oesophageal sphincter tone e.g. alcohol, tobacco, chocolate, anticholinergic and calcium channel-blocking drugs
Heavy meals
[a]Complicated interactions exist between these factors

ing the basal cranial nerve nuclei as occurs in bulbar and pseudobulbar palsy (see Ch. 9); this usually results from degenerative or vascular causes. The dysphagia of myasthenia gravis (see Ch. 9) is recognizable from its progressive occurrence late in the day.

Achalasia of the cardia. This syndrome is characterized by failure of the lower oesophageal sphincter to relax, due to neurological degeneration of Auerbach's nerve plexus in the oesophageal wall. The condition is associated with painful dysphagia, massive oesophageal dilatation and regurgitation; aspiration pneumonia is a real danger, and the condition causes profound weight loss and nutritional deficiencies. It may respond to drug therapy combined with mechanical dilatation, but surgical division of muscle fibres at the lower end of the oesophagus (Heller's operation) may also be of benefit.

Oesophageal spasm. This includes several ill-understood functional disorders with episodic dysphagia, especially while eating, and associated severe chest pain. Abnormal contractions in the oesophagus can be recognized by pressure manometry. Symptoms may be improved by muscle relaxant drugs e.g. diazepam.

Other oesophageal conditions

Hiatus hernia

In this condition, a hernia of the stomach occurs upwards through the diaphragmatic hiatus. The commonest anatomical form is illustrated in Figure 10.1. Here, the gastro-oesphageal junction is displaced into the thorax, resulting in a pouch of stomach above the diagram. It will be clear that an important component of the normal antireflux mechanism at the oesophagogastric junction has been lost, and hiatus hernia is an important contributory cause of reflux disease.

Oesophageal varices

In cases of portal venous hypertension as a result of, for example, liver cirrhosis, there may be dilatation of anastomoses between the portal and systemic venous circulations, particularly in the lower oesophagus and upper cardiac end of the stomach. These thin-walled vessels may bleed dramatically, but can also be the cause of slow occult blood loss with resulting iron deficiency.

Disorders of the stomach and duodenum

Anatomy and physiology

The four anatomical regions of the stomach are the fundus, body, antrum and pylorus

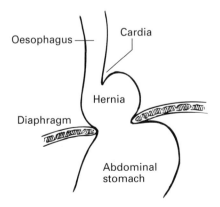

A

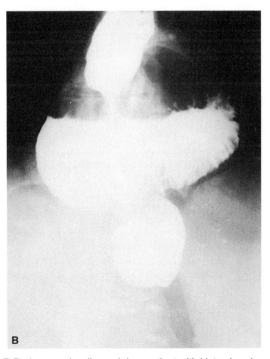

B

Fig. 10.1 **A** The relationship of a hiatus hernia to the diaphragm. **B** Barium meal radiograph in a patient with hiatus hernia.

(Fig. 10.2). It is situated mainly in the left upper abdominal cavity though in the intrathoracic position; this can, however, vary widely from individual to individual. The stomach is lined by a mucous membrane consisting of parietal cells producing hydrochloric acid and intrinsic factor, chief cells secreting pepsin, mucus-producing cells, and specialized cells producing the hormones gastrin and somatostatin which control secretion and motility of the stomach. Outside the mucosa are layers of muscle and connective tissue, and finally the peritoneal surface.

Entry of food and secretions to the duodenum is controlled by the pyloric sphincter; activity in the sphincter is induced by sympathetic activity and inhibited by parasympathetic impulses. The duodenum is around 35 cm long, and connects the pylorus with the proximal jejunum. It receives bile and pancreatic juice to mix with food. Its own secretions are alkaline, which, along with the pancreatic juice, raise the pH of intestinal contents to near neutral.

Functions of the stomach

Mechanical. The capacity of the stomach allows meals to be eaten intermittently. It has an important function in mixing swallowed food with secretions, and releases food through the pylorus into the absorptive area of the gut at a controlled rate.

Protective. The strongly acidic milieu of the stomach is lethal to most microorganisms, thus protecting the gut from colonization with bacteria and fungi. In addition, noxious substances can be ejected by vomiting.

Digestive. Pepsin begins the breakdown of proteins, although complete digestion does not take place until the semi-liquid meal reaches the intestine.

Haemopoietic. Intrinsic factor has a vital role in complexing with ingested vitamin B_{12} (extrinsic factor), and enables its subsequent absorption in the terminal ileum. In the absence of acid gastric juice, absorption of food iron is also impaired.

Investigations

The mainstays of gastric investigation remain radiological (visualization with radiopaque media, usually a barium meal) combined with endoscopy and biopsy. Measurement of gastric acid secretion, studies of emptying rate, and detection of *Helicobacter pylori* infection (see below) are also useful.

Gastritis

Acute gastritis usually results from chemical injury with non-steroidal anti-inflammatory drugs, or alcohol. The mucosa becomes oedematous, congested and haemorrhagic, and overt bleeding from erosions may occur. Healing is spontaneous within a few days. Chronic gastritis follows infection with *H. pylori*, and may also result from autoimmune processes; the latter may progress to gastric atrophy with loss of all acid, pepsin and intrinsic factor secretion as is found in Addisonian pernicious anaemia (see Ch. 7).

Peptic ulceration

This is the most important and widespread gastrointestinal disease. Chronic peptic ulcer may develop in any area exposed to acid gastric juice, especially in the duodenum and antrum of the stomach. It is commoner in males, with duodenal ulcer incidence peaking at a younger age than gastric ulcer.

The aetiology has been obscure for decades but clearly results from an imbalance between the erosive effect of gastric juice and the defence mechanisms of the mucosa. Predisposing factors include

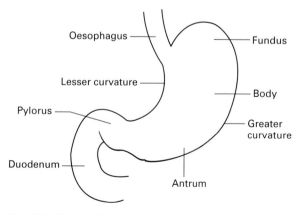

Fig. 10.2 The configuration of the normal stomach.

male sex, smoking, ingestion of corticosteroids and non-steroidal anti-inflammatory drugs, blood group O, a positive family history, and a dubious role for stress. While many patients have gastric acid hypersecretion, especially those with duodenal ulcer, this is not true of all.

The discovery of *H. pylori* in 1983 has led to much fertile research. This transmissible Gram-negative spiral bacterium is only found in gastric mucosa and has the extraordinary capacity of protecting itself from gastric acid by producing ammonia and thus creating a favourable local milieu for its survival. It is capable of inducing chronic gastritis, and is very strongly associated with both duodenal and gastric ulcers; infection also induces gastric hypersecretion. Eradication of infection from the antral mucosa with a 1–2 week course of antimicrobial drugs induces prolonged remission and healing in ulcer disease.

Clinical features

The classic symptoms include epigastric pain, which may radiate to the back; it is relieved by eating, and is thus generally worse when the patient is hungry or during the night. Distension, temporary relief from alkalis, and a remitting/relapsing course are also characteristic; vomiting and weight loss are less usual features. It is true, however, that the majority of patients do not show fully typical features, and it is not uncommon to find active peptic ulcers in patients with no complaints. Apart from mild epigastric tenderness, physical signs are few.

Complications

These may be life-threatening and include gastrointestinal bleeding with haematemesis or melaena, pyloric stenosis, perforation with localized or generalized peritonitis, or, in the case of gastric ulcer, malignant change (this last association is dubious).

Management

This includes avoidance of precipitating factors (see above), prescription of inhibitors of acid secretion including H_2 receptor antagonists (cimetidine or ranitidine) and proton pump inhibitors (e.g. omeprazole), antibiotic eradication of *H. pylori* infestation, antacids for symptomatic relief, and mucosal protection with sucralfate. Surgical intervention in uncomplicated peptic ulcer disease is indicated for failure of adequate medical measures; modern operations such as highly selective vagotomy combined with a drainage procedure are associated with fewer absorptive, motility, and other complications of older procedures. Surgery has a vital role in the emergency management of acute gastrointestinal bleeding and perforation, and in the treatment of pyloric stenosis.

Carcinoma of the stomach

This is a common malignancy worldwide that has been declining in the UK in recent decades. Perhaps the most important aetiological factor is pre-existing chronic gastritis and *H. pylori* infection; epidemiologically, overcrowding and easier transmission of this organism may explain the higher incidence of gastric carcinoma in lower socioeconomic groups. There is also an increased incidence associated with the gastric atrophy in pernicious anaemia patients. Other aetiological influences include blood group A, cigarette smoking, and the possibility of ingested carcinogens in the diet, especially nitrosamines.

These tumours are usually adenocarcinomas and commonly present as ulcerating growths; a minority may extend diffusely throughout the gastric wall without penetrating the mucosa. Spread occurs locally to adjacent organs and to lymph nodes, and also frequently to the liver and lungs.

Clinical features

The patients usually present with progressive weight loss and some abdominal pain; many also have nausea, anorexia, and early fullness on eating. Failure of general health and unexplained iron deficiency anaemia are common. The diagnosis should be suspected in all subjects presenting for the first time in middle age or elderly life with these complaints. Examination may show an abdominal mass, but relatively few have clinical evidence of hepatic, peritoneal or pelvic metastases until late on.

Management

Surgical resection of localized tumours offers the only hope for cure, but long-standing success occurs only in the minority. The disease is still fatal in 90% of cases. Palliative surgery is justified for the relief of symptoms such as severe gastric outlet obstruction. Single- or multi-agent chemotherapy combined with surgery continues under active investigation.

The duodenum is only rarely involved by malignant tumours. Gastroduodenal polyps may be associated with perioral pigmentation (Peutz–Jeghers syndrome; see Ch. 27). They may cause intestinal obstruction or undergo malignant transformation.

The small intestine and malabsorption

Anatomy and physiology

The small intestine is particularly adapted to complete the process of food digestion begun in the stomach, and in addition to undertake absorption of the bewildering array of essential substances derived from the diet; these include water and electrolytes, amino acids, simple carbohydrates and fats, and also vitamins, essential minerals and trace elements. In most cases, absorption does not simply involve passive diffusion of a food element across the mucosal cell but rather a series of quite complex adaptations and controls which are individual to that food constituent alone, e.g. vitamin B_{12}, iron, fats. In addition, the upper small intestine receives bile, essential for the emulsification and absorption of lipids, and pancreatic juice containing amylases, lipase and trypsin for the digestion of carbohydrates, fat and protein.

The mucosa is lined with tall columnar cells with a brush border on the luminal surface; these cells are formed in crypts and when mature, migrate up to their functional position on the villi, microscopic fronds of mucosa projecting into the lumen. Each villus contains stroma, lymphatics and blood vessels to carry away absorbed material. In addition, the mucosa is folded to increase the absorptive area many times. Outside the mucosa lie muscular layers and the peritoneal surface. The intestine enjoys a very active immune system (mucosal-associated lymphoid tissue; MALT), with T cells distributed widely throughout the mucosa, and also localized in the organized milieu of mesenteric lymph nodes and Peyer's patches. B cells are also numerous, and are responsible for the local system of secretory IgA production.

For many years the small intestine was one of the most inaccessible areas in the body to investigate; this has changed in modern times. The gut may be imaged by barium follow-through, best done via a tube positioned in the duodenum. Mucosal biopsy (single or multiple) can be obtained relatively easily by specially-adapted tubes using suction, after swallowing and positioning radiologically, or by endoscopy. Absorption and transit studies are also important.

Malabsorption

Patients with malabsorption present either through the systemic effects of deficiency, or with suggestive bowel symptoms, or through a combination of both. It is important always to consider underlying malabsorption in deficiency syndromes, especially in adults without intestinal complaints. The main clinical effects are summarized in Table 10.2; many patients, especially with

Table 10.2 Malabsorption of some food constituents

Malabsorbed food constituent	Clinical features
Carbohydrate	Gaseous distension Flatulence Frothy stools Abdominal pain
Protein	Wasting Short stature
Fat	Steatorrhoea (stools pale, bulky and offensive) Wasting Loss of fat-soluble vitamins A, D, E and K
Iron	Iron deficiency anaemia
Calcium and vitamin D	Osteomalacia
Thiamine	Neuropathy
Folic acid	Megaloblastic anaemia
Vitamin B_{12}	Megaloblastic anaemia

gluten enteropathy (see below), may present with stomatitis or aphthae (see Chs 19 and 26).

There are numerous causes of intestinal malabsorption, ranging from infestations and infections, anatomical variations such as short circuits and diverticulae, obstructive jaundice, pancreatic failure, and rapid transit, to mucosal disease, of which coeliac disease is the most important example. Chronic inflammatory bowel disease is discussed later.

Coeliac disease (gluten enteropathy)

This is the classic and most common malabsorptive disease, caused by sensitivity to ingested gluten, an important constituent of cereals, including wheat, rye and barley. The entire mucosa from the duodenum to the terminal ileum is affected. The damage results from interactions between gluten and T lymphocytes; the mucosa becomes heavily infiltrated with chronic inflammatory cells, the villi become stunted, and eventually a 'flat' atrophic mucosa results. In most cases, the lesion is fully reversible after gluten withdrawal from the diet. There is a strong linkage with genes encoded at the MHC class II D loci on the short arm of chromosome 6; for this reason the condition may run in families, and it clusters in geographical areas – it is particularly common in the West of Ireland.

Management involves replacement of all deficiencies, and the establishment of a gluten-free diet. This requires the input of a trained dietician to give advice and support to achieve the necessary lifestyle alterations, and to provide guidance about obtaining gluten-free products and their preparation. The publications of the Coeliac Society are very helpful for the patient in recognizing obscure sources of gluten. After introduction of the diet, the mucosa heals from distal to proximal, with the duodenum the last to recover; this will require around 3 months, and thereafter nutritional supplementation can be withdrawn. Diet should be lifelong since there is some evidence that the known small risk of supervening intestinal malignant lymphoma may be reduced by strict dieting. Failure of response to gluten withdrawal requires specialist investigation.

Repeat biopsy to confirm healing after gluten withdrawal is wise but not strictly necessary, except in obscure cases.

The colon and rectum

Anatomy and physiology

The colon extends from the ileocaecal valve proximally to the rectum and anus distally.

The colon receives around 1500 ml of semi-liquid material from the ileum daily, and reduces this to around 200–250 g of faeces by the reabsorption of water. Stool volume is also very dependent on the diet, especially its fibre content. Frequency of evacuation varies widely in normal individuals but is usually once every day or every 2 days. Altered bowel function should always be assessed against the pre-existing norm for any individual patient. The commonest symptoms are constipation and diarrhoea.

Other important bowel symptoms include colicky lower abdominal pain, the passage of blood or mucus per rectum, painful defaecation and tenesmus (painful ineffective straining at stool).

Investigation

Clinical assessment in patients with altered bowel function should include a careful general and abdominal examination, and digital examination of the rectum. Proctoscopy and rigid sigmoidoscopy still have an important place in the visualization of the rectum and sigmoid colon. Radiology by barium enema can give excellent pictures of the colon, especially if air is insufflated after barium evacuation (double-contrast enema). Flexible colonoscopy is increasingly the investigation of choice, and in most cases can visualize the colon to the ileocaecal valve or even higher; biopsy is an additional advantage of endoscopy.

Constipation

Constipation is usually defined as the infrequent or difficult passage of hard stools, and can be confirmed clinically by their presence in the rectum on clinical examination. Some causes are given in Table 10.3. Acute intestinal obstruction may present with total failure to pass faeces or flatus.

Diarrhoea

Diarrhoea is characterized by the increased passage of loose or watery motions; in malabsorption,

Table 10.3 Some causes of constipation
Poor muscle function and physical immobility, especially in old age
Low dietary fibre
Organic obstruction, often due to stricture formation
Carcinoma
Diverticular disease
Inflammatory bowel disease
Drugs
Anticholinergics
Antidepressants
Painful defaecation, e.g. anal fissure
Neuropsychiatric
Depression
Parkinson's disease
Metabolic – hypothyroidism
Functional – irritable bowel syndrome

Table 10.4 Some causes of diarrhoea	
Acute infections[a]	Pathogenic *Escherichia coli*
	Campylobacter spp
	Shigella spp – dysentery
	Salmonella spp
	Gastroenteritis, food poisoning
	Typhoid, paratyphoid
	Cholera
	Staphylococcus aureus food poisoning
	Viruses, e.g. rotaviruses, adenoviruses
	Cryptosporidium in HIV-infected patients
Chronic infection	Tuberculosis
	Amoebiasis
	Giardiasis
Drugs	Antibiotics
	Purgative abuse
Inflammatory bowel disease	Crohn's disease
	Ulcerative colitis
Diverticular disease of colon	
Malabsorption	
Iritable bowel syndrome	

[a]Clinical effects are induced not only by the presence of infectious organisms but also by the endotoxins they produce.

steatorrhoea also causes soft bulky stools which are often buttery and offensive. Some examples of causes of diarrhoea are given in Table 10.4.

Carcinoma of the colon

This is a very frequent malignancy, virtually confined to Western Europe and North America. In most cases the aetiology is unknown, although malignant change can supervene on pre-existing simple adenomatous polyps, in familial adenomatous polyposis (see Chs 12 and 26), or in patients with chronic inflammatory bowel disease. In these patients, regular colonoscopy is advisable, and occasionally prophylactic colectomy is performed. The geographical distribution suggests a pathogenic role for low fibre and high animal fat content in the diet.

Involvement is commonest in the rectum, less so in the sigmoid colon, and less frequently still in the right side of the colon. These tumours initially involve the bowel wall only, but later may spread locally outside the gut to the lymph nodes and liver. Patients commonly present with altered bowel habit, passage of blood or mucus, anorexia or weight loss, intestinal obstruction, or iron deficiency anaemia from chronic blood loss. Peritoneal involvement may produce ascites.

Treatment is by surgical removal, either with restoration of bowel continuity, or, if this is not possible, by removal of a segment of colon and the establishment of a permanent colostomy on the abdominal wall, draining into a colostomy bag.

The overall cure rate is around 25%, but in early cases without spread, can be as high as 80%. Early diagnosis is thus essential, and there is much current interest in population screening, e.g. by stool testing for occult blood.

Diverticular disease

The primary abnormality is the herniation of mucosa outwards through the bowel wall, usually at weak spots where blood vessels traverse the submucosa (Fig. 10.3). Involvement of the sigmoid colon is most frequent, but diverticulae can occur at any point. The condition increases with age over 30 years, and can be found in 50% of screened asymptomatic populations. Although the cause is not entirely clear, it is confined largely to western countries, and is probably associated with altered pressure effects in the colon resulting from the reduced stool volume of low-fibre diets.

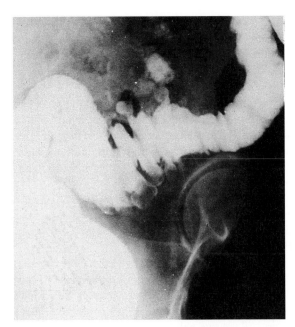

Fig. 10.3 Barium enema radiograph of a patient with diverticular disease. Note the outpouchings of barium. Unrelated calcified abdominal lymph nodes are also visible.

Clinical features

Symptoms may arise when inflammation occurs in the diverticula (diverticulitis). This may result in diarrhoea, rectal bleeding, local abscess formation or perforation with generalized peritonitis, and strictures with obstruction.

Management

Patients with uncomplicated diverticular disease should be given a high-fibre diet and reassured. Surgery may be required for the complications.

Inflammatory bowel disease

This condition exists in two main forms – ulcerative colitis and Crohn's disease. Both are characterized by chronic inflammatory changes of unknown aetiology in the gastrointestinal tract. Though both are usually considered together, most patients can be separated into one or the other on clinical and histological grounds.

Crohn's disease

The disease first received its definitive description in 1932 by Crohn, who recognized its predilection for the terminal ileum. The disease can affect any part of the gastrointestinal tract from the oral cavity to the anus, but classically it involves both the small and large bowel in discrete areas (skip lesions) and does not produce continuous involvement along the length of the gut. The bowel wall becomes thickened and often stenosed. Histologically it is heavily infiltrated with chronic inflammatory cells throughout all coats, from the mucosa out to the serosal surface, and is associated with oedematous thickening and hyperaemia. Characteristic non-caseating granulomas occur in around 60% of cases.

Clinical features due to local bowel involvement. Diarrhoea, abdominal pain and weight loss are characteristic; chronic blood loss may lead to iron deficiency anaemia, but overt rectal bleeding is less common. Spread of inflammation to the serosal surface may cause adhesions to adjacent structures, with the production of palpable abdominal masses, and fistulae to other bowel loops, to the urinary tract or to the abdominal wall. Fibrous strictures in the submucosa may lead to subacute or acute intestinal obstruction. Extensive small bowel involvement may lead to malabsorption with impaired nutrition, which can become gross; preferential involvement of the terminal ileum may lead to steatorrhoea on the basis of impaired bile salt reabsorption and to vitamin B_{12} deficiency. Acute cases involving the ileum may mimic acute appendicitis. Direct involvement of the mouth is described elsewhere (see Ch. 26).

Extraintestinal manifestations. Clinical abnormalities distant from the gut are common in both forms of chronic inflammatory bowel disease. These include recurrent aphthae, erythema nodosum and pyoderma gangrenosum, pyostomatitis vegetans (see Ch. 26), inflammatory eye complications (uveitis, conjunctivitis and episcleritis), sacroiliitis and ankylosing spondylitis, and various forms of liver disease. Not all these complications are necessarily associated with disease activity in the bowel.

Diagnosis. This is made by small bowel barium enema, which shows characteristic mucosal abnormalities, and by colonoscopy with biopsy. Rectal biopsy is often helpful even in patients without overt rectal involvement.

Aetiology. This remains unknown despite intensive investigation of dietary antigens, possible infective agents, local vascular factors and immunological disease; it generally commences in young adults, has an equal sex incidence, and is commoner in smokers.

Management. The disease runs a remitting and relapsing course, is potentially lifelong, and patients can never be regarded as definitely cured. A team approach, with nutritionists, physicians and surgeons, is best. The effects of malabsorption and malnutrition should be identified and corrected. Corticosteroids to suppress the inflammatory reaction are the mainstay of drug treatment. The benefit of 5-aminosalicylic acid (5-ASA) is less well defined than in ulcerative colitis, and formal immunosuppression with azathioprine or cyclosporin A needs further evaluation. Surgery may be required for strictures, fistulae, abscess or perforation. Maintenance of high morale is essential in this chronic debilitating condition.

Ulcerative colitis

Unlike Crohn's disease, this condition involves the colon only; the rectum is always affected, 40% of cases have sigmoid involvement, and pancolitis (involving the whole large bowel) occurs in 20%. The onset is typically between 20 and 40 years, and unlike Crohn's disease there is no recent increase in incidence.

The inflammatory process involves only the mucosa, which is initially hyperaemic, oedematous and granular. Infiltration of inflammatory cells affects the crypts, with the formation of microabscesses, and eventually ulceration of the overlying mucosa develops. In chronic cases, the mucous membrane becomes atrophic and featureless.

Clinical features. Although the disease may occasionally present in an acute or even fulminating form suggestive of a severe infective colitis, most patients have a more gradual course. Diarrhoea is the most prominent symptom, often by day and night, with rectal bleeding, passage of mucus and tenesmus; abdominal pain and the passage of pus are less common. Weight loss often occurs, and in cases with severe diarrhoea, loss of

fluid and electrolyte becomes an important feature. Iron deficiency anaemia may result from chronic blood loss, and protein loss from the inflamed mucosa may lead to hypoalbuminaemia with clinical oedema.

Extraintestinal manifestations are similar to those found in Crohn's disease. Complications in acute cases include massive haemorrhage, perforation or acute colonic dilatation, and in more chronic cases, strictures or supervening malignancy.

Diagnosis. The diagnosis is based on the appearance at endoscopy with biopsy confirmation. A characteristic barium enema is shown in Figure 10.4.

Aetiology. Again, the cause remains unknown despite investigation of the aetiological factors described above for Crohn's disease. Paradoxically, smoking appears to exert some protective effect against ulcerative colitis.

Management. Medical management is influenced by the acuteness or chronicity of the disease, and also by the extent of colonic involvement. Useful drugs include corticosteroids systemically or in retention enema, and 5-ASA containing drugs orally. Severe disease is danger-

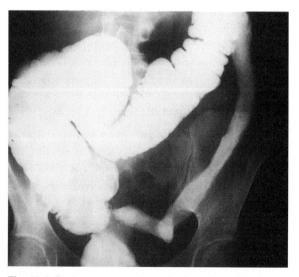

Fig. 10.4 Barium enema radiograph of a patient with chronic ulcerative colitis. Note the featureless 'tube-like' sigmoid and descending colon with loss of haustrations.

ous, and the patient requires hospital admission. After clinical remission is achieved, maintenance with 5-ASA drugs such as sulphasalazine is useful. Surgery is required for severe cases unresponsive to medical therapy and for chronic active disease where there is an additional risk of malignancy. For many years, operation involved total colectomy with permanent ileostomy; more recently, the preferred procedure is conservation of the lower rectum with the fashioning of an ileal pouch anastomosed to the remaining anal canal.

Irritable bowel syndrome

Many patients present with gut symptoms for which no organic cause can be determined and these are usually included under the general title of functional bowel disorder or irritable bowel syndrome. Up to half of patients attending specialized gastroenterology clinics are classifiable in this way. Despite quite extensive investigation into aetiology, no unitary hypothesis has yet emerged to explain the manifestations. However, some clinical features suggest a basis in abnormally reactive smooth muscle, with both intestinal hurry and stagnation, a possible lowered threshold to pain stimuli arising in the gut, dietary triggers and psychosomatic mechanisms altering autonomic function.

Symptoms include abdominal pain, constipation with low-volume pellety stools, diarrhoea and the passage of mucus, and often functional dyspepsia suggestive of upper gastrointestinal involvement as well. While all these features may individually suggest the possibility of significant organic disease, a diagnosis of irritable bowel syndrome is usually possible on clinical grounds alone, without the need for extensive invasive investigation.

Management consists of strong reassurance, dietary advice including increased fibre for those with constipation, and advice to avoid excess alcohol and the use of purgatives. Drugs should play only a minor and temporary role, and include antispasmodics and relaxants for pain, bulking agents for constipation, antinauseants, and antidepressants if indicated.

Gastrointestinal bleeding

Acute gastrointestinal bleeding

This is a common medical emergency. Bleeding from the oesophagus, stomach or duodenum presents through haematemesis (vomiting fresh red blood or blood altered to brown or black by contact with gastric juice) and/or melaena, the passage of tarry black, partially digested material in the stools. Red blood per rectum usually indicates a source distally in the large bowel, rectum or anus. Large-volume blood loss indicates erosion of a major vessel, artery or vein, and is frequently associated with clinical signs of shock (see Ch. 6). With a combined medical/surgical approach the majority of patients do well, but mortality rises significantly over the age of 65 years.

Chronic gastrointestinal bleeding

Chronic low-volume blood loss from the gut is also common, and unless from the rectum cannot be recognized by the patient. Such long-continued occult bleeding is a frequent cause of iron deficiency anaemia (see Ch. 7), and requires special stool testing to detect (faecal occult blood test). Any presentation with iron deficiency anaemia should prompt careful consideration of underlying undeclared gastrointestinal tract pathology.

Causes of gastrointestinal tract bleeding

These are summarized in Figure 10.5. The majority of these conditions are dealt with elsewhere in this text. Haemorrhoids are the commonest cause.

Haemorrhoids (piles)

Haemorrhoids occur as a result of distension or varicosity of the anal veins; these veins contain no valves, and the upright posture of humans, requiring drainage of blood upwards against gravity, ensures the uniqueness of the condition in our species. Haemorrhoids may lie outside the anal orifice or internally within the anal canal; clinical manifestations are most frequent with internal haemorrhoids. Some possible causes are shown in Table 10.5.

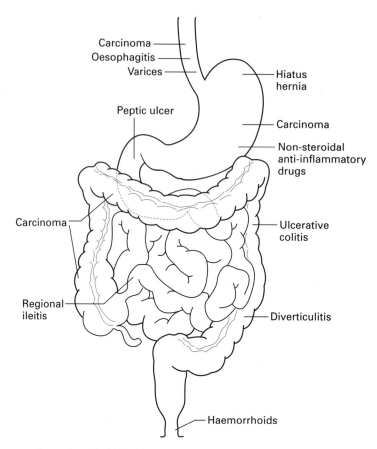

Fig. 10.5 The main sources of gastrointestinal blood loss.

Clinical features. Patients usually present with recurrent rectal bleeding, during or following defaecation; in chronic cases, iron deficiency anaemia is a characteristic feature. Eventually the haemorrhoids may prolapse transiently during defaecation, or even remain permanently prolapsed. Pain is usually not a prominent complaint unless prolapsed haemorrhoids become 'strangulated' by anal sphincter tone.

Management. It is important not to accept patients' proffered explanations of rectal bleeding as due to 'piles', and all patients should be properly examined and assessed to exclude more serious pathology in the rectum. Avoidance of constipation and the achievement of soft, regular stools may suffice in mild cases. Alternatively, the veins can be injected with sclerosant via a proctoscope, ligated or excised surgically.

Liver and biliary tract

Anatomy and physiology

The liver is the largest solid organ in the body, with a weight of around 1.5 kg in adult life. It

---

Table 10.5 Some possible causes of internal haemorrhoids

Familial – association of haemorrhoids and varicose veins
Straining, e.g. chronic constipation, urinary tract obstruction
Pregnancy
Portal hypertension – theoretically possible but a valid association is not supported by clinical experience

receives blood from the hepatic artery, and from the portal vein; the hepatic veins drain directly into the inferior vena cava. The biliary system collects bile from the liver, concentrates it in the gall bladder, and delivers it to the duodenum. The main right and left hepatic ducts unite to form the common bile duct in the liver hilum; this then passes down in close relationship to the head of the pancreas, and opens into the gut lumen through a small papilla in the duodenal wall, guarded by the sphincter of Oddi.

Microscopically, arterial and portal blood enter the liver lobule through the portal tracts. Blood can then pass along sinusoids between the plates of liver cells, and then drain by the central vein of each lobule. This arrangement allows a close relationship between blood and the hepatocyte surface, and facilitates exchange between them. The sinusoids are also lined by stationary macrophages (Kupffer cells). Biliary canaliculi run away from the hepatocytes, and coalesce into larger biliary vessels, situated again in the portal tracts.

The liver subserves a complex series of functions, which are summarized below.

Bile pigment metabolism

This involves the uptake by the liver of bilirubin derived from haemoglobin catabolism, its conjugation with glucuronic acid to render it water-soluble, and thereafter its secretion in the bile.

Bile salt synthesis

These salts are conjugates of cholic and chenodeoxycholic acids, and on reaching the gut via the bile, have an important role in emulsifying ingested fat and facilitating fat absorption. They are reabsorbed in the terminal ileum and re-excreted via the bile (enterohepatic circulation).

Protein metabolism

The liver synthesizes almost all the plasma proteins from absorbed amino acids and from muscle. It also regulates plasma amino acid levels by controlling gluconeogenesis.

Carbohydrate metabolism

Glucose derived from digested carbohydrate is stored as glycogen, the main glucose source in starvation. These functions are under the influence of insulin, corticosteroids, glucagon and catecholamines.

Lipid metabolism

The liver synthesizes and secretes lipoproteins, designed to carry the major plasma lipids in soluble macromolecular complexes. A rise in the plasma free cholesterol level is seen where there is obstruction to free bile flow.

Drug metabolism

Many drugs, particularly those which are fat-soluble and of high molecular weight, are altered and cleared by the liver, and care should always be taken in administering drugs to patients with liver disease. Conversely, there is an increasing number of drugs recognized to damage the liver through a wide variety of mechanisms.

Blood coagulation

Several important clotting factors (see Ch. 7) are synthesized in the liver under the action of vitamin K, and impaired coagulation is an important feature of liver disease (see also obstructive jaundice).

Investigation of liver disease

Clinical history and physical examination is as important as in all other systems, and must accompany interpretation of other tests.

Serum liver function tests (see Table 10.6)

Liver ultrasound

This is successful in assessing liver size, bile duct calibre, and the presence of gallstones and tumours.

Table 10.6 Biochemical tests of liver function

Mechanism	Serum concentrations
Tests reflecting impaired synthesis	↓ Albumin ↓ Coagulation factors (prolonged prothrombin time)
Tests reflecting diminished excretion (cholestasis)	↑ Bilirubin ↑ Alkaline phosphatase ↑ γ-Glutamyl transferase
Tests reflecting hepatic cell necrosis	↑ Aspartate aminotransferase ↑ Alanine aminotransferase

↑, increased; ↓, decreased.

Isotope scanning

This is also useful for assessing liver size, and the presence of space-occupying lesions greater than 2 cm in diameter.

Computerized tomography and magnetic resonance imaging

These provide excellent views of liver structure and the presence of tumours.

Contrast radiology

This is useful for demonstrating biliary tract disease. The common bile duct and pancreatic duct can also now be canalized endoscopically and good images obtained.

Liver biopsy

This is performed by a percutaneous needle technique usually under local anaesthesia; unfortunately it is often contraindicated by coagulation abnormalities. It is, however, an important diagnostic tool both for intrinsic liver disease and also for systemic diseases involving the liver.

Immunological testing

Useful serum antibodies include smooth muscle antibody, often positive in non-viral chronic active hepatitis, and antimitochondrial antibody found in primary biliary cirrhosis.

Jaundice (icterus)

This term is applied to the yellow coloration of patients with elevated serum bilirubin levels; the skin, mucous membranes and sclerae of the eyes are affected. Normally the serum bilirubin level must rise above twice normal for clinically detectable icterus to appear. Mild jaundice may thus be difficult to detect but as it deepens very profound shades of yellow or even green may appear.

Jaundice may occur in three ways:

Haemolytic jaundice

This occurs in haemolytic disease (see Ch. 7) where the increased load of unconjugated bilirubin derived from excess haemoglobin catabolism is beyond the capacity of the liver to conjugate and excrete it. This unconjugated bilirubin is attached to plasma albumin, and it does not appear in the urine (acholuric jaundice). Stools and urine are normal in colour, but the increased urobilinogen being formed in the gut is subsequently reabsorbed and excreted, and can be measured in the urine. The coexistence of anaemic pallor may result in a lemon-yellow skin colour.

Obstructive jaundice

This implies obstruction to the free flow of bile (cholestasis), and can either be intrahepatic, where liver disease itself is responsible, or extrahepatic in the main bile duct system. Cholestatic jaundice may also be produced by some drugs, e.g. chlorpromazine.

In such patients the stools are pale, and because conjugated bilirubin (water-soluble) can be reabsorbed from the blocked bile ducts, it appears in the urine. Since free excretion of bile salts is also impaired, defective fat digestion occurs with resulting steatorrhoea; bile salts can also be reabsorbed from the obstructed biliary system and cause severe generalized itching (pruritus). Vitamin K is fat-soluble, and the steatorrhoea of obstructive jaundice may lead to malabsorption of vitamin K and resulting impaired synthesis of vitamin K-dependent clotting factors (see Ch. 7).

Hepatocellular jaundice

Serum bilirubin levels rise both in acute hepatitis and in chronic liver disease, occasionally from failure of conjugation but usually from inability to excrete bilirubin after conjugation has occurred. Where a cholestatic element is present in the hepatocellular jaundice, pale stools, dark urine and pruritus may result.

Acute hepatitis

The commonest cause of hepatitis worldwide is viral infection, and liver disease due to infection with hepatitis A, B, C and D has already been discussed (see Ch. 5); in most cases these are self-limiting illnesses, but a minority of patients may progress to chronic active hepatitis or cirrhosis. Other infective agents associated with hepatitis include Epstein–Barr virus (glandular fever), the arbovirus agent causing yellow fever, and the causative agent of Weil's disease (*Leptospira icterohaemorrhagica*).

In developed countries, alcohol abuse is now a common cause of acute hepatitis either de novo or superimposed on pre-existing chronic liver disease. In addition, some drugs may induce hepatitis; important examples include accidental or deliberate overdose of paracetamol, and repeated exposures to halothane anaesthesia.

A few patients with hepatitis may progress to massive liver cell necrosis and fulminant hepatic failure. This life-threatening event requires inten-

sive support, and consideration of liver replacement therapy by transplantation.

Chronic liver disease

Harmful sublethal insults to the liver continued over a period of time lead to hepatic cirrhosis; pathologically this is characterized by fibrosis of the liver accompanied by regenerating nodules of hepatocytes. The liver eventually becomes shrunken and scarred, resulting in chronic hepatocellular failure, portal hypertension, and hepatic neuroencephalopathy.

Chronic hepatocellular failure

This is usually of gradual onset. The patients look well until late in the disease when muscle wasting and emaciation may become severe. Specific clinical features are indicated in Table 10.7.

Deep jaundice is a bad prognostic sign in chronic liver disease.

Ascites

Excessive fluid within the peritoneal cavity, an important sign of chronic liver failure, results from hypoalbuminaemia, increased portal venous pressure, and retention of salt and water. The quantity may be slight, but can become enormous, leading to gross abdominal distension (Fig. 10.6). Ascites may also result from infection such as tuberculosis, malignant involvement of the peritoneum, other causes of profound hypoproteinaemia, and right heart failure. Important diagnostic information can be obtained by needle aspiration for biochemical, bacteriological and cytological examination of the fluid.

Portal hypertension

In hepatic cirrhosis, narrowing of the sinusoids by the disease process results in impedance to the flow of portal blood through the liver. This in turn leads to portal venous hypertension, causing splenomegaly and, more importantly, the opening up of communications between the portal and systemic venous systems. Varicosities develop at these sites, principally at the lower end of the

Table 10.7 Some features of chronic liver disease

Clinical feature	Mechanism
Jaundice	Impaired bilirubin excretion
Oedema Ascites	Impaired protein synthesis, hypoalbuminaemia Secondary hyperaldosteronism
Spider naevi Testicular atrophy Gynaecomastia	Abnormal processing of endogenous oestrogen
Leuconychia ('white nails')	Hypoalbuminaemia
Bruising, bleeding	Impaired synthesis of coagulation factors
Hypoglycaemia	Reduced glycogen stores
Diarrhoea, steatorrhoea	Impaired bile salt excretion, fat malabsorption
Pruritus	Bile salt retention

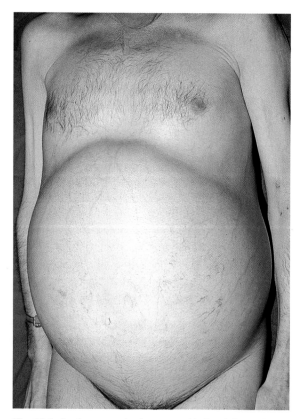

Fig. 10.6 Ascites occurring in a man with liver failure. Note the gross abdominal distention.

oesophagus, and catastrophic bleeding may follow if the portal pressure continues to rise.

Portal hypertension may also arise in patients with no liver pathology from obstruction or thrombosis of the portal vein itself.

Hepatic neuroencephalopathy

This syndrome results from two coexisting processes, i.e. significant reduction in functioning liver tissue, and diversion of blood via porta-systemic collaterals. The precise mechanism of the clinical neurological features is still debated, but is thought to be due to the products of protein digestion in the gut, unmodified by abnormally-functioning liver, reaching the systemic circulation. Such toxic substances appear capable of damaging brain metabolism. In susceptible patients, a high-protein diet, bleeding into the gut, catabolic processes such as trauma or infection, and an alcoholic binge are all important precipitants. Almost any neurological deficits can be produced, but apathy, disturbed consciousness, spatial disorientation, a flapping tremor of the hands, and even coma are characteristic. The syndrome is associated with a poor outlook.

Causes of chronic liver disease

Alcohol. Alcohol is a direct hepatotoxin, but liver damage is only likely at consumptions exceeding 20–30 units weekly. Factors increasing susceptibility include a genetic component, female sex, poor nutrition, and coexisting liver pathology. Liver function tests are unpredictable, but an elevated γ-glutamyl transferase level and macrocytosis with normal vitamin B_{12} and folate levels are useful diagnostic tools in the pre-symptomatic stage. There is no specific treatment, and withdrawal of alcohol is vital.

Chronic active hepatitis. This picture results mainly from chronic viral infection, and is especially associated with hepatitis B and C; in the former there is a particular risk of active inflammation progressing to cirrhosis. Treatment strategies include α-interferon, antiviral drugs such as ribavirin and liver transplantation.

There is also an autoimmune form of chronic active hepatitis, occurring mainly in women; this may be associated with autoimmune multisystem manifestations elsewhere. Antinuclear and anti-smooth muscle antibody tests are often positive. It can be treated with corticosteroids or azathioprine, but carries an unfavourable long-term prognosis.

Liver function tests are compatible with active liver cell necrosis.

Primary biliary cirrhosis. This is an autoimmune condition, initially causing inflammatory destruction of bile canaliculi, and then progressing to cirrhosis. It occurs predominantly in women, and the patients have a high incidence of antimitochondrial antibodies. The clinical picture and biochemical tests are dominated by evidence of intrahepatic cholestasis, and the patients thus present with obstructive jaundice, pruritus, steatorrhoea, and hypercholesterolaemia.

The course of the disease is slowly progressive; trials of immunosuppressive therapy have proved unrewarding, and definitive therapy is liver transplantation.

Rarer causes. Primary haemochromatosis is a genetic defect allowing absorption of inappropriate amounts of iron from the diet (see Ch. 7); much of the excess iron is stored in the liver and the patients present with hepatic cirrhosis in middle life. There is damage to other organs, including pancreatic islets and other endocrine glands.

Women are protected to some extent by the iron losses of menstruation. A regular venesection programme is the most effective means of iron removal.

Wilson's disease is a genetic defect associated with the accumulation of copper in the liver and nervous system (hepatolenticular degeneration). Patients usually present with juvenile hepatic disease, initially with a histological picture similar to chronic active hepatitis, but eventually progressing to cirrhosis. The neurological picture is dominated by movement disorders. Copper removal by chelating agents, e.g. penicillamine, should be introduced as early as possible.

Treatment of chronic liver disease

Much can be achieved by removing or modifying the underlying cause, and by treating individual manifestations of hepatic insufficiency as they arise. Crisis management is required for bleeding oesophageal varices, and for hepatic neuroencephalopathy.

The indications for liver transplantation are acute hepatic necrosis, e.g. after paracetamol overdose, and end-stage liver disease where pathology is confined to the liver alone, e.g. primary biliary cirrhosis. Carefully selected patients with other forms of chronic liver disease are also suitable. Alcoholic cirrhotics produce few candidates suitable for transplantation.

Hepatic tumours

Liver involvement in malignancy usually occurs because of metastasis from primary tumours elsewhere. These are principally carcinoma of the stomach, bowel, pancreas, lung and breast. In Europe, primary liver cancer is rare, although it can complicate hepatic cirrhosis of any cause; because of its association with chronic hepatitis B and C infection, however, its incidence is geographically much higher where these viruses are endemic. The prognosis of both primary and secondary hepatocellular carcinoma is poor.

Gallstones

Bile contains high concentrations of cholesterol, phospholipids and bile salts; stones probably arise because of supersaturation of the bile with one or other constituent; the relationship of cholesterol to bile salt concentrations appears to be critical. Risk factors include a positive family history, female sex, lower socioeconomic class, and the use of oral contraceptives.

Gallstones remain asymptomatic in the gall bladder, but stones migrating through the cystic or common bile duct give rise to biliary colic, an agonizing right-sided abdominal pain. Impaction of stones in the cystic duct may lead to acute cholecystitis, and in the common bile duct to obstructive jaundice with a risk of ascending infection (cholangitis).

Treatment is surgical, consisting of exploration and drainage of the common bile duct and cholecystectomy. Modern non-invasive approaches to gallstone disease include laparoscopic cholecystectomy, dissolution of stones by external lithotripsy or drugs (chenodeoxycholate), and the removal of common bile duct stones by retrograde endoscopy via the duodenum.

Cholecystitis

Acute cholecystitis results from obstruction of the cystic duct or common bile duct by gallstones. Infection, often with *Escherichia coli*, develops behind the obstruction, and the patient presents acutely ill with right hypochondrial pain, tenderness, fever and prostration; coexisting jaundice implies a stone in the common bile duct. Treatment is either by immediate cholecystectomy, or by conservative therapy with fluids, antibiotics and analgesics followed by cholecystectomy at a later date.

Chronic cholecystitis is often demonstrable histologically in gall bladders containing stones. It is conventional to attribute flatulent dyspepsia following fatty meals to this cause, but convincing proof is lacking.

Biliary tract tumours

Cancer is uncommon in the biliary tree; gallstones represent a weak risk factor. Tumours usually present with painless obstructive jaundice and pruritus. Surgery is technically difficult, and the results are poor.

Diseases of the pancreas

The endocrine function of the pancreas is dealt with in Chapter 13. This section is concerned purely with the exocrine or digestive portion of the organ, which makes up 99% of its bulk. Damage to the pancreas usually results in exocrine failure before endocrine function is affected.

The pancreas is situated retroperitoneally. The microstructure is acinar, and its secretions are channelled through the main pancreatic duct (conjoined with the common bile duct after leaving the pancreas) into the duodenum. The pancreatic juice is rich in bicarbonate, and contains enzymes concerned in the digestive breakdown of fats (lipase), protein (trypsin) and starches (amylase). Pancreatic failure is thus characterized by malabsorption, in particular affecting fats.

Acute pancreatitis

This is an acute inflammatory condition resulting in necrosis of the gland, causing release of its enzymes into the circulation; elevated levels of serum amylase are thus a useful diagnostic test. The patient is severely ill, with abdominal pain radiating through to the back, vomiting and collapse. The condition has many aetiological factors, but the majority of patients have biliary tract disease or abuse alcohol. Acute pancreatitis is a life-threatening condition, but fortunately the majority of patients settle after 48 h with supportive management. Recurrences can be reduced by identifying and removing the underlying cause.

Chronic pancreatitis

This is associated with destruction of pancreatic tissue. The inflammatory component is low-grade, but the gland eventually becomes fibrotic and atrophic. The majority of patients abuse alcohol, and biliary tract disease is less important than in acute pancreatitis.

Patients present with relapsing upper abdominal pain, gross steatorrhoea and malabsorption of the fat-soluble vitamins A, D, E and K. There may be coexisting alcoholic hepatic cirrhosis.

Management consists of forbidding alcohol, a low fat diet, and the use of oral pancreatic enzyme supplements.

Cystic fibrosis

Cystic fibrosis is a common autosomal recessive disorder caused by defective chloride transport, reflected by diminished sodium reabsorption from, and diminished water transport into, mucus secretions. This in turn leads to increased mucus viscidity, which 'clogs' the ducts of secretory glands, especially in the gut of the newborn and in the lungs and pancreas of older children and surviving adults.

The condition may thus present in the neonatal period with meconium ileus, i.e. intestinal obstruction on the basis of very tenacious meconium. The majority of patients survive infancy, to present later with failure to thrive, chest disease, and malabsorption on the basis of pancreatic insufficiency. The malabsorption can be managed by oral pancreatic enzyme replacement therapy. The pulmonary effects are more serious as a challenge to life.

Gene therapy for the condition is under active investigation.

Carcinoma of the pancreas

This is a major cause of mortality, the more so because symptoms usually only occur late in the disease. The aetiology is unknown, and there is no link with preceding pancreatitis; there is a statistical link with cigarette smoking and with diabetes mellitus.

The classic presenting symptom is painless obstructive jaundice with pruritus. Anorexia and weight loss, back pain from local invasion, and metastases in the liver are sadly often present before diagnosis can be made. Even with extensive surgery the late results remain poor.

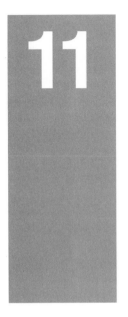

11 Disorders of the kidney and urinary tract

Introduction

A discussion of the anatomy, physiology, and investigation of the kidneys and urinary tract will be followed by consideration of the important disorders (Table 11.1).

Anatomy and physiology

The kidneys lie retroperitoneally, high in the posterior part of the abdomen, around the level of T12 to L1; each measures approximately 12 cm in length. A longitudinal section is shown in Figure 11.1. The naked eye can easily recognize the subdivisions of the parenchyma into cortex and medulla; the papillae project into the minor calyces, which unite to form major calyces and then the urinary pelvis itself. The latter merges into the ureter, conveying urine to the bladder. The hilum also contains the renal artery and vein to deliver and remove the abundant blood supply.

The functional unit of the kidney is the nephron (Fig. 11.2); there are around 1 million of these in each kidney. The glomerulus is a tuft of capillaries with an afferent and an efferent arteriole; it invaginates Bowman's capsule, the expanded end of the proximal renal tubule. A basement membrane lies between the capillary

Table 11.1 Disorders of the kidneys and urinary tract

Renal failure
Glomerulonephritis
Urinary tract infection
Renal calculus
Prostatic hypertrophy
Tumours
Polycystic kidneys

endothelium and the renal epithelium, this triad forming the 'glomerular sieve' and allowing intimate contact between the blood and epithelial cells. The tubule comprises the proximal convoluted tubule, the loop of Henle, and the distal convoluted tubule. Urine is carried by the collecting tubules to the calyces and renal pelvis.

Formation of urine

Glomerular filtrate

The differential resistance to flow in afferent and efferent arterioles leads to a high capillary pressure within the glomerulus. This favours the movement of water and other constituents from blood plasma to Bowman's space. A normal individual forms around 180 litres of glomerular filtrate daily, similar in composition to plasma except that it is free of fat and virtually free of protein.

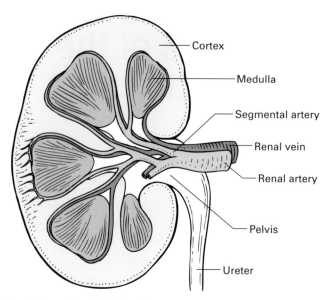

Fig. 11.1 The appearance of the kidney on longitudinal section.

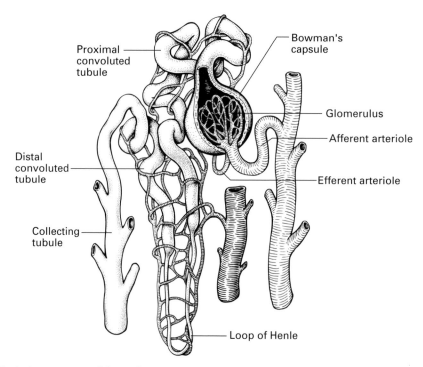

Fig. 11.2 The principal components of the nephron.

Tubular action

Glomerular filtrate is modified in the tubules as follows:

- the volume is reduced by reabsorption of water

- other substances of value (e.g. glucose and electrolytes) are wholly or partly reabsorbed
- certain substances can be secreted into the filtrate by the tubular cells e.g. hydrogen ions in the regulation of acid–base balance, and creatinine.

The average urine volume in 24 h is around 1000–1500 ml, but this varies very widely under physiological conditions. Urine does not normally contain sugar or protein.

Functions of the kidney

The functions of the kidney are described below.

Excretion of waste products of metabolism

Examples of excreted waste products of metabolism are urea, creatinine, urate, oxalate and phosphate.

Excretion of substances ingested in excess of requirement

Examples of substances that are excreted when ingested in excess are water, sodium, potassium and calcium.

Regulation of homeostasis.

Total body water. This is kept constant largely by the sensitivity of the hypothalamus to extracellular fluid osmolality. Any increase in the latter stimulates production of antidiuretic hormone (vasopressin) by the posterior pituitary; this acts on the distal tubule by increasing its permeability to water and thus enhances water reabsorption. In the absence of antidiuretic hormone (diabetes insipidus), the tubule becomes relatively impermeable to water, which is then excreted in excess.

Sodium. Most filtered sodium is reabsorbed in the proximal tubule iso-osmotically. Control of sodium excretion is exerted in the distal tubule, where reabsorption is under the active control of the renin–angiotensin system and aldosterone; these hormones promote sodium reabsorption. In addition, there is a powerful peptide from the atria of the heart that increases sodium excretion (atrial natriuretic peptide).

Potassium. This is also under the control of aldosterone, which acts on the distal tubule to increase potassium excretion.

Acid–base balance. This is achieved by appropriate reabsorption of bicarbonate in the proximal convoluted tubule and the secretion of hydrogen ions in the distal convoluted tubule. Respiration also has an important role in acid–base balance.

Hormone production

Some hormone-dependent renal functions are listed above. In addition, however, the kidney itself synthesizes several important hormones.

Erythropoietin. This hormone increases red cell differentiation and production by the bone marrow. Secretion is stimulated by renal hypoxia.

1,25-Dihydroxy vitamin D. This is formed by the kidney from 25-hydroxy vitamin D; failure of this conversion leads to a characteristic type of osteomalacia found in renal failure (renal osteodystrophy).

Renin/angiotensin. Renin production by the kidney is stimulated by reduced renal blood flow, leading in turn to increased production of angiotensin II; this promotes aldosterone secretion, sodium reabsorption and potassium loss. This system has an important role in renal hypertension and heart failure.

Drug excretion

The kidney excretes water-soluble drugs, mostly of low molecular weight.

Diagnosis of renal and urinary tract disorders

The principal symptoms include abnormalities of passing urine (micturition), the passage of increased (polyuria) or reduced (oliguria or anuria) amounts of urine, alterations in the urine itself such as haematuria, and pain arising in the kidney, ureters, bladder or urethra.

Signs include oedema, the presence of hypertension and its effects, anaemia, abdominal tenderness over masses arising in the kidneys, bladder distension and, in men, prostatic enlargement on rectal examination.

Urine

Much important information depends on careful examination of the urine, e.g. the urine volume in

24 h, the specific gravity, the appearance, chemical testing, especially for protein and sugar, microscopic examination of the deposit for blood and cells, and urine culture for infection.

Renal function

Useful information is obtainable from simple biochemical quantification of the plasma, especially the urea and electrolytes, bicarbonate levels and the hydrogen ion concentration.

Imaging

Plain radiography of the abdomen may show stones, but intravenous urography produces more informative pictures of the kidney, ureter and bladder, and is also helpful in assessing excretory function. Retrograde urography via a catheter passed into the ureters at cystoscopy is also useful.

Additional imaging can be obtained by ultrasonography, computerized tomography, arteriography, and radioisotope renography.

Endoscopy

Cystoscopy is the standard procedure for visualization of the lower urinary tract, especially of the bladder and prostate; it also allows biopsy. Needle aspiration of the prostate can also be performed at rectal examination.

Renal biopsy

Needle biopsy through the loin under local anaesthesia is useful in carefully selected cases, especially for the diagnosis of glomerular disease. Safeguards include ultrasound guidance, control of bleeding disorders and careful selection and preparation of the patients.

Renal failure (uraemia)

Uraemia literally means 'urine in the blood'. Clinical features are not likely to occur until the glomerular filtration rate has fallen below 20–25% of normal. It is convenient to consider the aetiology of renal failure in three categories, each of which may present in an acute or chronic form.

1. *Pre-renal uraemia.* Here, the cause lies outside the urinary tract itself. Most frequently this involves severe hypotension and failure of renal perfusion, usually due to a fall in cardiac output, e.g. in shock or heart failure (see Ch. 6). Treatment is to restore blood pressure and renal perfusion.

2. *Renal uraemia.* In this category, there is structural renal parenchymal disease, e.g. glomerulonephritis, diabetic nephropathy or exposure to nephrotoxic substances.

3. *Post renal uraemia.* It is important to recognize this type, since the causes are often reversible. Most commonly they are associated with obstruction, either to both ureters or bladder (e.g. pelvic malignancy or prostatic hypertrophy), or to the ureter of a single functional kidney. Treatment is by relief of the obstruction.

It is often possible to identify more than one cause in an individual patient, the accumulation of which causes the renal failure to declare itself, e.g. acute tubular necrosis (renal) following on severe hypotension (prerenal).

Chronic renal failure

The biochemical consequences of chronic renal failure can be understood by referring back to the section on renal function. Accumulation of nitrogenous end-products leads to apathy, confusion and drowsiness. The tongue may be brown coated, and the breath has an ammoniacal odour; stomatitis is quite frequent (see Ch. 26). There is a tendency to retain potassium, and the patient also develops metabolic acidosis with characteristic compensatory over-breathing (Kussmaul respirations). Anorexia, nausea and vomiting are common. The patient becomes anaemic because of erythropoietin lack, and renal osteodystrophy results from failure of 1,25-dihydroxy vitamin D production. Bleeding due to impaired platelet function is frequent (see Ch. 7).

Management depends on accurate diagnosis, especially to identify and remove reversible contributory causes. Patients can often be managed conservatively by metabolic control, especially by ensuring an adequate daily urine output and by controlling dietary sodium and protein intake. If this is insufficient to improve or maintain well-being and biochemical status, or if the chronic renal failure continues to progress, it becomes necessary to introduce renal replacement therapy with regular haemodialysis on an artificial kidney machine or by peritoneal dialysis; much better restoration to health can be achieved by renal transplantation, either with a cadaver kidney or from a sufficiently matched live donor.

Because of the haemorrhagic tendency of uraemia, it is best to time any dental extractions to follow recent dialysis, but after any heparin effect has worn off. It is important, also, to remember before prescribing that drug excretion is often impaired in renal failure, and that transplant patients may be on corticosteroids or other immunosuppressive drugs which may predispose to infections (see Ch. 26).

Chronic renal failure is the end result of a wide variety of progressive renal disorders, including chronic glomerulonephritis, renal involvement in diabetes mellitus and other multisystem disorders, toxic damage to the kidney, chronic pyelonephritis or polycystic disease of the kidneys.

Acute renal failure

This involves the rapid deterioration of renal function within hours or days. It can arise de novo or may be superimposed on a background of pre-existing chronic renal impairment, sometimes unrecognized. Again the causes may be prerenal, renal or postrenal. The biochemical abnormalities are similar to those already described, but more severe reductions in urinary output are characteristic (oliguria or anuria), and dangerous rises in serum potassium (which can cause cardiac arrest, see Ch. 6) become a problem. Haemodialysis or peritoneal dialysis are often life-saving, and if the precipitating cause can be treated promptly the prognosis is quite favourable.

GLOMERULONEPHRITIS

This is a complex topic, and the following is a simplified account. Many of the several glomer-ulonephritis-producing diseases have immunological mechanisms as their pathogenesis. The glomeruli can be damaged when native glomerular constituents become altered and generate an antibody response; alternatively, immune complexes may be formed elsewhere in the body, and are transported to the kidney and deposited there. In both instances, complement may be activated, and a variety of inflammatory mediators released locally, with consequent damage to the glomeruli.

Acute glomerulonephritis

This occurs classically as a reaction to preceding infection with *Streptococcus pyogenes* (e.g. sore throat, see Chs 5 and 8); somewhat similar features may follow virus infections including hepatitis B infection, and renal involvement in multisystem disorders. The characteristic features include an abrupt onset with headache, vomiting and loin pain. Facial oedema, especially in the mornings (Fig. 11.3), moderate hypertension, and urine containing blood and protein are characteristic. The urine is usually reduced in amount, and the blood urea level elevated. This picture is often described as an 'acute nephritic' picture.

The majority of cases completely recover after 3–4 weeks, although a minority may die of renal failure or the complications of severe hypertension. A few, especially in adult life, progress to chronic glomerulonephritis.

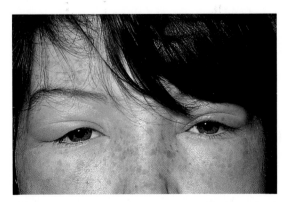

Fig. 11.3 Periorbital oedema in a patient with the nephrotic syndrome.

Nephrotic syndrome

The classic feature of the nephrotic syndrome is a heavy leak of plasma protein into the urine, which may be as much as 15–20 g in 24 h. This results in severe hypoalbuminaemia, in turn causing oedema which can be gross; ascites and pleural effusions are also common. The blood picture is usually normal, however, and there is no haematuria.

Several types of glomerular disease (distinguished by renal biopsy) can be associated with this presentation. In children, minimal-change glomerulonephritis is the commonest lesion, and is usually self-limiting. In adults, other varieties of glomerulonephritis and, especially, the glomerular lesion of diabetes mellitus predominate; the latter is associated with marked non-inflammatory thickening of the basement membrane, which becomes permeable to protein, and diabetes is currently the commonest cause of chronic renal disease in developed countries.

The oedema can be controlled by diuretics and a high-protein diet. Infusions of salt-poor albumin may be used to raise the serum albumin level, and corticosteroids or immunosuppressive drugs have a role. The protein leak also allows escape of circulating antibodies into the urine, and intercurrent systemic infection is often a problem.

Chronic glomerulonephritis

This may follow acute nephritis or the nephrotic syndrome; however, it is common for the diagnosis to be made in the absence of a clear preceding history of renal disease. The kidneys are small, scarred and granular, and there is a severe loss of functioning nephrons. The clinical picture is that of chronic renal failure, with anaemia and often associated hypertension. Management is as described for chronic renal failure, with appropriate drug therapy for any raised blood pressure.

Urinary tract infection

This is very common indeed; infections of the lower urinary tract make up the majority, usually with a mild illness associated with little constitutional upset. Unfortunately, especially in females, recurrent lower urinary tract infections are frequent. Ascending infection to involve the renal pelvis is less common. Factors predisposing to urinary tract infection are shown in Table 11.2.

Symptoms of acute infection include burning dysuria and increased frequency of small quantities of urine; the urine is cloudy because of pus, sometimes foul, and there may be haematuria. In acute pyelonephritis, there is additional loin pain, renal angle tenderness, bacteraemia and fever. On the other hand, much chronic infection is asymptomatic, and is only discovered on urine testing for other purposes. Diagnosis is reached by culture of cleanly voided samples (midstream specimen of urine) to identify the responsible organism (Table 11.3) and its antibiotic sensitivity. Treatment is with appropriate antibiotics and ensuring a high urinary output; all male patients, and all females with recurrent infections require investigation. Tuberculosis should be suspected when the urine contains leucocytes but appears sterile on ordinary culture.

Renal calculus (stone)

Normally urine contains many materials of low solubility in quite high concentrations; it is thus not surprising that supersaturation may easily occur. It is likely that the urine of normal individuals contains organic inhibitors of crystallization. Factors favouring the formation of stones include

Table 11.2 Factors predisposing to urinary tract infection
Female sex – short urethra
Incomplete bladder emptying – stagnant residual urine
Instrumentation, including catheterization
Pregnancy
Diabetes mellitus
Congenital urinary tract anomalies
Urinary tract stones

Table 11.3 Important urinary tract pathogens
Escherichia coli
Enterococci
Proteus spp.
Mycobacterium tuberculosis

concentrated urine as in hot climates, or conditions favouring increased concentration of solutes such as calcium oxalate and phosphate. The commonest stone type is that consisting of calcium oxalate, and the more easily understood metabolic stones are least common, e.g. uric acid stones in gout (see Ch. 14), cystine stones in the metabolic disease, cystinuria, and the increased stone formation found in the hypercalcaemia of vitamin D toxicity and hyperparathyroidism (see Ch. 13).

Stones may be asymptomatic when lodged in the kidney or renal pelvis; however, migrating stones, especially those traversing the ureter, are associated with renal colic (an extremely severe loin pain) and haematuria. Stones impacted in the ureter cause obstruction, leading to proximal dilatation of the renal pelvis (hydronephrosis) and eventual failure of the kidney. Bladder stones may often cause severe dysuria.

Conservative management includes the prescription of strong analgesics for colic, and ensuring a high urinary output. Stones may be removed from the ureter and bladder by cystoscopic techniques, although larger stones may require open surgical removal. External shock lithotripsy using ultrasound to shatter stones in selected cases has proved of very great benefit in avoiding surgery, and is a major advance in management.

Prostatic hypertrophy and carcinoma

Prostatic enlargement is very common in middle-aged and elderly men; this is usually due to benign hypertrophy and less commonly to adenocarcinoma. It is the most important cause of bladder outlet obstruction, and in addition to obstructive symptoms, may lead eventually to chronic back pressure with an enlarged bladder, bilateral hydronephrosis and renal failure. The obstruction may become suddenly severe, leading to complete inability to void any urine (acute retention). This constitutes a surgical emergency, and requires urgent catheterization.

Treatment is by transurethral prostatectomy using a cystoscope, and now increasingly by insertion of a small indwelling drainage tube (stent) across the obstructed section of urethra.

Tumours

Malignant growths of the urinary tract are relatively common; they affect the renal parenchyma, bladder mucosa or prostate. Tumours of the ureter are rare. The cardinal symptom is haematuria, which should always be conscientiously investigated, particularly by the use of ultrasound, computerized tomography, intravenous urography and cystoscopy.

Treatment of renal tumours is by surgical excision where possible; they are relatively resistant to radiotherapy and chemotherapy. Bladder tumours are often superficial, and can be treated by diathermy via a cystoscope, often for many years; extensive or invasive tumours may require radical cystectomy, the fashioning of an ileal bladder, and radiotherapy. Prostatic carcinoma is androgen-dependent, and is usually treated by antiandrogenic drugs.

Polycystic kidneys

This comprises a group of inherited disorders which result in the production of multiple large cysts in both kidneys; these can often be palpated through the abdominal wall. Many cases are asymptomatic, but enlargement of the cysts can cause progressive renal parenchymal damage with resulting chronic renal failure and hypertension. Genetic counselling and screening are now available.

Sexually transmitted diseases

Gonorrhoea and syphilis cause urethral and genital lesions. These are described in Chapter 5.

12 Dermatological disorders

Introduction

Disorders affecting the skin account for over 10% of medical practitioner consultations. Several skin diseases also affect the mouth, such as lichen planus (see Ch. 21) and vesiculobullous disorders (see Ch. 20), and the oral manifestations are considered in Part 2 of this book. Many skin diseases are treated with topical corticosteroids, which may cause atrophy or be absorbed and cause adrenal suppression (see Ch. 13).

In addition to a careful history and examination, patients with skin disorders may require other investigations, such as examination of skin scrapings for fungi, skin biopsy and patch testing for allergies.

The traditional method of identifying allergens in contact dermatitis and also in mucosal allergy (see Ch. 26) is to apply patch tests to clinically normal skin, usually of the back (Fig. 12.1). These are left in place for 48 h, when they are removed and the skin examined for redness, swelling or vesiculation immediately and 48 h thereafter (Fig. 12.2). This is usually done for the European Standard Battery of potential allergens with additions, e.g. dental materials where appropriate. The immediate sensitivity can also be assessed in this way using patches on the forearms, or with prick tests, though these are more relevant to asthma. Radioallergosorbent test (RAST) blood assays for some allergens and serum IgE levels are also helpful

The more important skin diseases are discussed under the headings shown in Table 12.1.

Autoimmune disorders

Several autoimmune disorders affect the skin and these are shown in Table 12.2. The main examples, pemphigus and pemphigoid, are discussed in Chapter 20. The others, the connective tissue diseases, are discussed in Chapter 14.

Dermatitis (eczema)

Dermatitis is synonymous with eczema, and several important forms are recognized (Table 12.3).

Table 12.1 Skin diseases
Autoimmune diseases
Dermatitis (eczema)
Facial dermatoses
Genetic disorders
Infections
Pigmentation disorders
Psoriasis and other papulosquamous diseases
Tumours
Vesiculobullous disorders

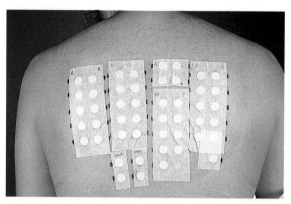

Fig. 12.1 Adhesive patches in place on the back of a patient undergoing patch testing.

Table 12.2 Autoimmune disorders

Pemphigus
Pemphigoid
Systemic lupus erythematosus (see Ch. 14)
Dermatomyositis (see Chs 9 and 14)
Scleroderma (see Ch. 14)

Table 12.3 Important forms of dermatitis

Allergic dermatitis
Atopic dermatitis
Dermatitis artefacta
Dyshydrotic eczema
Seborrhoeic dermatitis

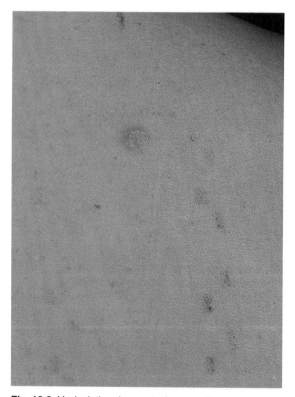

Fig. 12.2 Vesiculation demonstrating a positive result in a patient patch tested to nickel.

Allergic dermatitis (contact dermatitis)

Allergic dermatitis is caused by exposure to an allergen. It affects 1–2% of the population and often affects the hands and forearms of sufferers. It is an increasing problem among health care professionals using latex rubber gloves. Other causes

and areas commonly affected are shown in Table 12.4. Topical antibiotics are common causes, and should be avoided.

Treatment involves identifying the allergen either clinically or by patch testing, and its avoidance. Topical corticosteroids may produce clinical improvement.

Atopic dermatitis

Atopic dermatitis is a chronic itchy rash which is largely genetically determined and is often associated with asthma and hay fever (see Ch. 8). It affects 1–3% of the population, and is commonly seen in association with a positive RAST assay to pollens, cat and dog dander, house dust mite and food allergens. It is commonest in pre-school children.

Clinically, it is characterized by dry itchy skin, especially at elbow and knee flexures, with associated lichenification (skin thickening due to

Table 12.4 Sites and causes of allergic dermatitis

Site	Cause
Face	Cosmetics, soaps
Hands	Lanolin, latex, nickel
Mouth	Amalgam, toothpaste
Lips	Lipsticks
Neck and Ears	Nickel
Wrists	Nickel
Body	Nickel
Any	Topical antibiotics

scratching, resulting in accentuated skin markings) and an increased susceptibility to skin infection (Fig. 12.3).

Therapy involves control of the itch with antihistamines, topical corticosteroids and avoidance therapy, care of the dry skin with bath oils and emollients, and reduction of lichenification with tar preparations, Occasionally, photochemotherapy (pulsed ultraviolet A, PUVA) or systemic corticosteroids are required in severe cases.

Dermatitis artefacta

This is caused by, or deliberately aggravated by, the patient. Clearly, there are usually associated psychological problems, but even when one's suspicion is raised by bizarre clinical findings, diagnosis may be difficult and even psychological referral may be unsuccessful.

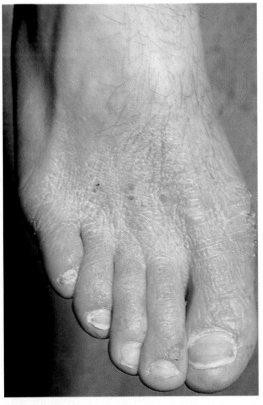

Fig. 12.3 Eczema on the foot. Note the excoriation and lichenification due to scratching. (Photograph courtesy of Dr A. Forsyth, Glasgow Royal Infirmary.)

Dyshydrotic eczema (pompholyx)

This is a common, poorly understood condition characterized by uncomfortable, deep-set, itchy papules or vesicles on the fingers and palms (cheiropompholyx) and occasionally also the feet (cheiropodopompholyx), often associated with contact dermatitis and stress. It is usually self-limiting.

Seborrhoeic dermatitis

Seborrhoeic dermatitis affects the face, scalp (dandruff) and anterior chest, and is associated with the surface yeast *Pityrosporum ovale*. Topical imidazole antifungals (shampoos) and topical corticosteroids provide temporary benefit. It may be severe in HIV-infected patients (see Ch. 5).

Facial dermatoses

This important group of diseases requires vigorous treatment due to the site affected, and the commonest causes are shown in Table 12.5.

Acne vulgaris

Patients with acne have blackheads, whiteheads (comedones) and pustules, mainly due to infected sebaceous glands, especially on their forehead, nose and chin, and sometimes on the chest, back or elsewhere (Fig. 12.4). Scarring may be severe in some people. It affects teenagers, especially girls, and may persist for 2–3 years, or more. It is less common nowadays, perhaps due to better hygiene and the increased use of 'spot creams'. The bacterium *Propionibacterium acnes* is found in the sebaceous glands of acne patients. Treatment involves topical peroxide preparations, systemic antibiotics (tetracycline or erythromycin), or, occasionally, hormone therapy in persistent acne or retinoids in older women.

Table 12.5 Facial dermatoses
Acne vulgaris
Lupus erythematosus (see p. 190)
Photosensitive eruptions
Rosacea

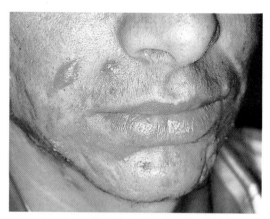

Fig. 12.4 Acne affecting the face of a young man.

Photosensitive eruptions

Photosensitive eruptions arise due to sensitivity to ultraviolet light. The patient may be sensitized by systemic lupus erythematosus or by drugs, such as phenothiazines, thiazide diuretics and antibiotics. The exposed skin surfaces are the affected areas. Treatment is by avoiding sunlight and relevant drugs.

Rosacea

Rosacea is characterized by sebaceous hyperplasia, vasomotor instability and facial flushing. It is commoner in females, and in severe chronic cases, especially in males, causes tissue hypertrophy, especially of the nose, which becomes red and bulbous (rhinophyma).

Genetic disorders

There is a genetic background in many skin disorders, but several are recognized as primarily genetic. These are shown in Table 12.6.

Ectodermal dysplasia

Ectodermal dysplasia is a rare sex-linked skin disorder characterized by sweat glands which fail to form, and thus heat control is defective (hypohydrotic ectodermal dysplasia); hypodontia or anodontia (teeth present may be of simple conical form); hair which is fine, blond and scanty (hypotrichosis); and absent eyelashes and eyebrows.

Table 12.6 Genetic disorders
Ectodermal dysplasia
Epidermolysis bullosa
Familial adenomatous polyposis coli (Gardner's syndrome)
Multiple basal cell naevi (Gorlin–Goltz syndrome)
Neurofibromatosis type 1 (von Recklinghausen's disease)
Sturge–Weber syndrome
Tuberous sclerosis
Peutz–Jegher syndrome

Epidermolysis bullosa

Epidermolysis bullosa is a group of rare bullous diseases affecting skin and mucosae with various forms of inheritance. Vesicles and bullae form in response to mild or insignificant trauma and may lead to disabling scarring. (see Ch. 20).

Gardner's syndrome (familial adenomatous polyposis coli)

Gardner's syndrome is an autosomal dominant trait characterized by multiple osteomas, skin fibromas and epidermoid cysts, and multiple polyps of the colon and rectum which almost invariably undergo malignant change (see Ch. 10 and 26).

Multiple basal cell naevi syndrome (Gorlin–Goltz syndrome)

The multiple basal cell naevi syndrome (Gorlin–Goltz syndrome) is inherited as an autosomal dominant trait, and consists of multiple basal cell naevoid carcinomas, odontogenic keratocysts and anomalies of the vertebrae and ribs and skull deformities, including calcification of the falx.

Neurofibromatosis, type I (von Recklinghausen's disease) (see Ch. 27)

Neurofibromatosis type I is an autosomal dominant condition consisting of tumours of the nerve sheath (neurilemomas or neurofibromas) in which sarcomatous change may develop, and patches of skin hyperpigmentation (café-au-lait spots).

Sturge–Weber syndrome

The Sturge–Weber syndrome (encephalotrigeminal angiomatosis) is characterized by an angioma in the face and also within the brain. Clinically, there are convulsions, and often hemiplegia and learning disability.

Tuberous sclerosis

Tuberous sclerosis is an autosomal dominant trait characterized by epilepsy, learning disability, and skin lesions in a butterfly pattern across the cheeks, bridge of the nose, forehead and chin.

Peutz–Jegher syndrome

This is characterized by intestinal polyposis and perioral pigmentation. It is discussed fully in Chapter 27.

Infections of skin

Infections of skin may arise due to viruses, bacteria or fungi, in addition to skin infestations (see Ch. 5). The more important disorders to be discussed are shown in Table 12.7.

Viral infections

Warts

Warts are benign cutaneous swellings due to human papillomaviruses. Common warts (verruca vulgaris) are particularly common in children, especially on the hands. They may be more numerous and resistant to treatment in the immunosuppressed, (e.g. those with HIV disease or renal transplant patients). Planar warts are flatter and frequently occur on the back of the hands and face. Plantar warts (verruca plantaris) are ingrowing on the soles of the feet due to pressure. Genital warts (condylomata acuminata) form large clusters and are transmitted sexually. Different warts are due to various human papillomavirus types, and so butchers' warts are caused by different types than those responsible for fishmongers' warts. Treatment is usually unnecessary for common warts, which resolve spontaneously. If treatment is required, topical application of salicylic acid is often effective.

Table 12.7 Skin infections and infestations

Viral	Herpes simplex (see p. 34)
	Herpes zoster (see p. 35)
	Warts
	Molluscum contagiosum
	Dermatological complications of HIV infection (see Ch. 5)
Bacterial	Impetigo
	Erysipelas
	Cellulitis
Fungal	Candidosis
	Dermatophyte infections
Infestations	Fleas
	Lice
	Scabies

Topical podophyllin may be helpful in more resistant cases. Cryotherapy is also effective in the management of warts.

Molluscum contagiosum

This condition, caused by a poxvirus, causes multiple umbilicated papules on the face, neck and trunk. Treatment requires pricking the lesions and applying iodine. It is common in patients with HIV infection.

Bacterial infections

Impetigo

This is a superficial highly contagious infection caused by either staphylococci or streptococci, which affects particularly children's hands and face, and can occur in outbreaks (Fig. 12.5). It is less common nowadays with improved hygiene, but can affect those with pre-existing dermatitis

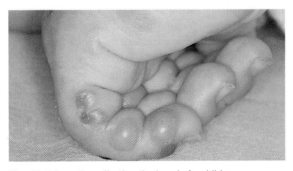

Fig. 12.5 Impetigo affecting the hand of a child.

such as eczema. It is either blistered or crusted, and is treated with topical antibiotics (such as fucidic acid) or systemic antibiotics.

Erysipelas

This is usually a streptococcal infection which infects the superficial lymphatics of the face or leg and causes a well-demarcated, unilateral spreading patch of redness, oedema and blistering. Treatment is with oral penicillin.

Cellulitis

This is a deeper infection than erysipelas and usually also streptococcal. It is a sign of spreading infection from, for example, a dental abscess or a skin wound and requires systemic antibiotic therapy.

Fungal infections

Candidosis

Candidosis is usually an oral infection, but also causes genital thrush. On the skin or nails it affects compromised patients or those at the extremes of age: it causes nappy rash in infants and intertrigo in moist skin folds in the obese or elderly. Cutaneous candidosis appears as a bright-red, glazed area. Treatment is with improved hygiene, drying and exposing skin folds along with topical or systemic antifungals.

Dermatophyte infections (tinea or ringworm)

Cutaneous lesions are more likely to be caused by dermatophytes which cause athlete's foot (tinea), nail infections and ringworm of the scalp and body. These fungi are not susceptible to nystatin or amphotericin, and miconazole or systemic griseofulvin or terbinafine are required. Topical methylated spirits as a desiccator or tea tree oil are good preventive measures for athlete's foot, used in conjunction with good hygiene.

Infestations

Scabies

Scabies is a common infestation with a mite, *Sarcoptes scabiei*, which is transmitted by close contact, particularly in bed, or to health care personnel. The mite burrows into the skin and lays eggs which cause an inflammatory response. An itchy rash develops, typically on the wrists and between the fingers (Fig. 12.6). Scabies is treated in the patient and family/partners with malathion or permethrin, and improved hygiene advised. The itch may persist for several weeks after elimination of the infestation.

Lice

There are three main types of lice:

- head lice (*Pediculus capitis*)
- body lice (*Pediculus corporis*)
- crab lice (*Pthirus pubis*) – found around the genitals.

Lice feed off the host's blood, and are transmitted by close contact or via discarded clothing. The bites can become itchy and bleed. Lice infestations are increasing in many areas, especially in vagrants, and head lice (nits) are particularly common in school children. Lice can, under appropriate circumstances, also transmit disease such as typhus (*Rickettsia prowazeki*). Treatment is with improved hygiene and the use of malathion and carbaryl.

Fleas

Fleas are parasites of man and other animals, living mainly on the hairy parts of the body, depositing eggs that can cause an itchy rash. They are transmitted to those in close proximity.

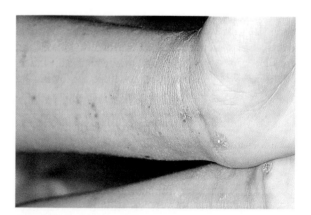

Fig. 12.6 Scabies affecting the forearms and wrists.

Rodent fleas in particular can act as vectors of plague (*Pasteurella pestis*) and typhus, and have been responsible for recent outbreaks of disease in India and other areas. Improved hygiene and malathion are indicated.

Pigmentation disorders

Pigmentation disorders are common, and those to be discussed are shown in Table 12.8.

Addison's disease (see Ch. 13)

The pituitary hormones melanocyte-stimulating hormone and adrenocorticotrophic hormone are increased in Addison's disease, which causes increased pigmentation in skin flexures and in the mucous membranes.

Chloasma

Pregnant women or those on the oral contraceptive pill may get hormonally-induced brownish pigmentation, especially of the face.

Freckles

Freckles or ephelides are areas where melanocytes produce increased melanin in sunlight. Treatment is sun avoidance.

Pigmented naevi (moles)

Several forms of naevi or moles exist, most of which are benign. Their importance is to distinguish them from malignant melanoma (see later).

Vitiligo

Vitiligo is characterized by areas of depigmentation, which is thought to be autoimmune in nature, and is often associated with systemic autoimmune diseases (Fig. 12.7).

Psoriasis and other papulosquamous diseases

The papulosquamous diseases include those shown in Table 12.9.

Psoriasis

Psoriasis is a common chronic inflammatory skin disorder causing pruritic erythematous papules and plaques, predominantly on the scalp, elbows and knees (Fig. 12.8), with the Koebner phenomenon (skin lesions appearing at sites of trauma, e.g. scratches or under watch straps), and pitting lesions of the nails. There is a strong genetic background and associations with stress and alcoholism. There may be an associated arthritis (see Ch. 14). Management may include photochemotherapy (PUVA), topical applications of tars, steroids or

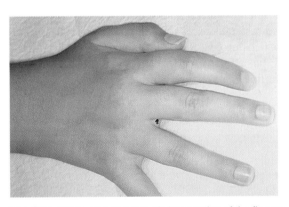

Fig. 12.7 Vitiligo showing loss of pigmentation of the fingers.

Table 12.8 Pigmentation disorders
Addison's disease
Chloasma
Freckles
Naevi
Vitiligo

Table 12.9 Papulosquamous diseases
Psoriasis
Lichen planus
Pityriasis
Darier's disease

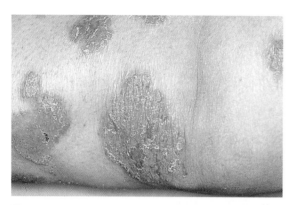

Fig. 12.8 Plaque psoriasis affecting a middle-aged woman.

retinoids, and in severe cases systemic medication with methotrexate, cyclosporin or retinoids.

Lichen planus

Lichen planus is a common itchy papular rash which affects chiefly the wrists, forearms and legs, and also shows the Koebner phenomenon (Fig. 12.9). The oral mucous membranes are frequently affected (see Ch. 21). The skin papules are violaceous, and have a white, lacy appearance (Wickham's striae). The rash is thus purple, pruritic and papular.

Therapy includes antihistamines for the itch, and resistant cases may require a short course of corticosteroids. Retinoids have also been reported to be effective. Skin lesions tend to be self-limiting, and resolve within 2 years.

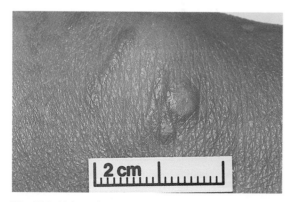

Fig. 12.9 Lichen planus of the skin showing a Koebner phenomenon.

Pityriasis

Pityriasis is characterized by red scaly macules on the trunk. It occurs in outbreaks in the spring and autumn, and is thought to be viral in nature. It is self-limiting but antihistamines can be given to help the itch.

Darier's disease (keratosis follicularis)

Darier's disease is a rare genetically determined keratinization of the hair follicles, which in severe cases is disfiguring and requires retinoid therapy (see Fig. 21.1).

Tumours of skin

The most important tumours of skin are shown in Table 12.10.

Basal cell carcinoma

Basal cell carcinoma or rodent ulcer is a locally destructive tumour which is commoner than either squamous cell carcinoma or malignant melanoma. It arises as a necrotic ulcer with a rolled margin in a light-exposed area usually on the upper cheek or inner canthus (Fig. 12.10). It does not metastasize, and can be treated by radiotherapy or surgery.

Bowen's disease

Bowen's disease is an intraepidermal carcinoma in situ which occasionally becomes invasive. It appears as an isolated scaly plaque usually on the trunk, clinically similar to psoriasis. A small number become malignant. The treatment is excision biopsy.

Table 12.10 Tumours of skin
Basal cell carcinoma
Bowen's disease
Keratoacanthoma
Malignant melanoma
Mycosis fungoides
Squamous cell carcinoma

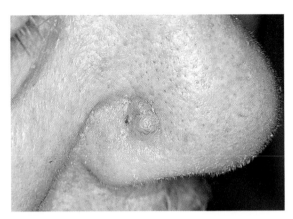

Fig. 12.10 A basal cell carcinoma on the side of the nose in a middle-aged farm worker.

Keratoacanthoma

This clinically resembles carcinoma but is self-healing.

Malignant melanoma

This is a tumour of melanocytes. Its incidence is increasing, which is thought to be due to increased sunbathing in the susceptible Caucasian populations. Clinically, melanoma may present as spreading lesions, as macules on the exposed skin of the elderly, as an ulcerated lesion, or a lesion on the sole of the foot or palm of the hand or peri-ungually. The depth of the lesion is inversely proportional to the prognosis. Current practice, therefore, is to perform excision biopsy of suspect lesions to establish the diagnosis and the lesional depth. Thick lesions are then widely excised. Moles of the skin are very common, but malignant melanoma is rare. There is no justification, therefore, for prophylactically removing moles

unless there are features such as darkening, rapid growth, ulceration or the appearance of satellite lesions.

Mycosis fungoides

This is a rare low-grade cutaneous T cell lymphoma (see Ch. 7) which affects the middle-aged or elderly, and may progress very slowly or even regress. Treatment is with photochemotherapy or superficial radiotherapy.

Squamous cell carcinoma

Squamous cell carcinoma is common, usually arises in sun-damaged skin and presents as a hyperkeratotic ulcer which metastasizes to local lymph nodes. Treatment is surgical excision.

Vesiculobullous disorders

The important vesiculobullous disorders are shown in Table 12.11.

These are all mucocutaneous in distribution. Most are characterized to a greater or lesser extent by cutaneous blisters (see Fig. 20.3). The main features and treatments are discussed in detail in Chapter 20.

Table 12.11 Vesiculobullous disorders
Pemphigus
Pemphigoid
Dermatitis herpetiformis
Linear IgA disease
Angina bullosa haemorrhagica (oval only)
Erythema multiforme
Epidermolysis bullosa

13 Endocrine disorders

Introduction

From ancient times it was believed that certain organs were capable of producing substances which could act on distant sites. These are now known to be hormones, secreted directly into the blood by endocrine glands. This chapter will be concerned particularly with disorders of these glands, although it must be appreciated that many hormones are produced from other organs, e.g. erythropoietin from the kidney, atrial natriuretic peptide from the heart. The sensitivity of modern hormone assays has contributed much to the understanding of endocrine pathophysiology.

Chemically, hormones are of two classes:

1. Molecules based on amino acids or peptides. The smallest of these are closely allied to neurotransmitters, e.g. adrenaline and dopamine, and illustrate the close relationship between endocrine glands and the nervous system. Larger peptides include insulin, parathyroid hormone, and luteinizing hormone.

2. Molecules derived from cholesterol precursors. These hormones are all based on the steroid nucleus, are lipid-soluble, and include corticosteroids, testosterone and progesterone.

Hormones are often transmitted through the blood attached to specific binding proteins, and abnormalities of these proteins may lead to problems in interpreting hormone assay results. Having reached the target cell, hormones may act either:

1. Through specific cell surface receptors. In general this process engenders a secondary messenger which then acts upon a range of substrates in the cell. Examples include adrenocorticotrophic hormone (ACTH), follicle-stimulating hormone (FSH), thyroid-stimulating hormone (TSH), antidiuretic hormone (ADH) and calcitonin.

2. Through intracellular receptors. The hormone enters the cell, and a hormone–receptor ligand is formed within the nucleus, which then binds to specific regions of DNA. This then codes for specific proteins important in cell function. Examples include thyroxine (T4) and all the steroid hormones (and vitamin D).

The functions of hormones are:

- cellular growth and differentiation
- maintenance of homeostasis, including fluid and electrolyte balance
- reproduction.

Regulatory feedback systems

This concept is fundamental to clinical endocrinology; most of the designated endocrine glands are under this form of control, largely based on the pituitary gland. Active secretion by a gland increases the plasma concentration of its hormone product, and this then inhibits secretion of the driving (trophic) hormone from the pituitary, allowing the gland in question to 'switch off'; when the plasma concentration of the hormone again falls, pituitary secretion of the stimulatory trophic hormone is 'switched on' once more, thus restoring plasma levels to normal.

In addition, pituitary activity itself is closely regulated by hormones produced in the hypothalamus; again a negative-feedback system operates to control the interactions of pituitary and hypothalamus. This 'double-loop' system allows a high degree of fine tuning of hormone secretion.

Endocrine disorders

Most endocrine disorders can be grouped according to hypo- or hyperfunction. These malfunctions can result either from intrinsic pathology within the endocrine gland itself, or by deficiency or excess of stimulating hormones from the pituitary gland. In addition, some non-endocrine malignant tumours are capable of producing substances which mimic the actions of hormones (ectopic hormone production).

The endocrine glands to be discussed are shown in Table 13.1. Reproductive endocrinology is considered after the pituitary gland, to facilitate clarification of this subject. Although usually not endocrine in aetiology, obesity is considered at the end of this chapter because of its link to diabetes mellitus. The recent discovery of the hormone leptin, which is involved in weight regulation, may establish an endocrine role in obesity.

The pituitary gland

The pituitary gland consists of two principal lobes, anterior and posterior. It derives from the fusion of a downgrowth from the floor of the third ventricle, and from an upward invagination of the primitive stomatodaeum (Rathke's pouch). The gland is enclosed in a bony cavity, the sella turcica; this is roofed over by a fibrous sheet, perforated only by the pituitary stalk, carrying nerve

Table 13.1 The endocrine glands

Pituitary
  Anterior
  Posterior
Thyroid
Adrenal
  Cortex
  Medulla
Parathyroid
Pancreatic islets (diabetes mellitus)
Testis
Ovary

fibres, the blood supply and venous drainage. The sella turcica is closely related on its lateral sides to the cavernous sinuses, cranial nerves III, IV and VI, and to the optic chiasma, which lies above. Pituitary tumours can therefore compress the optic chiasma, causing bitemporal hemianopia (see Ch. 9).

The two lobes are functionally quite separate.

Anterior pituitary gland

The anterior pituitary has a pivotal role in the control of several other endocrine glands by the production of trophic (stimulating) hormones e.g. adrenal cortex (ACTH), gonads (luteinizing hormone (LH) and follicle stimulating hormone (FSH)), thyroid (TSH) and breast (prolactin). It also produces growth hormone (GH), a 'primary' hormone of its own, with direct physiological effects on non-endocrine tissue. In addition to negative-feedback circuits from other glands (see above), production of pituitary hormones is also mediated by control from the hypothalamus by 'releasing' hormones e.g. thyrotrophin-releasing hormone (TRH) (Table 13.2).

Disorders of the pituitary are rare (Table 13.3); a short description of the more important diseases follows. Hyper- or hypofunction of other glands are described under their individual headings.

Growth hormone. GH functions largely by acting on the liver, to produce insulin-like growth factor (IGF_1); this in turn influences the growth of cartilage and soft tissues.

Failure of GH secretion during childhood is a recognized cause of dwarfism; such an individual is small, but usually of normal proportions.

Table 13.2 Anterior pituitary hormone control and release (simplified). Commonly used abbreviations are shown in brackets. Hypothalamic hormones are stimulatory except where shown. We do not attempt to distinguish between feedback inhibition acting on the pituitary or the hypothalamus

Hypothalamic hormone	Pituitary hormone	Target organ	Hormone product feedback inhibition
Gonadotrophin-releasing hormone (GnRH)	Luteinizing hormone (LH)	Ovary (hormone production Testis (hormone production)	Oestradiol Testosterone
	Follicle-stimulating hormone (FSH)	Ovary (gametogenesis) Testis (gametogenesis)	See text
Corticotrophin-releasing hormone (CRF)	Adrenocorticotrophic hormone (ACTH)	Adrenal cortex Skin melanocytes	Cortisol
Growth hormone-releasing hormone (GHRH)	Growth hormone (GH)	Liver[a] ↓ Insulin-like growth factor (IGF$_1$) ↓ Cartilage	Stimulated by hypoglycaemia
Somatostatin (inhibitory)			
Thyroid-releasing hormone (TRH)	Thyroid-stimulating hormone (TSH)	Thyroid	Thyroxine (T4)
Dopamine (inhibitory)	Prolactin	Breast (lactation)	

[a] See text.

Table 13.3 Causes of pituitary disease

Pathogenesis	Effect
Vascular Infarction or haemorrhage (Sheehan's syndrome[a]) Pressure from aneurysm	Hypofunction
Tumours (rarely malignant)	Hyperfunction from cell type involved Hypofunction from pressure of tumour on surrounding normal gland
Granulomas	Hypofunction
Irradiation	Hypofunction

[a] See text.

Excess GH production, acting before the epiphyses of the long bones have fused, results in gigantism – heights of 2–2.5 m may be reached.

Acromegaly (literally 'large extremities'), results from excessive GH secretion in adults, usually from a pituitary adenoma. The hands and feet become enlarged, and the facial features are coarse and heavy, especially the lips and nose (Figure 13.1). The mandible enlarges more than the maxilla, resulting in a prominent lower jaw, with widely spaced teeth and malocclusion. Dentures become ill-fitting. The frontal ridges are prominent, and the tongue enlarges. Increased sweating is an early feature of active acromegaly, and heart disease and diabetes mellitus are common complications. The pituitary tumour often

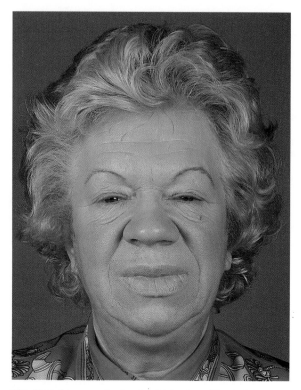

Fig. 13.1 Acromegaly showing thickening of the facial features and frontal bossing.

causes headache, and visual field defects (classically bitemporal heminopia) may occur when the growth breaks out above the sella turcica to compress the optic chiasma.

Diagnosis can be confirmed by serum GH and IGF1 assays, and radiology of the area may show an enlarged sella turcica and erosion of the clinoid processes; computerized tomography shows the tumour itself.

Treatment is by surgery through the nasal cavity, radiation therapy, or conservatively by administration of GH suppressants or antagonists, e.g. somatostatin or its analogue octreotide, bromocriptine.

Hyperprolactinaemia. Hyperprolactinaemia may result from a number of processes distant from the pituitary, including the use of certain drugs and other endocrine disorders; normal pregnancy is of course the most frequent cause. The commonest pituitary disease associated with hyperprolactinaemia is a microprolactinoma; this leads to unwanted milk secretion (galactorrhoea)

and erratic menstruation or lack of periods (amenorrhoea). Treatment is by administration of dopaminergic agents such as bromocriptine.

Panhypopituitarism (Simmond's disease). This usually presents clinically through combined failure of target endocrine glands, e.g. hypothyroidism, adrenocortical failure, depressed sexual function, and atrophy of the sexual hair and genitals. The condition most characteristically results from the necrosis of the hypertrophied gland in pregnant women who have suffered postpartum haemorrhage associated with shock (Sheehan's syndrome); such patients do not lactate or resume menstruation after delivery.

Posterior pituitary gland

The posterior pituitary secretes two hormones:

- oxytocin, which activates smooth muscle to promote uterine contraction, and to cause ejection of milk from mammary ducts
- arginine vasopressin (antidiuretic hormone (ADH)).

These hormones are first secreted in the hypothalamus, travel down neurons to the posterior pituitary, and are then stored until required.

Diabetes insipidus. This is the clinical syndrome resulting from failure of ADH secretion, and the consequent inability of the renal tubule to conserve water appropriately (see Chapter 11). The patient produces very large quantities of dilute urine – up to 10 litres daily – with resulting thirst and consumption of a large fluid volume to compensate. Denial of fluid except in controlled circumstances is dangerous, and results in rapid dehydration.

Diabetes insipidus is controlled by administration of the long-acting vasopressin analogue desmopressin (DDAVP), either by snuff taken intranasally or by injection in unconscious patients. Intravenous desmopressin is also used to treat mild haemophilia A or von Willebrand's disease, because it raises plasma levels of factor VIII/von Willebrand's factor, e.g. before surgery (see Ch. 7).

A clinically similar condition may result from resistance of the renal tubule to the action of ADH (renal diabetes insipidus); this occurs in hypercalcaemia and hypokalaemia.

Reproductive endocrinology

Introduction

Female reproductive medicine is considered separately in Chapter 16. Only the endocrine aspects are included in this section.

During intrauterine development, unless influenced by the presence of a Y chromosome, the primitive undifferentiated gonad will continue to develop into an ovary, and the external genitalia will be female. In males, the influence of the Y chromosome determines the evolution of testes, and the development of male external genitalia from 12–14 weeks gestation is dependent on the secretion of androgens from the primitive testes.

Males

The hormone function of the testes is controlled by LH from the pituitary (Table 13.2). Puberty is initiated by pulse doses of LH, mainly at night; later LH is secreted throughout the day, and plasma testosterone levels rise. This results in enlargement of the testes and external genitalia, increased muscular development, growth of long bones, establishment of male pattern body hair growth, laryngeal changes and sexual drive.

Clinically, androgen deficiency is unusual. It may result secondarily from pituitary disorders, general illness, malnutrition, or simply delayed puberty; in such cases LH and FSH levels will be reduced. Primary testicular endocrine failure may result from castration, bilateral orchitis, radiation and chemotherapy damage. In such cases, pituitary gonadotrophic hormone levels are elevated. A number of rare developmental defects (e.g. Klinefelter's syndrome) may also cause androgen deficiency.

Spermatogenesis is controlled by pituitary FSH, augmented by local testosterone secretion. Again, male infertility on the basis of hormone disorder is rare, and is more likely to result from primary testicular pathology, from spermatozoal dysfunction, or from disorders of ejaculation.

Females

On average, puberty occurs 2 years earlier in girls than in boys, with the onset of ovulation and menstruation. The hormonal regulation of this process is very complex, but depends on an inherent 28 day cyclicity within the ovary, hypothalamus and pituitary gland. Follicle maturation within the ovary is dependent on FSH; as the 14th day of the cycle approaches, there is a rise in oestrogen secretion from the follicle, initially inhibitory to the pituitary as expected, but finally inducing a surge of LH which stimulates ovulation, and induces the granulosa cells to form a corpus luteum. Meanwhile, the uterine mucosa is proliferating under the influence of oestrogen, and in the postovulatory phase the action of progesterone from the corpus luteum along with oestrogen converts the endometrium to the receptive secretory phase. The rise in progesterone levels during the second half of the cycle has an inhibitory action on the pituitary–hypothalamic axis, with a subsequent fall both in LH and FSH secretion. If fertilization does not occur in the optimum conditions pertaining in mid-cycle, the ovum is lost, and towards the end of the second 14 day period of the cycle the endometrium is shed as a menstrual period. Finally, both pituitary and ovarian hormone secretion returns to base levels.

If fertilization occurs, the blastocyst implants in the endometrium and then secretes its own LH-like hormone human chorionic gonadotrophin (hCG). This maintains the corpus luteum, and both progesterone and oestradiol secretion. In turn, this sustains the secretory structure of the endometrium. As pregnancy develops, a placenta is formed, which takes over the production of progesterone and oestrogen, and hCG secretion declines thereafter.

The menopause follows the recruitment and successful ovulation of the limited number of follicles present in the ovary from birth.

Ovarian failure. The principal manifestations of ovarian failure are disturbed menstruation, that is, amenorrhoea or oligomenorrhoea, and/or infertility.

Hypothalamic and pituitary causes are associated with low gonadotrophin levels, as well as low levels of oestradiol and progesterone. Amenorrhoea is thus characteristic of all types of pathological hypopituitarism (Table 13.3), and functional hypogonadotrophic hypogonadism may follow severe weight loss of any cause (characteristically anorexia nervosa). Hyperprolactinaemia of any cause is also associated with amenorrhoea, although the mechanism is not completely clear.

Where the ovary itself is responsible, oestrogen and progesterone levels are again low, but high levels of FSH and LH are present. This will result physiologically from the menopause, and also from failure of normal ovarian development (e.g. Turner's syndrome), premature ovarian failure as in the idiopathic form (low initial follicle number), after viral infection such as mumps, or following radiotherapy and cytotoxic drugs.

Treatment is that of the primary disorder, and hormone replacement where appropriate. Infertility associated with gonadotrophic failure may be treated in specialized centres by gonadotrophins or gonadotrophin-releasing hormone.

Thyroid gland

Structure and function

The thyroid is formed in early embryonic life from a tubular central downgrowth from the floor of the primitive pharynx – the thyroglossal duct. This enlarges at its lowest end to form the isthmus and medial parts of the future gland; the duct should become obliterated thereafter in its upper section, but may persist to form thyroglossal cysts, presenting in later life as central neck or tongue swellings. The adult gland consists of many secretory follicles containing colloid.

The thyroid contains 90% of body iodine, and the gland manufactures two hormones from the amino acid tyrosine combined with iodine; these are thyroxine (T4) and triiodothyronine (T3). Hormone production is stimulated by TSH from the pituitary. The main physiological function of thyroid hormone is to control the basal metabolic rate.

Thyroid function can be assessed by measuring the plasma levels of T3 and T4, and also by assay of TSH and the hypothalamic hormone TRH. The gland itself can be imaged isotopically (with radioiodine), by ultrasound, by plain radiography or by barium swallow.

Goitre

Thyroid enlargement (goitre) may have several causes (Table 13.4).

Simple diffuse goitres are very common, especially in young women, and often begin at the menarche or during pregnancy, suggesting a role for oestrogen. These goitres are soft, diffuse and seldom require therapy.

Multinodular goitres are also common. They may be due to iodine deficiency, but there are clearly other causes because iodine deficiency in western countries has largely been eliminated by iodized salt. Ingested dietary goitrogens may have a role. These patients are usually euthyroid but may occasionally become thyrotoxic due to a toxic adenoma. Pressure symptoms causing dysphagia may require partial thyroidectomy.

Thyroiditis may be viral or autoimmune (Hashimoto's disease); the latter is often associated with other organ-specific autoimmune diseases such as pernicious anaemia and commonly progresses to gland atrophy and hypothyroidism.

Thyroid neoplasms

These may cause pressure symptoms (dysphagia) and metastasize (e.g. to cervical lymph nodes and bone). Ultrasound or isotope scanning may show characteristic appearances; needle aspiration is usually diagnostic. Treatment is by thyroidectomy or high-dose radioiodine.

Hypothyroidism

The aetiology of hypothyroidism is summarized in Table 13.5. The commonest cause is undoubtedly autoimmune destruction of the thyroid gland. This usually simply causes atrophy, but may be preceded by a goitre with high serum levels of anti-thyroid antibodies (Hashimoto's disease).

Table 13.4 Some causes of goitre (thyroid enlargement)
Simple (non-toxic goitre, colloid goitre)
Multinodular goitre
Toxic goitre (thyrotoxicosis)
Thyroiditis
Neoplasm

Table 13.5 Causes of hypothyroidsm

Congenital (cretinism)	Now rare because of routine thyroid function screening at birth
Primary	Autoimmune thyroid disease
Secondary	Thyroidectomy Radiation (usually following previous radioactive iodine therapy for hyperthyroidism) Hypopituitarism-impaired TSH secretion

Clinical features. These can mostly be understood on the basis of low T4 levels. The patient becomes lethargic, and physically and mentally slowed; the skin is dry, and the weight increases despite a poor appetite (Fig. 13.2). The bowels are constipated, and intolerance of cold is marked; there is a consequent liability to hypothermia, which can cause a life-threatening coma. There is puffiness of the skin (myxoedema) periorbitally and in the supraclavicular fossae; at the wrists a similar phenomenon can be associated with the carpal tunnel syndrome. Deafness and bradycardia are common. Hypercholesterolaemia may predispose to ischaemic heart disease. It is important to distinguish simple obesity with depression from hypothyroidism.

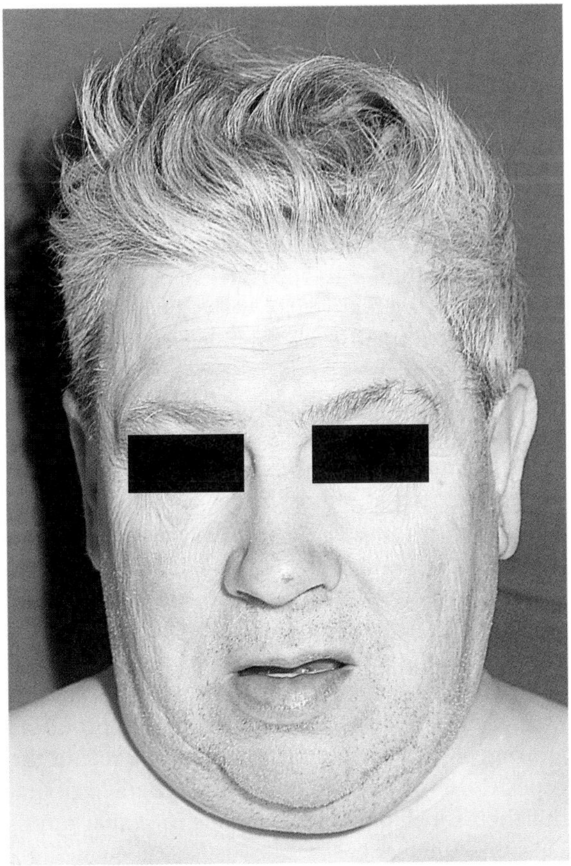

Characteristic biochemical features include reduced plasma T4 and T3 levels and a compensatory increase in the plasma TSH level, and a raised plasma cholesterol level.

Treatment. Treatment is by administration of thyroxine, given cautiously in small doses to begin with, especially in the elderly and in those with overt ischaemic heart disease. Treatment is lifelong since gland destruction is usually permanent.

Hyperthyroidism

The causes of hyperthyroidism are summarized in Table 13.6. The most important and frequent disorder is Graves' disease.

Graves' disease. This condition is commonest in women, and usually begins between 30 and 40 years of age. Autoantibodies against the TSH receptor on the thyroid cell surface mimic the actions of TSH, and stimulate gland activity. In addition, the characteristic eye features appear to result from related autoantibodies, directed

Fig. 13.2 A patient with hypothyroidism showing typical facies: the patient has thickened features, thinning of the hair and a lethargic expression.

Table 13.6 Cases of hyperthyroidism

Autoimmune – Graves' disease
Toxic adenoma
Inappropriate thyroxine therapy (e.g. for obesity) or self-administration of tablets

against the extrinsic orbital muscles and fat; the increased intraorbital volume leads to exophthalmos (Fig. 13.3).

The clinical features are attributable either directly to autoimmunity or to the peripheral effects of thyroid hormone excess; the latter can be divided into those dependent on an increased basal metabolic rate, and those which enhance the actions of catecholamines (Table 13.7).

Antithyroid drugs (e.g. carbimazole) block the synthesis of thyroid hormone, and are the treatment of choice especially where exposure to radioisotopes is inadvisable. Since spontaneous remission is possible, the drugs can be withdrawn after 1–2 years, and reintroduced if relapse occurs. Partial thyroidectomy is also effective, and in good hands the risks of damage to parathyroid glands or to the recurrent laryngeal nerves are minimized. Ablation of the gland by radioactive iodine, which is concentrated in the thyroid, is useful in older patients, and in those who are poor surgical risks. Postsurgical or postirradiation hypothyroidism is almost inevitable, and requires replacement therapy; hence all treated patients should have lifelong regular thyroid function tests.

Adrenal glands

The two adrenal glands are situated on the upper pole of each kidney. The adrenal cortex and medulla are of different embryological origin and function. The cortex synthesizes steroid hormones, and the medulla produces the catecholamines noradrenaline and adrenaline.

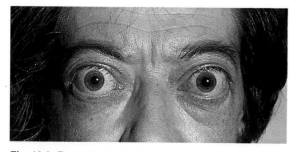

Fig. 13.3 Exopthalmos in a patient with hyperthyroidism: the whole of the iris is visible.

Table 13.7 Some features of Graves' disease

Autoimmune	Goitre
	Exophthalmos
Thyroid hormone excess	
Increased basal metabolic rate	Heat intolerance
	Weight loss with increased appetite
Sympathetic overactivity	Tachycardia, cardiac arrhythmias
	Diarrhoea
	Sweating
	Nervousness and irritability
	Excess activity in upper eyelids – lid retraction
	Tremor

Adrenal cortex

The adrenal cortex secretes hormones with the following functions:

1. *Carbohydrate metabolism.* The glucocorticoids, especially cortisone and hydrocortisone, are secreted in response to ACTH stimulation. They have an important role in glucose homeostasis by stimulating hepatic gluconeogenesis and by a catabolic action on muscle; this can be seen as an anti-insulin effect, tending to raise blood glucose levels. They inhibit the immune system, and also collagen synthesis. In their absence, responses to physiological stress are impaired. They also have a range of therapeutic usefulness well beyond the simple replacement of adrenal insufficiency, because of their immunosuppressive effects in supraphysiological doses.

2. *Sodium and potassium metabolism.* The main mineralocorticoid, aldosterone, acts on the renal tubule to promote sodium reabsorption and enhance potassium excretion (see Ch. 11). Its secretion is largely independent of ACTH, and is stimulated mainly by extracellular concentrations of sodium and potassium, and by angiotensin II (Fig. 13.4).

3. *Sex hormones.* The adrenal cortex produces androgens and oestrogens; these have a role in the production of secondary sexual characteristics, but their other possible functions in sexual physiology are unclear.

Adrenocortical failure (Addison's disease, hypoadrenalism). The mechanisms of adrenal

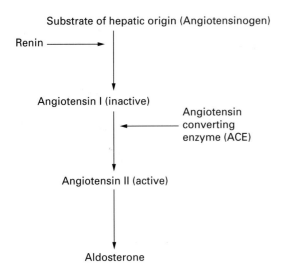

Substrate of hepatic origin (Angiotensinogen)

Renin ⟶

Angiotensin I (inactive)

Angiotensin converting enzyme (ACE)

Angiotensin II (active)

Aldosterone

Fig. 13.4 Renin is secreted in the kidneys by the juxtaglomerular cells of the afferent arterioles, which are sensitive to tubular concentrations of sodium. A fall in filtered sodium levels stimulates renin production, which in turn drives the series of reactions shown above. Aldosterone then enhances sodium reabsorption. Angiotensin II is also a powerful vasoconstrictor.

failure are summarized in Table 13.8. The clinical features are best understood by reference to the physiological functions of adrenal hormones described previously. The condition presents gradually with lethargy or depression; fatigue and dizziness are associated with hypotension and hypoglycaemia. Compensatory excess of ACTH and melanocyte-stimulating activity cause pigmentation of the skin, including areas not normally exposed to sunlight, and of the buccal mucosa, (see Chs 12 and 26). Alimentary complaints such as anorexia, weight loss and abdominal pain are common. Mineralocorticoid deficiency leads to hypovolaemia from sodium and water depletion, and the serum potassium level rises.

The particular danger to these patients lies in their inability to respond to physiological stress; they tolerate infection, anaesthesia and operative procedures very poorly, and exposure to these may lead to death from adrenal crisis. Hence, all diagnosed patients should carry a card or bracelet to identify their condition.

Diagnosis of adrenal insufficiency. Simple measurement of plasma electrolytes may show the characteristic combination of reduced sodium and increased potassium concentrations. Definitive tests include the simultaneous measurement of plasma cortisol (low, or low normal) and plasma ACTH (elevated) levels, or the demonstration of an impaired adrenal response to the administration of exogenous ACTH or a synthetic analogue (Synacthen).

In cases of hypoadrenalism of pituitary origin, endogenous ACTH levels will be low, and the Synacthen test should produce a satisfactory rise in cortisol secretion.

Management. Replacement therapy is with oral hydrocortisone once or twice daily; some patients require the addition of the mineralocorticoid fludrocortisone. Basal doses of hydrocortisone replacement should be increased promptly during infections or other physiological stresses, and prior to surgery, as prophylaxis of adrenal crisis.

Adrenal crisis. This may occur in any patient with unsuspected chronic adrenal failure, especially when precipitated by stress situations as previously described. Principal features include acute circulatory collapse, dehydration, hypoglycaemia, abdominal pain and vomiting. Bleeding into a hitherto normal gland (adrenal apoplexy) is characteristic of acute meningococcal septicaemia (see Ch. 5), and is a major cause of death in this disease. Treatment includes intensive and prompt

Table 13.8 Mechanisms of adrenocortical failure	
Primary	*Secondary*
Autoimmune (Addison's disease)	Hypopituitarism – failure of ACTH secretion
Tuberculosis	
Bilateral adrenalectomy	
Adrenal suppression from long-continued corticosteroid therapy	
Adrenal apoplexy (acute)	

administration of intravenous fluids and hydro-cortisone.

Adrenocortical excess (Cushing's syndrome). The causes of Cushing's syndrome are summarized in Table 13.9. The clinical features of Cushing's syndrome include obesity of the trunk, muscle wasting, especially of the limbs, thin skin with acne and striae, diabetes mellitus, hypertension, impaired wound healing and osteoporosis (see Fig. 13.5). Susceptibility to infection with *Candida* and reactivation of previously quiescent tuberculosis are features particularly of Cushing's syndrome due to corticosteroid therapy. Virilization in women is associated with hirsutism, and there is loss of libido in men. As expected, there is sodium retention and potassium loss; these features are particularly prominent in cases with ectopic ACTH secretion. Interpretation of biochemical and hormone assay results in Cushing's syndrome is often difficult in borderline cases, especially in patients with simple obesity and alcohol excess.

Definitive treatment is usually by surgical removal of the responsible tumour, either adrenal or pituitary. Preoperatively, or in patients unsuitable for surgery, steroid biosynthesis can be blocked by enzyme inhibitors such as metapyrone.

Patients taking high-dose corticosteroids (e.g. prednisolone) long-term develop adrenal atrophy, and are at risk of an adrenal crisis if treatment is stopped. They should therefore carry a steroid card to show any doctor or dentist. Corticosteroid therapy should not be interrupted by surgery or acute illness. Intentional corticosteroid withdrawal should be performed gradually, in order to allow endogenous adrenal function to recover; if it

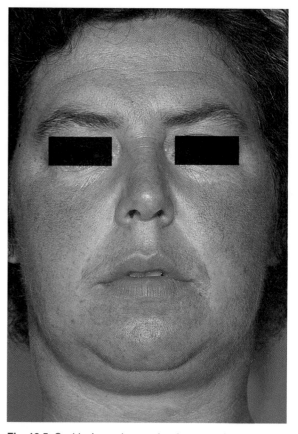

Fig. 13.5 Cushing's syndrome, showing moon face, hirsutism and a plethoric complexion.

does not, corticosteroid replacement therapy is required.

Conn's syndrome. This is caused by a rare tumour of the adrenal cortex, which produces excess aldosterone, causing surgically remedial hypertension, sometimes with hypokalaemia.

Table 13.9 Causes of Cushing's syndrome	
ACTH induced	Pituitary tumour ACTH therapy Ectopic ACTH secretion from non-endocrine malignant tumours, e.g. bronchus
Non-ACTH induced (autonomous adrenal)	Adrenal adenoma Adrenal carcinoma
High-dose corticosteroid therapy	Chronic therapy for immunosuppression, asthma, inflammatory bowel disease, autoimmune multisystem disorders, etc.

Adrenal medulla

Adrenaline is the major product of the adrenal medulla; it is of particular importance in the acute response to stress, leading to increased alertness, tachycardia, mobilization of glucose and fat, inhibition of insulin secretion, and a whole range of sympathetic autonomic responses. Its secretion is probably modulated by cortisol, which permeates the adrenal medulla from the cortex, and its peripheral actions are enhanced by T4.

It is a powerful vasoconstrictor, and tumours of the adrenal medulla (phaeochromocytoma) are a rare but surgically remediable cause of hypertension (see Ch. 6).

Parathyroid glands

The four parathyroid glands are situated behind the thyroid gland, and occasionally within the thyroid gland itself. Production of parathyroid hormone (PTH) is regulated independently of the pituitary by serum calcium and phosphate levels; it stimulates osteoclastic bone resorption, tending to raise serum calcium levels, and enhances renal excretion of phosphate.

Hyperparathyroidism

Overactivity of the parathyroid glands is commoner than previously suspected, owing to the routine measurement of serum calcium levels in many patients now attending hospitals and clinics. It is usually caused by an adenoma of one gland; less frequently there may be either adenomatous involvement of more than one gland, simple hyperplasia of all four glands, or, rarest of all, carcinoma.

Symptomatic cases may present with:

- hypercalcaemia (see Table 13.10 for causes and Table 13.11 for effects)
- renal disease (see Ch. 11), renal calculi, diffuse nephrocalcinosis resulting from hypercalciuria, and chronic renal failure
- bone disease (see Ch. 14), diffuse skeletal decalcification, and multiple cysts (osteitis fibrosa cystica).

The diagnosis is confirmed by the finding of increased serum calcium levels, reduced serum

Table 13.10 Causes of hypercalcaemia

Primary hyperparathyroidism
Inappropriate vitamin D intake
Extrarenal synthesis of Vitamin D, e.g. lymphoma, sarcoidosis
Widespread osteolytic bone lesions in malignancy, including myeloma
Ectopic PTH-like peptides – non-endocrine malignant tumours e.g. bronchus

Table 13.11 Effects of hypercalcaemia

Polyuria (nephrogenic diabetes insipidus)
Thirst
Confusion, coma
Anorexia, vomiting, constipation
Renal calcification
Acute pancreatitis

phosphate levels and an increase in bone alkaline phosphatase levels. The serum PTH levels are raised inappropriately for the serum calcium level.

Management is by detection of possible adenomas by imaging techniques and their subsequent surgical removal. It may be necessary to remove all four parathyroids if no localized adenomas can be demonstrated, with prophylactic vitamin D postoperatively to prevent tetany.

Hypoparathyrodism

This may result from surgical removal of the glands for hyperparathyroidism, or as a result of unintended injury during partial thyroidectomy. A primary form may result from an autoimmune process, analagous to Addison's disease of the adrenal cortex and Hashimoto's disease of the thyroid. The serum phosphate level is raised and the serum calcium level falls; the latter is particularly associated with neuromuscular hyper-excitability. Serum PTH levels are reduced or absent despite the low serum calcium level.

Tetany

Tetany is the classic manifestation of low serum calcium levels from any cause, including hypoparathyroidism, rickets/osteomalacia and malabsorption. Features include painful cramps and tingling in the extremities, spasms of the hands, leading to the classic 'main d'accoucheur' position, and fits. Psychiatric manifestations are a recognised complication.

Treatment in the short term consists of intravenous injections of 10 ml of 10% calcium gluconate; in hypoparathyroidism, the hypocalcaemia responds better to continued administration of oral 1,25-dihydroxy vitamin D.

Alkalosis of any cause may also cause tetany by reducing concentrations of ionized (but not total) calcium in the plasma. Overbreathing in anxious or hysterical individuals often leads to dramatic presentations with tetany in accident and emergency departments or dental surgeries (Fig. 13.6); this hyperventilation leads to the blowing off of excessive carbon dioxide with resulting alkalosis. The condition responds easily to reassurance, and to rebreathing from a closed bag held over the nose and mouth.

Diabetes mellitus (pancreatic islets)

Diabetes mellitus means the passage of excessive urine, 'sweet like honey'. The condition is characterized by chronic hyperglycaemia, resulting from failure of insulin secretion from the pancreas and/or resistance to the action of insulin at the tissue level. It is geographically widespread and frequent in all ethnic groups; it is thus a major drain on health resources, particularly taking into account the wide range of disabling disease complications which may arise.

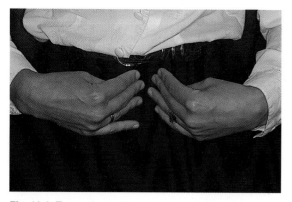

Fig. 13.6 Tetany due to hysterical overbreathing in an anxious dental patient.

Actions of insulin

Insulin is synthesized by the B cells in pancreatic islets of Langerhans and secreted into the portal blood; it reaches the general circulation after traversing the liver. Insulin has a wide range of anabolic actions involving ingested carbohydrate, protein and lipid, but its major primary effect is to enhance the uptake of blood glucose by the tissues, especially the liver and muscles.

Insulin secretion is stimulated by rises in blood glucose levels and suppressed in hypoglycaemia, ensuring that blood glucose levels are tightly controlled in health, despite the potentially enormous fluctuations induced by meals. In the fasting state, blood glucose levels vary between 3.0 and 6.0 mmol/l, but even after meals do not rise above 8.0 mmol/l in healthy individuals.

Where blood glucose concentrations exceed this upper level, the glucose load in the renal glomerular filtrate will exceed the capacity of the proximal tubule to reabsorb it (renal threshold), and glycosuria will result.

Aetiology and clinical forms of diabetes

Most diabetes mellitus is primary, but some cases are secondary to other diseases (Table 13.12). Primary diabetes is further subdivided into an insulin-dependent type (IDDM), where an absolute lack of insulin is involved, and a non-insulin-dependent type (NIDDM) due to a relative insulin lack compared to tissue insulin resistance (which is often increased by obesity). In general, IDDM predominates in young patients, and NIDDM in obese, older individuals, but either form can occur at any age. A comparison of IDDM and NIDDM is shown in Table 13.13.

The aetiology of primary diabetes is now becoming clearer, and is probably a mixture of genetic and autoimmune factors. Exposure to some viruses is capable of damaging islet cells in animals, but a link is harder to prove in humans.

Clinical presentation

While some patients with NIDDM present with classic complaints, many remain asymptomatic until routine blood or urine examinations suggest the diagnosis; indeed, some may present only

Table 13.12 Primary and secodary diabetes mellitus

Primary	IDDM
	NIDDM – obese or non-obese
Secondary	Pancreatic disease, pancreatectomy
	Acromegaly
	Corticosteroid therapy, Cushing's syndrome

when complications develop (see later). Patients with IDDM almost all present with symptoms of the uncontrolled diabetic state:

- polyuria, attributable to the osmotic diuretic effect of large concentrations of glucose in the urine
- intense thirst and polydipsia resulting from loss of fluid
- weight loss, often in the presence of a maintained appetite.

Diabetic ketoacidosis is a life-threatening metabolic emergency which may arise at any time during the course of diabetes, and is often the primary presentation in younger patients. Rapidly increasing hyperglycaemia and severe dehydration are associated with accelerated peripheral lipolysis leading to excessive circulating fatty acids, ketones in blood and urine, and severe metabolic acidosis with Kussmaul respiration (see Ch. 2). It is often precipitated by infection, metabolic stress, or interference with insulin administration. Disturbance of consciousness is common, and overt coma may occasionally result. Urgent hospitalization is required for treatment with intravenous infusion of insulin and fluids, intensive clinical and biochemical monitoring, and treatment of precipitating factors such as infection.

Diagnosis

In patients with symptoms, diagnosis is confirmed by an elevated blood glucose level. In asymptomatic patients, diagnosis can be made by two fasting venous levels greater than 6.7 mmol/l or two random levels greater than 10 mmol/l. An oral glucose tolerance test, measuring blood sugar levels over 2–2.5 h after ingestion of a standard glucose load, may be required in borderline cases. Glucose is capable of attaching itself to certain proteins non-enzymatically, including the β chain of haemoglobin; measurement of glycosylated haemoglobin levels is useful in monitoring control of diabetes, since these levels reflect the degree of hyperglycaemia over a period of time and not simply on the day of examination. Detection of glycosuria is useful confirmation, although this finding may occur in other conditions, such as a low renal threshold for glucose excretion. Ketonuria is present in ketoacidosis.

Complications of diabetes

These are a major cause of morbidity, thus, for example, 45% of all non-traumatic leg amputations are associated with diabetes, and diabetic retinal disease is now the commonest cause of blindness in the UK. Such complications tend to develop after diabetes mellitus has been present for some time, and are partly related to the quality of diabetic control.

Table 13.13 Comparison of IDDM and NIDDM

	IDDM	NIDDM
Genetic factors		
HLA subtypes	Strongly associated	Not associated
Chromosome 11	Associated	Not associated
Risk in siblings	Moderate	Strong
Autoimmunity	Good evidence	No evidence
Pathophysiology	Loss of islet cells	Partial loss of islet cells
	Insulin lack, no insulin resistance	Insulin resistance important
	Insulin therapy always required	Insulin therapy unusual
	Tendency to ketoacidosis	No ketoacidosis

The main complications are summarized as follows:

• Bacterial infections. Infections are commoner in diabetics than non-diabetics, partly due to subtle disturbances of immune function, and partly due to increased glucose in urine and body secretions. Minor infections such as staphylococcal boils, and candidal vaginitis or balanitis (penile infection) are often present at diagnosis. Abscesses due to *Staphylococcus aureus*, urinary tract infection and pulmonary tuberculosis are also strongly associated with diabetes.

• Cardiovascular disease (see Ch. 6). Ischaemic heart disease, cerebrovascular accidents and peripheral arterial disease especially involving the feet all have a high incidence in diabetic patients (Fig. 13.7).

• Eye disease – premature cataracts and microvascular retinal disease.

• Renal and urinary tract disorders – infection and microvascular renal disease.

• Neuropathy – sensory polyneuropathy, motor nerve root damage (radiculopathy), autonomic neuropathy and cranial nerve lesions.

Some of these mechanisms accumulate in certain anatomical sites; for example, the 'diabetic foot' is often a combination of peripheral arterial disease, ulceration resulting from foot anaesthesia and minor trauma, and infection. Gangrene may result, requiring toe, foot or leg amputation. Similarly, chronic renal failure in diabetics may be caused by the addition of chronic urinary tract infection and hypertension secondary to the specific microvascular glomerular lesion of diabetes.

Management

Diabetic clinic attendance. This ensures regular education of the patient and family, and supervision of the diet, weight and glycaemic control. It allows dieticians and specialists to involve patients in their own care, especially in the self-injection of insulin, to detect and initiate treatment of complications, and in general to provide an atmosphere where the innumerable questions arising from the disease can be asked and suitable support given. Such attendance is most important for patients with IDDM, especially children and

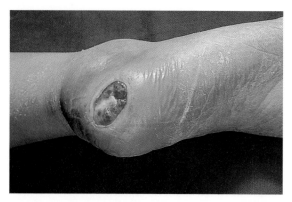

Fig. 13.7 An indolent, neuropathic ulcer on the heel of a patient with diabetes mellitus.

adolescents, for those with unstable disease and a tendency to develop ketoacidosis ('brittle diabetics'), and for those with complications. Other risk factors for vascular disease such as obesity, smoking and hypertension should receive appropriate attention. It is less important whether or not such facilities are sited in hospitals or the community; an 'open-door' daily availability for prompt help is an important feature of the best arrangements. 'Shared care' between community and hospital clinics is increasingly practised.

Dietary measures. A diet is designed to take account of the patient's ideal weight and the likely expenditure of energy on physical activity, especially during work; strong efforts may be required to reduce the weight of obese patients with NIDDM. Carbohydrates should be ingested in the unrefined form and not as simple sugars, and fats should be restricted. Excess alcohol intake is undesirable.

Medication. This may not be required at all in obese NIDDM patients, who become normoglycaemic on attainment of weight reduction. In other diabetics, dietary management must be supplemented either with oral hypoglycaemic agents or with insulin replacement therapy.

In general, oral hypoglycaemic agents are used in older NIDDM patients with no tendency to ketoacidosis. Sulphonylureas (e.g. glibenclamide or gliclazide), act by stimulating residual insulin secretion and biguanides (e.g. metformin) by increasing peripheral glycolysis.

Insulin therapy (with recombitant human

insulin, which has replaced bovine or porcine insulin) by subcutaneous injection is usually required for all patients with IDDM, and thus for all with a liability to ketoacidosis, for patients with NIDDM who have failed with diet and oral hypoglycaemics, and for the initial management of infective or traumatic crises. Since injected insulin can only approximate to the sensitive 24 h secretion of endogenous pancreatic insulin, peaks and troughs of insulin action are inevitable with routine subcutaneous injection once, twice or thrice daily. Alternative means of providing demand insulin by portable infusion devices remain under active investigation. Insulins are available in a wide variety of forms and durations of action, and tailoring of the appropriate preparations for an individual's needs is a skilled matter. Patients are educated in injection technique, and in monitoring their blood sugar levels (by a fingerprick sample and portable glycometer) or urine sugar levels.

Hypoglycaemia. While hypoglycaemia has a wide variety of causes, in clinical practice the most important is that occurring in diabetics on insulin replacement, or, less commonly, on oral agents. Hypoglycaemia occurs where there is inadequate matching of insulin to diet and to the energy consuming effects of exercise, or where an inappropriate regime is being used. Patients sometimes take their insulin but do not eat prior to attending the dental surgery, hence they are at risk of hypoglycaemia. The symptoms are both adrenergic (pallor, sweating, tremor, palpitation and pupillary dilatation), and neuroglycopenic (poor concentration, inappropriate or disinhibited 'drunk' behaviour, double vision, fits, decreasing consciousness and coma). Patients are often familiar with their own early hypoglycaemic symptoms, and can take appropriate action (e.g. taking sugar lumps or a glucose drink); elderly patients, those with autonomic neuropathy, and those on β-adrenergic blocking drugs may lose these warning symptoms.

If the patient cannot take rapidly absorbed sugars by mouth (e.g. owing to aggression or loss of consciousness), a rapid effect can be achieved by the intramuscular injection of glucagon, which raises blood sugar levels (0.5–1.0 unit). If there is no response, up to 50 ml of 50 g/dl glucose should be given intravenously (taking care to avoid extravasation of the injection, which may cause skin

ulceration). Response should be immediate, and no harm will accrue to patients with diabetic hyperglycaemia in the unlikely event of clinical confusion occurring.

Surgery in diabetes

The dental surgeon should liaise with the patient's diabetic clinic. Close monitoring of blood glucose levels and electrolytes is often required.

The following represents a basic plan of action for patients with NIDDM and IDDM:

NIDDM

1. Well-controlled patients on diet alone: treat as non-diabetics.

2. Patients on short-acting oral hypoglycaemics: omit drugs on day of surgery, treat as non-diabetic, and resume therapy next day.

3. Patients on long-acting sulphonylureas (e.g. chlorpropamide): stop drugs 3 days before surgery and substitute a short-acting oral preparation; then proceed as in 2).

4. Poorly controlled patients: restabilize on insulin before surgery; reconvert to oral hypoglycaemics postoperatively, or retain on insulin.

IDDM

1. Arrange 2–3 day hospital admission. Restabilize on short-acting insulin.

2. Schedule the operation early in the day. Omit breakfast and insulin; commence infusion of 500 ml of 10% dextrose, with 15 units of short-acting insulin and 10 mmol potassium chloride added to the pack. This should be infused at a rate of 100 ml/h. Added insulin can be modified according to blood sugar levels.

3. Continue infusion until the first meal is eaten; restart subcutaneous insulin 1 h before the drip is discontinued. Resume pre-operative regimen thereafter.

4. Consider parenteral or nasogastric feeding if normal nutrition is not resumed by 48 h.

Obesity

Endocrine disorders such as hypothyroidism, Cushing's syndrome and rare hypothalamic disorders contribute an insignificant proportion to the population frequency of overweight individuals. The majority are usually regarded as suffering from 'simple obesity', which is increasing epidemically in developed countries. The population prevalence rises with age in both sexes over the age of 16 years; in men the curve flattens off in late life, but continues to rise into old age in women. Overall, about 15% of men and 20% of women in the UK can be regarded as overweight, defined as a body mass index or BMI (=weight (kg)/height (m)^2) greater than 30. The prevalence in children is also increasing. The aetiology is complex, and includes interacting genetic, dietary and social factors, but clearly in all there is an imbalance between calorie intake and energy expenditure. Most obese patients have both an excessive intake over that required and decreased energy output from inadequate physical activity. It is clear, however, that some individuals are more prone to weight gain than others with a comparable energy intake.

It has been known for nearly a century from insurance statistics that overweight individuals have a decreased life expectation. Some of the metabolic changes accompanying obesity are shown in Table 13.14, and the clinical associations are summarized in Table 13.15. There is thus clear medical justification for encouraging weight reduction in obese patients.

Weight reduction is achieved mostly by reducing calorie intake, supplemented by increasing energy expenditure by exercise. Simply increasing

Table 13.14 Metabolic changes accompanying obesity

Decreased glucose tolerance
Decreased insulin secretion
Increased plasma insulin levels
Elevated plasma lipid levels (cholesterol, triglyceride)
Elevated plasma uric acid levels
Elevated blood pressure

Table 13.15 Clinical associations with obesity

Ischaemic heart disease
Diabetes mellitus (NIDDM)
Hypertension
Impaired pulmonary function
Increased surgical risks (anaesthesia, infection, venous thromboembolism, wound healing)
Osteoarthritis
Gallstones
Gout
Varicose veins, venous thromboembolism

exercise up to a level of 30 min walking daily or on alternate days, is appropriate. A strongly supportive team approach from doctor and dietician is needed, especially in maintaining determination and self-esteem. Voluntary self-help groups (e.g. Weight Watchers) are often valuable. Appetite-suppressant drugs, the use of T4 to increase the metabolic rate, jaw wiring to restrict food intake, and surgical gastroplasty to reduce stomach capacity and thus induce early satiety are rarely indicated. Leptin is a recently discovered hormone involved in weight regulation. Its therapeutic role remains experimental.

14 Musculoskeletal disorders

Introduction

These conditions include arthritis, connective tissue disorders, bone disorders and fractures. Each will be discussed in turn.

Arthritis

Taken together, joint disorders are responsible for enormous population morbidity, and have correspondingly severe effects economically both for the sufferer and for the community at large; it is estimated that in the UK there are 5 million sufferers from osteoarthritis and 0.5 million from rheumatoid arthritis. A description of the commoner conditions follows (Table 14.1). Some disorders may present with involvement of only one joint (monoarthritis), but presentations involving several joints are more frequent (polyarthritis).

Rheumatoid arthritis

Rheumatoid arthritis is a chronic disease, characterized primarily by inflammatory changes in the synovium; non-synovial joints are not involved. The disease has a predilection for peripheral (centrifugal) joints such as the hands, wrists, ankles and knees; the shoulders, hips and sacroiliac

Table 14.1 Arthritic disorders
Rheumatoid arthritis
Seronegative polyarthritis
Inflammatory arthropathies associated with:
specific bacterial infections
viral infections
Crystal arthropathies
Osteoarthritis
Arthritis in connective tissue disorders

joints are rarely affected, and spinal involvement is confined to the cervical spine and the apophyseal joints. The inflamed synovium becomes thickened and vascular, and is aggressively destructive to the whole joint, including cartilage and adjacent bone. The condition is three times more frequent in women than men, and can begin at any age, although middle age is usual.

Clinical features

The condition is usually of gradual onset, most typically starting symmetrically in the metacarpophalangeal and proximal interphalangeal joints of the hands. The involved joints become hot, swollen and painful; stiffness, worse in the morning or after inactivity, is characteristic. Function is limited at first by pain, then by joint destruction with or without ankylosis. Deformity is induced not only by arthritis itself but also by the stretching and rupture of tendons and ligaments around the affected joints. Typical hand deformities are illustrated in Figure 14.1.

Involvement of the temporomandibular joints may lead to pain on chewing and restricted jaw movements. The upper cervical spine is commonly affected; this is associated with pain and stiffness. Erosion of the odontoid peg with subsequent subluxation of the atlantoaxial joint is a potentially serious complication of rheumatoid arthritis, since compression of the cervical cord or vertebral arteries may lead to quadriplegia or sudden death; dentists and anaesthetists should always be aware of the dangers of manipulation of the neck, especially forced extension, in these patients. Hoarseness is a further unusual clinical feature. Although rheumatoid arthritis is predominantly an inflammatory polyarthritis, extra-articular manifestations are common, especially in patients with positive serology (Table 14.2). Of particular interest in oral medicine is Sjögren's syndrome, discussed more fully in Chapter 22.

Aetiology

Despite intensive investigation the aetiology remains uncertain. There is a strong genetic predisposition to the disease, and a high frequency of HLA class II alleles, especially DR4. T cells of CD4 phenotype (helper cells) probably have a significant role in mediating the inflammatory

Table 14.2 Some extra-articular associations of rheumatoid arthritis

Rheumatoid nodules
Anaemia, proportional to disease activity
Lung involvement
Sjögren's syndrome
Eyes, especially scleritis and episcleritis
Liver involvement
Splenomegaly and regional adenopathy
Myopathy with wasting
Arteritis
Amyloidosis

process. In addition, autoantibodies especially of IgM and IgG class may form immune complexes which could activate complement and potentiate or prolong joint inflammation and destruction through the action of inflammatory mediators. The search for an environmental factor such as infection has so far been unsuccessful.

Investigations

The erythrocyte sedimentation rate (ESR) is characteristically elevated, reflecting a rise in the serum acute phase protein concentration.

The demonstration of rheumatoid factor in serum is the key investigation, although this test may be positive in 4% of the normal population. The factor consists of IgM autoantibodies against Fc fragments of native IgG, and can be demonstrated by latex agglutination techniques; high titres are associated with erosive joint disease and with rheumatoid nodules.

Radiographs of affected joints may demonstrate erosions and periarticular osteoporosis. Aspiration of synovial fluid may provide useful serological confirmation, and is helpful in excluding infection in patients presenting with monoarthritis; synovial biopsy can be performed during the same procedure.

Management

Physical and general measures. Attention should be given to maintaining general nutrition. Acutely inflamed joints should be rested, and splinting is useful to control pain. Controlled exercise to prevent muscle wasting and preserve

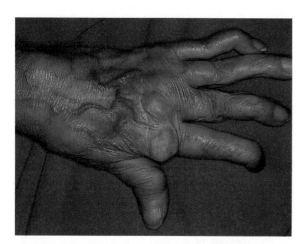

Fig. 14.1 Typical hand deformities in a patient with rheumatoid arthritis.

mobility is vital, and physical aids and appliances assist in keeping patients independent.

Drug therapy. Simple analgesics and the judicious use of non-steroidal anti-inflammatory drugs (e.g. ibuprofen) are the mainstay of treatment. Resistant cases may require the use of gold or penicillamine, and corticosteroids may be useful in some patients both for the arthritis, and also for the extra-articular manifestations.

Surgery. Patients should be managed with a combined medical–surgical approach, and in selected cases surgery is very successful in restoring function to affected joints; the procedures available include synovectomy, tendon reconstruction and repositioning, and replacement arthroplasty.

Course of rheumatoid arthritis

The condition is not always a crippling disease, and may burn out after a variable period. In approximately 25% of patients the condition may regress without permanent damage to joints; 40%, however, remain impaired, 25% have marked disability, and 10% may be reduced to a wheelchair existence.

Seronegative polyarthritis

This group of inflammatory polyarthritides is characterized by absence of rheumatoid factor in the serum, involvement of the sacroiliac joints, and by a peripheral inflammatory arthritis. The nodules characteristic of rheumatoid disease are not seen. The causes of seronegative polyarthritis are shown in Table 14.3, and these are discussed in turn.

Ankylosing spondylitis

This condition is five times commoner in men than women, and usually starts in the second or third decade. There is a strong association (90%) with HLA B27 phenotypes.

Initially the condition is dominated by sacroiliitis, with complaints of low backache radiating into the buttocks, and pronounced stiffness. The sacroiliac joints are tender on palpation and radiography shows sclerosis of the joint margins and obliteration of the joint space.

Table 14.3 Causes of seronegative polyarthritis

Ankylosing spondylitis
Psoriatic arthropathy
Inflammatory bowel disease
Reiter's syndrome and other reactive arthritides
Behçet's syndrome HLA B27 phenotypes.

The disease process may then affect the rest of the spine, including the neck; in advanced cases, there is calcification of the spinal ligaments with the formation of syndesmophytes (bamboo spine), and flexion becomes possible only at the hip joints. Involvement of the costovertebral joints impairs rib movement, and restrictive respiratory defects may predispose to recurrent chest infections. Peripheral joint involvement, especially in the lower limbs, is seen in 20% of patients.

The principles of therapy are as outlined for rheumatoid arthritis.

Psoriatic arthropathy

This common skin disease occurs in 1.6% of the population (see Ch. 12), and arthritis is a recognized complication in around 7% of these. The large limb joints may be affected as well as the sacroiliac joints, but the characteristic feature is involvement of the distal interphalangeal joints, often associated with nail dystrophy.

Inflammatory bowel disease

Activity in the arthritis tends to follow remissions and relapses in the bowel disease, and is often associated with other extra-articular manifestations (see Ch. 10). Joint destruction is rare.

Reactive arthritis, including Reiter's syndrome

This group of disorders consists of a sterile synovitis associated with infection elsewhere, either in the gut or urogenital tract (Table 14.4). Clinically, joint involvement usually shares the characteristic distribution of other seronegative arthropathies.

Reiter's syndrome is a particular clinical form of reactive arthritis and may be acquired either sexually, or after gastrointestinal tract infection.

Table 14.4 Infective causes of Reiter's syndrome

Gut	Urogenital tract
Campylobacter jejunii	Chlamydia spp.
Yersinia spp.	
Salmonella spp.	
(except S. typhi and S. paratyphi)	
Shigella flexneri	

The arthropathy is associated with a wide variety of extra-articular manifestations, some of which affect the mouth (Table 14.5); the defining associations of Reiter's syndrome are sterile conjunctivitis and urethritis. Reiter's syndrome is usually self-limiting, and the process resolves in the majority of patients by 6 months; a few patients go on to develop chronic inflammatory joint disease. There is no evidence that antimicrobial treatment against the underlying infection shortens the course. During active disease, management is on the principles described for rheumatoid arthritis.

The interval between infection and the onset of joint disease may vary from 3 to 30 days.

Inflammatory arthropathies associated with specific bacterial infections
(see Ch. 5)

Specific bacterial infections within joints may lead to arthritis (usually monoarthritis), most often after bloodborne spread from a primary infection elsewhere; important organisms include *Staphylococcus aureus*, *Neisseria meningitidis*, *Neisseria gonorrhoeae* and *Mycobacterium tuberculosis*. Treatment is by specific antimicrobial therapy.

Table 14.5 Extra-articular manifestations of Reiter's syndrome

Conjunctivitis
Urethritis
Circinate balanitis (inflammation of the glans penis)
Oral ulceration (see Ch. 26).
Plantar fasciitis
Keratoderma blenorrhagicum (horn-like skin lesions on the hands and feet)

Inflammatory arthropathies associated with viral infections

Certain viral infections are associated with a self-limiting sterile polyarthritis in a minority of affected patients; it is probable that arthropathy results predominantly from immune complex deposition in the synovium. These conditions include rubella and rubella vaccination, mumps, infective hepatitis and infectious mononucleosis.

Crystal arthropathies

These conditions are associated with the deposition of crystal aggregates in the synovium, and are usually caused by metabolic disorders.

Gout is the commonest of these; because of hyperuricaemia, crystals of urate accumulate in the joints (Fig. 14.2) and also in certain extra-articular sites such as ear cartilage (tophi) and the kidney. Joint inflammation occurs when there is ingestion of crystals by polymorphonuclear leucocytes; degranulation, followed by release of hydrolytic enzymes into the tissues. This leads to the further release of chemical inflammatory mediators.

Uric acid is derived from the physiological breakdown of purine bases, and most of this is normally excreted by the kidneys; hyperuricaemia may thus result either from increased production or impaired renal excretion of uric acid (Table 14.6). In classic primary gout, which can run in families, the mechanism is not completely clear,

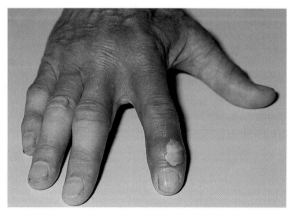

Fig. 14.2 Ulceration overlying a tophus in a patient with gout.

Table 14.6 Mechanisms of hyperuricaemia

Increased production	Impaired excretion
Rare enzyme deficiencies Increased turnover of nucleoproteins 　　Lymphoproliferative disorders 　　Myeloproliferative disorders 　　Chronic haemolysis	Classic primary gout (75–80%) Chronic renal failure Drugs, especially thiazide diuretics

but in the majority is probably due to an isolated renal lesion which reduces uric acid clearance; most patients with hyperuricaemia, however, do not develop clinical gout. Men are affected much more commonly than women. Other associations of gout include obesity, hypertension and polycythaemia.

The classic presentation of an acute episode involves a very painful arthropathy of the metatarsophalangeal joint of the great toe. Early attacks usually settle without residual joint damage, but eventually a chronic arthropathy can develop which may be disabling if large joints are affected. Chronic renal failure with or without hypertension is a serious complication resulting from parenchymal deposition of urate and from the obstructive effects of urate renal calculi.

Treatment of the acute attack is by immobilization and the use of non-steroidal anti-inflammatory drugs; thereafter the hyperuricaemia should be controlled by the long-term use of allopurinol, a metabolic inhibitor of uric acid production. Any underlying disorder should be treated appropriately.

Osteoarthritis

This commonest of arthropathies remains ill-understood; because its incidence increases with age, it has been too readily assumed to result from simple mechanical 'wear and tear' on the joints. The reality is certain to be more complex, involving altered mechanical stresses, imbalance in repair and remodelling mechanisms, and biochemical changes in the cartilage. Aetiological factors are shown in Table 14.7.

In established cases, the cartilage over the articular surfaces becomes fibrillated, thin and cratered, and may eventually disappear. Bone ends become thickened and sclerosed, exposed areas of bone become eburnated ('like ivory'), and bony outgrowths (osteophytes) appear round the joint margins. There may be an increase in synovial fluid. Although usually considered a non-inflammatory arthropathy, this is not entirely true since low-grade inflammatory changes can be seen histologically in the synovium.

Clinical features

The affected joints are painful, particularly after exercise, and may become troublesome at night in severe cases. Stiffness, later associated with joint instability, becomes progressively worse, and is particularly disabling if the lower limb joints are affected. Examination shows bony enlargement of the joints, some synovial thickening and effusion, and coarse crepitus on movement; signs of inflammation are generally absent.

Table 14.7 Factors contributing to the development of osteoarthritis

Strong associations	Weak associations
Increasing age Female sex Positive family history Previous joint damage (trauma, inflammatory arthritis, 　　congenital abnormalities, haemarthrosis (e.g. severe haemophilia)) Impaired sensation, e.g. peripheral neuropathy	Obesity Joint hypermobility Occupation

The pattern of joint involvement varies widely but is different from rheumatoid arthritis. Large joints like the hips, knees and shoulders are commonly affected, often asymmetrically, and spinal involvement is also frequent. A clinically distinct subgroup ('generalized osteoarthritis') involves the distal interphalangeal joints, which may show Heberden's nodes (Fig. 14.3), the apophyseal joints of the spine, and the knees; this form is commoner in women.

Diagnosis

This is usually easy to make on clinical grounds alone. The diagnosis can be confirmed by radiology, by the absence in the serum of elevated parameters of inflammation such as the ESR, and by the absence of rheumatoid factor in the blood.

Treatment

This includes the maintenance of muscle strength and mobility by physiotherapy, home aids, and the effective use of non-steroidal analgesics. Surgery using implant arthroplasty has transformed the disability of many patients, particularly at the hip and knee.

Connective tissue disorders (collagen vascular disorders)

This is a diverse group of diseases, including systemic lupus erythematosus (SLE), polymyositis and dermatomyositis, systemic sclerosis, Sjögren's syndrome, and the systemic vasculitides such as polyarteritis nodosa, Wegener's granulomatosis, and giant cell arteritis. Many of these conditions have a predilection for the female sex, involvement of several body systems (multisystem disorders), and an autoimmune pathogenesis. Although each exists in a readily diagnosable pure form, widespread overlap can occur, both in clinical manifestations and in the associated immunological phenomena. The aetiology remains unknown, though a role for involvement of major histocompatibility-complex genes is becoming clearer by recent findings in immunogenetics. Exposure to drugs, chemicals or viruses in the environment can precipitate some of these illnesses.

Systemic lupus erythematosus

This condition largely affects young women of child-bearing age, and runs a chronic course with exacerbations and remissions. Its classic multisystem involvement should lead to suspicion of the diagnosis in any patients presenting with simultaneous disease of more than one organ (Table 14.8).

Immunological features

Demonstrable serum autoantibodies in SLE include anti-DNA histone, anti-single-stranded DNA, and IgG anti-double-stranded DNA, which is thought to be associated with the pathogenesis of the disease. Anti-double-stranded DNA is the basis of most serological tests to confirm the diagnosis. Local organ damage probably results from fixation of immune complexes with the activation of complement.

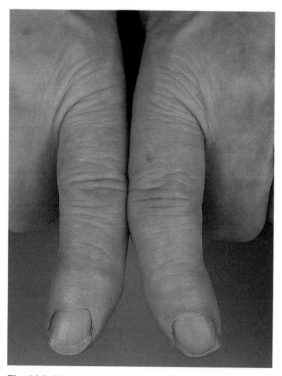

Fig. 14.3 Heberden's nodes on the fingers of a patient with osteoarthritis of the hands.

Table 14.8 Clinical manifestations of SLE

Skin	Classical facial 'butterfly' rash and other erythemas, alopecia, photosensitivity
Joints	Non-erosive polyarthritis
Kidney	Glomerulonephritis
Mucous membranes	Oral ulceration (see Ch. 26)
Nervous system	Polyneuritis, cerebritis (cerebral lupus)
Vascular	Raynaud's phenomenon, arterial and venous thrombosis
Heart	Pericarditis, endocarditis and myocarditis
Lungs	Pleuritis
Eyes	Anterior uveitis
Blood	Autoimmune haemolytic anaemia
	Autoimmune thrombocytopenia and neutropenia
Fever	

Additional autoantibodies against all three formed blood elements commonly cause anaemia, leucopenia and thrombocytopenia (see Ch. 7).

Treatment

Corticosteriods alone or in combination with other immunosuppressive drugs such as azathioprine or cyclophosphamide form the mainstay of therapy. A wide variety of therapies can also be used effectively in the management of target organ damage, e.g. antimalarials for skin and joint lesions, barrier creams for photosensitivity, analgesics for arthritis, and haemodialysis or transplantation for end-stage renal failure.

Systemic sclerosis

This is an uncommon multisystem disorder, affecting women three times more than men; the onset is usually around 30–60 years. It causes fibrosis both in the skin and internal organs, and also causes widespread damage to small blood vessels, particularly capillaries and arterioles; these show proliferation of the intima and thickening of the adventitia. When the process is confined to the skin alone, the term 'scleroderma' is applied (see Ch. 26); the clinical features of systemic sclerosis are shown in Table 14.9.

A benign variant of the condition is called CRST syndrome, i.e. subcutaneous calcinosis (C), usually affecting fingers and forearms, Raynaud's phenomenon (R), sclerodactyly (S), and telangiectasia (T).

The aetiology is unknown, although environmental toxins and drugs have been implicated; an immunological attack both on vascular endothelial cells and fibroblasts is likely. A number of autoantibodies have been identified, and correlations between these antibodies and particular

Table 14.9 Clinical features of systemic sclerosis

Skin	Thickened, tightened and atrophic, especially in the hands and face; late contractures
	Microstomia, puckering of lips, pinched face
	Telangiectasia of nail folds, arms, mouth, etc.
	Raynaud's phenomenon
	Calcification
Oesophagus	Dysphagia
Small bowel	Stasis, malabsorption
Renal	Chronic renal failure (main cause of death)
Lung	Interstitial fibrosis
	Pulmonary hypertension
Musculoskeletal	Myopathy, arthropathy

clinical manifestations are currently being explored. For example, 70% of patients manifest antinuclear antibodies, and anticentromere antibodies have a predictive value for the CRST syndrome.

Specific treatment is not available, and there is little controlled evidence of benefit from corticosteroids, other immunosuppressive drugs or plasmapheresis; penicillamine may have a role in inhibiting fibrosis. Management must consist mainly of ameliorating the clinical manifestations.

Systemic vasculitis

Primary systemic vasculitides are characterized by inflammatory changes confined to the blood vessels themselves; organ manifestations are secondary to these. Histologically, some conditions are associated with the formation of granulomas (see also Ch. 26). The clinical features depend largely on localization, the size of the blood vessels involved and the presence or absence of vaso-occlusive events (Table 14.10). Constitutional features are often present, with fever, weight loss, anaemia and an elevated ESR. Clinical presentations are understandably very variable, but the diagnosis should be suspected in any patient with a multisystem disorder.

The aetiology is largely not understood. Hepatitis B infection can be associated with polyarteritis nodosa, and there is less secure evidence of association with other microbial pathogens. A role for drugs and toxins has also been proposed. Circulating autoantibodies, especially antineutrophil cytoplasmic antibodies (ANCA) can be found in the majority of patients, and may have a pathogenetic role.

Treatment is by the use of corticosteroids and cytotoxic immunosuppressive drugs. Response is variable; dramatic and immediate benefit is strikingly shown in giant cell arteritis for example, whereas Henoch–Schönlein purpura not resolving spontaneously tends to be resistant to such therapy.

Table 14.10 Systemic vasculitides			
Blood vessel	With granulomas	Without granulomas	Main clinical features
Large	Takayasu's disease		Young oriental women Aortitis; rarer involvement of pulmonary arteries
	Giant cell arteritis (see Ch. 25)		Cranial arteritis Temporal headache Visual impairment/loss Jaw claudication Polymyalgia rheumatica
Medium		Polyarteritis nodosa	Widespread internal organ damage mainly to kidneys, gastrointestinal tract, nervous system (peripheral nerves and brain), arthralgia
		Kawasaki's disease	Childhood systemic vasculitis, especially coronary arteries
Small (arteriole and capillary)	Wegener's granulomatosis		Necrotizing vasculitis affecting upper respiratory tract (nasal ulceration, perforated septum) and lower respiratory tract, including the lungs Kidney (see also Ch. 26)
	Churg–Strauss's syndrome		Necrotizing vasculitis, mainly affecting the lungs; can present with asthma
		Henoch–Schönlein purpura (see Ch. 7)	Skin, joints, gastrointestinal tract, kidneys

Bone disorders

The rigidity of bone may give the impression of physiological inertness. On the contrary, bone is metabolically very active tissue, undergoing continuous remodelling by bone resorption and formation, even in the adult when growth has ceased. New bone is formed by osteoblasts, situated mainly in the periosteum; these cells synthesize the collagen matrix of bone, control bone mineralization, and respond in a complex way to various cytokines. Bone resorption is brought about by osteoclasts; their activity is enhanced by the action of parathyroid hormone (see Ch. 13) and by 1,25-dihydroxy vitamin D, and is suppressed by calcitonin (which is produced by the thyroid C cells).

Total bone mass is also influenced by genetic factors, race, physical exertion, good nutrition, maintenance of body weight, and, above all, by sex hormone levels. Males have a higher bone mass than females, and although both sexes progressively lose bone mass after young adult life, this process occurs very rapidly in women for the first 10 years after the menopause. This accelerated bone loss in women can be reduced by hormone replacement therapy (HRT).

Many bone diseases can be diagnosed clinically. Presentations are summarized in Table 14.11. Pathological fractures are further discussed in the next section. Relevant biochemical investigations include serum levels of calcium, phosphate, alkaline phosphatase and parathormone. Radiology of the skeleton by plain radiography is often helpful, and additional information can be gained by isotope bone scanning, and by radiological measurement of bone density and bone mass. On occasion, needle bone biopsy is helpful.

Osteomalacia

This condition is characterized by defective bone mineralization; it is described as rickets when the condition occurs in growing bone. Histology shows wide osteoid seams and inactive osteoblasts. It occurs in three main circumstances: deficiency of vitamin D or abnormal vitamin D metabolism accounts for the majority of cases (Table 14.12), but it can also complicate phosphate depletion, and chronic metabolic acidosis.

Biochemical investigation usually shows a low normal plasma calcium level (maintained by secondary hyperparathyroidism), a low phosphate level (also maintained by parathyroid activity) but an increased bone alkaline phosphatase level. Treatment is by oral administration of vitamin D tablets, often combined with calcium, and by exclusion and treatment of any underlying disorder.

Osteoporosis

This term is applied to loss of bone mass per unit volume. The chemical composition of bone is normal, there are no demonstrable metabolic changes, and routine blood biochemistry is normal.

Since there is progressive physiological loss of bone with age, clinical effects from osteoporosis are more common in the elderly, and especially if maximal bone mass has not been achieved earlier in life. A rise in population age is the main reason for the increased visibility of the condition, and women are particularly disadvantaged by the rapid loss of bone during the first 10 years after the menopause. Falls, very common in the elderly, often lead to presentations with osteoporotic fractures. The condition is thus responsible for a vast amount of morbidity, and there has been much recent interest in its prevention. Risk factors are shown in Table 14.13.

Treatment of established osteoporosis is unsatisfactory, and at best can usually only show further bone loss. Bisphosphonates increase bone density, but there is some doubt about the mechanical quality of the resulting bone; these drugs can be combined with generous dietary calcium. Prevention should be tackled on a wide scale, and there is now little doubt that HRT in postmenopausal women is effective, and although there may be a very small increased risk of endometrial or breast carcinoma, and of venous thrombosis, HRT also reduces the risk of ischaemic heart disease (see Ch. 6).

Table 14.11 Presenting features of bone disease

Deformity, e.g. kyphosis, scoliosis
Bone pain
Pathological fracture, e.g. of vertebrae or long bones
Associated metabolic abnormalities, e.g. hyper- and hypocalcaemia

Table 14.12 Vitamin D deficiency

Reduced intake/absorption	Poor dietary content of vitamin D Fat malabsorption – steatorrhoea
Skin synthesis impaired	Lack of exposure to sunlight Pigmented skin
Metabolism abnormal	Impaired renal activation of 25-hydroxyvitamin D to 1,25-dihydroxy vitamin D, e.g. chronic renal failure Interference by anticonvulsant drugs

Table 14.13 Risk factors for osteoporosis

Physiological	Pathological
Ageing	Alcohol
Female sex	Corticosteroid drugs, Cushing's syndrome
Early menopause	Multiple myeloma
Immobility	Diabetes mellitus
Underweight	Hypogonadism } rare causes
Childhood maturation failure	Thyrotoxicosis
	Smoking

Paget's disease of bone

This is a common condition, possibly affecting as many as 4% of the population over the age of 40 years. It is a chronic focal disease, and can affect any bone in the body; axial and heavy long bones are most often involved. Distribution is usually random and non-symmetrical.

After many years of obscurity, it now seems likely that it represents a slow virus disease, possibly due to the effect of persisting measles or respiratory syncytial virus infections. The osteoclasts are morphologically abnormal, and contain cytoplasmic and nuclear inclusions thought to be nuclear capsids. Chaotic bone resorption occurs, and this is balanced by increased activity in osteoblasts. Increased bone turnover is thus the hallmark of the disease. The clinical features are summarized in Table 14.14.

The diagnosis is radiological, and isotope bone scanning reveals 'hot spots' at the sites of active disease. Serum calcium and phosphate levels are normal but the alkaline phosphatase level is elevated, in keeping with increased osteoblastic activity.

Treatment was initially by the use of calcitonin, but this has been superseded by the new generation of bisphosphonates, especially etidronate or pamidronate.

Table 14.14 Clinical features of Paget's disease

Deformity, e.g. leg bowing, altered skull shape
Warmth over affected areas (increased vascularity)
Pathological fractures
Nerve entrapment in bony canals, e.g. deafness
Secondary osteoarthritis
Secondary osteogenic sarcoma

Skeletal dysplasias and other rarer connective tissue syndromes

These conditions are unusual, and diagnosis often requires specialist consultation. The main features are summarized in Table 14.15.

Fractures

A fracture may be defined as loss of continuity in a bone, and can vary from a simple crack to complete fragmentation (comminuted fracture). The force necessary to fracture normal bones is usually considerable, but can be negligible if bone

Table 14.15 Skeletal dysplasias and other rarer connective tissue syndromes

Disease	Main clinical features	Pathogenetic defect
Osteogenesis imperfecta	Brittle bones Multiple fractures Dwarfism Blue sclerae	Collagen gene mutations
Marfan's syndrome	Long limbs, increased height Joint hypermobility High arched palate Lens dislocation upwards Aortic dilatation	Dominant inheritance Fibrillin gene mutation
Ehlers–Danlos syndrome (see Ch. 7)	Hyperelastic skin (easy bruising) Joint hypermobility	Variable inheritance Abnormal collagen in some

Homocystinuria	Marfanoid body habitus
	Lens dislocation downwards
	Increased tendency to venous
	    thrombosis
		Autosomal recessive inheritance
		Deficiency of cystathionine β-synthetase;
		uncertain relationship to
		    clinical features

Achondroplasia	Short limbs	Autosomal dominant inheritance
		Failure of epiphyseal cartilage to
		    grow – membranous and periosteal
		    bone normal

Osteopetrosis (marble-bone disease)	Decreased bone marrow space,
	    leading to leucoerythroblastic
	    anaemia
	Bone deformity (metaphyses)
	Delayed tooth eruption
		Dominant inheritance
		Increased bone density, without
		    modelling or remodelling
		Subcategory associated with
		    carbonic anhydrase II deficiency

Fibrous dysplasia of bone	Mono-ostotic
	    Isolated bone cysts
	    Any bone affected
	Polyostotic (McCune–Albright syndrome)
	    Multiple cystic bone lesions
	    Pigmentation of skin
	    Sexual precocity, and other endocrine
	        associations
		Aetiology unknown – possible gene
		    disorder

strength is already compromised by disease (pathological fracture). Repeated small stresses applied to a single area of bone may result in fatigue fractures, e.g. the metatarsal heads in subjects whose occupation requires much walking on hard surfaces. It is worth remembering that although most fractures occur at the site of injury as a result of directly applied violence, a proportion follow indirectly from stresses applied at some distance away, e.g. fractured vertebrae may occur as a result of falls from a height on to the feet. Fractures are described as closed when the overlying skin is intact; open fractures occur when the skin is breached, allowing infection to gain access to the fracture site (compound fractures).

Diagnosis can usually be suspected clinically from an assessment of the history, and the findings of deformity, local tenderness, limitation of movement, and bruising or swelling. Because of the vascularity of the bone marrow, torn vessels at the fracture site can often lead to considerable bleeding – up to 2 litres in the case of large long bones – and this will be associated with shock, even without any evidence of external blood loss. Fractures must be confirmed radiologically for both clinical and medicolegal reasons.

Management

Fractures which are undisplaced and not subject to mechanical stresses during healing may require only simple support techniques. More often, any deformity requires manipulation and reduction under anaesthesia, followed by some form of fixation; this can be achieved either by external splintage, (usually by plaster of Paris), continuous traction, or internal fixation using screws and plates. In suitable sites, e.g. the tibia, the fractured bone can be held in position by pins inserted percutaneously and braced externally.

It is vital to minimize any period of immobilization to avoid muscle wasting and joint damage, and physiotherapy is an essential component both in the acute and convalescent phases in regaining optimum function. Prophylaxis of venous thromboembolism is important in immobilized patients (see Ch. 6).

15 Psychological medicine

Introduction

Psychological disease is very prevalent, and is one of the commonest reasons for general medical practitioner consultations. In addition, many outpatient clinics are dominated by complaints of 'functional' disorders with a strong psychological component (psychosomatic disease), e.g. chest pain, back pain, irritable bowel syndrome, globus hystericus, etc. A full discussion of functional facial pain syndromes is found in Chapter 26.

Psychological disease may be classified as shown in Table 15.1.

Minor psychological signs and symptoms can be regarded as exacerbations of normal. The point when personality traits such as worrying or anxiety become abnormal (i.e. disorders) is subjective. When symptoms interfere with behaviour, performance or interpersonal relationships they may be indicative of disease. Not only can

Table 15.1 Classification of psychological disease
Neurosis
Psychosis
Disorders of personality and behaviour
Chemical dependence
Learning disability

psychological disease complicate the clinical presentation of other diseases, it may in fact present as organic symptoms (somatization) or may complicate health care, including oral health care.

Neurotic disorders are exaggerated 'normal responses', which are usually manifestations of anxiety. Patients are, however, in touch with reality. In contrast, those with psychosis may be detached from reality and have bizarre thought processes. Thus, neurotic people may 'build castles in the air' but psychotics 'live in them'!

Traditionally, patients with depression were regarded as having either reactive 'neurotic' depression in response to adverse life events, or 'endogenous' depression as part of a manic–depressive psychosis. This distinction is no longer regarded as valid, because most depressive episodes are initiated or aggravated by adverse life events in predisposed individuals and because the management is the same.

Behaviour disorders or personality disorders such as sociopathic states, are considered later.

Finally, as mentioned above, organic disease may be complicated or be initiated by emotional factors and require treatment directed towards both the physical and psychological problems.

These conditions will now be discussed in turn.

Neurosis

Psychoneurosis, or 'nerves', as it is commonly called, is classified according to the symptoms, which are usually anxiety based or hysterical (Table 15.2).

Anxiety neurosis

Anxiety is a normal response to stress, e.g. before examinations. It may be exaggerated in 'worriers', and may be extreme and chronic. Sometimes it is associated with depression ('agitated' depression). Anxiety is characterized by increased autonomic activity and adrenaline release, leading to apprehension, dry mouth, palpitations, sweating, restlessness, headaches and diarrhoea. When anxiety is provoked by certain objects or situations it may be regarded as a phobia, e.g. arachnophobia (spiders) or claustrophobia (closed spaces). Such phobias are treated by desensitization. Chronic anxiety was traditionally treated with minor tranquillizers such as diazepam which caused chronic dependence problems. It is now managed mainly with simple counselling (often by the general medical practitioner), sometimes combined with short courses of either β-blockers or antidepressants. Cognitive behaviour therapy and psychotherapy are also useful treatments in selected cases.

Depression

Depression may or may not be associated with anxiety. It is characterized by many important symptoms (Table 15.3).

Sleep disturbance is characteristic, with the patient waking early with a troubled mind. The condition may present with functional headache (see Ch. 9) or facial pain, which deteriorates towards evening (see Ch. 26).

Table 15.2 Psychoneuroses

Anxiety
Simple depression
Hysteria
Obsessive neurosis
Post-traumatic stress disorders

Table 15.3 Features of depression

Sadness of mood
Sleep disturbance, e.g. early morning wakening
Loss of appetite
Loss of weight or gain in weight
Loss of libido
Loss of interest in daily life
Poverty of thought
Depersonalization (also seen in anxiety)
Atypical headache and facial pain
Suicidal thoughts
Delusions of worthlessness and guilt

Depression is most commonly reactive to adverse life events, the most severe of which are bereavement, house moving, separation, divorce and retirement. However, it may be endogenous. The main danger is of suicide, and questioning on suicidal thoughts is important in routine assessment.

Treatment is with antidepressants, and social, family and psychological treatment, including cognitive behaviour therapy. Tricyclic antidepressants (e.g. dothiepin) have been largely replaced by the selective serotonin reuptake inhibitors (e.g. fluoxetine), which usually have fewer side-effects, particularly in self-overdose.

Hysteria

Hysteria is a subconscious device used by the patient to resolve anxiety. This may take several forms such as paralysis of an arm ('conversion' hysteria) or amnesia as seen in dissociative reactions. Some hysterical patients may hyperventilate and this, by expelling carbon dioxide and changing the acid–base balance, may cause tetany and collapse (see Ch. 13).

Obsessive neurosis

Many of us have an obsessive personality and, for example, automatically line up rulers and pens with the edge of a desk. In extreme cases, however, obsessive neurosis leads to repetitive actions or compulsions and obsessional thoughts (nominations) which interfere with life. Examples include constant hand washing, or returning to the house on several occasions to check that the lights have been switched off or doors locked. Supportive psychotherapy is helpful. More active psychology treatments are best. Again, cognitive behaviour therapy is being used as is 'response prevention'. Drug therapy can also be effective in selected cases.

Post-traumatic stress disorders

These conditions occur after life-threatening experiences, e.g. car crashes, or after being exposed to disastrous events, such as plane crashes. Symptoms include irritability, loss of concentration and recurrent nightmares. The prognosis is not always good, but supportive psychotherapy is helpful. Cognitive behaviour therapy and antidepressants are also used.

Psychosomatic disorders

Most conditions, even when clearly organic in nature, are modified by the psychological status of the patient. Thus, the soldier wounded in battle may be unaware of an injury until the day is won. Several disorders such as dysmenorrhoea, alopecia, asthma and eczema are significantly influenced by emotional factors. A holistic approach to patient care will ensure that both the physical and emotional aspects of the patient's disorder are addressed.

Traditionally, psychological considerations are only taken into account once organic disease has been eliminated or treated. This is an inappropriate practice since psychological disease may produce greater morbidity than the organic component or even mortality in the form of suicide if the psychological aspects of the patient's complaints are ignored and management delayed.

Psychosis

Psychosis may be functional or organic in nature (Table 15.4).

Functional psychosis

Affective psychosis

Affective disorders are those which affect mood. Premorbid personalities exhibit mood swings, and

Table 15.4 Psychosis	
Functional	Affective – manic–depressive psychosis Schizophrenia
Organic	Acute – delirium Chronic – dementia

everyone is aware of individuals with cyclothymic personalities, who have large mood swings, and those with depressive personalities, who are always gloomy. Manic–depressive psychosis, however, is characterized by extreme swings of mood with manic episodes (Table 15.5) and deep depressive episodes. It is more common in women, and sometimes is seen in mother and daughter. The condition may be lifelong and require long-term prophylaxis with lithium – a mood-stabilizing drug. The cardiotoxicity and renal toxicity from this drug are a problem, and careful monitoring is required because of a narrow therapeutic window. Lithium therapy should therefore not be altered except by the patient's prescribing psychiatrist or medical practitioner. Electroconvulsive therapy under general anaesthesia is also used in some cases of manic–depressive psychosis, as are antidepressants and antipsychotics, as appropriate.

Schizophrenia

This is the most severe form of functional psychosis because it is attended by the most profound psychological derangement. Schizophrenia involves disorders of thought, particularly disjointed and distorted thought processes. There is also disorder of emotion, which is often incongruous or apathetic, and disorder of volition, with obstinacy or lassitude. Delusions and

Table 15.5 Symptoms of mania
Overactivity
Overtalkativeness
Decreased sleep
Increased energy (including sexual)
Increased sociability/familiarity
Distractibility

hallucinations are characteristic, and patients classically hear voices as an early symptom. Patients may also withdraw completely and become motionless and speechless (catatonic) (Table 15.6).

Major tranquillizers such as chlorpromazine are often required; depot intramuscular injections given at the clinic or by the community psychiatric nurse are useful. Non-drug treatments, such as family and work support, are important. Deterioration of the patient's personality over time is usual although by no means inevitable and some people recover after one episode.

Organic psychoses

These arise due to central nervous system disease, or physical illness arising elsewhere in the body.

Delirium

Acute organic states are called delirium, and are characterized by clouding of consciousness leading to disorientation in time and place. Hallucinations, especially visual, are characteristic. The best known is delirium tremens due to acute alcohol withdrawal. Other common causes include other drugs (overdose and withdrawal), infections, especially chest infections, which cause brain hypoxia, and neurological disorders including acute stroke (see Ch. 9).

Dementia

Chronic organic states are called dementia, and are characterized by an irreversible decline in mental capacity. Most obvious is intellectual deterioration, with short-term memory loss and slow laboured thinking. Characteristically, patients may still remember events from their earlier life. Degeneration is progressive, and eventually incontinence may ensue. The commonest cause is senile dementia due either to idiopathic neuronal atrophy (Alzheimer's disease) or cerebrovascular disease (after lacunar strokes, see Ch. 9). Correctable aetiologies, such as vitamin B_{12} or thyroxine deficiency, syphilis, hydrocephalus should be excluded. In younger persons, HIV infection, Creutzfeldt–Jakob disease and its new variant (see Ch. 5), and the genetic disorder Huntington's chorea (see Ch. 9) also occur although they are irreversible. Treatment is supportive. Considerable support is often required as patients can become totally dependent – in essence almost a reversal to infancy.

Disorders of personality and behaviour

Personality traits usually refer to the psychoneurotic trends described earlier. Character/personality disorders in contrast refer to serious problems of social adaptation, such as psychopathy, which is a term used to describe affectionless characters who often are incapable of feeling guilt or remorse. Criminal behaviour is sometimes a consequence, and such patients may then be detained within secure units. Treatment is difficult since the character disorder is usually lifelong.

Drug use and chemical dependence

Alcohol abuse still causes the most serious problems, because of accidents, trauma, liver disease, cardiomyopathy, neuropathy and self-neglect (e.g. leading to infections such as pneumonia). Treatment is with rehabilitation and abstinence, with or without the use of drugs which cause unpleasant side-effects if taken with alcohol, such as disulfiram.

Other drug use is increasingly widespread, particularly among teenagers and young adults. Nearly 50% of school children will take illicit drugs. The results of drug use, especially if this develops from 'recreational' to chemical dependence, may damage not only the individual but also the immediate family, other members of society and, in the case of the addicted pregnant mother, the fetus. Crime, violence and medical complications frequently follow. Injected drug use can be

Table 15.6 Features of schizophrenia	
Disorders of	Thought
Disorders of	Emotion
Disorders of	Movement

associated with particular problems due to blood-borne infections, notably hepatitis B and C and HIV (see Ch 5), *Staphylococcus aureus* endocarditis (see Ch. 6), and also venous thrombosis at injection sites. Sexually transmitted disease and poor compliance with health care are common in the drug-using population. The most common habits are use of alcohol, solvents and cannabis. Abuse of psychedelics (particularly ecstasy), heroin, methadone and cocaine is increasing.

Organic solvents are commonly abused by children and teenagers, and can cause neurological, respiratory, liver and cardiac effects, including dysrhythmias, which may be fatal. Benzodiazepine abuse is also common, the main effect being loss of memory. Barbiturates cause central nervous system and respiratory depression, which may be fatal. Opioids (narcotics) can cause respiratory depression, malnutrition and depression – sometimes culminating in suicide. Psychedelics (including ecstasy) stimulate, causing hallucinations and paranoia, a raised pulse rate and blood pressure, pyrexia, and dysrhythmias, which may be fatal. Cocaine can also cause hallucinations, paranoia, dysrhythmias, cerebrovascular accidents, respiratory depression and, sometimes, death.

Treatment of drug abuse requires extensive psychotherapy and rehabilitation.

Learning disability

Mentally challenged patients, or those with learning disability, have a neurological defect of some kind. Learning disability is the result of brain damage of many types, but genetic causes, birth trauma and, later, road traffic accidents are particularly important. Patients with brain damage often also have disabilities such as cerebral palsy, and epilepsy.

Most patients are 'high grade', with an intelligence quotient (IQ) between 50 and 75, and frequently live at home or in the community. More severely subnormal patients (IQ below 50), who are totally dependent on others, may require long-term care. Learning disability often also results in social incapacities and abnormal behaviour. Body-rocking and self-mutilation are common in the severely handicapped, especially in the barren environment of an institution. Pica (the ingestion of inedible substances) is also common.

Crime and sexual promiscuity are common, especially in the higher grades. Retribution often follows, because those with learning disability lack the resources to evade detection and often find themselves pregnant or in court, or both, at an early age.

Down's syndrome is the most common genetic cause, and is the result of a chromosomal anomaly; patients are also of short stature, and have impaired craniofacial, dental, immune and cardiac development, and often hepatitis B (see Ch. 5). Fragile X syndrome, the next most common chromosome anomaly, affects males, and manifests with autistic-like behaviour and learning disability.

Autism is a failure in interpersonal relationships, ritualistic behaviour, failed development of language and speech in children of normal appearance. Affected individuals are of normal intelligence, though they may appear to be mentally challenged.

Disorders of the female reproductive system

Introduction

A number of disorders occur within the female genital tract. These are shown in Table 16.1.

Subsequently, infertility, abortion, pregnancy and breast disease will be discussed. A separate consideration of reproductive endocrinology is found in Chapter 13.

Disorders of the vagina

Vaginal discharge

This is most commonly caused by a variety of infections, although retained foreign bodies (e.g. tampons) are another relatively common cause of a vaginal discharge. Vaginal candidosis is the commonest infection, and this may present with discharge as well as vaginal discomfort and irritation. Risk factors for vaginal candidosis

Table 16.1 Gynaecological disorders

Disorders of the vagina
Carcinoma of the cervix
Disorders of menstruation
Menopausal disorders
Disorders of the uterus
Ovarian tumours

include the same predispositions which are described for oral candidosis (see Ch. 22). Indeed, it is not uncommon for oral and vaginal candidosis to coexist. Other infective causes of vaginal discharge include *Trichomonas vaginalis* and gonorrhoea (see Ch. 5).

Carcinoma of the cervix and cervical intraepithelial neoplasia (CIN)

Carcinoma of the cervix occurs more frequently among women of lower socioeconomic groups, those with multiple sexual partners, cigarette smokers and those whose partners have genital warts (due to an association with specific human papillomavirus types, see Ch. 5). Invasive carcinoma of the cervix is invariably preceded by a premalignant stage which lasts for several years. Thus, every effort should be made to identify the abnormality at an early stage by cervical screening, when treatment is simple and effective. All sexually active women should be screened at regular intervals (two smears in the first year of sexual activity and at 3 year intervals thereafter). Screening is undertaken by examining exfoliated cells obtained by taking a cervical smear. The exfoliated cells are stained and examined for cytological evidence of cellular atypia, which is predictive of CIN. Suspicious smears which persist or frankly abnormal smears are indications for biopsy and histological examination to enable a definitive diagnosis to be made.

The classification of CIN is summarized in Table 16.2.

Again in contrast to premalignant lesions of the oral mucosa, the natural history of CIN is fairly well established. Thus, in the absence of treatment it is believed that most CIN III lesions will progress to invasive carcinoma. The risks for lesions graded as CIN I or II is slightly less clear, although it is estimated that 50% will progress to CIN III within 2 years.

Preinvasive carcinoma of the cervix is best assessed by colposcopy, where the cervix is visualized using a binocular microscope with ×10–60 magnification. Local application of iodine stains abnormal tissue and facilitates more appropriately targeted biopsy. Early abnormalities can be treated by cryotherapy, electrodiathermy or laser ablation. Invasive carcinoma of the cervix is treated by hysterectomy and removal of a cuff of the vagina. Some advocate radiotherapy prior to surgery.

Disorders of menstruation

A number of disorders of menstruation occur, and these are discussed in turn. In addition, non-menstrual bleeding may also occur for a variety of organic reasons or may be psychological in origin (dysfunctional uterine bleeding). Premenstrual syndrome (PMS) is also discussed.

Investigation of uterine bleeding may involve dilatation of the cervix and curettage of the lining of the uterus under anaesthesia ('D & C'). This procedure is also used for early termination of pregnancy and also evacuation of retained products of conception (incomplete abortion).

Table 16.2 Classification of cervical intraepithelial neoplasia

CIN I	Mild dysplasia
CIN II	Moderate dysplasia
CIN III	Severe dysplasia
	Carcinoma in situ

The onset of menstruation (menarche) occurs during puberty, and may occur at any time between the ages of 10 and $16\frac{1}{2}$ years. Conventionally the day of onset of menstruation is regarded as day 1 of the menstrual cycle. The length of the cycle is highly variable (22–35 days), but an average is 28 days from the start of one menstrual period to the start of the next.

During the course of the menstrual cycle the lining of the uterus undergoes cyclical structural changes, which can be divided into three phases (see Ch. 13):

- *Menstrual phase* – when the superficial layers of the endometrium are shed.
- *Proliferative phase* – this is characterized by proliferation of the endometrium to repair the destruction resulting from menstruation. These changes are primarily mediated by oestrogens.
- *Secretory phase* – during this phase the glands within the endometrium develop a more complex structure and begin to secrete mucus under the influence of progesterone. In this phase the lining of the uterus is prepared for implantation of the fertilized ovum.

During menstruation the superficial layers of the lining of the uterus are shed, and this is accompanied by bleeding. Thus the menstrual flow, or menses, consist of blood and fragments of the endometrium, including its secretions and tissue fluid. Characteristically the blood is unclotted, probably due to the presence of fibrinolysins within the tissue fluid. If clots are present it is usually a result of excess bleeding. The menstrual period itself lasts about 4 days on average, but with wide individual variation. The menstrual loss typically has a distinctive pattern – starting suddenly and gradually increasing until peak loss occurs during the second day. Thereafter the loss gradually declines to a watery tissue fluid. Blood loss at menstruation varies from 10 to 80 ml, with an average of 30 ml. Iron deficiency may ensue if blood loss is excessive. Normal menstruation may be accompanied by some discomfort in the pelvis, groin and lower back. The discomfort is most noticeable on the first day and subsides thereafter. Many women who suffer this discomfort resort to analgesics.

There are a variety of disorders of menstruation – amenorrhoea, oligomenorrhoea, dysmenorrhoea, premenstrual tension and menorrhagia.

Amenorrhoea

Amenorrhoea is a failure to menstruate, and clearly this occurs as a physiological event during pregnancy, prior to the menarche and also after the menopause. It is important to be aware that amenorrhoea is only a symptom and not a specific diagnosis. Pathological amenorrhoea is defined as a failure to menstruate for at least 6 months during the normal reproductive years in the absence of pregnancy.

Pathological amenorrhoea can be classified as primary, where menstruation has never occurred, and secondary, where menstruation has previously occurred. The majority of cases are endocrine disorders (including amenorrhoea following cessation of oral contraceptives), although occasionally an anatomical defect may be responsible.

Oligomenorrhoea

This term means infrequent menstruation, and is applied when the duration of the menstrual cycle exceeds the norm for that individual by 2 weeks. As with amenorrhoea it is a symptom and not a diagnosis. Oligomenorrhoea shares most of the same causes as amenorrhoea.

Menorrhagia

This term denotes excessive blood loss (>80 ml) during menstruation. Menorrhagia has a wide variety of causes, including fibroids, dysfunctional uterine bleeding, carcinoma, endometriosis and bleeding disorders, especially von Willebrand's disease. Short courses of the fibrinolytic inhibitor tranexamic acid are useful in the treatment of dysfunctional uterine bleeding or von Willebrand's disease (see Ch. 7). Iron deficiency anaemia is common.

Dysmenorrhoea

This means painful menstruation, and is a frequent symptom. Two types are reported – primary or spasmodic dysmenorrhoea and secondary dysmenorrhoea.

Primary or spasmodic dysmenorrhoea starts shortly after the menarche, achieving its maximal severity between the ages of 15 and 25 years, and thereafter symptoms decrease. It is characterized by a colic type pain, located deep in the suprapubic region, lower back, groin and thighs. The symptoms start several hours before menstruation, and are usually restricted to the first day. Primary dysmenorrhoea is probably an exaggerated form of the normal pain associated with menstruation, and is not due to any organic problem. There may be a significant psychological overlay in some cases. Primary dysmenorrhoea can be treated with mild analgesics or non-steroidal anti-inflammatory agents, although it is also clearly important to reassure the patient. Alternatively, effective treatment can be provided by suppressing ovulation with the oral contraceptive pill.

Secondary dysmenorrhoea develops in adult life and is uncommon before the age of 25 years. The pain of secondary dysmenorrhoea starts several days before menstruation and increases in severity as menstruation approaches. The pain is of a more constant nature, and is principally located in the pelvis and lower back. Factors implicated in the causation of secondary dysmenorrhoea include endometriosis (see below) and pelvic inflammatory disease. Treatment is aimed at the cause. However, in approximately half of those affected there is no evidence of an organic lesion, and the cause is often attributed to psychosexual problems.

Non-menstrual bleeding

This is defined as non-cyclical vaginal bleeding which has no obvious pattern. Empirically it can be classified as postcoital, intermenstrual or postmenopausal according to the temporal relationship of the bleeding. Postcoital bleeding is frequently due to a lesion of the cervix, while intermenstrual and postmenopausal bleeding are due to lesions of the endometrium.

In view of the diverse range of possible causes, non-menstrual bleeding always merits investigation. Indeed, a diagnosis of carcinoma involving the genital tract must be considered until proven otherwise.

Dysfunctional uterine bleeding

This is abnormal uterine bleeding in the absence of an organic cause. It is believed that the problem may have a psychological cause whereby emotional factors acting through the hypothalamus may upset the normal reciprocal release of gonadotrophins with resulting impaired ovarian steroid hormone production.

Premenstrual syndrome

Many are aware of the mood changes in the weeks leading up to menstruation. However, the changes are usually quite mild and do not have any significant impact on normal life. Indeed, these mild symptoms are often regarded as part of the norm. In contrast, in a small proportion of women the changes are much more marked and are associated with physical symptoms and adverse effects on interpersonal relationships, leading to major disruption in their lives. The common symptoms of PMS are summarized in Table 16.3.

PMS is commoner among women in the 30–45 year age group. Establishing a diagnosis relies on identifying a particular temporal pattern to the above symptoms. Thus, the symptoms should be maximal in the 2 weeks prior to menstruation and relieved by the onset of menstruation. In addition, the patient should be asymptomatic in the week after menstruation.

Many treatments have been advocated, including essential fatty acids, hormones, vitamins, diuretics and herbal remedies, although none is universally successful. Clearly the symptoms are very distressing for the individual, and affected patients should be treated sympathetically. Indeed, recognition of the problem as a genuine entity together with reassurance and explanation is frequently helpful.

Table 16.3 Symptoms of PMS	
Emotional	Physical
Tension	Abdominal bloating
Irritability	Breast swelling
Depression	and tenderness
Lethargy	Oedema
Mood swings	Headache
Aggression	Backache
Emotional lability	Nausea
Confusion	Weight gain

Menopausal disorders

Menopause refers to the cessation of menstrual periods and occurs on average at the age of 51 years (range 40–58 years). The term 'climacteric' is generally applied to the perimenopausal years when the majority of symptoms related to the menopause occur. Menstrual periods may stop suddenly or there may be a gradual lengthening of the cycle. Many women experience some physical or psychological complication. The principal endocrine effect occurring at the menopause is an abrupt fall in oestrogen levels followed by a gradual decline. The resulting oestrogen deficiency leads to atrophy of the mucosa of the genital tract, lower urethra and skin. This can lead to dryness of the vulva and vagina, with resulting irritation, dyspareunia (painful intercourse) and bleeding. Secondary bacterial infection may ensue, leading to vaginal discharge. In addition there is atrophy of the breasts and loss of the typical female body fat distribution. Thus the patient may perceive a loss of attractiveness, which can have significant psychological effects. Gradual osteoporosis with an associated increased susceptibility to fractures (especially the neck of the femur, vertebrae and distal forearm) are also features. Hot flushes are quite common, and occur as a result of cutaneous vasodilatation. In some cases they may be particularly severe.

Psychological disorders, particularly insomnia and depression, are common but frequently mild. Not surprisingly, concomitant psychological disorders may influence the patient's perceptions of the above physical symptoms. Oral dysaesthesia and atypical facial pain are common in this age group, although there is no substantive evidence of benefit from hormone replacement therapy.

As mentioned earlier, many women experience symptoms which are sufficiently severe to seek medical attention. Hot flushes and atrophic vulvovaginitis respond to hormone replacement therapy. The progression of osteoporosis is also prevented by hormone replacement therapy, although the situation is not reversed.

Disorders of the uterus

Fibroids

These are benign tumours which arise from the smooth muscle of the uterus. They are not infrequently multiple, and vary considerably in size from small, seed-like masses to massive tumours which may occupy much of the abdomen. In many instances, fibroids are asymptomatic, while the commonest presenting symptom is menorrhagia with heavier menstrual bleeding, which is often more prolonged. Bleeding associated with uterine fibroids may result in severe anaemia. Other presentations of fibroids include infertility, and with large tumours there may be pressure effects on the bladder, leading to urinary frequency. A further pressure effect of fibroids is on the venous system, contributing to varicose veins. Fibroids may be a cause of abdominal pain in some cases.

The natural history of fibroids is that they undergo atrophy after the menopause. However, if the fibroid is large this will simply reduce the size, and it will not actually disappear completely. In many cases, fibroids are left untreated, particularly if asymptomatic. Indications for surgery include menorrhagia, infertility and pressure symptoms.

Endometriosis

This is a condition where foci of functioning endometrium are found in sites other than the uterus. Sites affected include the ovaries and peritoneum; less commonly, deposits may be found in the bladder, wall of the bowel, abdominal wall and vagina. The ectopic endometrial tissue forms small cysts which respond to the cyclical secretion of oestrogen and progesterone, undergoing proliferation and then bleeding at the time of menstruation. As the blood is trapped within the cyst with the passage of each menstrual cycle, they slowly enlarge in size. The deposits may vary in size from minute pinhead spots to large cysts.

The aetiology of this condition is largely unknown, but it is thought to be due to retrograde menstruation. The incidence of endometriosis is difficult to determine as many cases are asymptomatic. Clinical symptoms do not correlate well with the severity of the disease. Indeed, extensive endometriosis may be asymptomatic while tiny deposits may give rise to marked symptoms. The commonest presenting symptoms are pain, which usually occurs around the time of menstruation, and menorrhagia. Other presenting features include dyspareunia and infertility due to ovarian malfunction or blockage of the fallopian tubes. Asymptomatic endometriosis does not warrant treatment. For symptomatic disease, treatment with an antiandrogen or surgery may be used.

Carcinoma of the uterus

Carcinoma of the uterus usually presents with postmenopausal bleeding. Hence the importance of full investigation of this complaint. It is rare prior to the menopause, and is most common in the two decades after the menopause. Diagnosis is by histological examination of tissue obtained by uterine curettage. Treatment in the early stages involves total hysterectomy with bilateral salpingo-oopherectomy. More advanced cases may be treated with palliative radiotherapy.

Ovarian tumours

An extensive range of tumours may affect the ovaries. The vast majority of these (94%) are benign cystic lesions. Small lesions are frequently asymptomatic; larger lesions may present with abdominal distension or pressure symptoms on the bladder, leading to urinary retention. Symptoms most frequently arise due to complications such as torsion of the tumour pedicle, spontaneous rupture or haemorrhage, all leading to sudden onset of pain. Some ovarian tumours secrete hormones, which may manifest as a disturbance of menstruation.

Malignant ovarian tumours present most commonly after the menopause. Modes of presentation include abdominal swelling, ascites, abdominal pain and vaginal bleeding. They are associated with a poor survival rate as they frequently present late. Spread occurs locally within the pelvis, with seeding into the peritoneum and lymphatic spread to the regional lymph nodes and uterus. Blood-borne metastases may also occur. Treatment depends on the stage of the tumour.

Infertility

Infertility is a common problem, affecting approximately 10% of young couples. Many couples will accept this without significant adverse effects on their life. However, for others it results in significant emotional turmoil. The time taken for a normal fertile couple to achieve conception is on average six cycles, although approximately 20% take longer than 1 year. Frequently there is no single factor which accounts for the couple's infertility, and a variety of factors may operate, which when combined make it less likely that the couple will conceive during any one cycle. Causes of infertility include defective ovulation, defective sperm production, blockage of the fallopian tubes, other gynaecological abnormalities such as fibroids, and sperm antibodies produced by the female or autoantibodies produced by the male. However, after thorough investigation no cause is identified in about 20% of couples.

Artificial aids to conception include artificial insemination and in vitro fertilization, when the ovaries are stimulated by drugs to produce ova which are then harvested and fertilized in the laboratory. Fertilized ova are then implanted into the uterus subsequently. Much ethical debate surrounds these fertility procedures.

Abortion

Abortion may be either spontaneous or 'therapeutic'.

Spontaneous abortion

Abortion is defined as the loss of a pregnancy before 24 weeks' gestation, and frequently the euphemistic term 'miscarriage' is used. Approximately 10–15% of all pregnancies terminate as spontaneous abortions during the first trimester, and most are believed to occur as a result of defects in the ovum or fetus, primarily chromosomal defects. In the majority of cases the aetiological factor is not recurrent, and therefore the prognosis for subsequent pregnancies is not affected. Abortion is classified according to the clinical findings at the time of presentation. Thus, several varieties of abortion are recognized: threatened abortion, inevitable abortion, incomplete abortion, complete abortion and missed abortion.

Diagnosis of a threatened abortion is made when there is bleeding from the uterus before week 24 of a pregnancy, the cervix remains undilated with no loss of the products of conception. Uterine contractions when present are slight. On an empirical basis, bed rest is often advised, although there is no objective evidence that this has any beneficial influence on the outcome. In the majority of cases the pregnancy will proceed satisfactorily.

Inevitable abortion is a progression from threatened abortion. The features are similar, and in addition there is dilatation of the cervix with increasingly painful contractions of the uterus. Shortly after the onset of symptoms there is loss of the products of conception. If all the products of conception have been passed, the abortion is termed complete. In the majority of patients only part of the products of conception are passed, and the abortion is thus considered to be incomplete. In the latter situation the retained products of conception should be evacuated from the uterus. Missed abortion is a situation where the fetus dies in utero but is not expelled spontaneously.

'Therapeutic abortion'

Therapeutic abortion is an issue in medicine with significant moral, ethical and religious dimensions which are clearly outside the scope of this text. The regulations governing legally induced abortion vary considerably in different countries. Under the present British Abortion Act various criteria must be met before a pregnancy can be legally terminated. These are summarized in Table 16.4.

Thus, indications for therapeutic abortion include the following:

- medical problems in the mother, e.g. severe cardiac or renal disease, or breast or cervical cancer

Table 16.4 Criteria for therapeutic abortion

Continuation of the pregnancy would involve a risk of injury to the physical or mental health of the pregnant woman greater than if the pregnancy were terminated

Continuation of the pregnancy would involve risk of injury to the physical and/or mental health of existing children of the pregnant woman greater than if the pregnancy were terminated

There is a substantial risk that if the child were born it would suffer from such physical or mental abnormalities as to be seriously handicapped

- severe psychiatric disease in the mother
- fetal anomalies, e.g. genetic or congenital defects, or rubella infection (see Ch. 5)
- social.

Currently, most 'therapeutic' abortions are performed for social or psychiatric reasons.

Termination of pregnancy is safest during the early weeks of pregnancy. Prior to 12 weeks' gestation the products of conception can be evacuated with a suction curette. After this period the procedure is more hazardous, and abortion is induced with prostaglandins which stimulate uterine contractions.

Pregnancy

Pregnancy produces marked changes in the maternal physiology designed to provide the fetus with adequate nutrition and the mother with the additional energy required for labour and subsequent lactation.

These changes can be discussed under a variety of headings:

- Hormonal changes. Progesterone synthesized by the corpus luteum and subsequently by the placenta results in increased temperature and decreased smooth muscle activity, with principal effects on the uterus, gut and ureters. High circulating levels of oestrogens promote breast and nipple growth, water retention and protein synthesis. Human placental lactogen promotes growth hormone and insulin release, and also stimulates growth of the mammary glands.

- Genital changes. The size of the uterus enlarges progressively, increasing from 50 to 950 g at term. There is also swelling and softening of the cervix together with an increased desquamation of cells from the vagina, which leads to an increased vaginal discharge.
- Cardiovascular changes. Cardiac output increases by approximately 30% in the early stages of pregnancy with no significant change thereafter. Blood pressure is slightly lower during the normal pregnancy. Venous engorgement leading to accentuation of varicose veins and haemorrhoids are common, partly as a result of smooth muscle relaxation and partly due to the high pressure in the pelvic veins due to pressure from the uterus on the inferior vena cava.
- Haematological changes. Blood volume increases by 50% during pregnancy. Plasma volume increases relative to red cell mass, leading to lower normal ranges for the haemoglobin level, haematocrit and red cell count: the 'physiological anaemia' of pregnancy (see Ch. 7). Iron and folate deficiency are common, and are prevented by routine oral supplements.

Diagnosis of pregnancy

In retrospect it is rarely possible to determine when ovulation occurred, and the last menstrual period is the only readily available marker. The duration of pregnancy is expressed as the gestational age of the fetus, and by convention is calculated from the first day of the last menstrual period. In an average menstrual cycle lasting 28 days, ovulation occurs at about the mid-point, i.e. day 14 of the cycle. Thus the gestational age is 14 days longer than the fetal age. The average length of gestation is 40 weeks or approximately 9 calendar months and 7 days.

Pregnancy may be suspected on the basis of the following physical symptoms: delayed menstruation, tenderness and fullness of the breasts, polyuria, tiredness and nausea. Diagnosis can be made on the basis of physical signs. The relevant signs are as follows: enlargement of the uterus (evident from 6 weeks), softening of the uterus, increased vascularity of the vagina, and pigmentation of the areolar tissue of the breasts. However, before 12 weeks this diagnosis is fraught with difficulty except in experienced hands. In the light of the unreliable nature of these assessments the accurate diagnosis of pregnancy relies on the detection of high levels of circulating human chorionic gonadotrophin. Using this test, pregnancy can be diagnosed as early as 25 days after ovulation. Commercially available tests can be purchased over the counter in chemist shops.

Symptoms in pregnancy

Pregnancy is accompanied by a wide variety of symptoms.

Nausea and vomiting

About 50% of pregnant women complain of these symptoms. This usually starts by the sixth week of pregnancy and normally ceases by week 12, although in a small minority of patients it may persist throughout pregnancy. The principal aetiological factor appears to be the effect of oestrogens on the chemoreceptor trigger zone, which induces nausea and vomiting.

Backache

This is particularly common during the third trimester, and the pain is located over the sacroiliac joints. The pain is due to relaxation of the ligaments and muscles supporting the joints, and is exacerbated by the change in posture which the woman adopts to cope with the increasing weight of the uterus.

Constipation

Gut motility is decreased throughout pregnancy, and the situation is exacerbated during the later stages by pressure from the uterus.

Reflux oesophagitis

Regurgitation of stomach contents occurs as a result of relaxation of the cardiac sphincter. There is also relaxation of the pyloric spincter, which allows reflux of bile into the stomach.

Micturition

During the early weeks of pregnancy there is increased frequency of micturition due to increased water excretion by the kidneys. Increased frequency is also a feature in the later stages of pregnancy as a result of direct pressure from the fetal head on the bladder. Stress incontinence affects over 50% of women. Thus, following 'stress' such as laughing or coughing a small volume of urine escapes.

Oedema

This is a normal physiological adaptation to pregnancy, and is caused by an increase in the extracellular fluid.

Fetal development

The major fetal organs (brain, limbs, heart, kidneys, etc.) develop between weeks 4 and 9 of pregnancy. By this time they are close to their final structural form, and undergo only minor changes thereafter. Thus, teratogenic agents acting during this period are likely to produce maximal damage and result in major anatomical defects. Teratogens acting before this period often cause death of the embryo, but after 9 weeks they are likely to produce lesser anatomical defects. Important tetratogens include the rubella virus (see Ch. 5) and drugs, including oral anticoagulants and thalidomide

Labour

This is defined as the spontaneous vaginal delivery of the infant within 24 h of the onset of regular spontaneous uterine contractions. Conventionally it is divided into three stages. The first stage of labour extends from the onset of regular contractions until the cervix is fully dilated. In a woman's first pregnancy this stage normally lasts up to 12 h although in subsequent pregnancies it lasts about $7\frac{1}{2}$ h. The second stage of labour is the time from complete dilatation of the cervix until delivery of the baby. Average times for this stage are 3/4–2 h in the first pregnancy and 1/4–3/4 h in subsequent pregnancies. The third and final stage is the delivery of the placenta, and this lasts approximately 15 min.

Episiotomy

This refers to an incision in the perineum, and is performed in an attempt to prevent uncontrolled tearing of the perineum during delivery of the baby. Indications for episiotomy include when tearing appears imminent, forceps delivery and for delivery of premature babies in fetal distress. The advantages of an episiotomy are that uncontrolled ragged tears are avoided, there is no damage to the sphincter of the rectum and the fetal head is subject to less pressure. Complications of episiotomy include bleeding, infection and, over a longer term, dyspareunia.

Forceps delivery

Obstetric forceps have two principal actions, namely traction and compression. Some forceps also allow rotation. Forceps may be used if there is a delay in the second stage of labour or there is fetal distress during the second stage. Unskilled use of forceps may be associated with damage to the mother (lacerations of the vagina and cervix, or rupture of the uterus) and/or fetus (intracranial haemorrhage, skull fracture, or facial nerve palsy due to inaccurate placement of the blades of the forceps).

Caesarean section

Caesarean section denotes removal of the child from the intact uterus by abdominal operation. In recent years the incidence has increased significantly, and 5–15% of labours end in caesarean

section. In some cases caesarean section is undertaken as an elective procedure. In this instance, indications include disproportion between the size of the fetus and the pelvis, situations where the placenta is positioned in the lower part of the uterus and therefore hinders a normal vaginal delivery, a history of previous caesarean section, or where some part of the fetus other than the head presents. Emergency section may be required as a result of fetal distress during the first stage of labour or haemorrhage. Caesarian section increases the risk of venous thrombosis, and prophylaxis is required after delivery (see Ch. 6).

Breast disease

Presenting symptoms relating to breast disease include pain, swelling, nipple discharge and nipple retraction. Common breast disorders include benign proliferative breast disease as well as benign and malignant neoplasms. These entities will be discussed in turn.

Benign proliferative breast disease (mastitis)

This is not a solitary entity and is a condition which encompasses a range of morphological changes. Accordingly the clinical features are variable. The condition is common, and at least 10% of women have clinically apparent disease, although a far greater proportion have histological evidence of the condition. The incidence of benign proliferative breast disease increases as the menopause approaches, and then sharply declines. In the 30–45 year age group the proliferative changes are characterized by fibroadenosis and epithelial hyperplasia, while in the 40–45 year age group, fibrocystic change and cystic hyperplasia predominate. While the condition is entirely benign it is of some importance. Firstly it may be a source of intermittent severe breast pain, secondly it may mimic breast cancer, and, finally, atypical epithelial hyperplasia is associated with an increased risk of breast cancer. Cystic change alone does not appear to be associated with any increased risk.

Benign neoplasms

Benign breast tumours include fibroadenomas, duct papillomas, adenomas and a variety of connective tissue tumours. Fibroadenomas are the commonest type, with a peak incidence in the third decade, although they can occur at any age from puberty onwards. They present as a well-defined, painless, freely mobile mass which is clearly demarcated from the surrounding breast tissue. During pregnancy they may increase in size rapidly. Treatment is by simple local excision.

Duct papillomas are less common, and most frequently present in middle-aged women as a blood-stained discharge from the nipple. The papilloma may be palpable as a small nodule, and pressure over the swelling will elicit the discharge. Adenomas and connective tissue tumours (haemangiomas, lipomas and leiomyomas) are much rarer lesions.

Breast cancer

This is one of the commonest malignant tumours affecting women. Indeed, it is estimated that each woman within the UK has a 1 in 10–14 risk of developing the disease. It accounts for 20% of all malignant tumours in the UK, and is the commonest cause of death for women in the age range of 35–55 years. A variety of factors are recognized which confer an increased risk: female sex, increasing age, early age at menarche, late age at first pregnancy, late age at menopause, nulliparity, previous history of benign breast disease and a family history of breast cancer. Indeed, several genes have been identified which are linked to a high risk of breast cancer in some families. Occasionally (<1% cases) breast cancer may affect males.

Tumours infiltrate locally, involving skin, and this may manifest clinically as ulceration and tethering. In addition, direct spread occurs by invasion of the underlying muscles of the chest wall. Metastatic spread occurs via lymphatics, most commonly to the axillary lymph nodes. Spread may also occur to other lymph node groups such as the supraclavicular and tracheobronchial nodes. Between 40 and 50% of patients will have axillary lymph node involvement at the time of initial presentation. Blood-borne metastasis occurs most commonly to bone and lungs; involvement of the pleura may lead to a pleural effusion. Spread to other organs such as the liver, brain and adrenal glands is also common. In general, breast cancer is a slowly progressive disease, and metastases may present as long as 20 years after apparently successful local treatment.

Malignant tumours may present as swelling within the breast, bloody discharge from the nipple or retraction of the nipple due to tethering. Accordingly these symptoms should not be disregarded. Occasionally the first presenting feature may be a sign of metastatic disease – axillary lymphadenopathy or distant metastasis (e.g. in the brain, bone or lungs).

Breast tumours are categorized into several different types based on the histological appearances. Most cases are invasive ductal carcinomas. Approximately 70% of malignant breast tumours express oestrogen receptors, and these tumours are more likely to respond to endocrine manipulation. Prognosis of breast cancer is dictated by a variety of factors: size and histological grade, presence or absence of metastasis, and the hormone receptor status.

In the past, breast cancer was treated by two principal methods: radical mastectomy, where the breast was removed completely together with the axillary lymph nodes, or by simple mastectomy, which involved removal of the breast alone followed by radiotherapy to the axilla. However, it became apparent that these mutilating surgical procedures provided a long-term cure for only a minority of patients, and this led to a more conservative approach to the local control of the disease together with the introduction of systemic therapy. Accordingly, current management of small tumours favours conservation of the breast by means of a simple 'lumpectomy'. At the time of surgery the axillary nodes are also sampled to look for metastatic deposits. Following surgery, radiotherapy to the breast and axilla may be given, depending on the lymph node status. Alternatively, a short course of chemotherapy may be given. These simpler operations appear to provide local control which is similar to that obtained by the more extensive mastectomy procedures. As mentioned earlier, some tumours express oestrogen receptors, indicating that they are functionally well differentiated. This has led to the development of drugs which act as oestrogen receptor antagonists (*e.g.* tamoxifen). Use of these drugs has been shown to improve long-term survival.

In several countries with a high incidence of breast cancer, screening programmes have been introduced in an attempt to identify disease at an early stage. These primarily rely on the technique of mammography. Various studies have strongly suggested that women whose tumours are identified by mammography have an improved survival. This relates to the fact that lesions are detected at an earlier stage and therefore the risk of metastasis is less. In contrast, women who do not have screening tend to present with tumours which are considerably larger and with an increased chance of metastasis having occurred already.

Currently in the UK, women between the ages of 50 and 64 years are invited to attend for mammographic screening every 3 years. Features suggestive of malignancy include microcalcification and localized increased density. Suspicious lesions are further investigated by careful clinical examination, ultrasound scanning, and cytological examination of aspirated cells from the lesion to confirm the diagnosis.

Oral medicine

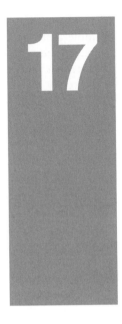

17 Introduction to oral medicine

Dentists, like their medical colleagues, may now use the courtesy title of doctor. This reflects the dental profession's desire to be perceived as respected health care workers with an increasingly wider remit in the management of oral disease, and not just dental disease. Historically, dental surgeons were trained as barber surgeons, and only subsequently aligned themselves with the medical profession. As a result, although the dental undergraduate curriculum has increasingly included medical subjects, dentistry has remained the only specialty of medicine to be studied at undergraduate level in the UK: to specialize in ophthalmology, dermatology or plastic surgery, one must first complete the medical undergraduate degree. Consequently, oral and dental disease is given very little coverage in the medical curriculum, as oral disease is clearly the remit of the dentist.

The definition of oral medicine, as defined by the General Dental Council, is:

Oral Medicine may be defined as the specialty of dentistry concerned with the health care of patients with acute or chronic, recurrent and medically related disorders of the oral and maxillofacial region, and with their diagnosis and medical management. It is also concerned with the investigation of the aetiology and pathogenesis of these disorders leading to understanding which may be translated into clinical practice. Oral Medicine is a clinical and academic specialty that is dedicated to the investigation, diagnosis, management and research into medically

related oral diseases, and the oral and facial manifestations of systemic diseases. These include diseases of the gastrointestinal, dermatological, rheumatological, and haematological systems, autoimmune and immunodeficiency disorders, and the manifestations of neurological or psychiatric diseases.

This places a great onus of responsibility on the aspiring dentist to be competent in the field of oral diagnosis, the management of oral soft tissue disease, the management of the oral manifestations of systemic disease and the dental care of those with special needs, i.e. those with physical, mental or medical disability. This is the realm of oral medicine, which is the interface between medicine and dentistry, and brings together the knowledge acquired in Part 1 of this book with a detailed knowledge of oral disease.

Oral soft tissue disease may be a largely local problem, and can be simply diagnosed and treated. For example, a candidal infection leading to denture-induced stomatitis may be a purely oral problem. The disease presentation and treatment may, however, be complicated by systemic illness or treatment such as diabetes or antibiotic therapy, and so a holistic approach to the management of oral disease is always required.

The influence of systemic disease on oral disease is alluded to throughout the text and cross-referenced with the general medical conditions in Part 1 of this text. Information on the impact of medical conditions on the delivery of oral health care is also included in Part 1.

Prescribing regulations

The *British National Formulary* (BNF) is produced in the UK to provide information on drug therapy for the guidance of health care professionals. The Dental Practitioners' Formulary, which can be found within the BNF, specifically lists and provides information on those drugs prescribable within the National Health Service by dentists. Dentists, however, may administer in their surgeries, or prescribe privately, any drugs within the BNF as long as the prescribing regulations are obeyed.

Particularly in the management of oral soft tissue disease, it may be necessary to prescribe medication which is not included in the Dental Practitioners' Formulary, for example a stronger topical steroid than hydrocortisone. In these circumstances, the dentist may either write a private prescription which can be taken directly to the pharmacist, or the prescription, in the form of a note, can be delivered by the patient to their general medical practitioner, who can, at his or her discretion, prescribe the medication on the dentist's behalf. This has the advantage of not only lowering the cost for the patient but also keeping the general medical practitioner informed of the patient's drug history. Useful information on each drug is provided in the Dental Practitioners' Formulary and the BNF, although often the Data Sheet Compendium should also be consulted.

Information on individual drugs and their prescription is given in the individual chapters of Part 2.

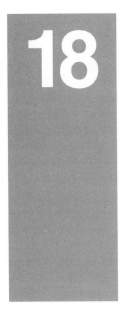

18 Clinical examination in oral medicine

Introduction

Clinical examination and history taking has been considered in Part I of this book from the standpoint of general medical problems. Clinical examination as part of the oral management of a patient has substantially the same principles, and is considered in detail here.

The clinical examination comprises two components, namely the history and the physical examination. Each is based on a thorough, methodical routine. It is widely accepted that the history is the more important of these two elements. Indeed, in many instances the history provides valuable pointers to the diagnosis. The art of obtaining a thorough, accurate history can be developed with practice, and comprises three main stages which are not necessarily mutually exclusive: first, a courteous approach to the patient; second, allow the patient to tell the story; third, a methodical questioning of the patient to elucidate details of the patient's history, if possible avoiding leading questions. This last element is also utilized to obtain information on the patient's medical, social and family history.

The same approach is used for all patient encounters and, with practice, the junior clinician's expertise will improve until he or she is able to deal with all the whims of daily practice in a confident and competent manner. While a variety of different schemes exist for obtaining a history, it is preferable to adhere to a particular format to ensure that information is obtained in an efficient manner.

Perhaps not surprisingly, many patients are apprehensive when confronted by a dentist or doctor, and therefore they may be easily disturbed if, for example, the clinician appears indifferent or unsympathetic to their problem. This may result in barriers to effective communication which will simply hinder the clinician. Therefore it is essential that the patient is made to feel the focus of the clinician's interest.

History taking

The elements of the history are shown in Table 18.1.

Presenting complaint

Any history should begin by allowing the patient to explain the nature of the problem or reason for attendance. This is recorded in the patient's own words. Often this can be elicited by a general question such as 'What is the problem?' or 'Why have you come to see us today?' or 'Please tell me

Table 18.1 Elements of the clinical history
Presenting complaint
History of the presenting complaint
Medical history, including drug history
Dental history
Social history

Table 18.2 Key features in a history of pain
Principal site affected
Radiation
Character
Severity
Duration
Frequency and periodicity
Precipitating and aggravating factors
Relieving factors
Associated features

about the problem'. This simple technique of an introductory question, allowing the patient to express his or her concerns, often aids in establishing a good rapport with the patient. If the patient has a variety of complaints, some attempt should be made to prioritize them and establish the patient's principal problem.

History of the presenting complaint

Having established the patient's principal complaint, further enquiry allows valuable clues leading to the diagnosis. It is important to determine the specific nature of the problem, e.g. pain, swelling, ulceration, etc. Several features should be elicited during this part of the history:

- When was the problem first noticed?
- What is the location of the problem?
- Are the symptoms continuous or intermittent?
- If the problem is intermittent, how frequently do episodes occur?
- Is the patient aware of any precipitating or relieving factors?
- Has the problem become more severe; is it improving or is it static?

Pain

If pain is the patient's principal complaint, it is essential to determine several key features in the history (Table 18.2). Almost all causes of pain can be assessed on the basis of these features.

Principal site affected. Is the pain localized or diffuse? Valuable information can be obtained by observing the patient when asked about the site of the pain. For example, patients frequently point with one finger when describing the pain associated with trigeminal neuralgia, whereas atypical facial pain is more diffuse.

Radiation. Two main aspects of radiation of pain should be considered: firstly, referred pain and, secondly, spread of pain as a consequence of extension of disease.

Character. Patients frequently use terms such as 'sharp', 'dull', 'aching', 'throbbing' or 'shooting' to describe pain, which may be helpful in pointing towards a specific diagnosis.

Severity. Clearly pain is a subjective experience, and patients vary so much in their ability to tolerate pain that the severity of pain may be a difficult feature to assess. Thus a mere statement of severity is often insufficient. In this situation the use of a simple rating scale is helpful. A useful technique is to ask the patient to rate the pain on a printed scale of zero to 10, where zero is equivalent to no pain at all and 10 is the most severe pain that the patient has experienced. This simple technique (visual analogue scale) provides the clinician with a reasonable assessment of the severity of the pain and may also be useful in monitoring the response to treatment. The effect of the pain on the normal sleep pattern is also useful information in assessing the severity of the problem.

Duration of pain. The approximate duration of each episode may provide pointers to the diagnosis. Thus, the excruciating pain of trigeminal neuralgia lasts for seconds while the pain associated with pulpitis lasts for a longer period.

Frequency and periodicity. In some conditions the pain may occur at specific times of day, e.g. the pain of myofascial pain dysfunction syndrome may be more severe on waking whereas the pain of periodic migrainous neuralgia frequently disturbs the patient's sleep at a specific time each night. In addition, patients should be asked if the pain occurs every day, and if there is a positive response to this question, how does the pain change during the day.

Precipitating, aggravating and relieving factors. The patient should be asked if he or she is aware of any factors which have an influence on the pain. Any positive responses to this question should be assessed for reliability to determine if this is a genuine effect or merely coincidence. If the patient is not aware of any factors which affect the pain it is prudent to ask a few suitable questions. It is important at this point to avoid leading questions, such that 'yes' or 'no' cannot form the full answer from the patient. Thus, 'Does posture have any effect?' is more appropriate that 'Does bending down make the pain worse?' However, with vague historians it may be necessary to resort to leading questions.

Associated features. Some types of pain may be associated with other signs which are of diagnostic value. Thus, periodic migrainous neuralgia is often accompanied by unilateral nasal stuffiness or lacrimation.

Medical history

The importance of obtaining an accurate and comprehensive relevant medical history for every patient cannot be overemphasized, and this should be undertaken before examining the patient. The use of a preprinted questionnaire is helpful, as it encourages more truthful responses to 'sensitive' questions (Fig. 18.1) However, the information obtained through the questionnaire should be verified by the clinician. The information gained in this part of the history may influence treatment. The medical history should also include details of drugs taken on medical advice or self-medication.

Dental history

The dental history should establish information on the pattern of attendance at the patient's general dental practitioner (*e.g.* regular or irregular attendance) as well as the patient's attitude to dental treatment. If the patient wears dentures it is useful to record details of their age and also information on denture hygiene measures.

Social history

Important information obtained in this section of the history should include the age of the patient, the patient's employment and what it involves, marital status, and dependants. These factors may have an impact on the patient's availability for treatment. Oral disease is influenced by tobacco use and alcohol consumption, and therefore this information should also be recorded.

At this stage the clinician should evaluate all the information obtained through taking the history. It is important to separate the relevant from the irrelevant material. This process will often lead the clinician to a provisional diagnosis or a differential diagnosis.

Physical examination

It is important to emphasize that the physical examination of the patient begins at the moment of first contact as valuable information can be obtained from the general demeanour of the patient. Does the patient appear fit and healthy? Is the patient relaxed or appear to be apprehensive or anxious? As well as an assessment of the overall demeanour of the patient it may be possible to observe general features of systemic disease in the fully clothed patient.

Examples include the following:

- rashes
- weight loss associated with cancer or HIV disease
- cyanosis from cardiorespiratory disease
- conjunctival pallor associated with anaemia
- conjunctival pigmentation due to jaundice
- joint deformities of arthritis.

Such signs may corroborate information obtained earlier in the medical history or may occasionally point towards previously unrecognized systemic disease.

Extraoral examination

The extraoral examination begins with inspection of the neck. This is best achieved by observing the patient from the front, noting any obvious asymmetry or swelling. The clinician should then

TITLE: MR/MRS/MISS/MS (Delete as Appropriate)

NAME _____

ADDRESS _____

_____

_____

DATE OF BIRTH _____

HOSPITAL NUMBER _____

BUSINESS TEL. NO. _____

HOME TEL. NO. _____

EMERGENCY CONTACT NO. _____

OCCUPATION _____

		YES	NO	DETAILS
1.	Are you an expectant or nursing mother?	☐	☐	_____
2.	Have you had rheumatic fever or St Vitus Dance (chorea)?	☐	☐	_____
3.	Have you had hepatitis, jaundice or tuberculosis?	☐	☐	_____
4.	Have you had any heart complaints, such as heart attack, high blood pressure, angina, heart murmur or a replacement heart valve?	☐	☐	_____
5.	Do you suffer from bronchitis, asthma or other chest condition?	☐	☐	_____
6.	Do you have diabetes?	☐	☐	_____
7.	Do you have arthritis?	☐	☐	_____
8.	(a) Are you receiving any tablets, creams, ointments from your doctor?	☐	☐	_____
	(b) Are you taking or have you taken steroids in the last 2 years?	☐	☐	_____
9.	Are you allergic to any medicines, foods or materials?	☐	☐	_____
10.	Do you suffer from epilepsy or are you prone to fainting attacks?	☐	☐	_____
11.	Have you ever bled excessively (eg. following a cut, tooth extraction or operation)?	☐	☐	_____
12.	Have you been hospitalised? If yes, what for and when?	☐	☐	_____
13.	Are you attending any other hospital clinics or specialists?	☐	☐	_____
14.	Do you suffer from blood disorders such as anaemia?	☐	☐	_____
15.	Do you have any other medical condition/special needs or disabilities?	☐	☐	

Doctor's Name and Address

_____

_____

Tel No. _____

Dentist's Name and Address

_____

_____

Tel No. _____

Date: Signature: Parent/patient:

Fig. 18.1 Medical history questionnaire.

proceed to palpate the neck for lymphadenopathy. Standing behind the patient the clinician palpates the superficial lymph node groups in the neck. This should be performed in an ordered manner, starting at the submental nodes and moving posteriorly to palpate the submandibular, posterior auricular and occipital nodes. The nodes of the deep cervical chain are then assessed by palpation. For a comprehensive examination of the cervical lymph nodes the neck should be fully exposed down to the level of the clavicles. Clearly within the confines of the dental surgery this may not be entirely practical.

Inspection should then be directed towards the face and major salivary glands, and the parotid glands palpated, noting any swelling or tenderness. Early enlargement of the parotid gland is characterized by outward deflection of the lower part of the ear lobe, which is best observed by looking at the patient from behind. This simple sign may allow distinction from simple obesity.

Both temporomandibular joints should be palpated simultaneously while asking the patient to perform a full range of mandibular movements including maximal opening and lateral excursions. Any restriction of movement or tenderness should be noted, together with any clicking, crepitus and locking.

The masseter muscle may be palpated bimanually by placing one finger intraorally and the index and middle fingers of the other hand on the cheek.

It is possible to palpate the origin of the temporalis muscle by asking the patient to clench. The insertion of the temporalis tendon can also be palpated intraorally by applying gentle pressure to the anterior border of the ascending ramus.

Medial pterygoid may be palpated distal to the lower wisdom tooth lingually. The lateral pterygoid muscle is not readily accessible to palpation, although it can be assessed by recording its response to resisted movement. The patient should be asked to open against resistance and also to move the jaw to one side while applying a gentle resistance force.

Intraoral examination

As with all components of the examination this should be conducted in a systematic fashion to ensure that no areas are overlooked. Complete visualization with a good source of light is essential. If the patient wears any removable prostheses these should be removed in the first instance, although it will be necessary at a later stage to replace the prostheses to assess fit, function and relationship to any oral lesion. All mucosal surfaces should be examined, starting away from the location of any known lesions. The labial mucosa, buccal mucosa, hard and soft palates, dorsal surface of the tongue, and floor of mouth should be examined in sequence. The lateral margin of the tongue should be inspected by gently holding the tip of the tongue in a gauze swab. This simple manoeuvre allows visualization of lesions which may otherwise pass unnoticed. The teeth present should be recorded, together with a brief assess-

ment of the gingival and periodontal status and the requirement for any dental treatment.

During this part of the examination the quantity and consistency of saliva should be assessed. Examine for the normal pooling of saliva in the floor of the mouth. Place the surface of a dental mirror against the buccal mucosa. The mirror should lift off easily; if it adheres to the mucosa, then xerostomia is present. The orifices of the parotid and submandibular glands should be identified. Gentle palpation of each gland in sequence should result in a free flow of clear saliva from the relevant duct orifice. Enlargement or tenderness of the submandibular salivary glands can be assessed by bimanual palpation. Briefly place the index finger of one hand medial to the lower border of the mandible. The other index finger is placed along the floor of the mouth, and enables the operator to detect any swelling or tenderness of the submandibular gland.

Examination of a swelling

Swelling is a common presenting feature, and it is important to record several specific features in the examination routine (Table 18.3).

Position. The anatomical position should be defined as accurately as possible.

Size. The size should always be measured and recorded. A diagram may be helpful. Thus, significant changes which may occur later can be recognized. In contrast, vague comments describing the swelling as medium or large are unhelpful.

Shape. Many swellings have characteristic shapes which point towards the diagnosis. Thus the swelling of the parotid gland associated with

Table 18.3 Important clinical features of a swelling

Position
Size
Shape
Colour and temperature
Tenderness
Movement
Consistency
Surface texture
Ulceration
Margin
Associated swellings

mumps fills in the space between the posterior border of the mandible and the mastoid process.

Colour and temperature. The skin overlying acute inflammatory lesions, such as an abscess, is frequently red and warm. Brown or black pigmentation may be due to a variety of causes such as melanoma. Purple or red may be due to purpura, an angioma or Kaposi's sarcoma.

Tenderness. Inflammatory swellings such as an abscess are characteristically tender, although clearly palpation must be gentle to avoid excessive discomfort to the patient.

Movement. The mobility of any swelling should be tested to determine if it is fixed to adjacent structures or the overlying skin/mucosa such as with a neoplasm.

Consistency. This may vary from soft and fluctuant to hard. Fluctuation refers to the presence of fluid within a swelling such as a cyst. This sign is elicited by detecting movement of fluid when the swelling is compressed.

Surface texture. The surface of a swelling may vary from a uniform smooth texture of a cyst to the grossly irregular such as papilloma.

Ulceration. Some swellings may develop superficial ulceration such as squamous cell carcinoma. The character of the edge of the ulcer and the appearance of the ulcer base should also be recorded. Ulcers should be examined for induration, which is indicative of malignancy.

Margin. The margins of the swelling may be well defined or poorly defined. This may give some indication of the underlying pathology. Thus, ill-defined margins are frequently associated with malignancy, whereas clearly defined margins are suggestive of benign growth.

Associated swelling. Some conditions are associated with multiple swellings of a similar nature, e.g. neurofibromatosis.

On completion of the history and clinical examination the clinician should be in a position to make a provisional diagnosis or list a differential diagnosis. Special tests or investigations such as a biopsy may be required to confirm or refine the diagnosis.

19 Oral ulceration

Introduction

An ulcer may be defined as a breach in the epithelium exposing the underlying connective tissue. Any condition which results in mucosal damage or loss may result in ulceration, and therefore many different conditions may present as oral ulceration. Oral ulceration is thus the commonest oral mucosal disorder.

Erosion is a term used to describe very shallow ulceration, and by convention is used to describe ulcerative forms of lichen planus. Atrophic patches are often mistaken for ulcers such as in geographic tongue but, since there is no break in the epithelium, these areas are not ulcerated and thus are not considered further in this chapter.

There are a large number of causes for oral ulceration. The important causes are shown in Table 19.1. Aphthae are the most common.

Aphthae

Classification

Recurrent aphthae or recurrent aphthous stomatitis are also commonly termed recurrent oral ulceration, and in the USA are called canker sores. Recurrent aphthae are the commonest oral mucosal disease, affecting up to 20% of the popu-

Table 19.1 Causes of oral ulceration

Aphthae
Carcinoma
Gastrointestinal disease
Haematological disease
Infections
Mucocutaneous disorders
Radiotherapy
Trauma

lation at some point in their lives, and 2% of the population suffer from aphthae at any particular time. Clinically, recurrent aphthae can be distinguished into three different types, and this forms the basis of the classification (Table 19.2).

> Recurrent aphthae are the commonest oral soft tissue disease

Clinical features

Minor aphthae

Minor aphthae are the commonest form of recurrent oral ulceration, and affect 85% of recurrent aphthae sufferers. The ulcers are less than 1 cm in diameter, usually only 2–3 mm in diameter (Fig. 19.1). They occur singly or in crops of up to 10 ulcers, which last from between 3 days to 2 weeks

Table 19.2 Classification of recurrent aphthae
Minor
Major
Herpetiform
Behçet's syndrome

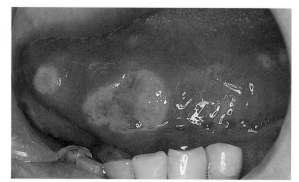

Fig. 19.2 Major aphthae affecting the tongue.

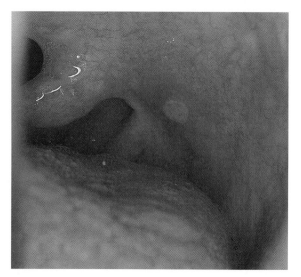

Fig. 19.1 Minor aphthous ulcer on the soft palate.

before healing spontaneously without a scar. The ulcers are round or oval with a regular erythematous halo and a grey or yellow base. The ulcers affect only the non-keratinizing mucosa, i.e. inside the lips, the buccal sulcus and buccal mucosa, the floor of mouth and under-surface of the tongue, and the soft palate. They may occasionally affect the dorsum of the tongue but never affect the attached gingivae or the hard palate.

Major aphthae

Major aphthae are a more severe form of recurrent oral ulceration. They are usually more than 1 cm in diameter, and have an irregular outline (Fig. 19.2). They are usually single and often affect the fauces. The ulcers are much more severe and may be deeper and have a tendency to bleed. They may last for several weeks or months before healing, and when they do they often heal with significant scar formation. Again the ulcers tend only to affect the non-keratinized mucosa,

and the hard palate and attached gingivae are spared. Major aphthae affect about 7% of the patient population.

Herpetiform aphthae

Herpetiform aphthae are so called because patients with these ulcers have a condition which looks similar to a primary herpes infection. The ulcers are 1–2 mm in diameter, and there may be 20–200 ulcers occurring simultaneously (Fig. 19.3). These ulcers last from a few days to 2 weeks before healing spontaneously without scar formation. Again they affect only the non-keratinizing surfaces. About 7% of the patient population suffer from herpetiform ulcers. Herpetiform ulceration can be distinguished from a primary herpes infection, firstly on the basis that

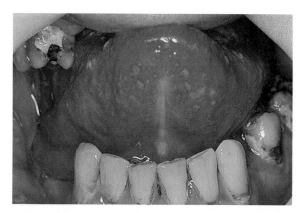

Fig. 19.3 Herpetiform aphthae affecting the under-surface of the tongue.

it is recurrent, and, secondly, in primary herpetic gingivostomatitis not only are the attached gingivae and the hard palate affected by the ulcers but often gingival ulceration dominates the clinical picture. This is not the case with recurrent herpetiform aphthae.

Behçet's syndrome

This is a rare condition in the UK and USA. Behçet originally described the triad of oral and genital ulceration associated with anterior uveitis, which is inflammation of the anterior chamber of the eye. Subsequently, however, Behçet's syndrome has been recognized to be a multisystem disorder in patients who have clinically recurrent aphthae. They also suffer from a range of problems affecting other systems, and these are shown in Table 19.3. The major criteria are of more significance in making the diagnosis of Behçet's syndrome than the minor criteria.

Aetiology

The aetiology of recurrent aphthae can be conveniently divided into host and environmental factors. The host factors determine the overall susceptibility of an individual to develop recurrent aphthae, whilst the environmental factors tend to distinguish the site and time of onset of individual ulcers. The most important host and environmental factors are shown in Table 19.4.

Host factors

Genetic factors are thought to be important in the development of recurrent aphthae for several rea-

Recurrent self-healing ulcers affecting exclusively the non-keratinizing mucosa are inevitably recurrent aphthae

Table 19.3 Diagnostic criteria in Behçet's syndrome

Major	Minor
Oral ulcers	Skin pustules
Genital ulcers	Neurological involvement
Eye problems	Arthritis
	Gut disease

Table 19.4 Aetiological factors in recurrent aphthae

Host	Environmental
Genetic	Trauma
Nutritional	Allergy
Systemic disease	Smoking
Endocrine	Infection
Immunity	Stress

sons. Although only 20% of the population suffer from recurrent aphthae, 50% of the fathers of patients with recurrent aphthae will have similar ulceration, as will 60% of their mothers. Twin studies also indicate a genetic component. Also, there is a weak HLA association with recurrent aphthae which is associated with the HLA types A2 and B12, with the relative risk for each of these being 3. There is, however, no demonstrable mendelian inheritance pattern in families who suffer from recurrent aphthae.

Behçet's syndrome shows HLA associations on the basis of the particular systems involved. Because the HLA type may predict those patients who will have eye involvement (HLAB5101), it is a useful test to carry out to discover whether an individual patient will be susceptible.

Nutritional deficiencies of iron, folic acid or vitamin B_{12} occur singly or in combination in approximately 20% of patients. The importance of this is that replacement therapy is often attended by a remission or marked improvement in the oral ulceration, particularly with vitamin B_{12} and folic acid replacement. The majority of these deficiencies are latent, i.e. there is no detectable alteration in the peripheral blood associated with these deficiencies, and therefore it is necessary to assay individual levels of ferritin, folic acid and vitamin B_{12} as well as carrying out a full blood count (FBC) (Table 19.5). The prevalence of nutritional deficiencies among patients with recurrent aphthae is not necessarily much greater than that in the normal population. However, patients who are genetically susceptible to recurrent aphthae or susceptible for other host or environmental reasons may develop severe or clinically significant ulceration when they become nutritionally deficient, and replacement therapy will reduce this susceptibility.

Table 19.5 Blood tests in recurrent aphthae
FBC
Film
Serum ferritin
Serum or whole blood folate
Serum vitamin B_{12}

Table 19.6 Systemic disease in aphthae
Menorrhagia
Chronic gastrointestinal blood loss (e.g. haematemesis)
Dietary deficiency
Malabsorption
Coeliac disease
Crohn's disease
Pernicious anaemia
Ulcerative colitis
Carcinoma of colon
HIV infection

> The majority of nutritional deficiencies in recurrent aphthae patients are latent

Patients without other susceptibilities to recurrent aphthae will not develop ulceration, even when they become quite anaemic.

Patients who have an iron, folic acid or vitamin B_{12} deficiency will not have such a deficiency without cause, and diet and systemic disease should be examined. Identification of a systemic disease and its successful treatment will often cause a remission or significant improvement in the patient's ulceration, either by eliminating the associated nutritional deficiency, e.g. the elimination of iron deficiency associated with menorrhagia or haemorrhoids, or it may directly improve the ulceration, as in patients with coeliac disease or ulcerative colitis. Systemic disease in patients with recurrent aphthae is often first discovered after investigation of nutritionally deficient patients, and occult systemic disease which was otherwise unsuspected may be discovered. The commonest systemic diseases identified in patients with recurrent aphthae are shown in Table 19.6.

Endocrine influences may also be important in the clinical presentation of recurrent aphthae, particularly female sex steroids. This is apparent from the observation that, firstly, women are more susceptible than men to develop recurrent aphthae. Secondly, 80% of women become ulcer-free during pregnancy, although these ulcers return after the baby is born, and also some women develop menstrually associated recurrent aphthae. In particular, 5% of females who suffer from recurrent aphthae have exclusive premenstrual ulceration, i.e. in the luteal phase of their menstrual cycle, and become ulcer-free at the start of menstruation. This indicates that the ulcers are dependent on sex steroid levels, and, indeed, experimental treatment of patients with injectable forms of contraception such as depot-progestogens often renders these women ulcer-free. This works by mimicking pregnancy by increasing the levels of progesterone, which has immunosuppressant properties.

The immune system is thought to be of central importance to the pathogenesis of recurrent aphthae. Lymphocyte-mediated damage to the prickle cell layer of the epithelium occurs during the early stages of recurrent aphthae, and in the pre-ulcer stage lymphocytes are the dominant cell type in the associated submucosa. The immunological events are complicated, and other immunocompetent cells such as macrophages, plasma cells, eosinophils and mast cells are also present in the area surrounding an aphthous ulcer, whilst polymorphs predominate in the base of an established ulcer. This is in addition to immunoglobulin, which has been demonstrated to be deposited both in the epithelium and in the basement membrane zone.

Significant alterations in the ratios of various types of helper and suppressor T cells occur during the natural history of an individual ulcer, indicating that immune alterations are important. It is now felt more likely that these immune alterations take place in response to an exogenous agent rather than as a result of autoimmunity, although an infectious agent responsible for recurrent aphthae has never been convincingly demonstrated. Aphtho-like ulcers may be seen in HIV disease.

Environmental factors

Trauma has been shown to initiate individual aphthous ulcers. Minor trauma such as injection of a local anaesthetic solution during dental treatment has been demonstrated to create quite large aphthous ulcers in susceptible individuals.

Mild trauma can trigger an aphthous ulcer

Other traumas such as damage with sharp foods or a toothbrush can also cause inappropriately severe ulceration in susceptible individuals. Interestingly, abrasion of the surface of an established ulcer seems, however, to encourage healing, probably by removing the adherent ulcer base containing both antigen and polymorphs. Thus, patients who complain of ulceration in response to trauma may not be suffering from simple traumatic ulceration, particularly if this is a frequent event, but may be suffering from traumatically induced recurrent aphthae. The exact diagnosis may be difficult to establish, particularly in patients with new or replacement dentures. Their ulceration associated with the denture periphery may be purely traumatic in nature or may be traumatically induced recurrent aphthae.

Allergy, particularly dietary allergy, is another important initiating factor in some patients who suffer from recurrent aphthae (see Ch. 26). Thus, an individual who suffers from oral ulceration may get this in response to ingesting certain foods. The common foods involved are shown in Table 19.7. These foods can be identified by asking the patient to keep a diet diary which will catalogue those foods persistently ingested before the patient develops ulceration. Foods may be identified more objectively by patch testing, where this facility is available. Patients usually develop fresh ulceration within 12–24 h of ingesting the suspect food or may get an exacerbation of the pain in a pre-existing ulcer. Dietary avoidance is often attended by clinical improvement.

Smoking is negatively associated with recurrent aphthae, such that it is unusual for people who smoke to develop recurrent aphthous ulceration, or their ulceration may be significantly improved as a result of continued cigarette smoking! Often patients first develop recurrent aphthae when they cease the smoking habit, although smoking is obviously not a credible therapeutic measure.

Table 19.7 Common dietary allergens in aphthae patients

Cheese
Chocolate
Nuts
Tomatoes
Citrus fruits
Benzoates
Cinnamon aldehyde

Early suggestions that smoking had a beneficial effect as a result of increasing mucosal keratinization are unlikely to be accurate since patients can suppress individual ulcers in their prodromal stage by smoking a single cigarette, and this suggests that the immunosuppressive effects of cigarette smoke are more important. Interestingly, patients with recurrent aphthae tend not to develop oral carcinoma, and patients with oral carcinomas do not give a history of recurrent aphthae, suggesting that the two conditions tend to be mutually exclusive, and it is interesting that smoking is associated with oral carcinoma and negatively associated with recurrent aphthae.

Patients with aphthae are usually non-smokers

As mentioned previously, no infectious agents have been shown to be responsible for causing recurrent aphthae, although several research papers indicate that patients have an abnormal immunological response to cell wall-deficient forms of *Streptococcus sanguis*, and certain histological features suggest that herpetiform ulcers could potentially have a viral aetiology. Microbial heat shock proteins have also been implicated.

Antiseptic or antibiotic mouthwashes, and occasionally antiviral agents, have been shown to have a beneficial effect in recurrent aphthae. Although the mechanism of action of these agents is unclear it certainly does not prove an infectious aetiology for recurrent aphthae.

Many patients complain that stress aggravates their oral ulceration, and this could be true for a number of reasons: stress could mediate its effect directly on to the oral mucosa by cells called Merkel cells which have neurological connections, or individuals may have their immune status modified by stressful situations. Also, stressed individuals, such as students working for exams, may damage their mucosa more readily with parafunctional habits such as nail biting or pencil chewing, or indeed stress itself may make the discomfort associated with individual ulcers more apparent and difficult to deal with. There is no objective evidence that stress causes ulceration, although it seems likely since so many patients make the association. Regardless, anxiolytic agents do not have therapeutic benefit and cannot be recommended as a form of treatment.

Treatment

The treatment of patients with recurrent aphthae can be divided into those treatments designed to prevent the appearance of new ulcers and those treatments designed to provide symptomatic relief where ulcers arise despite attempts to prevent them. The range of preventive treatments available for recurrent aphthae is shown in Table 19.8.

As mentioned above, haematinic replacement and dietary avoidance may cause a dramatic improvement in the clinical symptoms in recurrent aphthae, and if a haematological deficiency or a dietary allergen is identified, then this should be the mainstay of preventive therapy.

Tetracycline topically appears dramatically effective in reducing the number of ulcers seen in approximately half the patients who use it, although it is not possible to predict those patients who will respond. A tetracycline mouthwash can be prescribed most conveniently as a mouthwash made from tetracycline capsules which can be opened and the powder contents mixed in a teaspoonful of water. This is held in the mouth four times daily and then expectorated. This does not appear to be associated with candidal overgrowth

Table 19.8 Preventive therapy for recurrent aphthae

Haematinic replacement
Dietary avoidance
Tetracycline mouthwash
Systemic corticosteroids
Colchicine
Thalidomide

even with long-term use. Patients should be instructed to use the mouthwash four times daily for a month regardless of their ulcer experience, and if improvement is noticed they can then use the mouthwash only at the onset of ulceration until healing occurs.

Systemic corticosteroids are reserved for the most severe cases when the severity of ulceration significantly interferes with the patient's ability to eat, talk and work. Systemic corticosteroid therapy is effective if large enough doses are used, although the systemic side-effects of corticosteroid therapy (adrenal suppression, hypertension, etc.) are usually unacceptable.

Colchicine, which is used in gout, is an inhibitor of polymorph chemotaxis, and is sometimes effective in severe recurrent aphthae, although the blood must be monitored for potential side-effects.

Thalidomide, which is thought to act by inhibiting tumour necrosis factor, appears dramatically effective in severe forms of aphthae, although it has been removed from the market because of congenital defects in the offspring of pregnant women who took the drug (phocomelia). Thalidomide also can cause a peripheral neuropathy in a dose-dependent fashion, but apart from this is safe in non-child-bearing patients. Thalidomide is now only prescribable on a named-patient basis, and careful safety monitoring is always required. Thalidomide is the last resort, but can be dramatically effective in some patients.

Systemic corticosteroids, colchicine and thalidomide are also used in Behçet's syndrome, and colchicine seems particularly effective in some of these patients, since they display enhanced polymorph chemotaxis.

Preventive therapy is only effective or appropriate in a minority of patients, and therefore the majority of recurrent aphthae patients must rely on symptomatic therapy for relief. The main symptomatic therapies for recurrent aphthae are shown in Table 19.9. Chlorhexidine or benzydamine mouthwashes as required provide some symptomatic relief, although these are insufficient for the majority of patients. If pain is a particular problem, a topical lignocaine spray applied directly on to ulcers to allow eating or sleep may

Table 19.9 Symptomatic therapy for recurrent aphthae

Chlorhexidine mouthwash
Benzydamine mouthwash
Topical lignocaine spray
Topical steroids
   Triamcinolone in dental paste
   Beclomethasone inhaler spray
   Prednesol mouthwash
   Betamethasone mouthwash

provide symptomatic benefit. Topical steroids remain the mainstay of symptomatic therapy: triamcinolone in dental paste is effective if applied directly to a dried ulcer, especially at night (the ulcer being dried with a paper napkin before application). This requires some patient dexterity, and therefore may be unsuitable for patients who are not motivated, and indeed ulcers may be inaccessible if they are far back in the mouth. Also, dental paste is not appropriate for tongue lesions since the paste is easily rubbed off. The majority of aphthous ulcers, however, occur in the buccal sulcus and labial sulcus, and therefore triamcinolone is suitable for most patients. For tongue ulcers, ulcers far back in the mouth, or for patients who are less dextrous, a beclomethasone inhaler spray puffed twice daily directly on to an ulcer, especially in the early stages, is as effective as triamcinolone in dental paste, and many patients prefer this form of topical steroid. Prednesol and betamethasone mouthwashes three times daily, which are made up by dissolving a tablet in a spoonful of water, deliver steroids to all parts of the mouth easily but are also significantly more absorbed through the mucosa even if expectorated after use, and may cause adrenal suppression. These mouthwashes should therefore only be used intermittently and for short periods of time.

Carcinoma

Oral squamous cell carcinoma is one of the most important differential diagnoses since, if unrecognized, it will ultimately be fatal. A detailed consideration of the known aetiology and the clinical features is given elsewhere (see Ch. 21), but the important factors relating to carcinoma as a differential diagnosis of oral ulceration are considered further in this chapter.

Firstly, all ulcers persisting for more than 3 weeks without healing should be biopsied if clinical doubt exists as to whether or not they are malignant. Ninety per cent of oral carcinomas occur on the lateral borders of the tongue or the floor of mouth, and ulcers persisting in this region should be regarded with suspicion. This area, of course, is not visible to clinical inspection whilst the tongue is lying on the floor of mouth and across the lower teeth, and the trough on either side of the tongue should be inspected routinely or during every clinical examination. The differential diagnosis and appropriate clinical features are discussed in detail in Chapter 21, but regardless, clinical features may be misleading: chronic inflammation with associated scarring resulting from chronic trauma may appear remarkably similar to a carcinoma, and biopsy not only indicates the diagnosis in these cases but may also permit healing of a chronic traumatic ulcer.

> All undiagnosed ulcers lasting more than 3 weeks should be biopsied to exclude carcinoma

Gastrointestinal disease

As mentioned in the above section on recurrent aphthae, a number of gastrointestinal diseases may be associated with or exacerbate recurrent oral ulceration, and these are shown in Table 19.10. All of these conditions may give rise to recurrent aphthous ulcers, and in addition the inflammatory bowel diseases (Crohn's disease and ulcerative colitis) may manifest in the mouth with fairly pathognomonic lesions. Gastrointestinal diseases leading to oral problems are considered further in another chapter.

Haematological disorders

The oral manifestations of haematological diseases are discussed in detail in Chapter 26. They are, however, an important cause of oral ulceration, and are considered from that point of view here.

Table 19.10 Gastrointestinal causes of oral ulceration

Pernicious anaemia
Coeliac disease
Crohn's disease
Ulcerative colitis

Main haematological causes of oral ulceration are shown in Table 19.11. As mentioned in the section on recurrent aphthae, nutritional deficiencies of iron, folic acid or vitamin B_{12} may lead to oral ulceration, although this ulceration is exacerbated by the nutritional deficiencies per se and not by the anaemia which is often seen concurrently.

Leukaemia is an uncommon but important cause of oral ulceration. Patients with leukaemia seldom present with oral ulceration but more usually with hyperplastic gingivae, pallor, haemorrhage and lymphadenopathy, as discussed elsewhere. Similarly, malignancies of plasma cells uncommonly cause oral ulceration.

Neutropenia, either in isolation or as part of a pancytopenia, is an important cause of oral ulceration and gingivitis, and is often also associated with bacterial infection, particularly pharyngitis. It is usually seen secondary to drug therapy, and is an important reason for stopping the drugs when it occurs in consultation with the patient's physician. Pancytopenia or neutropenia can be diagnosed by doing a differential white cell count as part of an FBC. Cyclic neutropenia is an unusual condition where the neutrophils disappear from the patient's blood every 21 days. It is necessary to

repeatedly measure the FBC on a daily basis in order to diagnose this disorder.

Chemotherapy for either solid tumours or the haematogenous malignancies is also an important cause of oral ulceration, and this is particularly so with the folic acid antagonists such as aminopterin (methotrexate). Severe oral ulceration seen after treatment with these folic acid antagonists can be prevented by getting the patient to use a folinic acid mouthwash three times daily after the chemotherapy has been administered.

Infections

Infections are a very significant cause of oral ulceration, and Chapter 22 is devoted to oral infections. The infectious causes of oral ulceration are shown in Table 19.12. The characteristic clinical features of the viral infections are discussed elsewhere, as are the bacterial infections. Bacterial causes of oral ulceration are uncommon, and it is unlikely these will be diagnosed clinically. It is only after microbiological investigations that the true cause of such ulcers come to light.

Fungal infections do not commonly cause oral ulceration, and the systemic mycoses which can cause oral ulceration are rare in the UK.

Mucocutaneous disorders

Mucocutaneous (skin) disorders are an important cause of oral ulceration, and the main causes are summarized in Table 19.13. A more detailed

Table 19.11 Haematological causes of oral ulceration

Nutritional deficiencies
  Iron
  Folic acid
  Vitamin B_{12}
Leukaemia
  Lymphocytic
  Myeloid
Plasma cell tumours
Marrow aplasia
  Pancytopenia
  Neutropenia
Chemotherapy

Table 19.12 Infectious causes of oral ulceration

Viral	Herpes simplex virus I and II infection
	Herpes zoster
	Coxsackie virus infection
	Epstein–Barr virus infection
	Cytomegalovirus infection
	HIV
Bacterial	Tuberculosis
	Syphilis
	Gonorrhoea
Fungal	Systemic mycoses

Table 9.13 Mucocutaneous causes of oral ulceration

Pemphigus
Pemphigoid
Lichen planus
Erythema multiforme

consideration of these disorders is given in Chapter 20, but it is important to appreciate the differences in clinical presentation of these ulcers compared with more common forms of recurrent oral ulceration, so that the possibility that the patient has a mucocutaneous disorder is recognized and the patient is appropriately investigated in order to make the diagnosis.

Many mucocutaneous disorders are also vesiculobullous disorders but only occasionally present as blisters, more commonly presenting as mucosal ulceration. In these circumstances the ulcer is shallow and clinically resembles an erosion rather than a deep punched-out ulcer. The clinical differences between intra- (pemphigus) and subepithelial (pemphigoid) bullous disorders are subjective, and patients must be investigated by biopsy to establish the nature of the disorder. In addition, vesiculobullous disorders tend to cause erosions and ulcers which do not heal until treatment is implemented, with the exception of angina bullosa haemorrhagica, which is discussed in Chapter 20.

Erosive lichen planus and associated conditions such as lichenoid reactions and lupus erythematosus can present as eroded areas in isolation, but are usually associated with surrounding areas of mucosal keratosis. These are discussed fully in Chapter 21.

Radiotherapy

Radiation for head and neck malignancy is an increasingly important cause of oral ulceration associated with radiation mucositis (Fig. 19.4). If the mucositis is severe, sloughing with resultant ulceration can continue for several weeks. The slowness to heal is aggravated by a diminished blood supply in the area which occurs as a result of endarteritis obliterans associated with radia-

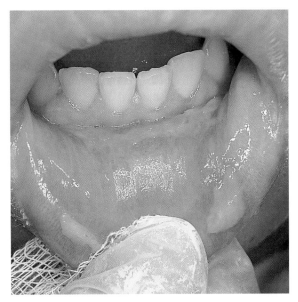

Fig. 19.4 Radiation mucositis in a child.

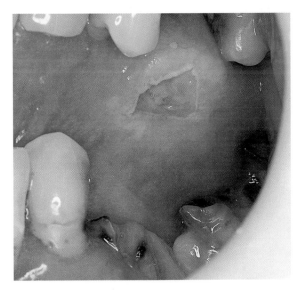

Fig. 19.5 Traumatic ulcer of the tongue caused by a broken tooth.

tion. The ulcers are non-specific but tend to become superinfected, and patients should be treated with analgesic therapy and antiseptic mouthwashes such as chlorhexidine. Tendency to infection may be aggravated by reduced salivary function caused by the radiotherapy.

Trauma

Traumatic ulcers usually have an obvious cause such as a sharp tooth or ill-fitting denture (Fig. 19.5). They may also occur after damage to the mucosa while it is anaesthetized during dental treatment. Chemical irritation may also damage the mucosa and lead to ulceration. Removal of the cause usually leads to uneventful healing. Chronic ulcers may, however, be slow to heal, and should be biopsied if malignancy is suspected. As mentioned previously, frequent 'traumatic ulcers' may be aphthous in nature. Traumatic ulcers can be treated, if symptomatic like aphthae, in order to promote healing.

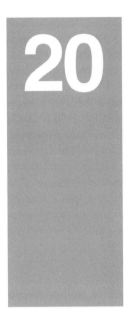

20 Vesiculobullous disorders

Introduction

Dermatological disorders very frequently manifest in the mouth. Mouth symptoms may antedate the appearance of skin lesions, or indeed dermatological disorders may be restricted to the mouth. The important dermatological disorders which affect the mouth are the keratoses such as lichen planus and lupus erythematosus which are discussed in Chapter 21, and the vesiculobullous disorders, which are considered in detail here.

Vesiculobullous disorders are so called because the characteristic lesion is a vesicle or a bulla (blister). Vesicles, by common usage, are small blisters (under 5 mm in diameter), and are characteristically caused by a viral infection (see Ch. 22). Bullae are larger blisters, and are the characteristic lesion seen in the mucocutaneous, vesiculobullous disorders discussed below. Mucosal bullae are very fragile, and often burst after a very short time to leave a ragged erosion which is clinically characteristic. They are therefore considered an important part of the differential diagnosis of oral ulceration, and a clinical comparison of oral ulcers is considered in Chapter 19. When blisters are seen clinically this suggests a vesiculobullous disorder, and the patient should be investigated appropriately. Vesiculobullous disorders can affect the gingivae, especially the anterior gingi-

vae, and occasionally this is the only clinical manifestation (desquamative gingivitis). A full consideration of desquamative gingivitis is found in Chapter 21.

There are a large number of vesiculobullous disorders which affect the mouth and these are shown in Table 20.1. Lichen planus also occurs in a bullous form and this is discussed in Chapter 21.

Clinical features and aetiology

Pemphigus

Pemphigus is an organ-specific, autoimmune disease characterized by intraepithelial bullae affecting the skin and mucous membranes. Pemphigus is the only important group of diseases among the vesiculobullous disorders which cause intraepithelial bulla formation. There are several

Table 20.1 Vesiculobullous disorders
Pemphigus
Pemphigoid
Dermatitis herpetiformis
Linear IgA disease
Angina bullosa haemorrhagica
Erythema multiforme
Epidermolysis bullosa

different types of pemphigus, but the important ones are pemphigus vulgaris, pemphigus vegetans, and the benign familial form of pemphigus, Hailey–Hailey disease. Pemphigus vulgaris is the commonest form of pemphigus, although it is much less common than pemphigoid in the UK. It is more prevalent in the USA, however, and is commoner among certain ethnic groups such as Jews and others with origins around the Mediterranean and Asia.

Pemphigus vulgaris is a chronic relapsing condition characterized by blister formation on the skin and mucous membrane, and is inevitably fatal in the absence of treatment. In over 50% of patients the appearance of bullae and ulceration in the mouth antedates the appearance of skin lesions, which appear as fluid-filled blisters which burst to leave a ragged ulcer or erosion (Fig. 20.1). Other mucosal surfaces such as the eye, nose and genitalia can also be involved. The site of intraepithelial splitting in pemphigus vulgaris is suprabasal, as discussed below. Rubbing the skin can cause blister formation (Nikolsky's sign) but this is not specific to pemphigus vulgaris and can occur in any vesiculobullous disorder.

> The bullae in pemphigus are intraepithelial

Pemphigus is an organ-specific autoimmune disease in which patients have antibodies to proteins in the desmosomes which bind the prickle cells together. Antibodies to desmoglein are the most important. Destruction of the desmosomes and the intercellular cementing substance causes separation of individual epithelial cells, which results in individual rounded cells being present within a bullae, called Tzanck cells. This process is called acantholysis, as opposed to acanthosis, which is a thickening of the prickle cell layer. The class of antibody involved in pemphigus is usually IgG or IgM, and the C3 component of complement is sometimes involved as well.

Pemphigoid

Pemphigoid occurs in two distinct clinical forms. Mucous membrane pemphigoid (cicatricial) and bullous pemphigoid. Mucous membrane pemphigoid may cause significant mucosal damage, particularly to the eyes as a result of scarring of bullous lesions, leading to its name cicatricial (Fig. 20.2). Interestingly, patients with mucous membrane pemphigoid are also prone to glaucoma, which further jeopardizes their vision. This appears to be unrelated to the use of corticosteroids for treatment.

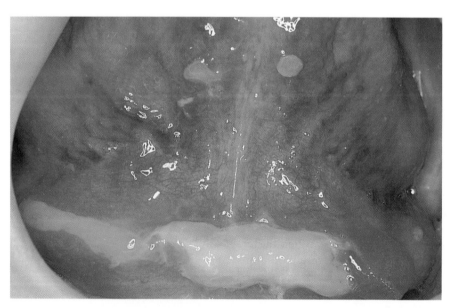

Fig. 20.1 A burst bulla sublingually in a patient with pemphigus.

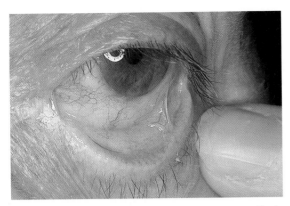

Fig. 20.2 Mucous membrane (cicatrial) pemphigoid affecting the eye, showing conjunctival scarring.

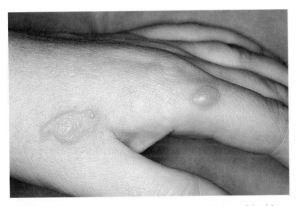

Fig. 20.3 Skin bullae in a patient with bullous pemphigoid.

The bullae in pemphigoid are subepithelial

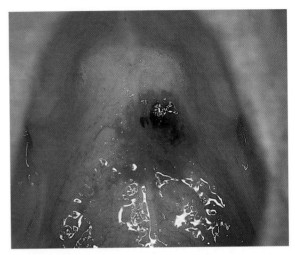

Fig. 20.4 A blood-filled palatal bulla in a patient with angina bullosa haemorrhagica.

Bullous pemphigoid, on the other hand, has a predisposition for the skin (Fig. 20.3) rather than the mucosal surfaces, although the mucosa can be affected also in bullous pemphigoid, and these disorders form a spectrum of disease rather than two distinct disease entities. Pemphigoid is a more benign condition than pemphigus, and does not lead to death in the absence of treatment, although, as stated above, can cause significant morbidity, especially due to blindness.

Patients with pemphigoid have antibody directed against various proteins in the basement membrane zone, and this causes damage resulting in the full thickness of the epithelium lifting off the submucosa. Again, the class of antibody is usually IgG or IgM, and C3 is also involved. Thus, pemphigoid is also an autoimmune disease which is tissue-specific.

Dermatitis herpetiformis

Dermatitis herpetiformis is characterized by an itchy, vesicular rash affecting the skin, although the majority of patients also have oral lesions. Dermatitis herpetiformis is a difficult clinical diagnosis to make, and the diagnosis is usually made on biopsy examination, as discussed below.

Dermatitis herpetiformis is characterized by deposition of IgA in a granular pattern along the basement membrane zone. Patients with dermatitis herpetiformis all have gluten-sensitive enteropathy (coeliac disease) (see Ch. 10), which may, or may not, be severe enough to cause clinical symptoms of malabsorption or villous atrophy on microscopic examination of the small bowel. All patients, however, have an allergy to α-gliadin, and a gluten-free diet is therefore an integral part of treatment.

Linear IgA disease

Linear IgA disease is another entity in the spectrum of vesiculobullous disorders which is difficult to distinguish clinically from pemphigoid or dermatitis herpetiformis. Again, a definitive diagnosis is based on biopsy findings, as discussed below.

Linear IgA disease has many of the characteristics of pemphigoid, but instead of having IgG or IgM deposited along the basement membrane zone, patients display a linear band of IgA along the basement membrane zone on immunofluorescence (see below). Linear IgA disease may therefore be part of a spectrum of diseases which encompasses dermatitis herpetiformis and pemphigoid.

Angina bullosa haemorrhagica

Angina bullosa haemorrhagica describes blood blisters affecting, usually, the soft palate. In this condition the patient develops usually a large blister 1–3 cm in diameter on the soft palate which is blood filled and is either burst by the patient using a pin or with their tongue leaving a large, empty balloon of skin (Fig. 20.4). In this respect, angina bullosa haemorrhagica is clinically similar to the other bullous disorders such as pemphigus and pemphigoid. In contrast to these, however, blistering in angina bullosa haemorrhagica tends to heal quickly, and usually resolves completely within a week. The patient may then go several months without a recurrence, and the condition is never severe but causes the patient significant concern, particularly in the absence of a diagnosis by a doctor or dentist. It has been suggested that angina bullosa haemorrhagica is more common in people who use steroid inhalers for asthma, although this has never been confirmed.

> The blisters in angina bullosa haemorrhagica heal in 1 week

The aetiology of angina bullosa haemorrhagica is unknown. There is no identifiable immunological damage to the tissues, and the lesions seem to heal uneventfully.

Erythema multiforme

Erythema multiforme sometimes affects only the mouth but usually affects the skin as well. In its severe form it is called the Stevens–Johnson syndrome, when the mouth, eyes, genitalia and skin may be involved, although the distinction between the two terms is unclear and they tend to be used synonymously. The oral mucosa looks severely inflamed, but the features are non-specific (Fig. 20.5), and usually a biopsy is required in order to confirm the diagnosis. Crusting of the lips is very characteristic of erythema multiforme, and lip involvement may cause significant morbidity (Fig. 20.6). The skin lesions are also bullous in nature, but because of the thickness of the epidermis, blistering is less obvious, and the lesions often appear like targets, although these can become quite large (Fig. 20.7). Classically,

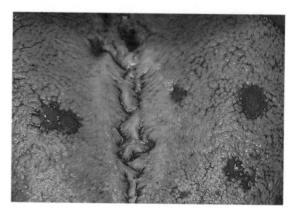

Fig. 20.5 Erythema multiforme lesions on the tongue.

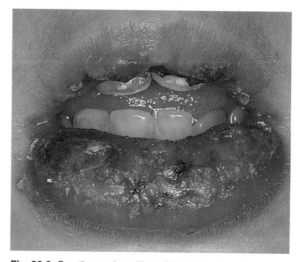

Fig. 20.6 Crusting and swelling of the lips in erythema multiforme.

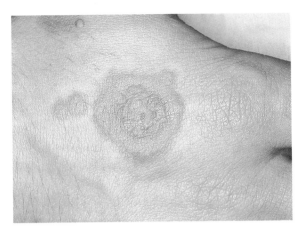

Fig. 20.7 Target lesions on the hand of a patient with erythema multiforme.

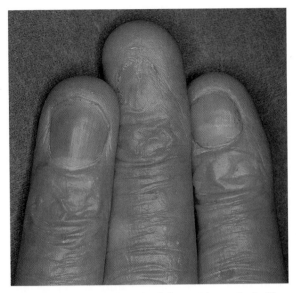

Fig. 20.8 Paper-like skin and nail damage in a patient with epidermolysis bullosa.

erythema multiforme regresses after 2 weeks, even without treatment, although a significant number of patients have constant or recurrent lesions unless they are treated aggressively.

Erythema multiforme is thought to be an immune complex disorder which arises as a result of an immune response to an outside agent such as herpes simplex virus or various drugs. Some patients develop erythema multiforme as a response to having a recurrent herpes labialis lesion. Patients may also develop erythema multiforme in response to the ingestion of certain foodstuffs to which they have an adverse response. In many patients with erythema multiforme, however, no cause is found, and treatment must be empirical.

Epidermolysis bullosa

Epidermolysis bullosa comprises a group of rare hereditary vesicular disorders which involve the skin and sometimes the oral mucous membranes and other mucosae. The vesicles arise usually at sites of normal friction or following trauma, but may occasionally occur spontaneously. The bullae rupture to leave a raw, painful surface and healing on the skin may sometimes be associated with exuberant keloid scar formation, contraction and/or pigmentation. A paper-like skin is characteristic (Fig. 20.8). Diagnosis is not usually a dental problem since most patients are born with the condition, and only those who have the milder

forms survive to adult life. In these patients, however, even routine dental care can cause significant damage to the mucosa, which is then slow to heal (Fig. 20.9).

Diagnosis

The diagnosis of vesiculobullous disorders can sometimes be made on clinical grounds alone,

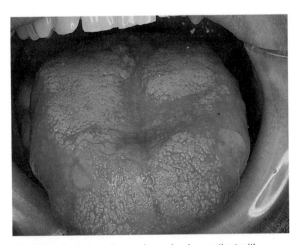

Fig. 20.9 Oral ulceration and scarring in a patient with epidermolysis bullosa.

e.g. a typical history in angina bullosa haemorrhagica is diagnostic. Also, lip crusting and cutaneous target lesion formation clinically confirms the diagnosis of erythema multiforme. Epidermolysis bullosa is usually diagnosed at a young age, and the patient's parents are aware of the diagnosis. In the remainder of these disorders under consideration here, or when the clinical features are atypical, diagnosis must rely on the demonstration of characteristic histological features or pathognomonic immunopathological features.

Histopathological criteria

An intact bulla (if possible) or tissue alongside an erosion (perilesional tissue) should be biopsied.

Because of the fragile nature of bullae, the opportunity to biopsy the intact bulla occurs infrequently, although biopsying perilesional or intact mucosa often causes epithelial splitting at a level specific to the disease due to the trauma of the biopsy. Thus, classically, pemphigus vulgaris is characterized by a suprabasal split in the epithelium with associated acantholysis (Fig. 20.10), although, when a bulla has burst, the histological features often become non-specific. Even in the case of pemphigus vegetans it is sometimes difficult to distinguish artifactual splitting from pathology.

A non-artifactual split of epithelium along the basement membrane zone suggests a diagnosis of pemphigoid (Fig. 20.11), although in a bulla of

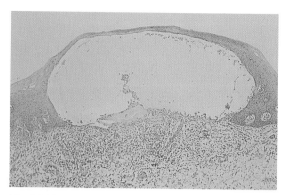

Fig. 20.11 An H & E stained section of a subepithelial bulla in pemphigoid.

any age, seeding of individual epithelial cells along the basement membrane zone often makes it difficult to distinguish pemphigoid from pemphigus. In addition, it is not possible to distinguish pemphigoid from linear IgA disease, or indeed angina bullosa haemorrhagica, without immunofluorescent testing.

If clinical doubt exists in erythema multiforme, affected tissues should be biopsied, and the immune complex nature of the disease characteristically results in a perivascular distribution of inflammatory and immune cells histologically suggesting the diagnosis.

> Immunofluorescence is usually performed on a frozen section

Immunofluorescence

The class and pattern of deposition of antibodies in the autoimmune vesiculobullous disorders is characteristic and diagnostic. The majority of diagnoses of vesiculobullous disorders rely on this technique. Immunofluorescent staining of antibody is achieved in two ways: direct and indirect immunofluorescence. In direct immunofluorescence, in vivo bound antibody is visualized directly on biopsy tissue which has been made into a frozen section and flooded with animal antihuman fluorescein-tagged antibody (Fig. 20.12). In this way, both the site and class of antibody within the patient's tissues can

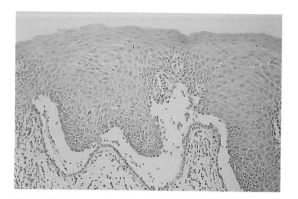

Fig. 20.10 A haematoxylin and eosin (H & E) stained section of pemphigus vulgaris showing suprabasal splitting and acantholysis.

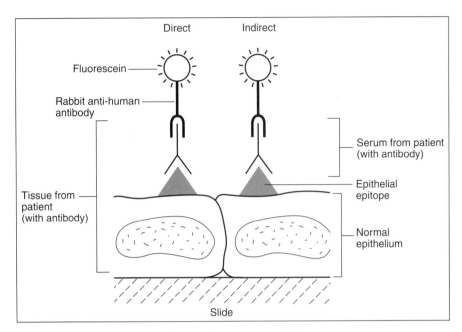

Fig. 20.12 A diagram showing direct and indirect immunofluorescence techniques.

be visualized under an ultraviolet microscope (Fig. 20.13). In indirect immunofluorescence, serum from the patient, which potentially contains circulating antibody against the target within the epithelium such as the basement membrane zone, is flooded on to a piece of normal mucosa, and if the abnormal antibody is present it will adhere to the target tissue, e.g. the basement membrane zone (Fig. 20.12). Subsequently, this section is washed, flooded with animal antihuman class-specific immunoglobulin, and again the class and distribution of the abnormal antibody give the diagnosis.

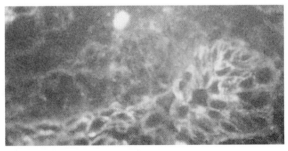

Fig. 20.13 Basketweave immunofluorescence due to intercellular binding in pemphigus.

Characteristic immunofluorescent findings, using both direct and indirect techniques, are shown in Table 20.2. It is interesting that in bullous pemphigoid, indirect immunofluorescent findings are often positive when the direct immunofluorescence test is negative. Also, although circulating immune complexes can be demonstrated by other means in erythema multiforme, immunofluorescence in this condition is unreliable.

Treatment

Pemphigus vulgaris, in the absence of treatment, is inevitably fatal, although the condition can usually be controlled by the use of high doses of systemic corticosteroids with or without steroid-sparing agents such as azathioprine or cyclophosphamide. Pemphigus vegetans tends to be less severe, but may require similar treatment.

Pemphigoid is usually a milder condition than pemphigus, and although treatment with systemic steroids is sometimes necessary to induce a remission, disease activity can usually be controlled by the use of topical steroids such as a beclomethasone spray or a betamethasone mouthwash.

Table 20.2 Immunofluorescence in vesiculobullous disorders

Disease	Direct	Indirect	Location
Pemphigus	G, M, C3+	G,M,C3±	Suprabasal
Pemphigoid			
Mucous membrane	G, M, C3+	G, M, C3±	BMZ
Bullous	G, M, C3±	G, M, C3+	BMZ
Dermatitis herpetiformis	A+ (granular)	–	BMZ
Linear IgA disease	A+ (linear)	–	BMZ
Angina bullosa haemorrhagica	–	–	–
Erythema multiforme	–	–	–
Epidermolysis bullosa	G,C3±	–	–

BMZ, basement membrane zone.

A prerequisite to the successful treatment of dermatitis herpetiformis is the placement of the patient on a gluten-free diet, since all patients with dermatitis herpetiformis have clinical or subclinical gluten-sensitive enteropathy. Patients with dermatitis herpetiformis may also benefit from treatment with dapsone or sulphonamides such as sulphapyridine. Steroids are seldom necessary in this condition. Linear IgA disease, on the other hand, is treated in a similar way to pemphigoid.

Angina bullosa haemorrhagica is a mild self-limiting condition, and the patient usually requires only reassurance. If the patient wishes, symptomatic therapy, then chlorhexidine or benzydamine hydrochloride mouthwash, should be given.

The mainstay of treatment in erythema multiforme, if the precipitating cause cannot be identified, is systemic steroids with or without steroid-sparing agents, depending on the severity of the condition. If the patient suffers from erythema multiforme intermittently, then steroids should be instituted within 24 h of onset in order to try and inhibit the full expression of the disease. In view of the observation that many patients have erythema multiforme in response to recurrent herpetic lesions, a therapeutic trial of aciclovir therapy (400 mg twice daily) may be used to eliminate herpes simplex as an aetiological factor.

The management of epidermolysis bullosa relies on protecting the individual from unnecessary friction or trauma, which can result in severe damage to the epithelium. Extreme care should be taken during routine dental treatment, and operators should avoid the use of procedures which will dry or stretch the mucosa, such as the use of cotton wool rolls. Some patients with epidermolysis bullosa obtain clinical improvement from the use of phenytoin.

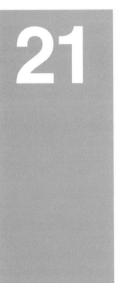

21 White patches and premalignant and malignant lesions of the oral mucosa

Introduction

Generally, if the mucosa becomes thickened then it will become white. For this reason, white patches are the end-organ effect of a wide range of disease processes, which are shown in Table 21.1.

A white patch is a particularly important clinical presentation, since it has been observed for over a century that carcinomas are more likely to arise in a pre-existing white patch. Some white patches are not premalignant whilst others have quite a high risk, which makes their differentiation most important. For example, white sponge naevi or traumatic white patches are not premalignant, while idiopathic leukoplakia is premalignant but in an unpredictable way.

A premalignant lesion is defined as 'a morphologically altered tissue in which cancer is more likely to occur than in its apparently normal counterpart', while a premalignant condition is defined as 'a generalized state associated with a significantly increased risk of cancer'. Examples are summarized in Table 21.2.

However, it must be emphasized that oral cancers may arise de novo with no recognizable pre-existing clinical abnormality.

In general, in order to fully understand as much as possible about a white patch it is necessary to biopsy it in order to characterize the nature of the lesion and to assess the degree of epithelial dysplasia. Biopsy will distinguish most white patch disorders, the most important and common being lichen planus and leukoplakia. Lichen planus is a specific disorder, as discussed elsewhere, with specific histological features which must be satisfied to make the diagnosis. In con-

Table 21.1 White patch lesions of the oral mucosa

Developmental/hereditary
Infective
Traumatic (frictional/smoking)
Dermatological
Idiopathic
Neoplastic
Other

Table 21.2 Premalignant lesions and conditions

Premalignant lesion	Premalignant condition
Leukoplakia	Oral submucous fibrosis
Erythroplakia	Sideropenic dysphagia
Discoid lupus erythematosus	Syphilis
Dyskeratosis congenita	
Chronic hyperplastic candidosis	
Lichen planus	
Chronic immunosuppression	

trast, leukoplakia is a clinical diagnosis with no specific histological criteria, and is thus a diagnosis of exclusion. Both are clinically associated with the occasional development of carcinoma. Malignancy arises in about 1% of those with lichen planus over a 5 year period (see below). The reported prevalence of malignant transformation in leukoplakia is variable but probably in the region of 2–4% over a 5 year period. Assessment of the degree of epithelial dysplasia relies on the presence histologically of several features relating to nuclear and cellular derangement (Table 21.3).

The severity is assessed on the individual features of epithelial dysplasia and also on the degree of involvement of the epithelium, with mild dysplasia restricted to the lowest third of the epithelium and severe dysplasia affecting the full thickness. Epithelial dysplasia can thus be graded semi-objectively according to severity as shown in Table 21.4.

Intraepithelial neoplasia of the uterine cervix is associated with a number of aetiological factors such as human papillomavirus infection and smoking. The condition progresses predictably through increasing levels of dysplastic change to invasive carcinoma. Cervical screening with smears thus allows prevention of cervical neoplasia. Unfortunately, the progression of intraoral epithelial dysplasia is not predictable in this way. Only up to 4% of white patches become malig-

nant during follow-up, and many carcinomas arise de novo from clinically normal epithelium. Generally, however, oral lesions displaying moderate or severe dysplastic change are more at risk of progressing to carcinoma, and serious consideration should be given to removal of these lesions when practical.

Tobacco use is an overarching factor in the aetiology of white patches: white patches are far more common among smokers and tend to regress on cessation of the habit. Because of this, white patches are often less sinister amongst smokers, who nevertheless should be counselled to stop their habit.

As alluded to above, moderately or severely dysplastic lesions are at increased risk of malignant transformation. Biopsy sampling may not be representative, however, and it is therefore difficult to be confident regarding the malignant potential of any lesion. Careful follow-up is therefore mandatory, and patients with persistent white patches should be reviewed every 3–6 months, and, if any sinister change is observed clinically, then rebiopsy is warranted to ensure early diagnosis of any malignant lesion.

Individual white patch lesions will now be considered in turn.

Developmental hereditary white patches

A variety of hereditary disorders present as white patch lesions affecting the oral mucosa, and are known as genokeratoses (Table 21.5). In general they are all relatively uncommon.

Darier's disease (dyskeratosis follicularis)

This is a rare autosomal dominant skin disorder with oral involvement in up to 50% of cases. The

Table 21.3 Histological features of epithelial dysplasia	
Nuclear	Hyperchromatism
	Increased and abnormal mitoses
	Pleomorphism
	Prominent nucleoli
	Increased nuclear:cytoplasmic ratio
Cellular	Abnormal keratinization
	Basal cell hypertrophy
	Disturbed maturation
	Drop-shaped rete pegs
	Loss of intercellular adhesion
	Loss of polarity

Table 21.4 Severity of epithelial dysplasia
Mild
Moderate
Severe
Carcinoma in situ

Table 21.5 Developmental/hereditary white patches
Darier's disease
Dyskeratosis congenita
Pachyonychia congenita
White sponge naevus

disease becomes increasingly severe in adult life. The skin lesions which frequently affect the shoulders and upper arms manifest as multiple heavily keratinized papules which ulcerate, crust over, coalesce and may become secondarily infected (Fig. 21.1). Retinoids may be indicated.

Dyskeratosis congenita

This is a rare inherited condition characterized by oral leukoplakia, dystrophic changes affecting the nails, and pigmented skin lesions. The leukoplakia ultimately undergoes malignant transformation.

Pachyonychia congenita

This is a rare autosomal dominant inherited trait characterized by white patch lesions affecting the oral mucosa, grossly thickened nails (pachyonychia), palmar and plantar hyperkeratosis, and hyperhidrosis (increased sweating).

White sponge naevus

This is a rare autosomal dominant disorder due to expression of an abnormal keratin gene. Most commonly the lesions achieve maximum severity during adolescence. Clinically the affected mucosa appears white, thickened and spongy to the touch (Fig. 21.2). The lesion may affect the oral mucosa, oesophagus, rectum or vagina.

Infective white patches

Infective white patches occur for a variety of reasons (Table 21.6). Infective causes of white patch lesions involving the oral mucosa (candidosis, syphilitic leukoplakia, hairy leukoplakia and papillomas) are discussed in Chapter 22.

Traumatic white patches

Trauma to the oral mucosa may result in white patch lesions. Traumatic keratoses can be classified on the basis of the nature of the trauma – mechanical, chemical or thermal. This classification, therefore, includes frictional and smoker's keratosis, which are important diagnoses since they can usually be recognized clinically and histologically and generally run a benign course.

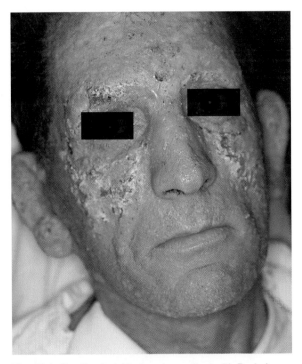

Fig. 21.1 Crusting facial lesions in a patient with Darier's disease.

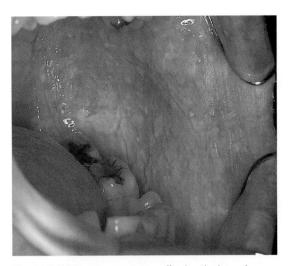

Fig. 21.2 White sponge naevus affecting the buccal mucosa. Other family members were also affected.

Table 21.6 Infective oral white patches

Candidosis
Candidal leukoplakia
Hairy leukoplakia
Papillomas
Syphilitic leukoplakia

Mechanical

Chronic irritation as a result of low-grade friction commonly leads to hyperkeratinization and a thickening of the epithelium. Chronic friction may be caused by cheek biting, irritation from a sharp tooth cusp, chewing on edentulous ridges or wearing ill-fitting dentures. The lesions of frictional keratosis appear as dense white lesions on the oral mucosa (Fig. 21.3). Diagnosis of a frictional keratosis relies on the identification of an obvious source of chronic irritation which correlates with the size and site of the lesion, and the lesion should resolve following elimination of the source of trauma. The lesions of frictional keratosis are inconsequential and are not associated with an increased risk of malignant transformation.

Chemical

Patients may place an aspirin tablet adjacent to a painful tooth in the mistaken belief that this will relieve their symptoms. Used in this way, aspirin causes epithelial necrosis, sloughing, ulceration and bleeding if the area is traumatized (Fig. 21.4). Thus a mixed appearance of white patch and ulceration may be seen. The typical aspirin burn resolves within 7–10 days. Similar effects may be produced by other medication such as teething gels and iron tablets if held in contact with the oral mucosa for prolonged periods.

In contrast, low-grade chronic chemical irritation is more likely to produce hyperkeratosis, such as results from tobacco use. Thus, lesions occur in those who smoke, chew or inhale tobacco as snuff.

Similar lesions may also be seen in those who chew betel nut.

Thermal

Patients who smoke tobacco in the form of cigarettes or cigars, or use a pipe, may develop white patch lesions, both thermal and chemical factors contributing to the aetiology. In cigarette smokers, lesions may develop on the lips, and in pipe smokers common sites for such lesions are at the junction of the hard and soft palates or the dorsal surface of the tongue where the hot smoke

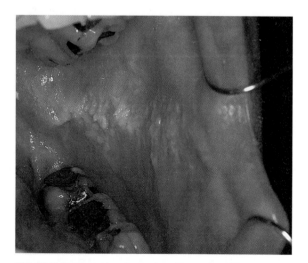

Fig. 21.3 Frictional keratosis along the occlusal line.

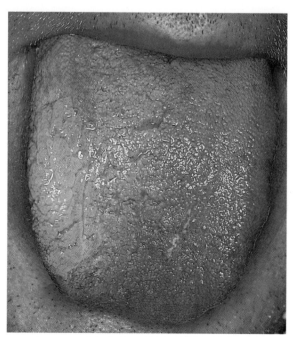

Fig. 21.4 An aspirin burn on the side of the tongue.

constantly impinges on the tissues or on the buccal mucosa (Fig. 21.5). Nicotinic stomatitis is a specific lesion affecting the palate, and occurs most commonly among pipe smokers. The palatal mucosa has a diffuse grey/white multinodular appearance with a small red dot in the centre of each nodule which represents a dilatated minor salivary gland duct orifice (Fig. 21.6). In extreme examples the affected area of the palate may assume a fissured or cracked appearance. Nicotinic stomatitis is a benign lesion which regresses if smoking is stopped.

Management of keratoses involves removal of the source of irritation. Failure of the lesion to resolve once the source has been eliminated should force a reconsideration of the diagnosis.

Dermatological lesions

Dermatological lesions frequently involve the mucous membranes of the mouth and other mucosal surfaces. Vesiculobullous lesions are considered in Chapter 20. Those which present as white patches include lichen planus and lichenoid reactions, and lupus erythematosus, both in its systemic and discoid forms.

Lichen planus and lichenoid reactions

Lichen planus and lichenoid reactions are in essence probably part of the same disease spectrum, with lichen planus considered a disease of unknown aetiology, and lichenoid reactions occurring in response to well-recognized precipitants, most commonly drugs and amalgam or mercury. There is undoubtedly some overlap between the two conditions, and in many instances it may be impossible to differentiate between them either on clinical features or on the basis of the histology. Some reports suggest that lichenoid reactions are more commonly asymmetrical, although there is no objective evidence to support this comment.

Lichen planus is a relatively common immunologically mediated mucocutaneous disorder of unknown aetiology. Females are more commonly affected and the peak age of incidence is among those in the fifth and sixth decades. Oral lesions are present in approximately half of those presenting with skin manifestations, whereas skin lesions are present in only 10–30% of those presenting with oral disease. The cutaneous lesions of lichen planus are discussed in Chapter 12.

Clinical features

Oral lesions of lichen planus can assume a variety of different clinical forms (Table 21.7). However, different types may often coexist in the same patient, and it may be difficult to differentiate some clinical types. The lesions can affect any part of the oral mucosa, although buccal mucosa

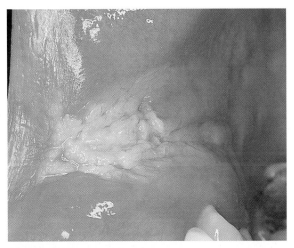

Fig. 21.5 Smoker's keratosis affecting the buccal mucosa.

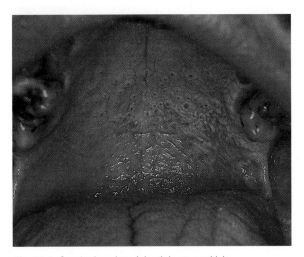

Fig. 21.6 Smoker's palate (nicotinic stomatitis).

Table 21.7 Clinical types of oral lichen planus
Reticular
Papular
Plaque
Atrophic
Ulcerative or erosive
Bullous
Desquamative gingivitis

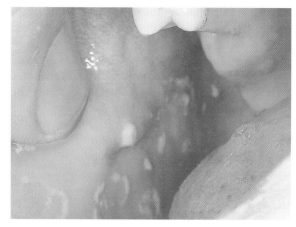

Fig. 21.8 Papular lichen planus on the buccal mucosa.

and the lateral margins of the tongue are most commonly involved. A bilaterally symmetrical distribution is almost invariable.

Reticular lichen planus, the commonest variant, is characterized by a fine lacy network of white striae (Fig. 21.7), frequently asymptomatic, although some patients may report a mild burning sensation due to the epithelial atrophy.

Papular lesions present as small white papules usually on the buccal mucosa (Fig. 21.8), and are frequently asymptomatic.

Plaque lichen planus is similar to leukoplakia, although radiating white striae may be observed at the periphery of the lesion (Fig. 21.9). Again this is often asymptomatic. It is seen particularly on the dorsum of the tongue.

Atrophic lesions are characterized by a diffuse erythematous glazed appearance, and there may be radiating white striae at the edges of the lesions (Fig. 21.10).

Ulcerative or erosive lesions are believed to arise as a result of trauma to the atrophic variant.

In extreme cases the entire dorsum of the tongue may be ulcerated, giving rise to severe pain and difficulty in eating.

Bullous lichen planus is the least common variant, and presents as subepithelial bullae, presumably due to extensive liquefactive degeneration at the basement membrane zone (Fig. 21.11).

Desquamative gingivitis

Desquamative gingivitis is a clinical diagnosis with features of full-thickness gingivitis associated with desquamation of the attached gingivae (Fig. 21.12). It may be due to a variety of disorders, the

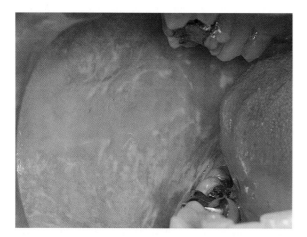

Fig. 21.7 Reticular lichen planus affecting the buccal mucosa.

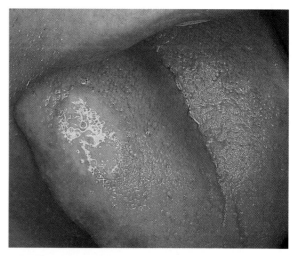

Fig. 21.9 Plaque lichen planus on the tongue.

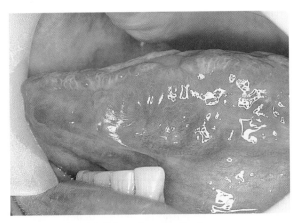

Fig. 21.10 Atrophic lichen planus on the tongue.

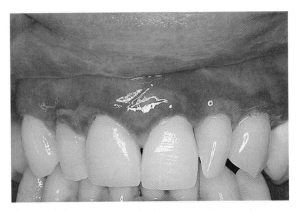

Fig. 21.12 Desquamative gingivitis in a patient with lichen planus.

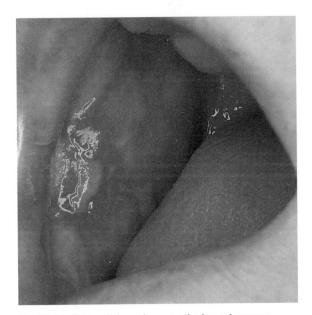

Fig. 21.11 Bullous lichen planus on the buccal mucosa.

Table 21.8 Causes of desquamative gingivitis

Lichen planus (Fig. 21.12)
Vesiculobullous disorders (especially pemphigoid) (Fig. 21.13)
Plasma cell gingivitis (allergic gingivitis)

---

commonest of which is lichen planus (Table 21.8).

Patients complain of gingival tenderness and sometimes bleeding on brushing. The condition is frequently misdiagnosed as plaque-induced marginal gingivitis, and the patient erroneously encouraged to brush more vigorously and hence cause exaggerated desquamation. Diagnosis of the underlying cause requires biopsy, including immunofluorescence to exclude pemphigoid if other concurrent mucosal lesions are absent. Biopsy should be away from the gingival margin

since chronic gingivitis will inevitably be present, and the lymphocyte infiltrate seen in chronic gingivitis will complicate the histological picture and make the biopsy diagnosis more difficult if the underlying pathology is lichen planus.

Plasma cell gingivitis is an archaic term for allergic gingivitis, which is most commonly due to toothpaste allergy, particularly to the more modern tartar control formulations. In the absence of patch-testing facilities, patients should be asked to empirically change to a non-allergenic toothpaste or to use bicarbonate of soda for brushing their teeth in order to exclude allergy as a precipitating factor. If this fails to improve the clinical situation then patch testing is warranted (see Ch. 26).

> Allergic gingivitis is most commonly due to toothpaste allergy

Treatment of desquamative gingivitis is as for other forms of intraoral lichen planus (see below), but problems of trauma from eating and brushing may prevent improvement. Splints or veneers may

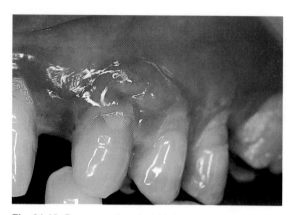

Fig. 21.13 Desquamative gingivitis in a patient with pemphigoid.

Table 21.9 Aetiology of Lichen planus	
Exogenous factors	*Systemic factors*
Dental materials	Drugs
Amalgam, mercury	Graft versus host disease
and gold	HIV infection
Food allergens	Liver disease
Infection	
Candida	
Bacterial plaque	
Stress	

be used to protect the affected gingivae and also act as a vehicle for delivery of topical corticosteroid creams or pastes (Fig. 21.14).

Aetiology

While the aetiology of lichen planus is unclear, a wide variety of factors have been implicated. These are summarized in Table 21.9. Numerous studies have suggested that amalgam and/or mercury itself are involved in the aetiology. In many patients, lesions of lichen planus develop closely related to adjacent amalgam restorations – so-called contact lesions. On patch testing, sensitivity to amalgam can be demonstrated in a significant proportion of patients with lichen planus. Moreover, resolution of lesions occurs following replacement of amalgam restorations with an alternative restorative material in some patients, even in those who are patch test-negative. Lichen planus may also develop in response to other dental materials, including gold. In some patients, lichen planus may develop following exposure to dietary allergens such as the flavouring agent cinnamon aldehyde. A further consideration of the allergic aspects of lichen planus is found in Chapter 26.

> Lichen planus lesions may resolve when amalgams are removed

A large number of drugs have been shown to induce lichenoid lesions, notably non-steroidal anti-inflammatory drugs, β blockers, α-methyldopa, antimalarials, sulphonamides and penicillamine. Drug-induced lichenoid lesions are frequently erosive rather than reticular. The exact mechanism whereby drugs induce this type of lesion is unclear, although it has been suggested that it may be a type IV hypersensitivity reaction.

Several studies have investigated a possible infective aetiology for lichen planus, although the results have not been convincing. Nevertheless, empirical antimicrobial therapy and oral hygiene may induce symptomatic improvement, presumably as a result of reducing the bacterial and/or fungal load within the mouth. Thus, the use of chlorhexidine may be helpful. Several studies have demonstrated an increased prevalence of candidal infestation in patients with lichen planus,

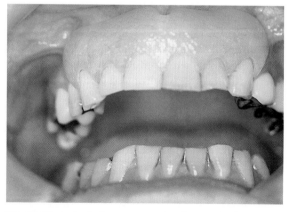

Fig. 21.14 A gingival veneer covering the attached gingivae in the upper anterior region in a patient with desquamative gingivitis.

and symptomatic as well as clinical improvement has been reported following antifungal therapy. This is particularly relevant if the patient is concomitantly receiving topical or systemic corticosteroids.

Stress is frequently reported as an important factor contributing to the aetiology, although convincing evidence is lacking.

Several systemic diseases have been investigated as possible aetiological factors. Early studies suggested a possible relationship with diabetes mellitus, although as both diabetes and lichen planus are common conditions the relationship appears to be coincidental rather than causative. Alternatively, patients may develop lichenoid reactions to hypoglycaemic drugs. Recent studies have demonstrated a high prevalence of hepatitis C virus infection among patients with lichen planus. This appears to affect only patients from Mediterranean countries and the Far East, probably related to specific HLA types. Lichenoid lesions may be seen in relation to HIV infection and graft versus host disease.

Diagnosis and management

If the onset of the lesion coincides with the start of drug therapy it is possible that the lesion is a lichenoid drug reaction, and consideration should be given to altering the patient's drug therapy in consultation with his or her general medical practitioner. Similarly, if the lesions are adjacent to amalgam restorations, sensitivity to amalgam may be an important factor, and replacement of the restorations with another material may be indicated.

An incisional biopsy is helpful in confirming the diagnosis, although it rarely allows absolute distinction between lichen planus or a lichenoid reaction. Some have suggested that a positive 'string of pearls' effect on indirect immunofluorescence supports the diagnosis of a lichenoid reaction, but the effect is non-specific.

If no precipitating factor can be identified, treatment is empirical and aimed at relieving symptoms. Non-erosive lichen planus is often asymptomatic, and no active treatment is indicated other than reassurance to the patient and regular review. Occasionally patients report a mild

burning sensation, and a chlorhexidine mouthwash may be helpful in relieving these symptoms.

In contrast, erosive forms of lichen planus often present a significant management challenge. As mentioned earlier, empirical antimicrobial therapy is frequently associated with an improvement in the level of the patient's symptoms. Thus, a chlorhexidine mouthwash is of potential benefit for mild symptoms. Similarly antifungal therapy, topically or systemically, may be beneficial in view of the higher prevalence of *Candida* carriage and infection among patients with lichen planus.

> Erosive lichen planus is usually symptomatic and thus requires treatment

---

Corticosteroids are the mainstay of treatment of lichen planus, and this may be associated with an increase in *Candida* carriage; hence the rationale for use of an antifungal agent as an adjunct. A variety of different preparations can be used, as summarized in Table 21.10.

Azathioprine may be used in extreme cases as a corticosteroid-sparing agent. Numerous other treatments have been advocated for resistant cases, including cyclosporin, dapsone and retinoids, although the evidence for efficacy of these treatments long-term is unclear.

Oral lichen planus as a potentially malignant lesion

Most cases of oral lichen planus run an entirely benign course. However, malignant transformation has been reported in a small proportion of cases. It has been suggested that malignant trans-

Table 21.10 Treatment preparations for oral lichen planus	
Topical	Hydrocortisone pellets
	Triamcinolone acetonide paste
	Betamethasone mouthwash
	Beclomethasone inhaler
Systemic	Prednisolone
Intralesional	Triamcinolone acetonide

formation is more common in erosive lesions or lesions affecting the gingivae or tongue, although the overall risk remains unclear. Several studies have estimated the risk as approximately 1% of patients over a 5 year period.

> Malignant transformation occurs in 1% of oral lichen planus cases

Lupus erythematosus

Systemic lupus erythematosis (SLE) is an important systemic autoimmune disease which is discussed in detail in Chapter 14. The oral manifestations and implications for oral health care are considered in Chapter 26. The condition is included here since it is clinically very similar to lichen planus. Oral lesions are seen in up to 20% of patients with SLE, and typically present as symmetrically distributed erythematous areas, erosions or white patches. Clinically there may be some difficulty differentiating them from lichen planus, and in some cases histological examination may also be inconclusive. The palate is a commonly affected site for lupus erythematosus but not lichen planus (Fig. 21.15) and lesions are frequently difficult to manage. Corticosteroids are the mainstay of treatment, although the lesions are often only responsive to unacceptably high doses. Concomitant therapy with azathioprine may allow a reduction in the dose of steroids.

Sjögren's syndrome may also be a feature of SLE.

In discoid lupus erythematosus (DLE), oral lesions most commonly affect the buccal mucosa, alveolar ridge and vermilion of the lip. Lesions are characterized by a central atrophic area surrounded by fine, white striae radiating perpendicular to the edge of the lesion (Fig. 21.16). The histological features of DLE are indistinguishable from SLE, and the two conditions can only be distinguished on serological grounds (anti-DNA antibodies are only seen in SLE) and the extent of systemic involvement.

Idiopathic white patches

This includes leukoplakia, which, as stated previously, can be a premalignant lesion. Leukoplakias may be homogeneous in appearance (Fig. 21.17) or non-homogeneous. These latter lesions may be speckled leukoplakias (Fig. 21.18) verrucous or nodular. Non-homogeneous lesions have a greater malignant potential.

> Non-homogeneous leukoplakias are more likely to turn malignant

Not only does the type of lesion affect the malignant potential, site is also of paramount importance: hard palatal leukoplakias in smokers have a low malignant transformation rate while

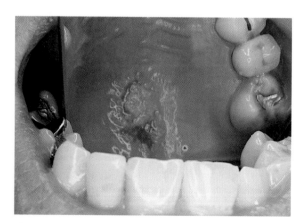

Fig. 21.15 Lupus erythematosus affecting the hard palate.

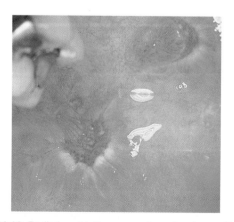

Fig. 21.16 Radiating striations around an ulcer in a patient with lupus erythematosus.

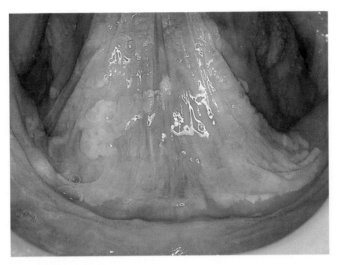

Fig. 21.17 A homogeneous sublingual keratosis.

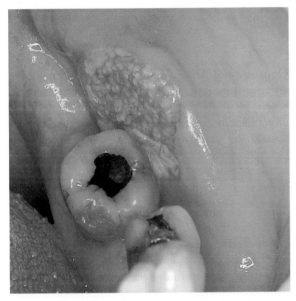

Fig. 21.18 Speckled leukoplakia affecting the buccal sulcus in a pipe smoker.

those on the soft palate may be more sinister. The most worrying site is the lateral border of the tongue and floor of mouth, which is where the majority of intraoral carcinomas arise. Early reports that up to 40% of floor of mouth leuko-plakias become malignant are highly exaggerated. Floor of mouth and lateral border of tongue leukoplakias should, however, be followed closely.

As alluded to earlier, lesions showing moderate or severe dysplasia should be removed if practical. When panoral or extensive dysplastic lesions exist, retinoids can be used, although the evidence for their efficacy is lacking. Topical cytotoxic drugs are unhelpful and should not be used. Close vigilance of dysplastic lesions is essential.

Leukoplakia

Leukoplakia is defined as 'a white patch or plaque which cannot be characterized clinically or pathologically as any other disease and is not associated with any physical or chemical agent except the use of tobacco' (World Health Organization).

Leukoedema

This term describes a faint whiteness of the mucosa almost as though the patient has just drunk some milk and some has remained in the mouth. It is due to mild keratosis and is of significance.

Erythroplakia (Fig. 21.19)

Erythroplakia is 'a bright red velvety plaque which cannot be characterised clinically or pathologically as being due to any other condition' (World Health Organization). Most are potentially malignant.

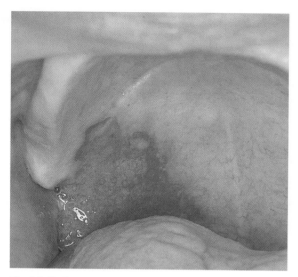

Fig. 21.19 Erythroplakia affecting the soft palate.

Neoplastic lesions

The overwhelming majority of malignant tumours in the mouth are squamous cell carcinomas arising from the oral mucosa. The minority of other malignant tumours include a wide range, such as sarcomas, malignant melanoma and tumours arising from the minor salivary glands. These are discussed in other chapters. The remainder of this discussion relates to squamous cell carcinoma.

The incidence of oral squamous cell carcinoma varies considerably throughout the world. In the UK and in most developed countries in the western world, oral cancer accounts for only 1–4% of all malignancies. In contrast, in some parts of India oral cancer represents 30–40% of all malignant tumours. Globally it has been estimated that oral cancer is the fourth commonest malignancy among men, and the sixth commonest among women. Oral cancer is more common among males, although there has been a dramatic reduction in this sex difference during the last 50 years. Thus, 50 years ago there were approximately five times as many cases among men compared to women, whereas currently the male:female ratio is only 2:1. In the UK there are approximately 2000 new cases per annum with almost 1000 deaths annually.

In common with many other malignancies, oral cancer predominantly affects patients over the age of 40 years, with more than 90% of cases occurring in this age group. Nevertheless, in recent years there has been an increase in the number of relatively young individuals, particularly males, with oral cancer. Thus, clinicians should have an awareness that malignant tumours may affect any age group. Oral cancer may affect any part of the oral mucosa, although there are particular sites of predilection with significant geographic variations. Thus, in the UK the commonest sites are the lip and tongue, followed by the floor of the mouth (males), the buccal mucosa (females) and the alveolus. In India, carcinoma of the buccal mucosa is the commonest site, which reflects the habit of chewing tobacco.

Aetiological factors

Numerous factors may be involved in the aetiology of oral cancer. These are summarized in Table 21.11. Alcohol and tobacco habits are the main factors.

Alcohol

Consumption of alcohol in excess is considered an important risk factor for oral cancer. Moreover, when alcohol and tobacco are combined the effects are not simply additive, and these factors appear to act synergistically, with a resultant marked increase in overall risk (Fig. 21.20).

Tobacco

This is the single most important aetiological factor, accounting for over 75% of cases. A wide variety of studies have demonstrated that the relative risk of oral cancer increases with increasing consumption and cumulative duration of tobacco use. Overall, cigar or pipe smoking is less of a risk than cigarette smoking. The synergistic effects of alcohol are mentioned above.

Betel nut chewing/smokeless tobacco

Chewing betel nut with added tobacco accounts for the very high incidence of oral cancer in South-East Asia.

> Smoking and alcohol act synergistically to increase the risk of malignancy

Table 21.11 Aetiological factors in oral cancer

Alcohol and tobacco
Betel nut chewing/smokeless tobacco
Immunosuppression
Infection
   Candidosis
   Syphilis
   Herpes simplex
   Human papillomavirus infection
Nutritional status
Occupational factors
Ultraviolet light

Immunosuppression

There is an increased incidence of lip cancer among renal transplant recipients, and, as discussed in the section on immunosuppression, HIV-seropositive patients have an increased risk of various tumours.

Infection

Chronic infection in the form of candidal leukoplakia or syphilitic leukoplakia can result in oral carcinoma, although this is extremely rare. This is suggestive evidence for a role for viruses including herpes simplex virus and human papillomaviruses in the aetiology of oral cancer.

Nutritional status

Sideropenic anaemia is associated with an increased risk of tumours of the mouth, pharynx and oesophagus, and in experimental studies iron deficiency has been shown to have an adverse effect on the structure and function of the oral epithelium. This is discussed further in Chapter 7.

Occupational factors

The development of oral cancer as an occupational hazard, for example lip cancer among workers using radioactive luminous paint, is now a thing of the past, although outdoor workers are at risk (see below).

Ultraviolet light

There is a well-established link between lip cancer and exposure to sunlight. Thus, there is an

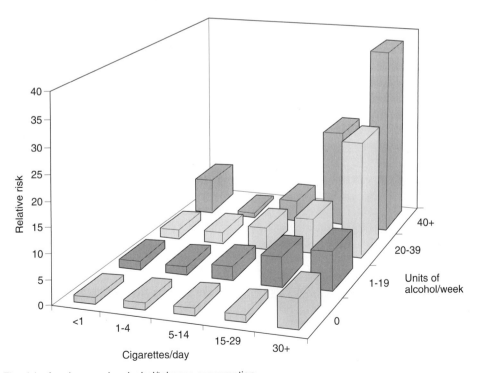

Fig. 21.20 The risk of oral cancer by alcohol/tobacco consumption.

increased incidence of active cheilitis and lip cancer among fair-skinned males who work outdoors. Melanin pigmentation affords some protective effect, and this accounts for the differing incidence among certain racial groups.

Clinical features

Oral squamous cell carcinoma can present in a variety of different ways. Clearly, early diagnosis is important, as this is associated with an improved survival. A high index of suspicion is required for any mucosal lesion for which no cause can be identified or which fails to respond to treatment.

Early lesions are frequently asymptomatic, and may present as a painless solitary ulcer (Fig. 21.21), an exophytic growth (Fig. 21.22), a white patch, an area of erythroplakia, a speckled patch (Fig. 21.23) or, in the case of lip cancer, a chronic crusted lesion. Pain is rarely a prominent early feature, which often results in patients failing to notice lesions until they are more advanced.

A high index of suspicion is desirable, and routine examination of the floor of mouth and lateral borders of the tongue by lingual displacement ensures that lesions will not be missed (Figs 21.24 and 21.25).

Prognosis

The prognosis for oral cancer relies on the TNM (tumour, nodes, metastases) classification for clinical staging (Table 21.12).

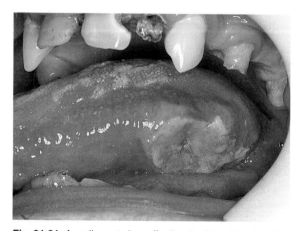

Fig. 21.21 A malignant ulcer affecting the lateral border of the tongue.

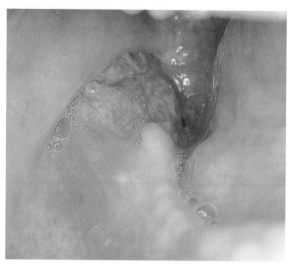

Fig. 21.22 An exophytic carcinoma affecting the retromolar area.

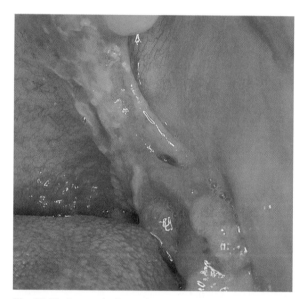

Fig. 21.23 An exophytic carcinoma arising in an area of speckled leukoplakia.

Treatment

Treatment is usually surgical with or without radiotherapy. Chemotherapy is rarely effective. Despite enormous advances in surgical techniques over the last few decades, the prognosis for oral cancer has not improved although the aesthetic consequences of surgery are better.

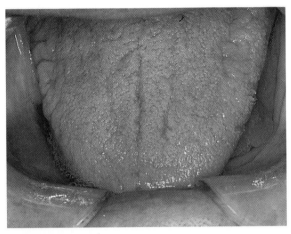

Fig. 21.24 Patient with a sublingual carcinoma with the tongue at rest.

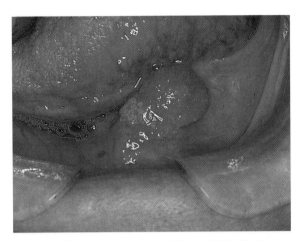

Fig. 21.25 The same patient as in Figure 25.24 with the tongue elevated.

Table 21.12 TNM and clinical staging of head and neck cancer (American Joint Committee on Cancer Staging)

a	TNM staging
TX	Primary tumour cannot be assessed
T0	No evidence of primary tumour
Tis	Carcinoma in situ
T1	Tumour ≤ 2 cm in greatest dimension
T2	Tumour > 2 cm but ≤ 4 cm
T3	Tumour > 4 cm
T4	Tumour invades adjacent structures (e.g. cortical bone, deep muscle of tongue, maxillary sinus, skin)
NX	Regional lymph nodes cannot be assessed
N0	No regional lymph node metastases
N1	Metastasis to single ipsilateral lymph node ≤ 3 cm
N2	Metastasis to single ipsilateral lymph node > 3 cm but ≤ 6 cm, to multiple ipsilateral lymph nodes (none > 6 cm), or to bilateral or contralateral lymph nodes (none > 6 cm)
N2a	Metastasis to single ipsilateral lymph nodes > 3 cm but ≤ 6 cm
N2b	Metastases to multiple ipsilateral lymph nodes (none > 6 cm)
N2c	Metastases to bilateral or contralateral lymph nodes (none > 6 cm)
N3	Metastasis to lymph node > 6 cm
MX	Presence of distant metastasis cannot be assessed
M0	No evidence of distant metastasis
M1	Distant metastasis

b	*Clinical staging*	
Stage	TNM	
0	TisN0M0	
I	T1N0M0	
II	T2N0M0	
III	T3N0M0	
	T1–T3N1M0	
	T4N0–N1M0	
IV	Any TN2–N3M0	
	Any T and N, and M1	

Stage I tumours have an excellent prognosis, whilst stage III and IV tumours have a very poor prognosis. Early investigation, when the lesion is small, is vitally important.

Other white patches

Skin grafting within the mouth is becoming more prevalent with modern microvascular surgical techniques. This should be borne in mind and enquired about since grafts appear white within the oral cavity (Fig. 21.26).

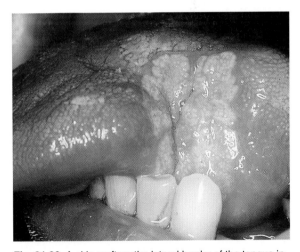

Fig. 21.26 A skin graft on the lateral border of the tongue in a patient who had a carcinoma removed.

22 Oral mucosal infections

Introduction

The oral mucosa is the target of a number of infectious processes caused by a range of organisms which are considered here under the headings viruses, bacteria and fungi. Parasites very rarely infect the oral tissues. Oral mucosal infections may occur as the primary disease process, or superinfection may complicate other conditions of the oral mucosa, such as candidal superinfection in lichen planus. Even in conditions which are primarily infectious, systemic factors may complicate the clinical picture or alter the severity, such as HIV, diabetes, corticosteroid therapy or cigarette smoking. Severe and intransigent infections of the oral mucosa are characteristic in HIV disease, and these are alluded to in this chapter, although the oral manifestations of HIV disease are considered elsewhere (see Ch. 23).

Viruses

The main viruses causing oral mucosal infections are the large herpes group of viruses, but oral mucosal infections can also be caused by coxsackieviruses, human papillomaviruses and others. These will be discussed in turn.

Herpesviruses

These viruses are a group of DNA viruses which cause a range of oral and systemic diseases. Viruses included in this group and the diseases which they cause are shown in Table 22.1.

Herpes simplex viruses

There are two types; herpes simplex type 1 (HSV-1) and herpes simplex type 2 (HSV-2). Classically, HSV-1 causes oral disease, whereas HSV-2 causes genital disease. The viruses are very similar however, and both can cause oral or genital disease, although there are differences in recurrence rates.

Primary exposure to HSV in the mouth causes acute herpetic gingivostomatitis (Fig. 22.1). The virus causes a viraemia, fever, malaise and lymphadenopathy. All surfaces of the mouth, including the hard palate and the attached gingivae, may be involved, initially with a vesicular rash which ulcerates and often becomes superinfected. The illness lasts for 10–14 days before resolving spontaneously. The individual is unwell for the first week and then the symptoms improve and healing is usually uneventful. In the early stages, oral discomfort may prevent eating and drinking, and this, in combination with fever and malaise, may lead to dehydration.

Table 22.1 Classification of human herpesviruses

Name	Herpesvirus	Disease
Herpes simplex virus 1 (HSV-1)	I	Gingivostomatitis, herpes labialis
Herpes simplex virus 2 (HSV-2)	II	Genital herpes
Varicella – zoster virus (VZV)	III	Chickenpox/shingles
Epstein – Barr virus (EBV)	IV	Glandular fever
		Hairy leukoplakia
Cytomegalovirus (CMV)	V	Glandular fever-like illness
Human herpesvirus 6 (HHV6)	VI	–
Human herpesvirus 7 (HHV7)	VII	–
Human herpesvirus 8 (HHV8)	VIII	Kaposi's sarcoma

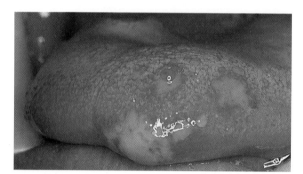

Fig. 22.1 Lingual ulcers in a patient with primary herpetic gingivostomatitis.

The diagnosis is usually made on clinical grounds, and confirmation is academic since the infection is self-limiting except in immune defects. The diagnosis can be confirmed however, by direct immunofluorescence of vesicular fluid to detect the virus using specific antiserum, by inoculation of cell culture, or by showing a threefold rise in the convalescent antibody titre over that seen in the acute phase.

The primary infection may be mild and subclinical in the majority of young children who are exposed to it, though the condition may be severe and debilitating, and in an immunocompromised individual may lead to severe illness and sometimes to herpetic hepatitis or encephalitis, which may be fatal in the absence of treatment. Serological studies of populations indicate that some >50% of 20-year-old patients have been exposed to HSV.

Oral infection arises from direct contact with secretions from an individual who has either a primary or recurrent HSV infection. Infection may also be contracted from asymptomatic individuals who have previously had primary HSV infection and who asymptomatically shed virus in their saliva on an intermittent basis.

Direct inoculation of the fingers or skin with virally contaminated secretions or fluid can lead to local infection, e.g. a herpetic whitlow causes a severely painful lesion of the finger and was a recognized occupational risk among dentists before the routine use of rubber gloves for treating patients (Fig. 22.2).

HSV is a neurogenic virus, and on recovery from the primary infection the virus may become latent within the trigeminal ganglia or basal ganglia of the brain, and may subsequently, be reactivated to cause a secondary infection (Fig. 22.3). Indeed, HSV has now been shown to be a cause of Bell's palsy (see Ch. 25).

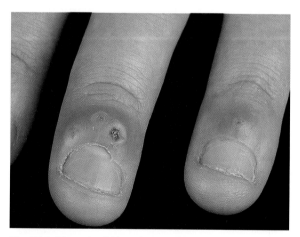

Fig. 22.2 Herpetic whitlows in a patient with herpetic gingivostomatitis.

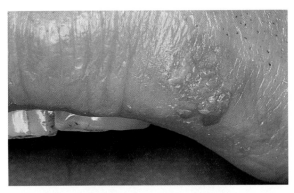

Fig. 22.3 Herpes labialis or 'cold sore' affecting the upper lip.

Primary genital HSV infection follows a similar clinical course to oral HSV infection, although infection of the genital mucous membranes is through sexual contact. Vesicular mucositis ensues, and the virus subsequently becomes dormant within the dorsal root ganglia.

Once the primary oral infection has resolved, the individual is immune from further primary infections, although reactivation of the virus, due to some stimulation, can cause a recurrent herpes labialis lesion. Recurrent herpes labialis lesions have a prodromal phase of approximately 24 h where there is a prickling sensation on the vermilion border followed by vesiculation with pain and occasional lymphadenopathy which lasts for several days before the lesion becomes crusted and healing ensues. The main factors involved in reactivation of the virus are shown in Table 22.2. Recurrent herpetic lesions also occur beyond the vermilion border, and may occur on the skin of the face, particularly in response to nerve trauma during dental treatment, e.g. during removal of impacted wisdom teeth.

Table 22.2 Reactivation of HSV
Trauma
Chemicals
Heat
Hormones
Sunlight
Emotion
Immunosuppression
Concurrent infection

Recurrent herpes labialis occurs in some 50–75% of individuals affected orally with HSV-1. The recommended treatment is 1% penciclovir cream.

> Herpes labialis arises from reactivation of latent HSV

Intraoral recurrent herpes also occurs, and recurs always in the same area with a painful crop of small ulcers often affecting the hard palate.

The treatment of primary herpetic gingivostomatitis comprises supportive therapy in the form of oral fluids, analgesia such as paracetamol, which is also antipyretic, and an antiseptic mouthwash such as chlorhexidine, sodium perborate or hydrogen peroxide. If the patient is seen within 72 h of the onset of the infection, aciclovir can be prescribed if the clinical severity warrants it at a dose of 200 mg five times daily for 5 days in adults and 100 mg five times daily for 5 days in those individuals less than 2 years old. Although aciclovir therapy can shorten the clinical course of the primary infection, there is no evidence that it reduces the incidence of recurrent herpetic lesions.

Varicella – zoster virus (VZV)

Like human HSV-1 and HSV-2, VZV is a neurogenic DNA virus which causes a primary infection in the form of chickenpox. Thereafter the virus remains dormant within the nerve tissue until reactivation in the form of shingles.

Chickenpox arises in an epidemic form after direct contact within infected individuals who have either chickenpox or shingles, and causes an acute vesicular rash associated with fever, malaise and lymphadenopathy. The vesicles burst to leave itchy crusted lesions which heal by scarring. Aciclovir is not justified except in immunocompromised individuals, and does not protect against the subsequent development of shingles.

Shingles usually arises as a result of reactivation of VZV in the nerves supplying a dermatome in individuals who have been immunosuppressed for some other reason, such as a concurrent illness. Shingles causes severe pain, vesiculation and subsequent ulceration within the distribution of one dermatome, and commonly occurs on the trunk on one side. It may also occur as a unilateral rash within the distribution of the trigeminal nerve. Often a unilateral rash develops along the distribution of one of the three branches of the trigeminal nerve affecting the skin of the face (Fig. 22.4), and when the ophthalmic division is involved, corneal ulceration may occur. Exclusively intraoral ulceration, vesiculation and ulceration may also occur, associated with significant pain. The diagnosis is made on the unilateral appearance of the ulceration, which usually affects one-half of the hard palate (Fig. 22.5) or one side of the tongue.

> Shingles may be exclusively intraoral

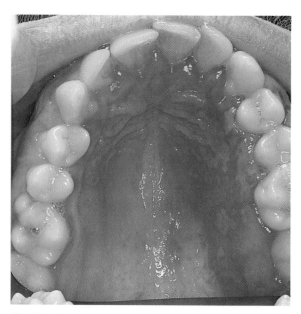

Fig. 22.5 Unilateral palatal ulceration in a patient with herpes zoster.

Shingles is a self-limiting condition, and heals with some scarring after 2–3 weeks. Shingles is a significantly painful condition, and the pain may persist after resolution of the infectious process, leading to a condition called postherpetic neuralgia. This pain arises more commonly with advancing age, and is also more intransigent in the elderly. Patients over the age of 80 years are extremely likely to develop postherpetic neuralgia, and in these cases it is likely to be persistent indefinitely. The pain of postherpetic neuralgia is extremely difficult to control, although carbamazepine and concurrent antidepressant therapy tends to provide partial relief.

VZV is less sensitive to aciclovir than HSV, and therefore the appropriate therapeutic regime for aciclovir is to use 800 mg five times daily for 7 days if the episode of shingles is seen within 72 h of onset. Systemic aciclovir may reduce the duration of the infective episode, and may reduce the pain during the acute phase, and there is now evidence that aciclovir treatment reduces the prevalence of postherpetic neuralgia.

> Systemic aciclovir reduces the prevalence of postherpetic neuralgia

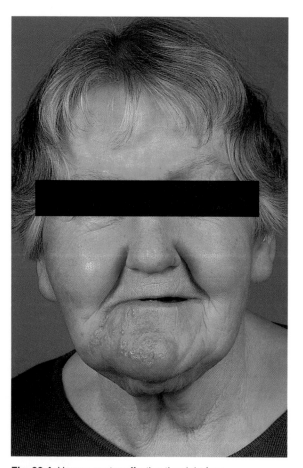

Fig. 22.4 Herpes zoster affecting the right face.

Epstein–Barr virus (EBV)

EBV is an interesting herpesvirus which is associated with a number of disease processes. In contrast to HSV and VZV, which are neurogenic, EBV has a predilection for infecting B lymphocytes. This infection of the B lymphocytes with the virus causes them to become activated and produce their own antibody, and not necessarily antibody against EBV. The virus is thus a polyclonal activator.

A primary infection with EBV causes glandular fever or infectious mononucleosis. In this infection the B lymphocytes become activated to non-specifically produce antibody, and the body then produces activated suppressor cells to dampen down this process. These large activated suppressor cells are the mononuclear cells which give mononucleosis its name, and are the basis of the monospot (Paul–Bunnell) tests. Clinically, the infection is characterized by fever, malaise and lymphadenopathy associated with a petechial rash at the junction of the hard and soft palate. The symptoms, however, are often non-specific, and may persist for months without clinical improvement. After clinical resolution of the infection, EBV persists, and may be shed asymptomatically in saliva.

Treatment of glandular fever is symptomatic, and if ampicillin is given inappropriately for the treatment of the patient's sore throat then a non-allergic rash may develop, presumably as a result of inappropriate antibody production by the polyclonally activated B cells. Such an ampicillin rash, as is seen in glandular fever, does not recur on subsequent administration of ampicillin once the acute infection has resolved.

Hairy leukoplakia occurs as a corrugated keratosis affecting the lateral borders of the tongue, and occasionally other intraoral sites, in individuals who are immunosuppressed, especially those with HIV disease. Hairy leukoplakia is discussed in detail in Chapter 23. Hairy leukoplakia has been shown to be due to an infection of the oral epithelium with EBV, and it is thought that this arises from autoinoculation of the virus into the mucosa of the lateral borders of the tongue when it is secreted in saliva in immunosuppressed individuals. Demonstration of EBV in biopsy tissue from hairy leukoplakia is a prerequisite to making a definitive diagnosis.

> EBV causes infectious mononucleosis, hairy leukoplakia, Burkitt's lymphoma and nasopharyngeal lymphoma

A combination of the continuous stimulation of B cells when they are infected by EBV, and the concurrent systemic condition causing immunosuppression, can lead to a neoplastic proliferation of B cells, which is the case in Burkitt's lymphoma seen in African children concurrently infected with EBV and malaria. EBV has also been shown to be implicated in the aetiology of nasopharyngeal carcinoma, which is common in the Far Eastern countries. A link has now also been made with lymphomas.

Cytomegalovirus

Cytomegalovirus has not been shown to cause any specific illnesses although it is associated with a glandular fever-like illness in childhood. It is found, on occasion, in severe atypical oral ulceration in people with HIV disease.

Human herpesviruses 6, 7 and 8

These three herpesviruses have been discovered in recent years. Human herpesvirus 8 has been demonstrated in Kaposi's sarcoma in patients who are HIV infected. Human herpesviruses 6 and 7 have not been shown to be associated with any specific oral disease processes.

Coxsackie viruses

Coxsackieviruses are RNA viruses, and it is various types of Coxsackie A virus which cause herpangina or hand, foot and mouth disease

Herpangina is a Coxsackie A virus infection which usually occurs in children, and is characterized by a herpes-like oropharyngitis, where the ulceration is predominately on the tonsil, soft palate and uvula (Fig. 22.6). The mild illness is associated with fever and malaise, but symptoms persist for only a few days. Serological testing is available but is usually not clinically justified. There is no specific treatment.

Hand, foot and mouth disease is also caused by a coxsackie A virus, and it also occurs predomi-

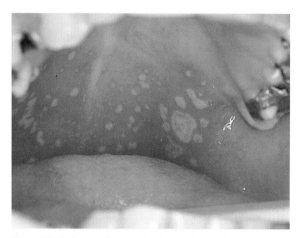

Fig. 22.6 Soft palatal ulceration in a patient with herpangina.

nately in children, although can be transmitted within families. The condition is also characterized by ulceration some 2–5 mm in diameter affecting the gingivae, tongue, cheeks and palate (Fig. 22.7). It is also associated with vesicles and ulcers on the palms and soles (Fig. 22.8). The symptoms may persist for as long as 2 weeks, and again can be confirmed serologically if there is clinical doubt. There is no specific treatment.

Human papilloma viruses

There are an increasing number of human papillomavirus (HPV) types which have been identified, and all are associated with different clinical entities. The common wart or verruca vulgaris is usually associated with HPV types 2 and 4. Warts can occur in the mouth, particularly in children who have autoinoculated themselves by biting finger or hand warts (Fig. 22.9). Warts can be treated by cryosurgery or simply removed surgically. Condyloma acuminata or venereal warts usually occur in the anogenital region, but can also be seen on the oral mucosa. They are associated with HPV types 6, 11 and 60. Focal epithelial hyperplasia, or Heck's disease, is a rare condition caused by HPV types 13 and 32, and causes plaques or polypoid lesions on the lower lips and buccal mucosa of certain ethnic groups, especially native North American Indians and Inuits.

HPV has been clearly associated with carcinoma of the uterine cervix, and an association

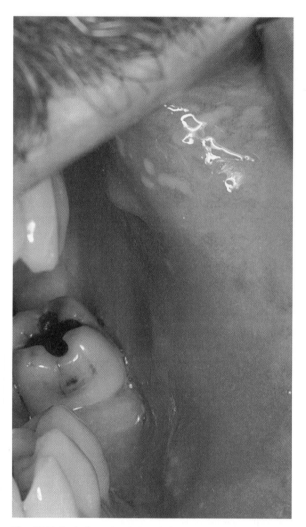

Fig. 22.7 Oral ulceration in hand, foot and mouth disease.

between HPV and oral carcinoma has been suspected but not proved.

Bacteria

Apart from the common dental diseases, caries and periodontal disease, and their sequelae, e.g. abscesses, bacterial infections in the mouth are surprisingly uncommon, and if properly diagnosed usually treated easily with antibiotics. Diagnosis may not, however, always be easy. The bacterial infections to be discussed are shown in Table 22.3.

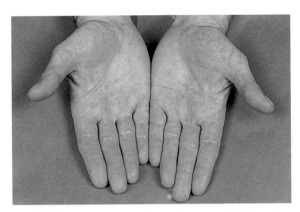

Fig. 22.8 Palmar lesions in hand, foot and mouth disease.

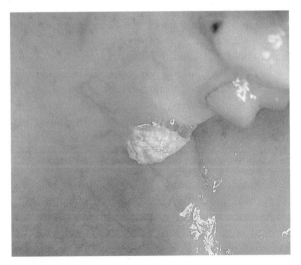

Fig. 22.9 A viral wart on the palate.

Table 22.3 Oral bacterial infections
Acute ulcerative gingivitis
Actinomycosis
Bacterial stomatitis
Gonorrhoea
Syphilis
Tuberculosis

Acute ulcerative gingivitis

This condition, also called Vincent's gingivitis, or acute necrotizing ulcerative gingivitis in the USA, is characterized by interdental and marginal ulceration covered in a slough, and the condition typi-cally bleeds readily and has a characteristic feotor oris. There may be an associated metallic taste or cervical lymphadenopathy. It is thought to be due to opportunistic infection with a mixture of organ-isms, especially spirochetes, fusiform bacilli and rods. It occurs in individuals predisposed by smoking, poor oral hygiene, or a medically com-promised state. It occurs chronically in HIV dis-ease. Treatment with oral hygiene measures is successful, but it is common practice to also give metronidazole 200 mg three times daily or peni-cillin 250 mg four times daily for 5 days.

Acute ulcerative gingivitis can progress to a necrotizing stomatitis in individuals with lowered resistance. This is seen most commonly in HIV disease, but classically occurs in malnourished children in Africa, so-called noma or cancrum oris, or those with an intercurrent infection such as primary herpes.

Actinomycosis

Classically, this infection with *Actinomyces* spp. presents as multiple submandibular sinuses with associated fibrosis arising from an intraoral infec-tion with endogenous organisms. This advanced presentation is rare nowadays with improved medical care, and the infection usually presents as a persistent abscess. Diagnosis relies on the demonstration of sulphur granules in the pus and a 'caput medusae' on Gram staining which has a Gram-positive centre surrounded by radiating Gram-negative filaments. Treatment requires prolonged therapy, e.g. with amoxycillin for 6 weeks.

Bacterial stomatitis

It is doubtful if streptococcal stomatitis actually occurs, but staphylococcal mucositis is occasion-ally seen in medically compromised patients, when it presents as a magenta red mucositis which responds to flucloxacillin therapy (Fig. 22.10).

Syphilis

Syphilis may present in the mouth as a primary chancre, secondary syphilis, as mucous patches or snail track ulcers, and as a gumma or as a

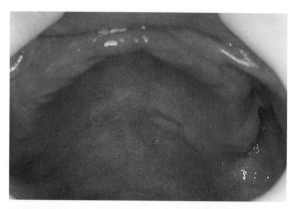

Fig. 22.10 Mucosal erythema affecting the soft palate as well as the denture-bearing area in a diabetic with staphylococcal mucositis.

syphilitic leukoplakia in the tertiary form of the disease. Congenital syphilis presents as a saddle nose and notched (Hutchinson's) incisors and mulberry molars. Oral syphilis is such a rare presentation nowadays that clinical diagnosis is unlikely, and the diagnosis is usually suggested by histology, serology or dark-ground microscopy of smears.

Tuberculosis

Primary tuberculosis in the mouth is very rare, but secondary lesions from coughing up infected sputum may cause oral lesions, usually in the form of a chronic ulcer on the dorsal surface of the tongue. Diagnosis requires biopsy, necessary for any chronic ulcer, and demonstration by the pathologist of tubercle bacilli in the tissues. This was traditionally done using a Ziehl–Neelsen stain for acid- and alcohol-fast bacilli, but more laboratories are now using the polymerase chain reaction as a molecular technique to look for the infectious agents. A general consideration of tuberculosis is found in Chapter 5.

The granulomatous appearance of the histology is similar to other 'non-infective' diseases such as sarcoidosis and Crohn's disease, although caseation is often also present in tuberculosis.

Tuberculosis occasionally presents as an enlarged cervical lymph node, and should be included in the differential diagnoses of neck swellings.

Patients diagnosed as having tuberculosis need referral to an infectious diseases specialist for specific antituberculous therapy.

Fungal infections

Fungal infections of the oral mucosa are most often due to *Candida* species and are particularly prevalent among denture wearers. Other mycoses such as blastomycosis, histoplasmosis or paracoccidioidomycosis are seen mainly in the Americas. They present usually as chronic ulcers.

Candidal infections

Candida spp. are part of the normal commensal flora in about half of the population. The commonest is *C. albicans*, but other commonly identified species include *C. glabrata*, *C. tropicalis* and *C. krusei*. They are all potentially pathogenic, and can cause infection when the person becomes predisposed in some way. The main predisposing factors are shown in Table 22.4, and these should be considered in anybody who presents with oral candidosis.

Candidal infections present in a number of different ways, and these are classified in Table 22.5.

As discussed below, denture-induced stomatitis and angular cheilitis may occasionally be due to infections with organisms other than *Candida* spp., and are therefore sometimes called *Candida-associated lesions*.

The individual candidal infections will be considered in turn.

Table 22.4 Factors predisposing to candidosis	
Local factors	*General factors*
Antibiotics	Immunosuppressive drugs
Dentures	Extremes of age
Steroids	Endocrine
Xerostomia	Diabetes
Drugs	Cushing's disease
Radiotherapy	Immunodeficiency
	Hereditary
	Acquired – HIV disease
	Nutritional deficiencies
	Iron
	Smoking

Table 22.5 Presentations of candidosis

Pseudomembranous candidosis
Erythematous candidosis
    Antibiotic stomatitis
    Denture-induced stomatitis
    HIV disease
    Median rhomboid glossitis
Chronic hyperplastic candidosis
Chronic mucocutaneous candidosis
Angular cheilitis

The white plaques in pseudomembranous candidosis can be scraped off

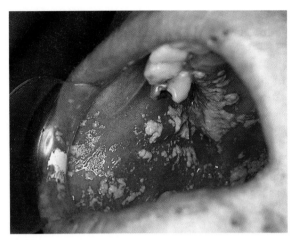

Fig. 22.11 Pseudomembranous candidosis in an alcoholic.

Pseudomembranous candidosis

This condition, also called thrush, usually occurs in an acute form, but may be chronic in the immunocompromised such as those with HIV disease. Indeed, the majority of those with HIV infection will eventually develop pseudomembranous candidosis, and it is the commonest presenting feature of HIV infection. Pseudomembranous candidosis also occurs in the extremes of life when the individual has defective defences: 5% of neonates develop thrush. In the 'normal' adult population, pseudomembranous candidosis is rare, and a cause such as HIV infection, undiagnosed diabetes or corticosteroid or antibiotic therapy should be considered.

Clinically, pseudomembranous candidosis appears as white curd-like spots or plaques on an erythematous mucosa (Fig. 22.11), especially the palate and fauces. In contrast to intraoral keratoses, the plaques seen in pseudomembranous candidosis can be removed by scraping, leaving a raw bleeding surface. The curd-like plaques comprise desquamated epithelial cells and candidal hyphae, which can be stained with potassium hydroxide or Gram stain to confirm the diagnosis, although this is rarely necessary. Culture is of little value in the diagnosis of candidosis since it only demonstrates the presence of *Candida* spp. which would be expected in half the population. To demonstrate infection, hyphae must be visualized in a smear. Culture of the candida, however, allows identification of the species. This is important in recurrent or in intransigent infections, since some species are more difficult to eliminate. Samples for cultures can be obtained from swabs of the mucosa or denture or by using a saline rinse which is washed around the mouth before being expectorated back into the bottle and sent to the laboratory for culture. For example, *C. krusei* is resistant to fluconazole. Pseudomembranous candidosis must be differentiated from other forms of intraoral white patches, which are discussed in Chapter 21.

Treatment of pseudomembranous candidosis involves eliminating the infection with antifungal therapy and looking for an underlying cause.

In uncomplicated pseudomembranous candidosis such as that seen after broad-spectrum antibiotic therapy, simple topical antifungal therapy in the form of amphotericin or nystatin is curative within about 1 week, and systemic antifungal therapy is rarely necessary. In individuals with a chronic immunocompromised state, systemic antifungal therapy such as fluconazole may be required, and long-term antifungal prophylaxis may be needed. This may, however, lead to fungal resistance, especially to the azole antifungals, and this is becoming a major problem in the management of individuals with HIV disease.

Erythematous candidosis

Candidal infection causes mucosal erythema, and this may present in a number of distinct clinical ways such as antibiotic stomatitis, denture-induced stomatitis, a mucosal erythema seen in HIV disease, which is similar to pseudomembranous candidosis without the white plaques, and median rhomboid glossitis. These will be discussed in turn.

Antibiotic stomatitis. This is a form of erythematous candidosis which arises as a result of the normal bacterial flora being eliminated by broad-spectrum antibiotic therapy. This results in generalized mucosal erythema, and may also be associated with a sense of dryness and discomfort. A topical antifungal such as amphotericin or nystatin used for 1 week is usually curative. A similar clinical appearance can arise due to bacteria such as staphylococci causing a mucositis, and if antifungal therapy does not cause rapid improvement, then a microbiological swab should be taken to identify the causative agent.

Denture-induced   stomatitis. Denture-induced stomatitis, or chronic erythematous candidosis, occurs as mucosal erythema under the fitting surface of an upper complete or partial denture in up to 50% of denture wearers. It may be associated with a dry or metallic taste in the mouth, but is usually asymptomatic, and is undiagnosed until the patient is examined by a dental practitioner. It has been classified by Newton into three distinct forms. Type 1 is a pinpoint erythema on the hard palate which may be due to trauma from the denture (Fig. 22.12). Type 2, which is the commonest form, is a diffuse erythema which covers the whole of the surface of the palate covered by the fitting surface of the denture (Fig. 22.13). This may be misdiagnosed as acrylic allergy, which is in fact extremely rare. Type 3 is a hyperplastic form of denture-induced stomatitis, and is characterized by papilliferous overgrowth of the palatal mucosa, especially in the vault of the palate (Fig. 22.14). It tends to be the sign of a more long-standing denture-induced stomatitis.

The treatment of denture-induced stomatitis is complicated, and if the underlying predisposing factors are not corrected, then the condition will return after treatment. The most important factor in the management of denture-induced stomatitis is oral hygiene. The dentures should be removed at night and stored in an antiseptic solution such as hypochlorite, which is ideal for soaking acrylic

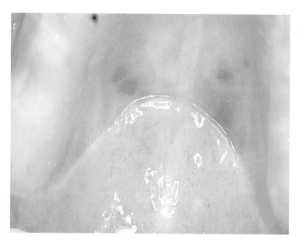

Fig. 22.12 Newton's type-1 denture stomatitis.

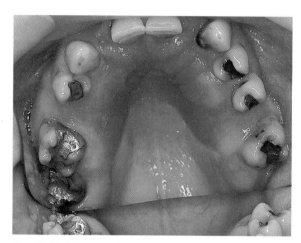

Fig. 22.13 Diffuse erythema affecting the whole of the denture bearing area in Newton's type-2 denture stomatitis.

dentures, but is corrosive for metal dentures, and in these circumstances chlorhexidine mouthwash can be used instead. The dentures should be scrubbed with soap and water to remove any plaque, and then dried and coated with a topical antifungal cream before reinsertion if topical antifungals are used in treatment. Just as important is the care of the mucosal surface, and patients should be encouraged to brush their palatal mucosa gently night and morning with a toothbrush, which will improve the blood supply and keratinization of the mucosa and prevent relapse of the condition. Patients should also be encouraged not to eat a high-carbohydrate diet, and

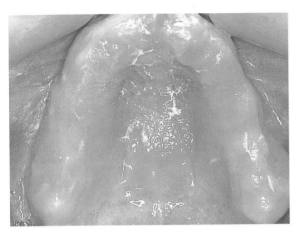

Fig. 22.14 Papillary hyperplasia in Newton's type-3 denture stomatitis.

Erythematous candidosis in HIV disease. This presents usually as a localized area of erythema, commonly on the palate (Fig. 22.15), and is seen in the absence of obvious predisposing factors. It is less clinically obvious than pseudomembranous candidosis, and is often underdiagnosed. It should be treated, however, in the same way as pseudomembranous candidosis in those individuals who have HIV disease.

Median rhomboid glossitis. Median rhomboid glossitis presents as an amorphous smooth red patch in the centre of the dorsum of the tongue anterior to the circumvallate papillae (Fig. 22.16). It used to be thought that it may be

should be prescribed appropriate antifungal therapy. This can either be in the form of amphotericin or nystatin lozenges sucked four times a day for 1 month used in association with cream applied to the fitting surface of the denture, or patients may use miconazole oral gel placed inside the fitting surface of the denture before insertion. An alternative form of therapy is to use a systemic antifungal agent such as fluconazole, which is secreted in saliva and has a half-life of 30 h, making it ideal for once-daily treatment. It improves compliance and does not suffer from the problems of bad taste and poor patient compliance which one finds with topical antifungal therapy. The patient should be prescribed 50 mg of fluconazole daily for 1–2 weeks. This, if combined with appropriate oral hygiene measures as described above, is usually curative unless there is some underlying systemic predisposing factor.

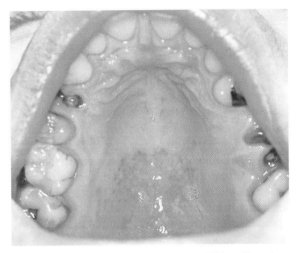

Fig. 22.15 Erythematous candidosis in an HIV positive patient.

> Recurrence of denture stomatitis can be reduced by brushing the palate

Denture trauma also contributes to the development and persistence of denture-induced stomatitis, and patients who present with chronic erythematous candidosis should have their dentures assessed and replaced if they are ill-fitting.

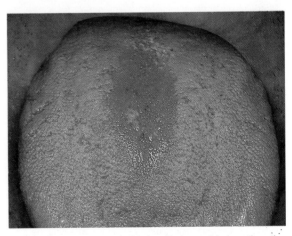

Fig. 22.16 Median rhomboid glossitis in an elderly asthmatic.

a lingual thyroid or a persistent tuberculum impar, but is now recognized as a form of erythematous candidosis, and biopsy will reveal candidal hyphae penetrating into the superficial epithelium. It is seen particularly in patients who are smokers or who use steroid inhalers for asthma. In steroid inhaler users there is also sometimes an erythema of the soft palate. Such individuals should be instructed to rinse their mouth with water after using their steroid inhaler if therapy is going to be successful without these adverse effects.

The condition is usually asymptomatic, and often reassurance is all that is required. If treatment is required, response to topical antifungals is usually slow, and systemic azole antifungal therapy in the form of fluconazole 50 mg each morning for 2 weeks is the preferred mode of therapy.

Chronic hyperplastic candidosis

This condition, also called candidal leukoplakia, presents as a white patch lesion classically inside the commissures of the lips bilaterally (Fig. 22.17) which on biopsy reveals penetration of candidal hyphae into the hyperkeratosis demonstrated using a periodic acid–Schiff (PAS) stain. There is also a varying level of epithelial dysplasia present, and candidal leukoplakia should be treated with antifungals initially and then in the same way as other forms of premalignant white patch.

Whether candidal leukoplakia arises as a result of candidal infestation of a pre-existing leukoplakia or whether it arises as a hyperkeratotic response to fungal infestation is not known. It occurs almost exclusively among smokers, and although systemic antifungal therapy causes clinical improvement, the condition will recur if the patient does not stop smoking. If the patient ceases his or her smoking habit, the condition may regress spontaneously.

> Candidal leukoplakia often regresses if the patient stops smoking

Chronic mucocutaneous candidosis

Chronic mucocutaneous candidosis is a condition characterized by candidal infections which occur both in the mucous membranes (Fig. 22.18) and the skin, including the nails. Chronic mucocutaneous candidosis is extremely rare.

Because of the deep-seated nature of chronic mucocutaneous candidosis, systemic antifungals are required for its treatment.

Angular cheilitis

The sores at the angle of the mouth seen in angular cheilitis may be weeping or encrusted. The

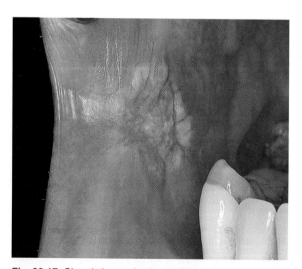

Fig. 22.17 Chronic hyperplastic candidosis affecting the commissure in a smoker.

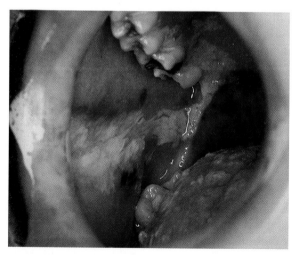

Fig. 22.18 Mucocutaneous candidosis in a patient with polyendocrinopathy showing intraoral candidal leukoplakia and pigmentation due to Addison's disease.

aetiology is multifactorial, including skin folding due to age or the reduced vertical dimension of the dentures, diabetes mellitus, nutritional deficiency of iron, folic acid or vitamin B_{12}, and an infection either with *Candida* species, when it tends to be a weeping angular chelitis, associated with denture-induced stomatitis (Fig. 22.19), or with staphylococci (Fig. 22.20), which may also be found in the anterior nares, or, more rarely, streptococci. The potential mixed nature of the infection has implications for treatment, and in addition to treating the intraoral infection, patients should be given miconazole gel or cream empirically in the first instance, as this is effective

not only against *Candida* species but also against staphylococci and streptococci. If the condition does not respond rapidly to this therapy, patients should have their blood screened and also have swabs taken from the angles of their mouth and intraorally to identify the causative agent, and more specific treatment with either a polyene antifungal topically or fucidin for bacterial infection. Nasal carriage of staphylococci may also need treatment with topical fucidin. Replacement dentures are helpful if the vertical dimension is reduced, although it is often difficult, even with increasing the vertical dimension of dentures, to eliminate the angular fold in older people.

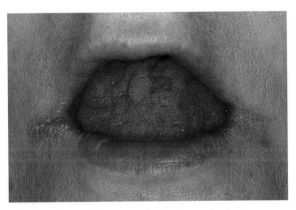

Fig. 22.19 Candidal angular cheilitis in a patient with denture stomatitis.

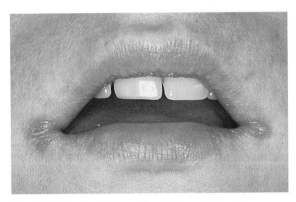

Fig. 22.20 Crusted lesions in a dentate patient with staphylococcal angular cheilitis.

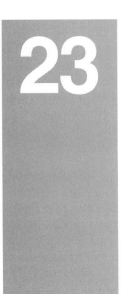

23 Immunodeficiency

Introduction

Immunodeficiency disorders may be classified as either primary or secondary. In general, all are characterized by an increased susceptibility to infections. Primary immunodeficiencies are uncommon, genetically determined, severe disorders often resulting in death at an early stage. They are classified according to the limb of the immune system which is principally affected, although some primarily affect more than one limb (Table 23.1). Clearly the different limbs of the immune system do not function autonomously, and defects primarily affecting one part of the immune system frequently have effects on other parts of the immune system.

Primary immunodeficiencies may present with ulcers, periodontal disease and recurrent herpes. In contrast to the other primary immunodeficiency states, selective IgA deficiency is a relatively common problem. This disorder is characterized by IgA deficiency in both serum and exocrine secretions, including saliva, while other immunoglobulin classes are either normal or elevated.

Secondary immunodeficiencies are acquired, and may develop secondary to a wide variety of underlying causes, and again principally affect one limb of the immune system. Examples of causes of secondary immunodeficiency states are shown in Table 23.2, but HIV infection is one of the more important.

Table 23.1 Primary immunodeficiencies	
Predominantly B cell defects	X-linked infantile hypogammaglobulinaemia (Bruton's syndrome) Common variable immunodeficiency
Predominantly T cell defects	Congenital thymic aplasia (Di George syndrome)
Combined B and T cell defects	Severe combined immunodeficiency Ataxia telangiectasia Immunodeficiency with thrombocytopenia and eczema (Wiskott–Aldrich's syndrome)
Selective immunodeficiencies	Selective IgA deficiency Complement component deficiencies

Table 23.2 Secondary immunodeficiencies

Malignancy	Hodgkin's disease
	Acute leukaemia
Infection	HIV-related disease
	Tuberculosis
Deficiency states	Malnutrition
	Iron deficiency
Autoimmune disease	Systemic lupus erythematosus
	Rheumatoid arthritis
Miscellaneous	Diabetes mellitus
	Neutropenia
	Chronic renal failure

HIV disease

A general consideration of HIV infection can be found in Chapter 5.

Oral lesions associated with HIV infection

Oral lesions have been an important component of the spectrum of disease seen in HIV infection since the early days of the HIV pandemic. Indeed, many of the patients who originally presented with what is now recognized as AIDS (acquired immunodeficiency syndrome) presented with evidence of oral disease, in particular oral candidosis. At present there are almost 40 different lesions reported in association with HIV infection. A preliminary classification divided these lesions into six broad categories largely based on aetiology. Thus the following categories were recognized: fungal, bacterial and viral infections, neoplasia, neurological conditions and lesions of unknown aetiology. However, this was a rather inflexible classification, and as our knowledge increased it was realized that some conditions which were in the original classification were not truly lesions associated with HIV infection and that the patients' HIV status was purely coincidental. The current classification divides lesions into three broad categories based on the strength of the association with HIV infection. Thus, three categories are now recognized:

Group I   Lesions strongly associated with HIV infection
Group II   Lesions less commonly associated with HIV infection

Group III   Lesions seen in HIV infection

This classification is much more dynamic, and as our knowledge continues to increase it is likely that some lesions will disappear from the classification. Equally, it is likely that other novel lesions will be added to the classification (Table 23.3).

Oral candidosis

Two types are commonly encountered among HIV-seropositive patients – pseudomembranous and erythematous. Candidosis is one of the commonest oral manifestations of HIV infection, and may affect over 90% of patients at some stage during their illness. Pseudomembranous candidosis typically presents as soft, white or yellow curd-like plaques on the oral mucosa which can be removed by gentle scraping to reveal an erythematous or punctate bleeding mucosal surface. The plaques comprise desquamated epithelial cells, necrotic material, yeast cells, hyphae and inflammatory cells. The lesions may be relatively inconspicuous, affecting small areas of the oral mucosa or there may be extensive mucosal involvement (Fig. 23.1). Previously classified as an acute infection, pseudomembranous candidosis may persist in HIV-infected patients for prolonged periods. The diagnosis is essentially clinical, although demonstration of *Candida* hyphae within the plaques provides support for the diagnosis.

In contrast, erythematous candidosis is a more subtle lesion, presenting as red lesions, most commonly affecting the dorsal surface of the tongue and the palate (see Fig. 22.15). Occasionally the buccal mucosa can be affected. The lesions on the dorsal surface of the tongue present as areas of depapillation. Once again the diagnosis is largely based on clinical appearance, although demonstration of *Candida* or a response to antifungal therapy provides support for the diagnosis.

Lesions of pseudomembranous and erythematous candidosis may coexist in the same patient. Both pseudomembranous and erythematous

Candidosis is one of the commonest presenting features of HIV infection

Table 23.3 Oral lesions in HIV infection

Group I – lesions strongly associated with HIV infection
Candidosis
    Erythematous
    Pseudomembranous
Hairy leukoplakia
Periodontal disease
Linear gingival erythema
Necrotizing (ulcerative) gingivitis
Necrotizing (ulcerative) periodontitis
Kaposi's sarcoma
Non-Hodgkin's lymphoma

Group II – lesions less commonly associated with HIV infection
Ulceration not otherwise specified
Necrotizing (ulcerative) periodontitis
Salivary gland disease
    Xerostomia
    Unilateral or bilateral salivary gland swelling
Thrombocytopenic purpura
Viral infections
    Herpes simplex virus
    Human papillomavirus
        Condyloma accuminatum
        Focal epithelial hyperplasia
        Verruca vulgaris
    Varicella – zoster virus
        Herpes zoster
        Varicella
Melanotic hyperpigmentation
Bacterial infections
    Mycobacterium avium-intracellulare
    Mycobacterium tuberculosis

Group III – lesions seen in HIV infection
Bacterial infections
    Actinomyces israelii
    Escherichia coli
    Klebsiella pneumoniae
Epithelioid (bacillary) angiomatosis
Cat scratch disease

Group III – lesions seen in HIV infection
Drug reactions
    Ulcerative
    Erythema multiforme
    Lichenoid
    Toxic epidermolysis
Fungal infections
    Cryptococcus neoformans
    Geotrichum candidum
    Histoplasma capsulatum
    Mucoraceae (mucormycosis/zygomycosis)
    Aspergillus flavus
Neurologic disturbances
    Facial palsy
    Trigeminal neuralgia
Recurrent aphthous stomatitis
Viral infections
Cytomegalovirus
Molluscum contagiosum

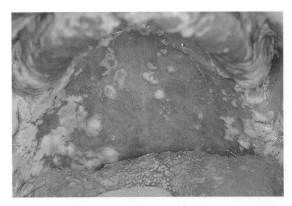

Fig. 23.1 Pseudomembranous candidosis in an HIV-positive patient.

candidosis are markers of poor prognosis in HIV-infected patients. Although pseudomembranous and especially erythematous candidosis are highly suggestive of HIV disease, it must be remembered that other causes of immunosuppression can also lead to these infections, for example diabetes mellitus or corticosteroid therapy (see Ch. 26).

Hairy leukoplakia

Hairy leukoplakia was originally described among male homosexuals who were subsequently shown to be HIV-seropositive. For several years the lesion was considered to be pathognomonic of HIV infection, although it has now been reported in patients who are immunosuppressed for other reasons. Thus, hairy leukoplakia is simply a manifestation of immunosuppression, and can be seen in patients who are immunosuppressed following solid organ transplantation, patients on cytotoxic therapy for acute leukaemia and also in patients receiving corticosteroid therapy. Typically, hairy leukoplakia is characterized by bilateral, vertically corrugated white patch lesions on the lateral border of the tongue (Fig. 23.2), although the clinical appearances are variable. It may affect the ventral surface of the tongue, where it assumes a more confluent appearance with loss of the corrugated ridges. Less commonly it may also affect the entire dorsal surface or other sites, although when it is present at these unusual sites it usually co-exists on the lateral margin of the tongue. The histological features of hairy leukoplakia include

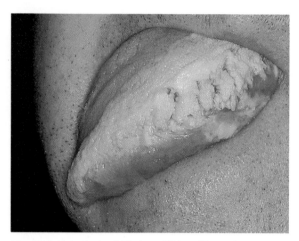

Fig. 23.2 Hairy leukoplakia in an HIV-positive patient.

an irregular surface layer of parakeratin, acanthosis and koilocyte-like (vacuolated) cells in the prickle cell layers. In approximately two-thirds of cases, candidal hyphae are present in the surface layer, although there is a striking lack of an associated chronic inflammatory cell infiltrate in the lamina propria. The vacuolated cells are sites of Epstein–Barr virus replication, which is now regarded as the causative agent of this unusual condition. Definitive diagnosis of hairy leukoplakia is by demonstration of Epstein–Barr virus within the lesion, and this can be accomplished by a variety of techniques including in situ hybridization or the polymerase chain reaction.

Hairy leukoplakia is usually an asymptomatic lesion; occasionally patients may report some discomfort or are concerned about the unsightly appearance of the lesion. Superinfection with *Candida* may give rise to some discomfort, and empirical treatment with an antifungal agent may relieve the patient's symptoms. As hairy leukoplakia is caused by Epstein–Barr virus replication within the epithelium, treatment with high-dose systemic aciclovir will cause some regression of the lesion, although when treatment is discontinued the lesion will inevitably recur. Other treatments which have been advocated include surgical excision, cryotherapy and topical application of podophyllin.

Like oral candidosis, hairy leukoplakia is a marker of poor prognosis among HIV-seropositive patients.

> Hairy leukoplakia is a marker of poor prognosis in HIV-seropositive patients

Kaposi's sarcoma (KS)

Prior to the advent of HIV infection, KS was known to occur in several different groups – elderly Jewish males of eastern European or Mediterranean descent, an endemic form in Africa and, less commonly, following renal transplantation. In the early years of the 1980s a dramatic increase in the incidence of this tumour was observed in some parts of the USA, and this led to the early recognition of HIV infection. KS is the commonest tumour associated with HIV infection. HIV-associated KS is a multifocal tumour which can affect any tissue system. Skin is the most commonly affected site, although approximately half will have oral involvement. Early KS lesions present as purple/violaceous macular lesions which are frequently asymptomatic. Later lesions may become raised and/or ulcerated, at which time they may become painful. Typical sites of involvement in the mouth include the palatal mucosa (Fig. 23.3), particularly overlying the greater palatine foramen, and the anterior maxillary gingivae. Rarely, KS may present as a non-pigmented lesion. KS occurs almost exclusively in those who have contracted HIV sexually, and is uncommon in those who have acquired HIV infection by other means. This led to the concept that KS was due to

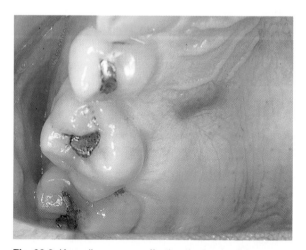

Fig. 23.3 Kaposi's sarcoma affecting the hard palate.

coinfection with another transmissible agent, and this has subsequently been characterized as human herpesvirus 8. Definitive diagnosis of KS is by histological examination. Treatment options for symptomatic lesions include local excision, cryotherapy, radiotherapy, or intralesional chemotherapy with vinblastine or vincristine. In patients with widespread lesions, systemic chemotherapy may be helpful.

> Kaposi's sarcoma is due to a coinfection with human herpesvirus 8

Non-Hodgkin's lymphoma (NHL)

As the survival of HIV-infected individuals continues to increase there has been an increase in the number of cases of NHL. NHL is characterized by a rapidly enlarging rubbery swelling which may subsequently ulcerate (Fig. 23.4). Sites of predilection within the oral cavity include the palate, tonsillar fossa and the gingivae. NHL occurs more commonly among male intravenous drug abusers. Despite aggressive therapy with cytotoxic agents, survival rates are poor.

Periodontal manifestations

A variety of periodontal lesions have been reported in association with HIV infection. At times the nomenclature has been rather confusing, although more recently this has been rationalized:

- linear gingival erythema
- necrotizing (ulcerative) gingivitis
- necrotizing (ulcerative) periodontitis
- necrotizing (ulcerative) stomatitis.

Linear gingival erythema is described as a well-demarcated band of intense erythema along the gingival margin (Fig. 23.5). The erythema is not associated with plaque accumulation and does not respond to conventional oral hygiene measures. Some have suggested that this may be associated with a *Candida* infection, although this remains unclear at present.

Necrotizing (ulcerative) gingivitis is characterized by painful ulceration of the interdental papillae, which may extend along the gingival margin (Fig. 23.6). Associated features include sialorrhoea, halitosis and spontaneous gingival bleeding. Patients may have generalized malaise, low-grade pyrexia and regional lymphadenopathy. Treatment requires intensive oral hygiene measures together with systemic metronidazole, although as the underlying immunosuppression persists it may subsequently recur.

Necrotizing (ulcerative) periodontitis is a distinct form of periodontal disease characterized by a painful, rapidly progressive loss of attachment and alveolar bone (Fig. 23.7). Occasionally this process

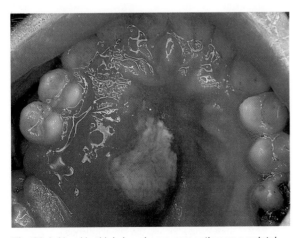

Fig. 23.4 Non-Hogkin's lymphoma presenting as a palatal swelling.

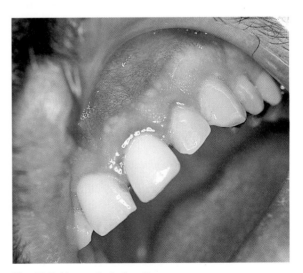

Fig. 23.5 Linear gingival erythema.

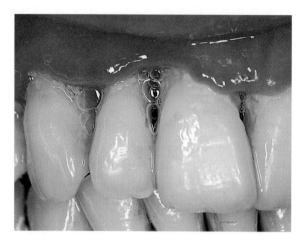

Fig. 23.6 Ulcerative (necrotizing) gingivitis.

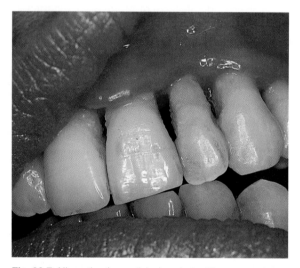

Fig. 23.7 Ulcerative (necrotizing) periodontitis.

may spread into the contiguous tissues, leading to extensive necrosis of soft tissue with exposure and sequestration of dead bone fragments – so-called necrotizing (ulcerative) stomatitis.

HIV-associated salivary gland disease (HIV-SGD)

HIV-SGD is characterized by swelling of one or more of the major salivary glands and/or xerostomia. The condition has some parallels with Sjögren's syndrome, as the patients complain of salivary gland swelling and xerostomia; some also report xerophthalmia. Moreover, the histological features are similar. HIV-SGD occurs more frequently in HIV-infected children compared to adult populations, and in children it is a marker of a good prognosis.

Other oral lesions

Other oral lesions seen in HIV disease include infections such as herpes simplex and herpes zoster infections. These may be much more severe than in immunocompetent individuals.

Human papillomavirus infections can cause extensive wart or condyloma formation which requires treatment with either conventional surgery or cryosurgery (Fig. 23.8).

Oral ulceration may be severe and intransigent in HIV disease. The ulcers often appear non-specific, and may be due to a variety of causes such as cytomegalovirus infection or syphilis, or may mimic aphthae.

Treatment then is often empirical, and as a last resort thalidomide is beneficial.

Squamous cell carcinoma

An increased number of oral carcinomas are seen nowadays in HIV-infected patients, and this almost certainly should be added to the list of oral manifestations. These carcinomas arise de novo and not in pre-existing hairy leukoplakias.

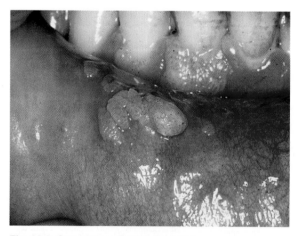

Fig. 23.8 Condyloma affecting the labial mucosa.

24 Salivary gland disorders

Introduction

A number of disease processes involve the salivary glands, and these may present as swellings, too little saliva (xerostomia), too much saliva (sialorrhoea or ptyalism) or other conditions such as necrotizing sialometaplasia or salivary fistulae. These will be discussed in turn.

Salivary gland investigation is of key importance in the proper diagnosis of salivary gland disease, and so the types of investigations available are discussed first.

Salivary gland investigations

Salivary flow rates (sialometry)

Measurement of salivary flow rates is a relatively simple, non-invasive technique, and may assess either resting or stimulated flow. Flow rates may either measure total production of mixed saliva by simply spitting into a container over a fixed time interval or alternatively, the flow rates of the major glands can be assessed independently. Most commonly the latter technique is applied to measurement of the parotid gland flow rate by placing a modified Carlsson–Crittenden cup over the parotid gland duct orifice (Fig. 24.1). Submandibular flow rates can also be measured

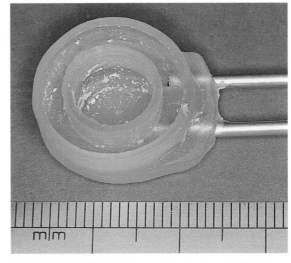

Fig. 24.1 A modified Carlsson–Crittenden cup. Suction is applied to the outer ring, holding it in place with the inner chamber over the parotid orifice.

using a similar principle, although this generally requires either cannulation of the duct or construction of a custom-made appliance which fits over the orifices of the ducts, and is rarely done.

Measurement of flow rates assesses the functional capacity of the salivary glands. The major drawback of this particular investigation is that the results are non-specific, and there is considerable variation in reference ranges which are quoted in the literature. In addition it is important to standardize the stimulus. It may have a role in assessing individual patients on a longitudinal basis, although due to significant diurnal variation it is important that the investigation is undertaken at the same time of day. Overall its main use lies within research applications.

Sialochemistry

Analysis of the constituents of saliva has been applied to a variety of conditions, including Sjögren's syndrome. Several abnormalities have been reported, but they are not consistent, and this may reflect the variation in concentration which occurs with flow rates as well as diurnal variations. Accordingly, this particular investigation is not used. Saliva can be used as a medium for measuring drug, antibody and hormone levels in situations where frequent sampling is required, or in young children to avoid venepuncture.

Plain radiography

Plain films can be helpful in demonstrating calculi in the major salivary gland ducts or glands (Fig. 24.2). However, a proportion of calculi are radiolucent, and these can only be demonstrated by sialography.

Sialography

This investigation demonstrates the structural pattern of the salivary gland duct system, principally the parotid or submandibular glands. The technique involves infusion of a radiopaque contrast medium into the main duct. The main duct is cannulated, and the contrast medium is introduced at a fixed rate while continuously monitoring the pressure within the system. This technique prevents excessive filling pressures developing which may promote gland damage. Appropriate radiographic views are then taken; usually two views in different planes.

Sialography demonstrates structural abnormalities of the duct system, including mucus plugs, calculi, areas of stricture or duct dilatation, and chronic inflammatory conditions (Fig. 24.3). The use of sialography to demonstrate salivary gland neoplasms has been superseded by more sensitive techniques such as computerized tomography

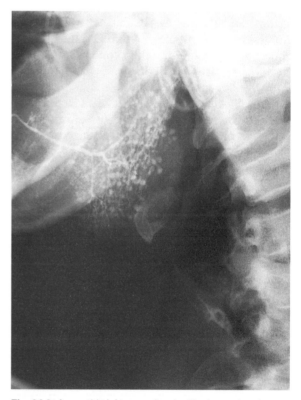

Fig. 24.3 A parotid sialogram showing the 'snowstorm' appearance of punctate sialectasis in a patient with Sjögren's syndrome.

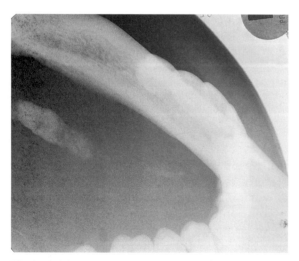

Fig. 24.2 A lower occlusal radiograph showing a sialolith in the submandibular duct.

(CT) scanning and magnetic resonance imaging.

Sialography is contraindicated in the presence of acute infection and if there is a history of allergy to iodine, as this is the principal constituent of the contrast medium.

Scintiscanning

The basis of this investigation is that several tissues have the functional capacity to concentrate a suitable radioisotope after it is administered intravenously. The salivary glands, along with the thyroid, concentrate iodine, although technetium-99m is used in preference because of its shorter half-life and lower radiation dose to the tissues (Fig. 24.4). Following an intravenous injection of the radioisotope, the salivary glands are scanned at regular intervals with a gamma camera, which plots the rate of concentration of the radioisotope into the glands. Thereafter the secretory capacity of the glands can be measured by orally administering a stimulant such as citric acid. The main uses of this investigation are as follows:

- to determine impaired function of one particular major gland by comparison with the others, as occurs in chronic infection, or
- to observe a generalized decrease in function in all major glands, as may occur in Sjögren's syndrome.

Salivary gland biopsy

Biopsy of a parotid gland has hazards of damage to the facial nerve, the production of a salivary fistula, and facial scarring. For these reasons, biopsy of minor salivary glands is usually chosen. The glands selected are the labial glands in the lower labial mucosa since they are easily biopsied through a simple incision inside the mouth (Fig. 24.5).

It has been shown that changes in the major salivary glands are also reflected into minor glands in Sjögren's syndrome. Thus, a focal lymphocytic sialadenitis in a minor gland biopsy is suggestive of Sjögren's syndrome affecting the major glands (see later).

Salivary gland swellings

Salivary gland swelling, which may be painful, especially if the swelling is acute, may be due to several disease processes (Table 24.1).

Bacterial infections

Bacterial sialadenitis

Historically, acute suppurative infections of the salivary glands were quite common among hospital patients, particularly following surgery to the

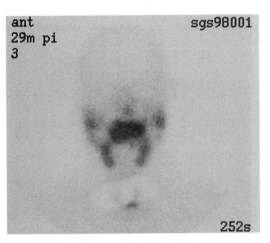

Fig. 24.4 A technetium scan showing uptake by the major salivary glands.

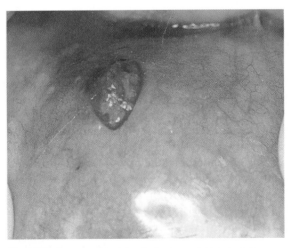

Fig. 24.5 A mucosal incision in the lower labial mucosa showing the minor salivary glands protruding through the wound.

Table 24.1 Causes of salivary gland swelling

Bacterial infection
    Ascending sialadenitis
    Recurrent parotitis of childhood
Duct obstruction
    Major gland
    Minor gland
Systemic infections
    Mumps
    HIV parotitis
Sjögren's syndrome
Sarcoidosis
Sialosis
Drugs
Neoplasms

gastrointestinal tract due to dehydration. Improved perioperative care, greater attention to fluid balance and an increasing use of prophylactic antibiotics has led to a dramatic reduction in the incidence of bacterial sialadenitis among surgical patients. Bacterial infections of the salivary glands are now most commonly secondary to a structural abnormality within the duct system such as calculi, mucus plugs or duct strictures. The reduced flow which arises as a result of these abnormalities allows ascending infection from commensals within the oral cavity. The organisms most commonly isolated include *Staphylococcus aureus* and *Streptococcus viridans*.

Suppurative infections of the major salivary glands most commonly affect the parotid glands, and present as painful swelling of the affected gland. The gland is tender to palpation, and there may be associated cervical lymphadenopathy. On intraoral examination, pus may be seen exuding from the duct orifice.

An uncontaminated sample of pus should be obtained by aspiration from the duct and submitted for culture and antibiotic sensitivity. This type of sample is preferable to a swab, which will inevitably be contaminated by the oral flora. Prompt antimicrobial therapy should be instituted with flucloxacillin, or erythromycin if the patient has a history of penicillin allergy.

> Flucloxacillin is the drug of choice for suppurative infections of the major glands

As mentioned earlier, suppurative infections of the salivary glands are commonly secondary to a structural abnormality. Clearly, if a calculus is present this should be removed at an early stage to encourage free drainage of pus. Once the acute phase has settled, sialography should be performed to identify any predisposing structural abnormality.

Of course, acute infection and inflammation in itself causes structural damage due to scarring. Sialography may itself produce some improvement in flow due to the mechanical flushing of the gland. To prevent further episodes of infection in a structurally damaged gland however, patients should be encouraged to take a salivary stimulant in the morning such as lemon juice or orange juice, and to 'milk' the gland by massaging it with their fingers.

Occasionally a gland becomes so badly damaged that excision of the gland should be considered. This is uncomplicated in the case of the submandibular gland but problematic in the case of the parotid gland, which is difficult to remove without damaging the facial nerve, especially when the gland is damaged and fibrosed. Simply tying off the parotid duct is not usually successful, and causes much pain and swelling. Usually the decision in these cases is to persist with aggressive antimicrobial therapy and stimulating the affected gland as described above.

Recurrent parotitis of childhood

This is an uncommon condition characterized by repeated episodes of bacterial sialadenitis. The predisposing factors are unknown. Sialography demonstrates the characteristic features of sialectasis. The patient should be encouraged to stimulate the gland to prevent recurrences, as suggested in the previous section, but may still require repeated courses of antibiotics when recurrences occur. The condition normally resolves at puberty or in early adult life.

Duct obstruction

Major gland duct obstruction

Salivary duct obstruction is usually by a calculus in the submandibular duct. Strictures, mucus plugs or neoplasms are occasional causes. Rarely, patients present with 'physiological' duct obstruction due either to duct spasm or an abnormal passage of the parotid duct through the buccinator or in relation to the masseter muscles (the so-called buccinator window syndrome).

A history of painful salivary gland swelling just before or at mealtimes is a classical feature of obstruction, but, in older patients, this history is not always obtained. There may be dull pain over the affected gland, referred elsewhere.

> 20–40% of salivary calculi are radiolucent

Salivary calculi affect the submandibular gland more commonly than the parotid, with over 75% of calculi occurring in the submandibular gland and duct. Less commonly, calculi may form in the sublingual gland or ducts of minor glands. Calculi may be present without any symptoms. However, obstruction to the outflow of secretion is accompanied by swelling of the affected gland and pain. These symptoms are more severe at meal times, when secretion is stimulated. Clinically the calculus may be evident on palpation in the floor of the mouth; multiple calculi involving one gland are not uncommon. Calculi which develop within the duct tend to be smooth and elongated, conforming to the shape of the duct lumen. In contrast, calculi forming within the gland itself tend to be more irregularly shaped. Plain radiographs may demonstrate radiopaque calculi (see Fig. 24.2). Approximately 20% of calculi affecting the submandibular gland are radiolucent, whereas 40% of those in the parotid are radiolucent. Sialography should help differentiate the various causes of major duct obstruction. Extraductal causes of obstruction may be clinically obvious or evident only on sialography or CT combined with sialography.

Salivary calculi are frequently asymptomatic and a chance finding on routine examination. However, on occasion, obstruction may be complicated by an acute suppurative process with accompanying systemic features such as pyrexia and malaise.

Treatment during the acute phase includes general supportive measures such as antibiotic therapy, analgesics and antipyretics.

Obstructions are overcome by removal of the obstruction (such as a calculus), or duct dilatation. To remove a stone, the duct should be ligated temporarily between the stone and the gland to prevent the calculus being pushed distally. The duct is then incised longitudinally, and the stone removed. The wound can be left open.

The term 'ranula' is applied to a swelling in the floor of the mouth which often arises from a mucous extravasation cyst involving the sublingual gland. Clinically the swelling resembles a frog's belly (Fig. 24.6).

Minor gland duct obstruction

The term 'mucocele' describes a 'cystic' lesion arising in connection with minor salivary gland tissue. Two main types are recognized – extravasation mucoceles accounting for approximately 90% of cases, and the far less common retention mucoceles. This distinction is based on histological examination: a retention cyst is lined by salivary duct epithelium whereas an extravasation mucocele is lined by macrophages which wall off the irritant mucus from the surrounding submucosa.

The most common site for an extravasation mucocele is the lower lip, although the buccal mucosa and floor of mouth are less frequent sites. Most occur in young patients. Clinically the lesion presents as a discrete, painless, translucent

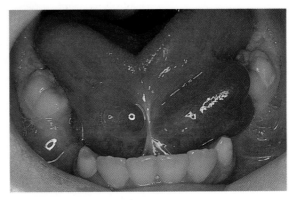

Fig. 24.6 A ranula.

submucosal swelling, and there may be a history of trauma to the area (Fig. 24.7).

Retention mucoceles affect an older age group, typically over 50 years of age, and almost never affect the lower lip. The treatment of mucoceles is surgical excision with the affected underlying minor gland. As an alternative to surgical excision, some advocate cryosurgery.

Systemic infections

Mumps (acute viral sialadenitis)

This is an acute, infectious illness caused by a paramyxovirus that primarily affects the salivary glands, most commonly the parotid glands. The virus has an incubation period of 2–3 weeks, and is transmitted by direct contact or droplet spread. The onset is usually acute, and characterized by bilateral swelling of the parotid glands although unilateral involvement may be present in the early stages. Submandibular glands may also be affected. The salivary gland swelling is frequently painful, and associated features may include trismus, headache, malaise and fever. The swelling is maximal within a couple of days, and resolves within a further 7 days. Many cases may be subclinical and pass unrecognized. The testes and ovaries may also be affected, particularly in adults, although sterility is rare. The virus less commonly affects the pancreas, liver, kidney and the nervous system.

The diagnosis is primarily based on the clinical features, although it can be confirmed by demonstrating a fourfold rise in antibody titres between acute and convalescent serum. Specific antiviral agents are not available, and therefore treatment is symptomatic, involving bed rest, antipyretic agents, adequate hydration and simple analgesics. As the virus is shed in saliva during the acute stage of the illness, isolation may be appropriate. Vaccination is now available and performed in childhood (see Ch. 5).

Several other viruses can rarely cause parotitis, including Coxsackie viruses, echovirus, parainfluenza viruses and HIV.

HIV parotitis

Occasionally, patients with HIV disease develop salivary gland swelling. This is discussed in Chapter 23.

Sjögren's syndrome

This is a common cause of chronic bilateral parotid swelling, and is discussed fully under the section on xerostomia.

Sarcoidosis

This rare cause of salivary gland swelling is diagnosed only on biopsy. The other features of sarcoidosis are discussed in Chapters 8 and 26.

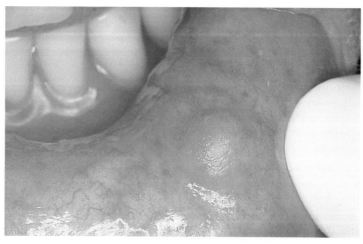

Fig. 24.7 A mucocele affecting the lower lip.

Sialosis

This condition is a benign, non-inflammatory, non-neoplastic, usually bilaterally symmetrical, painless enlargement of the salivary glands. The aetiology is unknown, but a variety of associated precipitating factors are recognized, as shown in Table 24.2. A common factor is autonomic neuropathy.

The clinical picture is characterized by soft painless enlargement of the involved glands, most commonly the parotids (Fig. 24.8). The diagnosis is essentially one of exclusion based on the history and clinical features. Investigation should routinely exclude predisposing causes such as diabetes and excess alcohol consumption. Clearly if there are other features to suggest a diagnosis of acromegaly, then appropriate investigations should be undertaken.

Drugs

As alluded to in the previous section, some drugs such as phenylbutazone may produce sialosis and salivary gland swelling.

Salivary gland neoplasms

Salivary gland neoplasms usually present as swellings. They are relatively uncommon, and account for only 3% of all tumours. Tumours affecting the major glands are more common than those of the minor glands, and account for 80–85% of cases. Of the tumours occurring in the major glands, approximately 90% arise in the parotid and about 10% in the submandibular. Tumours arising in the sublingual gland are rare (Table 24.3). The distribution of tumours in the minor glands is shown in Table 24.4.

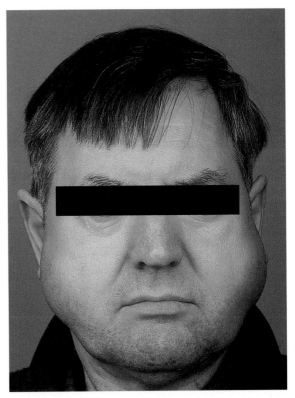

Fig. 24.8 Sialosis occurring in an alcoholic.

Table 24.3 Major salivary gland tumours

Tumour location	Occurrence (%)
Parotid	90
Submandibular	10
Sublingular	Rare

Table 24.4 Minor salivary gland tumours

Tumour location	Occurrence (%)
Palate	60
Upper lip	20
Other sites	20

Table 24.2 Factors associated with sialosis

Cirrhosis
Alcohol abuse
Diabetes mellitus
Acromegaly
Anorexia nervosa
Bulimia
Cystic fibrosis
Drugs (phenylbutazone, iodine)

While only a minority of tumours arise in the minor glands, the proportion of malignant tumours is considerably higher than in the major glands. Tumours arising in the sublingual gland are almost invariably malignant.

A large number of different tumour types are now recognized and have been classified by the

World Health Organization. The more important types are listed in Table 24.5.

Salivary gland tumours present as swelling of the affected area. In general, a prolonged history of painless swelling suggests a benign process, while rapid enlargement, pain or facial nerve involvement is more indicative of malignancy. The treatment of choice is surgical excision, as salivary gland tumours are relatively resistant to radiotherapy.

The more important salivary gland tumours will now be considered in turn.

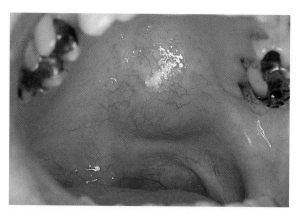

Fig. 24.9 A pleomorphic salivary adenoma arising in a palatal minor salivary gland.

Pleomorphic adenoma

This is the commonest salivary gland neoplasm, and most arise in the parotid gland. Most arise during the fourth to sixth decades, although they may occur at any age. They present as a slow-growing, painless, rubbery nodule often in the lower pole of the parotid. Intraorally, the commonest sites affected are the palate (Fig. 24.9) and upper lip. In the palate they may give the appearance of fixation to underlying bone, although there is no actual invasion. Histologically the tumours are poorly encapsulated, and therefore treatment is by excision with a margin of surrounding normal tissue. Fortunately, most affecting the parotid gland are superficial, and a superficial parotidectomy without disturbing the facial nerve is curative.

> Pleomorphic adenomas are the commonest salivary gland neoplasms

Table 24.5 Salivary gland tumours

Pleomorphic adenoma
Warthin tumour (adenolymphoma)
Oxyphilic adenoma (oncocytoma)
Other adenomas characterized and classified according to cell type and pattern
Ductal papilloma

Mucoepidermoid carcinoma
Acinic cell carcinoma
Adenoid cystic carcinoma
Carcinoma arising in pleomorphic adenoma
Polymorphous low-grade adenocarcinoma

Warthin tumour

This is the commonest monomorphic adenoma, and occurs almost invariably in the parotid gland. The tumour occurs with a male preponderance, and most commonly between 55 and 65 years. It presents as a painless, slow-growing mass, and may be bilateral or multifocal in the same gland in up to 10% of cases. The swelling is frequently soft or cystic in consistency, and there may be some fluctuation in size. Treatment is by simple excision.

Oncocytoma

This is an uncommon tumour which predominantly occurs among elderly females and most commonly presents in the parotid. Treatment is by excision.

Carcinoma ex pleomorphic adenoma

Malignant change in a pleomorphic adenoma is relatively uncommon, and appears to occur only if the tumour has been allowed to grow over a long period. Clinical features which may signify malignant change include rapid change in size of a previously slow-growing lesion, pain, fixation to skin or underlying structures, and facial nerve palsy. Treatment involves radical excision, but the prognosis is poor, with only a 50% 5 year survival.

Mucoepidermoid carcinoma

Most arise in the parotid gland, although the relative incidence in the minor glands, principally the palate, is higher. Frequently the tumour presents in a similar manner to that of a pleomorphic adenoma, although some may be associated with pain and ulceration. Various different histological patterns are recognized, although the behaviour cannot be predicted with any degree of certainty. Overall 5 year survival is approximately 70%.

Acinic cell carcinoma

This is an uncommon tumour, mostly arising in the parotid gland. Peak incidence is in the fifth and sixth decades with a female preponderance. Several histological patterns have been reported, but again it is difficult to predict the clinical behaviour.

Adenoid cystic carcinoma

This tumour type occurs principally in middle-aged or elderly patients. It predominantly affects the minor salivary glands of the palate. Clinically it presents as a slow-growing mass similar to a pleomorphic adenoma, although pain and ulceration are more common. Perineural invasion and spread is a characteristic feature. Distant metastases to lung, bone and brain occur, although this tends to be a late feature.

Xerostomia

This is the commonest symptom relating to the salivary glands. Some patients complain of a dry mouth, although in many cases there is no objective evidence to support this symptom, and the underlying problem in such cases may be related to psychological disease. Xerostomia has a wide range of possible causes (Table 24.6), although drugs are the most commonly implicated.

Developmental causes

The congenital absence of major salivary glands is a rare occurrence. Any of the major glands may be absent either unilaterally or bilaterally, and the situation gives rise to xerostomia.

Table 24.6 Causes of dry mouth

Developmental	Aplasia or agenesis
Iatrogenic	Drugs Irradiation
Salivary gland disease	Sjögren's syndrome Sarcoidosis HIV salivary gland disease
Dehydration	Diabetes mellitus Renal failure Haemorrhage Diabetes insipidus
Psychogenic	

Iatrogenic causes

Drug-induced xerostomia

Drugs which commonly cause a dry mouth are those with anticholinergic or sympathomimetic activity. A wide range of drugs can give rise to this problem, and the common classes of drugs involved are shown in Table 24.7.

Xerostomia as a complication of irradiation

The major salivary glands are often included in the fields of radiotherapy to malignant tumours of the head and neck, and not surprisingly xerostomia is a common complication. This is particularly true of tumours of the oropharynx and nasopharynx. There is a direct correlation between the total radiation dose and the degree of damage. Salivary flow is reduced within a week of radiotherapy, and the saliva has increased viscosity. If the degree of damage is not severe, some function may return after several months. Unfortunately, the effects are often irreversible due to severe damage and fibrous replacement of acinar tissue.

Table 24.7 Drugs causing xerostomia

Tricyclic antidepressants
Monoamine oxidase inhibitors
Antihistamines
Diuretics
Antipsychotics
Antiparkinsonian agents

Salivary gland disease

As discussed previously, sarcoidosis and HIV disease may not only cause salivary gland enlargement but may also produce xerostomia. By far the commonest and most important salivary gland disease causing xerostomia is Sjögren's syndrome.

Sjögren's syndrome

Sjögren's syndrome is a chronic multisystem autoimmune inflammatory disorder of unknown aetiology characterized by lymphocytic infiltration and destruction of acinar tissue in the exocrine glands, most importantly the salivary and lacrimal glands. Middle-aged and elderly females are predominantly affected with a female:male ratio of approximately 9:1. It is classified into two types: primary Sjögren's syndrome (SS-1), comprising dry eyes and a dry mouth, and, more commonly, secondary. Sjögren's syndrome (SS-2), comprises a triad of dry eyes, dry mouth and a connective tissue or autoimmune disorder. Rheumatoid arthritis is the commonest connective tissue disorder seen in secondary Sjögren's syndrome, although others such as primary biliary cirrhosis, systemic lupus erythematosus, progressive systemic sclerosis and mixed connective tissue disease may occur as part of the triad.

As well as affecting the salivary and lacrimal glands, Sjögren's syndrome may also involve other exocrine glands, thereby giving rise to a variety of problems such as nasal dryness, tracheitis, pancreatitis and vaginal dryness. In addition, a wide range of extraglandular manifestations may be observed as part of the syndrome, as shown in Table 24.8.

The oral symptoms of Sjögren's syndrome are primarily a consequence of xerostomia, and include:

- xerostomia
- difficulty eating and swallowing dry foods
- oral discomfort
- difficulty controlling dentures
- taste disturbances
- swelling affecting the major salivary glands.

Clinically the mucosa may appear dry (Fig. 24.10) with an absence of the normal pooling of saliva in

Table 24.8 Extraglandular manifestations of Sjögren's syndrome

Joints	Arthritis
Cutaneous	Purpura
	Raynaud's phenomenon
Neurological	Central and peripheral neuropathies
Haematological	Anaemia, leucopenia, thrombocytopenia
Immunological	Autoantibodies
	Hypergammaglobulinaemia
Endocrine	Thyroiditis
Drug allergies	

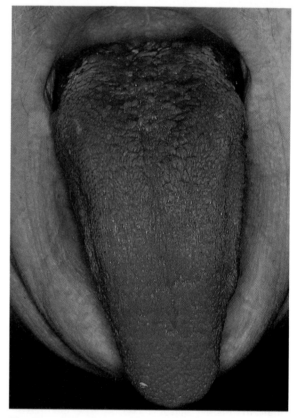

Fig. 24.10 The dorsal surface of the tongue in a patient with xerostomia due to Sjögren's syndrome.

the floor of the mouth. In more severe cases the dorsal surface of the tongue may appear erythematous, with a characteristic lobulated and fissured appearance, as well as varying degrees of depapillation (Fig. 24.11).

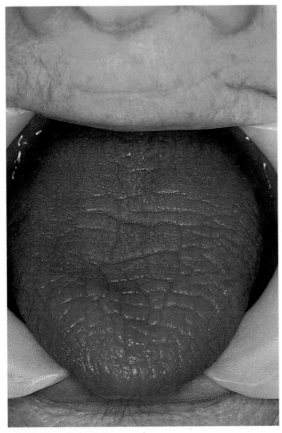

Fig. 24.11 Lobulation of the lingual mucosa in a patient with long-standing xerostomia.

Lymphomas are more common in primary Sjögren's syndrome

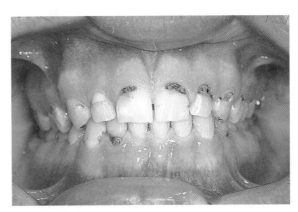

Fig. 24.12 Extensive smooth surface caries in a patient with xerostomia.

Common complications of Sjögren's syndrome relate primarily to the lack of saliva, and include dental caries, often severe and involving sites not usually susceptible to decay (Fig. 24.12), candidosis and bacterial sialadenitis. Variable, painless swelling affecting the major salivary glands, usually the parotid glands, is a common finding, and in some cases this may be very severe, with associated swelling of the regional lymph nodes. Patients with Sjögren's syndrome are at an increased risk of developing a B cell malignant lymphoma. Lymphoma appears to be more common among patients with primary Sjögren's syndrome. Lymphoma typically presents late in the disease process and frequently manifests as rapid persistent enlargement of one of the major salivary glands.

There is no single investigation which will confirm or exclude a diagnosis of Sjögren's syndrome,

and the diagnosis is usually made by the presence of a combination of clinical features and results of laboratory investigations. This concept is enshrined in the European classification criteria for Sjögren's syndrome shown in Table 24.9.

The typical results obtained from salivary gland investigations in Sjögren's syndrome are shown in Table 24.10. A comparison of the features of primary and secondary Sjögren's syndrome are shown in Table 24.11.

Because of the problems which arise in patients with xerostomia, it is necessary to institute a number of measures to minimize the damage caused by a lack of saliva. These include:

- *Control of dental caries.* Daily use of fluoride rinses or gels and limitation of sucrose intake.
- *Control of periodontal disease.* Meticulous oral hygiene phase therapy and regular use of 0.2% chlorhexidine mouthwash.
- *Prevention of candidosis.* Dentures should be kept out at night and soaked in sodium hypochlorite solution or chlorhexidine. Some advocate the prophylactic use of topical antifungal agents on a regular basis, although evidence for the efficacy of this approach is lacking.
- *Bacterial sialadenitis.* Acute episodes should be treated with an appropriate antibiotic according to the bacterial sensitivity.

Table 24.9 European classification criteria for Sjögren's syndrome

I. **Ocular symptoms** – a positive response to at least one of the following three questions:
(i) Have you had daily, persistent, troublesome dry eyes for more than 3 months?
(ii) Do you have a recurrent sensation of sand or gravel in the eyes?
(iii) Do you use tear substitutes more than three times a day?

II. **Oral symptoms** – a positive response to at least one of the following three questions:
(i) Have you had a daily feeling of a dry mouth for more than 3 months?
(ii) Have you had recurrently or persistently swollen salivary glands as an adult?
(iii) Do you frequently drink liquids to aid in swallowing dry food?

III. **Ocular signs** – objective evidence of ocular involvement defined as a positive result in at least one of the following two tests:
(i) Schirmers' test ($\leq$ 5 mm in 5 min)
(ii) Rose Bengal score $\geq$ 4

IV. **Histopathology** – a focus score >1 on labial gland biopsy
A focus is defined as an agglomerate of at least 50 mononuclear cells; the focus score is defined by the number of foci in 4 mm^2 of glandular tissue

V. **Salivary gland involvement** – objective evidence of salivary gland involvement, defined as a positive result in at least one of the following investigations:
(i) Salivary scintigraphy
(ii) Parotid sialography
(iii) Unstimulated salivary flow ($\leq$ 1.5 ml in 15 min)

VI. **Autoantibodies** – the following autoantibodies present in serum:
Antibodies to Ro (SS-A) and/or La (SS-B) antigens

In patients without any potential associated connective tissue disorder the presence of any four of the above six items is indicative of primary Sjögren's syndrome

In patients with a connective tissue disorder, item I or item II together with any two other items from III, IV and V is indicative of secondary Sjögren's syndrome

Table 24.10 Salivary gland investigations in Sjögren's syndrome

Investigation	Result	Comment
Sialometry	Reduced flow	Non-specific
Scintiscanning	Reduced uptake of radioisotope	Non-specific; may occur as a consequence of chronic infection
Sialography	Sialectasis	Non-specific; may occur as a consequence of chronic infection
Labial gland biopsy	Focal lymphocytic infiltrate Acinar atrophy Periductal fibrosis Duct dilatation	Fairly specific if overlying mucosa normal

- *Salivary substitutes.* A variety of salivary substitutes are available based either on mucin or methylcellulose. Their effects are transient, and many patients derive equal benefit from frequent sips of water. The advantage of commercially available salivary substitutes is their convenience.
- *Salivary stimulants.* Salivation can be stimulated only in those with some remaining salivary function.

Table 24.11 Comparison of primary and secondary Sjögren's syndrome

Feature	Primary	Secondary
Connective tissue disorder	Absent	Present
Oral involvement	More severe	Less severe
Recurrent sialadenitis	More common	Less common
Ocular involvement	More severe	Less severe
Lymphoma	More common	Less common
Rheumatoid factor	50%	90%
Anti-Ro (SS-A)	5–10%	50–80%
Anti-La (SS-B)	54–73%	2–6%
Salivary duct antibody	10–36%	67–70%

Oral infections are more common in Sjögren's syndrome

Those with absolute xerostomia have no salivary function to stimulate. Salivation in those with some function can be stimulated by chewing sugar free gum or sucking diabetic sweets. Glycerine and lemon should be avoided in dentate patients due to the low pH, which may accelerate progression of caries. Even in edentulous patients, glycerine and lemon should be used sparingly as low pH also promotes the growth of *Candida* species. Drugs with cholinergic effects such as pilocarpine and pyridostigmine may also be used to stimulate salivary flow. The use of these drugs may be limited by other cholinergic side-effects, and they should be used with caution in patients with a history of hypertension, asthma or peptic ulceration.

Dehydration

Occasionally patients complain of a dry mouth due to dehydration. This may imply an underlying disease process such as diabetes or haemorrhage, or may be an inevitable consequence of a pre-existing disease state, e.g. renal failure.

Psychological causes

Xerostomia may be a perceived rather than a real problem, or may be a consequence of a chronic anxiety state with associated autonomic overactivity (see Ch. 13).

Chronic anxiety may cause xerostomia

Sialorrhoea

Excessive saliva or sialorrhoea is a much less common complaint than xerostomia. Sialorrhoea may be a feature of acute ulcerative conditions in the mouth such as primary herpetic gingivostomatitis or acute ulcerative gingivitis. In addition, many patients report excess saliva after wearing dentures for the first time. In some cases there is no actual increase in salivary flow, and the problem occurs as a result of impaired muscle coordination, pharyngeal obstruction or difficulty swallowing. In these cases the underlying condition is usually related to neuromuscular disorders such as cerebral palsy or Parkinson's disease. In many cases no organic cause can be identified, and the condition may reflect an underlying psychological problem (see Ch. 13). Clearly, if an underlying psychological cause is suspected then treatment should be aimed at managing this. In theory, anticholinergic agents should be helpful in controlling symptoms of excess saliva, but their other side-effects limit their actual value. For patients with drooling, a variety of surgical procedures have been developed which principally involve redirecting the submandibular gland ducts towards the oropharynx.

Other conditions

Necrotizing sialometaplasia

This is a relatively uncommon condition of unknown aetiology, although it may be due to ischaemia. Males are more commonly affected, and the lesion predominantly affects smokers. The condition usually affects the minor glands of the palate, and the presenting features are rapid onset of ulceration, often leading to the formation of a crater-like defect with induration of the margins (Fig. 24.13). Some patients report a history of altered sensation involving the affected area prior to the onset of the ulceration. Clinically the lesion may be mistaken for malignant disease, and even the histopathology can mimic carcinoma. The lesion resolves spontaneously after several weeks.

Salivary fistula

A salivary fistula is an abnormal communication between the salivary gland or ducts and skin or mucous membrane. Trauma to the major glands may (rarely) cause a persistent fistula. The treatment is surgical. Sialography of the fistula is helpful in surgical planning.

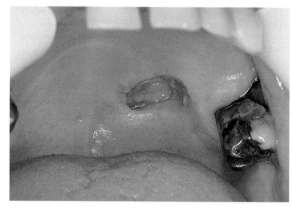

Fig. 24.13 A crater-like ulcer of the soft palate in a patient with necrotizing sialometaplasia.

Pain and neurological disorders

Introduction

Orofacial and dental pain are common problems in dental practice. Indeed, the majority of presenting symptoms are pain related, and many patients will only attend for clinical consultation with their dentist when in pain.

Odontological pain

Odontological pain may be pulpal or periodontal in origin, and the diagnosis and management of such 'toothache' is a core skill of the dental practitioner. Often the diagnosis of dental pain requires investigation to localize the origin of the pain despite the detailed history and clinical examination. Such investigation may involve vitality testing and radiography before embarking on the removal of 'suspect' restorations in the area of the pain. Even in the event of the painful stimulus being of dental origin, the clinical symptoms and signs may be altered and confused by patients' behaviour patterns in response to their symptoms. Such confounding problems include anxiety, fear, hypochondriasis and personality disorders.

The various types of odontological pain are shown in Table 25.1, and are now discussed in detail.

Table 25.1 Causes of odontological pain (alphabetically listed)

| Acute necrotizing gingivitis |
| Cracked tooth |
| Dentinal pain |
| Food impaction |
| Lateral periodontal abscess |
| Mucosal pain |
| Periapical periodontitis |
| Pericoronitis |
| Periodontal pain |
| Pulpal pain |

Acute necrotizing gingivitis

This causes soreness and pain localized at the gingival papillae and margin, usually accompanied by profuse gingival bleeding. In the early stages some patients may complain of a feeling of tightness around the teeth. A metallic taste is sometimes experienced, and usually there is halitosis. Fever and malaise are sometimes present. Examination shows necrosis and ulceration of the gingival papillae with different degrees of gingival marginal destruction.

Cracked tooth

Teeth can crack under trauma and can give rise to severe pain, which is worse on biting. The cause of pain if often difficult to ascertain.

Dentinal pain

This is sharp and deep, usually evoked by an external stimulus and subsides within seconds. Natural external stimuli are normally evoked by food and drinks which are hot, cold, sweet, sour and sometimes salty. Although extreme changes in temperature (e.g. hot soup followed by ice-cream) may cause pain in intact, non-affected teeth, pain evoked by natural stimuli usually indicates a hyperalgesic state of the tooth. The pain may be poorly localized, often only to an approximate area within two to three teeth adjacent to the affected tooth. Sometimes the patient is unable to distinguish whether the pain originates from the lower or the upper jaw. Pain from affected posterior teeth is more difficult to localize than that from anterior teeth. However, patients rarely make localization errors across the midline.

Food impaction

This causes localized pain that develops between or in two adjacent teeth after meals, especially when food is fibrous (e.g. meat). The pain is associated with a feeling of pressure and discomfort, may gradually disappear until being evoked again at the next meal, or may be relieved immediately by removing the impacted food. There is a faulty contact between two teeth, and often food trapped between them; the gingival papilla is tender to touch and bleeds easily. The adjacent teeth are usually sensitive to percussion.

Lateral periodontal abscess

This pain is similar to that of acute periapical periodontitis, well localized and with swelling and redness of the gingiva. However, the swelling is usually located more gingivally than in the case of the acute periapical lesion. The affected tooth is sensitive to percussion, and is often mobile and slightly extruded, and there is a deep periodontal pocket. Probing the pocket may cause pus exudation and subsequent relief from pain. The tooth pulp is usually vital.

Mucosal pain

This can be either localized or diffuse. Localized pain is usually associated with an erosion or ulcer.

Diffuse pain may be associated with a widespread infection, mucositis, mucosal atrophy or erosion, a systemic underlying deficiency disease or other factors, and is usually described as 'soreness' or, sometimes, 'burning'.

Mucosal pain may be aggravated mechanically or by sour, spicy, salty or hot foods.

Periapical periodontitis

This is spontaneous, and moderate to severe in intensity, lasting long periods of time (hours). Pain is exacerbated by biting on the tooth and, in more advanced cases, even by closing the mouth and bringing the affected tooth gently into contact with the opposing teeth. In these cases, the tooth feels 'high' (extruded) and is very sensitive to touch. Frequently there has been preceding pulpal pain. Periodontal pain, although of a more continuous nature, is usually better tolerated than the paroxysmal and excruciating pain of pulpitis; localization of periodontal pain is usually precise, and the patient able to indicate the affected tooth. The improved ability to localize the source of pain may be attributed to the proprioceptive and mechanoreceptive sensibility of the periodontium that is lacking in the pulp. However, although localization of the affected tooth is often precise, in up to half the cases the pain is diffuse and radiates into the jaw on the affected side.

During examination the affected tooth is located readily by means of tooth percussion. The tooth is usually non-vital, and the periapical buccal vestibular area often tender to palpation. In more severe cases there is swelling of the face, associated with cellulitis and, sometimes, malaise. Usually, when the face swells, pain diminishes in intensity due to rupture of the pus through the periosteum of the bone around the affected tooth and the consequent decrease in pressure at the tooth apex.

Pericoronitis

Acute pericoronal infections are common, related to incompletely erupted teeth partially covered by flaps of gingival tissue (operculum), particularly lower third molars. Pain is spontaneous, and may be exacerbated by closing the mouth. In more severe cases, pain is aggravated by swallowing, and there may be trismus.

Examination shows an operculum that is acutely inflamed, red and oedematous. Frequently, an opposing upper tooth indents or ulcerates the oedematous operculum, and the ipsilateral draining cervical lymph nodes may be swollen. Occasionally, fever and malaise are associated.

Periodontal pain

This is more readily localized than is pulpal pain; the affected teeth are often tender to pressure.

Pulpal pain

This is spontaneous, strong, often throbbing and is exacerbated by temperature change and pressure on a carious lesion. When pulpal pain is evoked it outlasts the stimulus (unlike stimulus-induced dentinal pain) and can be excruciating for many minutes. Localization is poor, and the pain tends to radiate or refer to the ipsilateral ear, temple and cheek but does not cross the midline.

Pain may be described by patients in different ways, and a continuous dull ache can periodically be exacerbated (by stimulation or spontaneously) for short (minutes) or long (hours) periods.

Pain may increase and throb when the patient lies down, and in many instances wakes the patient from sleep. The pain of pulpitis is frequently discontinuous and abates spontaneously; the precise explanation for such abatement is not clear.

Non-odontological pain

Occasionally, no dental cause can be found to explain the symptoms which may be due to a range of pathological conditions affecting the orofacial region such as sinusitis or neuralgia. These organic pain disorders will be considered at the end of this chapter.

Functional pain syndromes

The cause of orofacial pain may be functional (psychogenic) in nature when no organic stimulus

to pain can be identified. If the presenting features resemble toothache, then the patient may present with expectations of a dental cause being identified, thus putting severe pressure on the dental practitioner to diagnose a non-existent dental cause. Psychological disease may often complicate or precipitate functional facial pain syndromes, making diagnosis and management more difficult. It is important, therefore, to be familiar with those features of functional pain which are characteristic, in order to aid the diagnostic process. The three main functional pain syndromes which present as facial pain are temporomandibular disorders, atypical facial pain and oral dysaesthesia, and these will be discussed in turn later.

Functional pain is not restricted to the face and mouth region. All medical specialties have patients with functional pain syndromes who must be distinguished from those with organic disease. These include globus hystericus (functional dysphagia), chest pain, irritable bowel syndrome, some forms of back pain, and dysfunctional uterine bleeding.

As alluded to earlier, psychological and personality factors also dictate how 'ill' a patient is with a certain disease, the so-called 'illness behaviour pattern'. This pattern may be quite abnormal and hypochondriacal in a chronic pain sufferer. Also, adverse life events such as bereavement, divorce, house moving or stress at work can aggravate the symptoms of a disease, especially if the patient is already anxious or depressed, and patients may (even subconsciously) use their illness to attract sympathy, help or support. A particular precipitating factor may be anger by the patient, who may perceive the pain to be someone else's fault; for example, injury after a road traffic accident or a difficult extraction is more likely to become self-perpetuating. The opportunity for litigation or compensation may further exaggerate the symptoms! Regardless, the ability to feel pain often becomes facilitated by its own chronicity: the neurological pathways seem to become 'opened up' as a result of constant stimulation, often to the extent that the pain becomes spontaneous.

Other general factors dictate the sort of patient who presents with functional pain: over 80% of functional facial pain patients are women.

The specific features of the functional facial pain syndromes will now be discussed in detail.

Temporomandibular disorders

The commonest disorder is the temporomandibular joint pain dysfunction syndrome. This term is unfortunate since the joint itself is not usually involved or symptomatic. Temporomandibular pain dysfunction is called by several different names, and these are shown in Table 25.2. Typically the patient, who is a young woman in her teens or twenties, will have unilateral or bilateral facial pain in the preauricular area or masticatory muscles. Sometimes there is a clicking joint on one or both sides, and occasional locking may be a problem. The patient may have restricted jaw movements (trismus) and headaches. The symptoms may be worse on waking, and there may be a history of clenching or bruxing.

On examination, the patient may have some facial swelling or puffiness and tenderness of the masticatory muscles. There may be deviation towards the affected side on jaw opening, and the patients usually over-open their jaws, occasionally tending to sublux or dislocate their joint. There may be evidence of tooth faceting due to grinding, and there may be malocclusion, but this is seldom contributory to the symptoms since temporomandibular disorders are no less frequent in orthodontically corrected patients than in other populations. Many clinicians will subject such patients unnecessarily to 'occlusal adjustment' which, in fact, often makes matters worse by reinforcing an organic aetiology rather than a functional one. Indeed, studies have shown that 'sham' occlusal equilibration (pretending to grind the occlusion) is as effective as actual grinding, implying that the effect is a placebo response.

The aetiology of temporomandibular pain dysfunction is complex and variable, but muscle spasm is common. Any injuries such as dislocation or trauma may cause an acute arthritis or muscle pain. The patient then protects the jaw with muscle spasm, which causes more pain, and a vicious circle ensues. Normally this can be switched off by analgesia or reassurance, but can become self-perpetuating if muscle tone is increased and the pain threshold reduced due to pyschological considerations. Thus, a patient who is anxious or 'uptight', such as before exams, may develop masticatory muscle stiffness and pain. Persistence of the symptoms beyond 6 months implies a more serious and intransigent problem with an associated 'abnormal illness behaviour' pattern.

Diagnosis of the condition relies on the history and the clinical examination. Radiography is only justified if the temporomandibular joints are obviously painful or clinically involved.

Management involves explanation of the nature of the disorder and reassurance that the abnormality is functional rather than involving a physical abnormality. If the condition is acute and painful, non-steroidal anti-inflammatory drugs can be given for 10–14 days to allow recovery. If the condition is severe and associated with significant muscle spasm and trismus, then diazepam 5 mg three times daily for 3–7 days will cause resolution of the acute symptoms.

Occlusal splint therapy is the first-line treatment for more chronic problems. The mechanism of action is probably largely placebo, but the splint also interferes with grinding or clenching. A soft lower splint is the least intrusive and is more likely to fit than an acrylic splint! The splint should be worn at night for as long as the patient feels benefit. Patients should be reviewed every 2–3 months. Three-quarters of patients presenting with temporomandibular disorders will respond to the above measures and require no further treatment.

The remainder will continue to suffer intractable symptoms and will require psychotropic therapy, as discussed later.

Table 25.2 Synonyms for temporomandibular disorders

Costen's syndrome
Craniomandibular disorders
Facial arthromyalgia
Myofascial pain dysfunction
Temporomandibular joint pain dysfunction syndrome
Mandibular pain dysfunction

Atypical facial pain

Atypical facial pain is so called because it presents as pain often masquerading as toothache, but is atypical in its cause. There are several other terms used to describe atypical facial pain (Table 25.3), but they are all a spectrum of the same disorder.

Table 25.3 Atypical facial pain syndromes

Atypical facial pain	Facial Pain
Atypical odontalgia	Localized to one tooth
Atypical periodontalgia	Functional periodontal pain

The patient with atypical facial pain may present with symptoms suggestive of toothache or sinusitis, and so these organic diagnoses must be excluded before a diagnosis of atypical facial pain is made: you cannot diagnose functional pain in a tooth which has a periapical radiolucent area! The features which suggest atypical facial pain as a diagnosis are, firstly, chronicity: the patient often has had 'toothache' for months or years without remission – organic toothache seldom lasts more than a few days. The pain may be intermittent however, but is always very chronic. Also, analgesics have a limited benefit (and have often not even been tried), and the patient may not complain of food or drink making pain worse, as in typical toothache. Dental investigation or treatment, especially extraction, worsens rather than helps the pain, which then moves to the extraction socket or the adjacent tooth. Even when a patient has been successfully treated and is asymptomatic, dental treatment may cause a relapse, requiring a further course of treatment. The patient is usually female and the peak incidence is in the fifth decade. Occasionally, there is a history of chronic pain due to toothache, endodontics, or a difficult extraction at the site where the functional pain is localized.

A serious attempt must be made to identify a dental cause for the pain, but when no obvious or other organic cause exists, further destructive dental investigation should be stopped and the patient treated for functional pain with psychotropic therapy, as discussed below.

Trigeminal neuralgia is discussed in the next section of the chapter. However, it should be noted that the pain of trigeminal neuralgia, although it is fleeting in nature, is part of a chronic condition which seems in many patients to facilitate pain perception, and some patients subsequently develop atypical facial pain superimposed upon the trigeminal neuralgia. Such patients, usually with long-standing trigeminal neuralgia, complain not only of stabbing bursts of pain but also a background constant pain, and require treatment both for their trigeminal neuralgia to relieve the lancinating pain and also pyschotropic therapy to manage their atypical facial pain.

Oral dysaesthesia

The last syndrome of functional facial pains is oral dysaesthesia. It may present as a sore or burning tongue, lips or mouth, and historically goes under several terms (Table 25.4).

It may also present as an unpleasant taste or any other unpleasant sensation.

Oral dysaesthesia is the commonest cause of a burning tongue or mouth, but other conditions can also cause these symptoms, and so must be eliminated as a cause (Table 25.5).

Even if mucosal diseases, such as geographic tongue, are present (which are often asymptomatic), a functional dysaesthesia should be considered since it often complicates organic symptoms.

The features of the discomfort are often characteristic, and suggest a diagnosis even in the presence of other conditions: patients are almost always women between the ages of 40 and 70 years. The burning sensation is usually minimal on waking in the morning (unless it is particularly

> Organic pain must be excluded before making a diagnosis of atypical facial pain

> Constant toothache for months or years is most probably atypical facial pain

Table 25.4 Synonyms for oral dysaesthesia

Burning mouth syndrome
Glossopyrosis
Glossodynia
Stomatopyrosis
Stomatodynia

Table 25.5 Possible conditions that mimic oral dysaesthesia

Allergy
Candidosis
Diabetes
Geographic tongue
Haematological deficiency
Mucosal disease
Xerostomia

severe). The condition then deteriorates throughout the day, often after inserting dentures. This leads the patient erroneously to attribute the discomfort to denture wearing, although removing the dentures provides minimal relief. The condition worsens throughout the day, and reaches a crescendo in the evening, relief being provided only by eating, drinking or sucking sweets which causes a thought deviation from the symptoms in hand. Social contact also distracts the patient from the symptoms, although such symptoms often provide an excuse to avoid stressful social contact or confrontation. The patient is often cancerphobic, and has often been told that the condition is 'all in your mind'. Despite the severity of the symptoms the patients are not prevented from sleeping, are never wakened by the symptoms and are usually asymptomatic on waking. Sleep disturbance, however, is usual, especially early morning wakening, and this implies the presence of a depressive illness. Patients usually deny any depressive symptoms, however, but can often relate the onset or a deterioration in their problem to an adverse life event such as a bereavement.

> Oral dysaesthesia is the commonest cause of a burning tongue

Management involves the identification of any organic conditions contributing to the symptoms such as haematinic deficiency, although this is a rare cause. Patients should be screened for haematological deficiencies and diabetes. Clinical examination will exclude candidosis, mucosal diseases such as lichen planus, and denture design faults. Xerostomia may be due to drugs, autoimmune disease or smoking, but may also be due to chronic anxiety, and this may be part of the oral dysaesthesia syndrome. Psychotropic treatment of functional oral dysaesthesia, however, should not be delayed unnecessarily since psychological disease also causes significant morbidity and mortality.

Management requires control of the syndrome with reassurance and psychotropic therapy. The use of such therapy is now discussed for oral functional pain disorders in detail.

Psychotropic treatment of functional facial pain syndromes

The treatment of functional pain syndromes requires a psychological and pharmacological approach. Reassurance that the clinician has confidence in the diagnosis is extremely helpful since patients have usually already been inappropriately informed of the fanciful or imaginary nature of their symptoms. Cancerphobia is a component of many facial pain syndromes, and reassurance on the lack of a detectable pathology is important. In establishing the diagnosis it is necessary to broaden the agenda of the questioning to enquire about wider psychological issues such as sleep disturbance and adverse life events. This requires a degree of skill and sensitivity. Initially, enquiring whether the symptoms disturb sleep is a way of shifting the line of questioning to sleep patterns. This process of widening the scope of the relevant issues is called reattribution, and the important components of this process are shown in Table 25.6.

In addition to explaining the patient's symptoms within a wider context, the patient must have realistic expectations of the treatment outcomes: if the patient expects a bottle of tablets to cure the disease, then the treatment is doomed to failure.

Psychotropic medication involves the use of antidepressant therapy. Many patients are reluc-

Table 25.6 Exploring the psychogenic basis to disease

Make the patient feel understood
Broaden the agenda
Explore links to life events
Link symptoms to psychological factors

tant to take such medication, especially when they are trying to resist accepting a psychological component for their symptoms. Just as aspirin has antiplatelet effects as well as being a painkiller, so tricyclic antidepressants have effects other than on depression – some are analgesic – and this must be explained to the patient. Tricyclic antidepressants block the transmission of neuropathic pain, and hence are more effective at relieving pain in functional pain syndromes than the classic analgesics. Tricyclic antidepressants also improve sleep patterns without being 'sleeping pills', and most are also anxiolytic and hence reduce muscle tension. In addition, these drugs are antidepressant and will improve mood if the patient is depressed. In these ways, tricyclic antidepressants are beneficial to the facial pain patient, and this should be fully explained. The most popular drug used is dothiepin, which is a tricyclic antidepressant with anxiolytic but minimal sedating properties. Patients should be started on 25 mg nocte, and the dose increased weekly until the patient has morning drowsiness, which disappears within half an hour. The average dose is 50–75 mg at night. While on the medication, patients should be reassured about the reversible nature of their dry mouth and warned that their weight may increase. Those with high blood pressure should have their blood pressure monitored. It should be explained that although sleep may improve rapidly, pain relief and mood may take 3–4 weeks to improve and that the medication will only facilitate self-motivation to become well.

The commonest cause of treatment failure is not taking the tablets (the patient will then not complain of drowsiness or oral dryness), or an inability to take the tablets. Reinforcement of the need for treatment usually overcomes the problem, but if side-effects, or perceived side-effects, prevent the patient from taking the medication then selective serotonin reuptake inhibitor antidepressant tablets should be used instead (although these drugs tend to have a poorer painkilling effect). They do, however, cause less side-effects, and may be all that the patient can tolerate.

The aim of treatment is to achieve small but steady improvements rather than cure, and the majority of patients should be well after 6 months of therapy. Most can be taken off medication after 1 year, but a hard core of patients with intractable 'abnormal illness behaviour' and chronic pain will still be symptomatic, and treatment failure must be accepted. These patients should be given support without encouragement to become dependent: allowing the patient to derive gain from too frequent visits will only perpetuate them 'enjoying ill health'.

All the above therapies must be provided in conjunction with the patient's general medical practitioner, who will require expert dental advice to fully manage such a chronic pain patient.

If more significant psychological disease is suspected or the patient exhibits psychotic behaviour, then a formal psychiatric referral may be required.

Organic facial pain syndromes

Trigeminal neuralgia

Trigeminal neuralgia is a relatively common condition characterized by an intense pain in the distribution of one or more branches of the trigeminal nerve. Females are more commonly affected than males, and the age of onset is generally over 40–50 years. The attacks of pain are unilateral, brief, excruciating, and frequently described as like an electric shock or a lancinating type pain. The pain most frequently affects mandibular or maxillary divisions although in severe cases more than one division may be involved. Involvement of the ophthalmic division is uncommon. The pain can often be precipitated by simple touch, washing or shaving the affected area. In some instances a cold wind may be sufficient to trigger the pain. Intraoral trigger zones may be present, and the pain may be precipitated by eating, chewing or even toothbrushing. In such cases the pain may be misdiagnosed as an odontogenic problem. In the initial stages, the disease recurs intermittently, with remissions often lasting weeks or months, although, as time progresses, the remissions become increasingly short. As well as the episodic acute pain, patients frequently describe a continuous dull background ache, as described in the previous section on atypical facial pain.

Clinical examination may be difficult as the patient not unnaturally wishes to avoid unnecessary initiation of the pain. The diagnosis is essentially based on the history, and clinical examination is usually normal unless a trigger spot is identified. The presence of abnormal neurological signs such as muscle weakness or anaesthesia should prompt a thorough neurological assessment, as similar pain can be a manifestation of underlying pathology such as an acoustic neuroma or tumour of the posterior cranial fossa. Similarly, pain suggestive of trigeminal neuralgia in a patient under the age of 40 years should be regarded with a high index of suspicion, as the pain may be a presenting feature of a demyelinating process such as multiple sclerosis, and such patients should be referred for further investigation.

> Trigeminal neuralgia in a patient less than 40 years should be referred for further investigation

The treatment of choice for idiopathic trigeminal neuralgia is carbamazepine, an anticonvulsant successful in approximately 70% of patients. Treatment should be started with a low dose of, say, 200–300 mg daily in divided doses, and gradually increased at 3 day intervals until control of the pain is achieved. Most patients obtain satisfactory control of their symptoms on doses less than 600–800 mg daily. In some cases a higher dose (up to 1600 mg) may be required. Carbamazepine therapy is generally well tolerated, although a variety of side-effects are reported, most commonly sedation, nausea, vertigo, ataxia and an erythematous, pruritic skin rash. Less common but important adverse effects include blood dyscrasias and hepatic dysfunction; regular monitoring of full blood count and liver function tests is considered mandatory.

Patients who do not respond to carbamazepine can be treated with other membrane-stabilizing agents such as phenytoin and sodium valproate, although these drugs are generally less successful. Other treatment options are summarized in Table 25.7. The surgical procedure of microvascular decompression is based on the premise that the pain of trigeminal neuralgia is triggered by blood vessels pressing on the main root of the trigeminal nerve as it enters the pons. The procedure has a

Table 25.7 Management of trigeminal neuralgia

Medical	Carbamazepine
	Phenytoin
	Sodium valproate
	Baclofen
	Clonazepam
Surgical	Peripheral
	Cryotherapy
	Alcohol/phenol nerve block
	Ganglion
	Alcohol/phenol injection
	Balloon compression
	Radiofrequency
	thermocoagulation
	Central
	Microvascular
	decompression
	Rhizotomy
	Tractotomy

high success rate although there is significant risk of morbidity or mortality.

Glossopharyngeal neuralgia

This is a similar condition to trigeminal neuralgia, although is considerably less common. The pain has the same characteristics as trigeminal neuralgia, and the patient reports severe paroxysmal pain in the tonsillar region or oropharynx. Unlike trigeminal neuralgia, the age of onset is often below 50 years. The pain may radiate to the ear, and is frequently triggered by chewing, swallowing or coughing. Treatment with carbamazepine is usually successful. Pain similar to glossopharyngeal neuralgia may be a presenting feature of nasopharyngeal carcinoma, and therefore patients warrant careful ear, nose and throat examination to exclude malignancy.

Giant cell arteritis

This condition is a granulomatous vasculitis of unknown aetiology occurring chiefly in those over the age of 60 years. Females are more commonly affected. The extradural arteries are principally affected, although other branches of the proximal aorta may also be involved. A burning-type headache is an almost invariable feature, centred over the superficial temporal and/or occipital arteries. The affected vessels may be visibly swollen and tender, and touching the overlying skin may elicit pain. Other branches of the external carotid artery supplying the muscles of mastication and tongue may also be affected, leading to pain on eating (jaw claudication), difficulty opening the mouth, and pain on protrusion of the tongue. Occasionally, ischaemic necrosis of the tongue or lip may develop. Visual loss due to retinal vasculitis may develop in up to 25% of cases, hence the importance of the diagnosis. Systemic features such as malaise, weight loss, fever and generalized limb pain may also be features of the condition. Indeed, up to half of patients with giant cell arteritis have features of polymyalgia rheumatica.

The erythrocyte sedimentation rate (ESR) is usually substantially elevated in giant cell arteritis, although very rarely it may be normal. The levels of acute phase proteins such as C-reactive protein may be elevated. Normochromic normocytic anaemia is also a feature. Diagnosis is confirmed by temporal artery biopsy. A 1–2 cm segment is excised, as the characteristic granulomatous changes may be patchy.

In view of the high risk of blindness, it is important to commence treatment without delay. In a patient with typical features, treatment may be started before temporal artery biopsy. Systemic corticosteroids (prednisolone 40–60 mg daily) produce a rapid reduction in the severity of the symptoms. Indeed, a characteristic feature of the condition is that the headache may subside within hours of the initial dose. The dose of steroid is tapered off according to the improvement in the patient's symptoms and a fall in the ESR.

Periodic migrainous neuralgia (cluster headache)

Periodic migrainous neuralgia is an uncommon condition which is characterized by episodic facial pain centred over the maxilla. The cause still remains obscure. Males are more commonly affected than females, with a ratio of 6:1. The attacks of pain always occur on the same side and have a burning or pulsatile character, most commonly centred in and around the eye. Each attack lasts from 30 to 90 min; the pain is typically at night and sufficiently severe to disturb sleep, and patients often report restlessness and a compulsion to walk about. During each episode, patients may report ipsilateral lacrimation, conjunctival redness or rhinorrhoea. Attacks frequently occur at the same time each day, often in the early hours of the morning. Patients may have a number of individual attacks during a 24 h period. Attacks may be precipitated by alcohol, although this is by no means a universal finding. Treatment includes avoidance of alcohol if this is a recognized precipitant. Indomethacin is frequently helpful in controlling symptoms, while other agents such as β blockers and calcium channel blockers, sumatriptan or oxygen inhalation may also be used.

Angina pectoris

Angina, which means choking, typically manifests as central chest pain pectoris, and the characteristic features are described elsewhere in this text. A small minority of patients with angina report radiation of the pain to the left mandible and, less commonly, the teeth, tongue or palate. Very rarely these sites may be the only feature which resembles toothache. The pain in these cases may be precipitated by exercise.

Tension headache

A large percentage of chronic and recurrent headaches are attributed to 'tension' within the muscles of the scalp, although convincing evidence to support this concept is lacking. Nevertheless, regardless of the aetiology, the condition is benign. Frequently, patients complain of a tight band sensation, pressure sensation behind the eyes or a throbbing feeling. The pain may radiate to the forehead, temples or the back of the neck. Males and females are equally affected, although females present more often for treatment. While the entity is poorly defined, there appear to be associations with stress, anxiety and depression. Clinically there are no abnormal physical signs other than tenderness in the muscles of the back of the neck and scalp, management involves firm reassurance, avoidance of obvious precipitants, simple analgesics and relaxation.

Migraine

Migraine is a common problem which may affect up to 10% of the population. The cause is unknown, although it is believed to be associated with vasodilatation or oedema of the blood vessels leading to stimulation of nerve endings adjacent to affected vessels. It is relatively common around puberty, during the menopause and premenstrually. Some patients report a variety of precipitants, including chocolate, cheese, bananas, and some red wines – all contain tyramine. The oral contraceptive pill may also trigger attacks.

Several different types of migraine are recognized, ranging from intermittent attacks similar to tension headaches to severe headaches which may mimic cerebral ischaemia, although the distinction between each variant is perhaps rather artificial. Each attack is characterized by prodromal symptoms followed by the headache itself with a variety of associated features. Most, with the exception of common migraine and classic migraine, are uncommon.

Common migraine. This is the usual variant, with vague prodromal symptoms and recurrent headache with accompanying nausea and malaise. It may be impossible to differentiate from tension headache.

Classic migraine. Prodromal symptoms are often visual with field defects related to the distribution of the arteries affected. Transient aphasia (inability to speak), numbness and vague weakness may also occur. Associated nausea is common. These prodromal symptoms may last for an hour or more, and are initially followed by a localized headache which becomes generalized. There is an increase in the intensity of the nausea, and vomiting ensues. After several hours the attack resolves.

Management. Management of migraine includes the following:-

- *General.* Avoidance of dietary precipitants, although this is frequently unhelpful. Stopping the oral contraceptive pill or changing to an alternative preparation may be useful.
- *During each attack.* For mild episodes, simple analgesics together with an antiemetic may be helpful. More severe episodes can be treated with a serotonin receptor agonist such as sumatriptan.

- *Prophylaxis.* A variety of agents have been advocated, although none is universally successful. These include pizotifen, β-blockers, calcium channel blockers and clonidine.

On the basis that some patients report headaches on waking, it has been suggested that migraine may be related to parafunctional activity such as tooth grinding or clenching habits. Accordingly, some have advocated the use of occlusal splints in these patients. At present there is no convincing evidence to support this treatment.

Sinusitis

Maxillary sinusitis usually causes a dull, persistent pain in the maxilla principally at the medial margin of the orbit. The pain may be exacerbated by bending forwards, and radiates to the upper molar and premolar teeth as well as the zygomatic bone. The upper posterior teeth on the affected side may be tender to percussion due to the close proximity of their roots to the lining of the antrum.

Frontal sinusitis is characterized by frontal headache radiating to the area behind the eye. During the acute stage there may be associated swelling of the upper eyelid and tenderness on palpation over the supraorbital ridge.

Diagnosis is clinical, although radiographs showing sinus opacity or mucosal thickening or a fluid level are confirmatory. Acute sinusitis may successfully be treated with antimicrobials, although chronic sinusitis is often complicated by long-standing nasal congestion from whatever cause, and decongestants or topical corticosteroids may be required to improve symptoms.

Tumours of the sinuses or nasopharynx can also cause facial pain.

Other local causes of orofacial pain

Jaws. Pain can be caused by acute infection, malignancies and direct trauma to the jaw. Lesions such as cysts, retained roots and impacted teeth are usually painless unless associated with infection or fracture of the jaw. Odontogenic and other benign tumours of the bone do not normally produce pain, but malignant tumours usually produce deep, boring pain, sometimes associated with paraesthesia or anaesthesia.

Radiation therapy may result in severe pain due to infection and osteomyelitis associated with osteoradionecrosis.

Salivary glands. Pain from salivary glands is localized to the affected gland, may be quite severe, and may be intensified by increased saliva production such as before and with meals. The salivary gland is swollen and sensitive to palpation. In acute parotitis, mouth opening causes severe pain, and thus there is a degree of trismus. Salivary flow from the affected gland is usually reduced. Pain may be associated with fever and malaise. In children, the most common cause is mumps. In adults, pain from salivary glands results usually from blockage of a salivary duct by a calculus.

Pressure on the mental nerve. Rarely, pain is caused by pressure from a denture on the nerve which comes to lie on the crest of the ridge as the alveolar bone is resorbed in the edentulous mandible. Either the denture should be relieved from the area or, rarely, it is necessary to resite the nerve surgically.

Eyes. Pain from the eyes can arise from disorders of refraction, retrobulbar neuritis (e.g. in multiple sclerosis) or glaucoma (raised intraocular pressure), and can radiate to the orbit or frontal region.

Ears. Middle ear disease may cause headaches. Conversely, oral disease may cause pain referred to the ear, particularly from lesions of the posterior tongue.

Neck. Neck pain, usually from cervical vertebral disease, especially cervical spondylosis, very occasionally causes pain referred to the face.

Neurological causes of facial pain. Sensory innervation of the mouth, face and scalp depends on the trigeminal nerve, so that involvement of this nerve can cause orofacial pain or, indeed, sensory loss – sometimes with serious implications.

Facial neuralgia caused by tumours or other lesions. Any lesion affecting the trigeminal nerve, whether it be traumatic, inflammatory or neoplastic (e.g. a nasopharyngeal or antral carcinoma), may cause pain. These tumours are often carcinomas which infiltrate various branches of the trigeminal nerve and can remain undetected for long periods. Nasopharyngeal carcinoma often presents late, with facial pain, paraesthesia, ipsilateral deafness and/or cervical lymph node enlargement (Trotter's syndrome).

Severe facial pain suggestive of trigeminal neuralgia but with physical signs such as facial sensory or motor impairment can result from cerebrovascular disease, multiple sclerosis, infections such as AIDS, or neoplasms.

Herpetic and postherpetic neuralgia. Herpes zoster (shingles) is often preceded and accompanied by neuralgia (see Ch. 5), which may persist after the rash has resolved. Postherpetic neuralgia causes a continuous, burning pain that affects mainly elderly patients and may be so intolerable that suicide can become a risk.

Frey's syndrome (auriculotemporal syndrome). This is a paroxysmal burning pain, usually in the temporal area or in front of the ear, associated with flushing and sweating on eating caused by aberrant regeneration of postganglionic parasympathetic nerve fibres along sympathetic pathways to the blood vessels and glands of the affected region. This misdirection is initiated by damage to the parasympathetic axons by a traumatic procedure, most commonly parotid surgery. No specific treatment is available, but the condition tends to improve over time.

Neurological disorders

Facial palsy

The common causes of facial paralysis are strokes (upper motor neuron lesions) and Bell's palsy (lower motor neuron lesion). Occasionally, a temporary facial palsy follows the administration of an inferior alveolar local analgesic if the solution tracks through the parotid gland to reach the facial nerve.

The facial nerve neurons supplying the lower face receive upper motor neurons only for the contralateral motor cortex, whereas the neurons to the upper face receive bilateral upper motor neuron innervation. Upper motor neuron facial palsy, therefore, is characterized by unilateral facial palsy, with some sparing of the frontalis and orbicularis oculi muscles because of the bilateral cortical representation. Furthermore, although voluntary movements are impaired, extrapyramidal influences can still act, and the face may still move with emotional responses, for example, on laughing. There may also be a paresis of the ipsilateral arm, or arm and leg, or some aphasia, because of more extensive brain damage.

In contrast, lower motor neuron facial palsy is characterized by total unilateral paralysis of all muscles of facial expression, both for voluntary and emotional responses, but no hemiparesis.

In facial palsy, the forehead is unfurrowed, and the patient unable to close the eye on that side. Upon attempted closure, the eye rolls upward (Bell's sign). Tears tend to overflow on to the cheek (epiphora). The corner of the mouth droops, and the nasolabial fold is obliterated. Saliva may dribble from the commissure. Food collects in the vestibule on the affected side, and plaque accumulates on the teeth. Depending on the site of the lesion, other features such as loss of taste may be associated (Table 25.8).

Facial weakness is demonstrated by asking the patient to close the eyes against resistance, to raise the eyebrows, or to raise the lips to show the teeth or to try to whistle. The following diagnostic tests are also necessary:

- a full neurological examination is required, looking particularly for V, VI and VII nerve signs, hemiparesis, etc.
- hearing loss should be tested for, discharge from the ear and other signs of middle ear disease looked for
- blood pressure should be measured (to exclude hypertension), and urinalysis performed (to exclude diabetes)
- Lyme disease (tick-borne infection with

Borrelia burgdorferi) 'or HIV' must occasionally be excluded.

Bell's palsy

The commonest lower motor neuron lesion is Bell's palsy, caused by inflammation in the stylomastoid canal, which may be immunologically mediated and usually associated with herpes simplex or other virus infection. The onset of paralysis is acute over a few hours.

> Patients with Bell's palsy seen in the first 72 h should be treated with corticosteroids and aciclovir

Most patients recover within a few weeks, but the after effects in others can be so severe and distressing that all patients should be treated with corticosteroids and aciclovir if seen within 72 h of onset. The eye should be protected with a pad, since the corneal reflex is impaired and corneal damage may occur.

In chronic cases, where there is no recovery after months or years, it may be necessary to use a splint or fascial graft to prevent drooping at the commissure, or other manoeuvres such as facial–hypoglossal nerve anastomosis in an attempt to overcome the cosmetic deformity.

Ramsay–Hunt syndrome

Severe facial palsy with vesicles in the ipsilateral pharynx and external auditory canal (Ramsay–Hunt syndrome) may be due to herpes

Table 25.8 Differentiation of upper from lower motor neuron lesions of the facial nerve

Feature	Upper motor neuron lesions	Lower motor neuron lesions
Emotional movements of face	Retained	Lost
Blink reflex	Retained	Lost
Ability to wrinkle forehead	Retained	Lost
Drooling	Uncommon	Common
Lacrimation, taste or hearing	Unaffected	May be affected

zoster affecting the geniculate ganglion of the seventh nerve.

Bilateral facial palsy

Bilateral facial palsy is rare, but may be seen in HIV infection, the Guillain–Barré syndrome, sarcoidosis, arachnoiditis and brain tumours.

Abnormal facial movements

Facial dyskinesias

Facial dyskinesias are abnormal movements of the tongue, facial or jaw muscles usually associated with extrapyramidal disease such as athetosis or drugs such as phenothiazines with extrapyramidal effects.

Botulinum toxin or antiparkinsonian drugs such as benzhexol help to control these reactions.

Facial tics

Facial tics are benign spasms (habit spasms) such as blinking, grimacing, shaking the head, clearing the throat, coughing or shrugging, worsened by emotion or tiredness. Most resolve spontaneously.

Hemifacial spasms

Hemifacial spasm (clonic facial spasm) is spasm of the angle of the mouth or the eyelid, and is worse towards evening. Many cases are idiopathic, but some indicate a brain lesion.

Benign fasciculation

Benign fasciculation and myokymia (spontaneous intermittent twitching) of the lower eyelid are quite innocuous.

Facial myokymia

Facial myokymia – continuous, fine, worm-like contractions of one or more of the facial muscles – especially around the mouth or eyes, is rare. It is frequently associated with multiple sclerosis or other neurological disorders, and patients must therefore be referred for a neurological opinion.

Facial sensory loss

Lesions of a sensory branch of the trigeminal nerve may cause anaesthesia in the distribution of the affected branch. Facial sensory loss may be caused by intracranial or, more frequently, by extracranial lesions of the trigeminal nerve. It may lead to corneal, facial or oral ulceration (Fig. 25.1).

Lesions involving the ophthalmic division cause corneal anaesthesia, which is tested for by gently touching the cornea with a wisp of cotton wool twisted to a point. Normally, this procedure causes a blink but, if the cornea is anaesthetic (or if there is facial palsy), no blink follows, provided that the patient does not actually see the cotton wool.

Lesions of the sensory part of the trigeminal nerve initially also result in a diminishing response to pin-prick of the skin and, later, complete anaesthesia. It is important in patients complaining of facial anaesthesia to test all areas, but particularly the corneal reflex. If the patient complains of complete facial or hemifacial anaesthesia, but the corneal reflex is retained or there is apparent anaesthesia over the angle of the mandible (an area *not* innervated by the trigeminal nerve), then the symptoms are probably functional (non-organic).

Extracranial causes of sensory loss

The mandibular division or its branches may be traumatized by inferior alveolar local analgesic

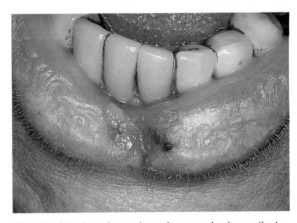

Fig. 25.1 Lip ulceration and scarring occurring in a patient with sensory loss to the area.

injections, fractures or surgery (particularly osteotomies or surgical extraction of lower third molars). Occasionally the mental foramen is close beneath a lower denture, and there is anaesthesia of the lower lip on the affected side, as a result of pressure from the denture. The lingual nerve may be damaged, especially during removal of lower third molars, particularly when the lingual split technique is used. Osteomyelitis or tumour deposits in the jaws may cause labial anaesthesia.

Nasopharyngeal carcinomas may invade the pharyngeal wall and infiltrate the mandibular division of the trigeminal nerve, causing pain and sensory loss and, by occluding the eustachian tube, deafness (Trotter's syndrome).

Damage to branches of the maxillary division of the trigeminal may be caused by trauma (middle-third facial fractures) or a tumour such as carcinoma of the maxillary antrum.

Intracranial causes of facial sensory loss

Common intracranial causes of facial sensory loss are multiple sclerosis, brain tumours and syringobulbia. Since other cranial nerves are anatomically close, there may be associated neurological deficits.

In posterior or middle cranial fossa lesions, there may be other neurological features such as ataxia.

Benign trigeminal neuropathy

This is a transient sensory loss in one or more divisions of the trigeminal nerve which seldom occurs until the second decade. The corneal reflex is not affected. The aetiology is unknown, though some patients prove to have a connective tissue disorder.

Psychogenic causes

Hysteria, and particularly the hyperventilation syndrome, may underlie some causes of facial anaesthesia.

Management of patients with facial sensory loss

In view of the potential seriousness of facial sensory loss, care should be taken to exclude local causes, and a full neurological assessment should be undertaken. If the cornea is anaesthetic, a protective eye pad should be worn and a tarsorrhaphy (an operation to unite the upper and lower eyelids) may be indicated, since the protective corneal reflex is lost and the cornea may be traumatized.

26 Systemic disease: oral manifestations and effects on oral health

Introduction

Oral lesions and symptoms are usually the result of local disease, but can be the earliest indication of, or in some instances may be the main features in, patients with systemic disease. Oral manifestations can sometimes lead to the diagnosis. Alternatively, systemic disease may require oral health care to be modified for the patient's or operator's safety. Many systemic diseases can produce oral manifestations, and these are noted throughout both sections of this book. Oral disease is largely considered in a problem-orientated way in Part 2 of this book, which is appropriate since, for example, constant exposure of mucosal lesions to moisture, trauma and a complex flora presumably explains why so many different lesions break down to produce mouth ulcers. Thus, ulcers can result from diseases of different systems and different aetiologies. These are considered in Chapter 20.

In this chapter, however, oral manifestations of systemic disease are considered in a systematic way which can be cross-referenced with the individual systemic diseases covered in Part 1 of the book.

Furthermore, drugs used in the treatment of systemic disease can sometimes have effects on the mouth or salivary glands, or dictate modification of oral health care. For example, a patient with HIV infection might have oral lesions caused by the disease and/or have a dry mouth secondary to treatment with dideoxyinosine and/or protease inhibitors (see Ch. 5). Indeed, there are surprisingly few diseases, or their treatments, which are not capable of causing some oral signs or symptoms or affecting oral health care.

However, in practical terms the problem is not often serious because routine restorative and orthodontic care under local anaesthesia can be carried out on most patients without any significant hazard. The major problems are with patients who have bleeding tendencies, allergies, are on corticosteroids, or have cardiac disease.

Not only can systemic diseases affect the mouth but, conversely, systemic disease can originate from the mouth, usually as a consequence of infection. The main example is infective endocarditis, but oral microorganisms can, albeit rarely, cause a variety of metastatic or systemic infections. Immunocompromised patients are at special risk.

The oral manifestations of systemic conditions and their effects on oral health care are now covered under the headings shown in Table 26.1.

Blood disorders

Haematological disease is common, and may be the cause of serious complications or oral symp-

Table 26.1 Oral manifestations of systemic conditions

Blood disorders – haemorrhagic diseases
Cardiovascular disease
Endocrine disorders
Gastrointestinal disorders
Granulomatous disorders
Immunological disorders
Infections
Liver disease
Neurological disorders
Nutritional deficiencies
Pregnancy
Psychiatric disorders
Renal disease

toms. Haematological diseases and their investigation are considered in detail in Chapter 7. The conditions to be discussed here are shown in Table 26.2.

Anaemia

The only oral sign of anaemia per se is mucosal pallor, but this is not obvious until the haemoglobin level drops below 8 g/dl. Several oral manifestations arise indirectly however. The main complication for oral health care is the risks from general anaesthesia, when a shortage of oxygen can be dangerous. A haemoglobin estimation and indices should be carried out when a patient has suggestive signs in the mouth or is to undergo oral surgery.

Haemolytic anaemias

The most important diseases in this group from an oral point of view are sickle cell disease and trait and the thalassaemias.

Sickle cell disease. Patients with sickle cell disease or trait are abnormally susceptible to

Table 26.2 Haematological diseases

Anaemia
  Haemolytic
  Aplastic
  Dyshaemopoietic
Lymphoreticular malignancy
Myeloproliferative disorders
Plasma cell tumours
Porphyria

infection, particularly pneumococcal or meningococcal, and osteomyelitis. Sickling crises can be precipitated (Table 26.3), and painful crises caused by blockage of blood vessels and bone marrow infarcts can affect the jaws, particularly the mandible. They can cause severe pain, and the infarcted tissue forms a focus susceptible to infection. Salmonella osteomyelitis is a recognized hazard.

Sickle cell anaemia should be suspected in black patients, particularly in those of Afro-Caribbean origin, and investigated, if anaesthesia is anticipated. If the haemoglobin concentration is less than 10 g/dl, then the patient is probably a homozygote with sickle cell disease, and hospitalization is necessary for anaesthesia. In those with sickle cell trait the main precaution is that general anaesthesia, if unavoidable, should be carried out with full oxygenation.

In sickle cell disease the oral mucosa may be pale or yellowish due to haemolytic jaundice. Radiographic changes can be seen in the skull, and sometimes the jaws, where extramedullary erythropoiesis causes premaxillary expansion and anterior open bite. Occasionally, sensory nerve loss is also a problem.

Regular oral health care and prompt antibiotic treatment of infections are important. Painful bone infarcts should be treated with non-steroidal anti-inflammatory analgesics, and fluid intake should be increased. Patients with sickling disorders are more likely to have pain which is indistinguishable from toothache – presumably due to pulpal infarcts. These patients should therefore be treated with analgesics in the first instance unless an obvious carious lesion is present. Admission to hospital is required for severe painful crises not responsive to analgesics.

> Patients with sickling disorders are more likely to have toothache-like pain

Table 26.3 Factors precipitating sickling crises

Hypoxia (particularly from poorly-conducted anaesthesia)
Dehydration
Infections (including oral infections)
Acidosis and fever

The thalassaemias. Thalassaemia major (usually homozygous β thalassaemia) is characterized by severe hypochromic, microcytic anaemia, great enlargement of liver and spleen, and skeletal abnormalities due to extramedullary erythropoiesis (see Ch. 7). There is failure to thrive and early death if repeated transfusions are not given. Regular transfusions are life-saving and prevent the development of bony deformities, but lead to increasing deposition of iron in the tissues. Haemosiderosis is the main cause of complications.

Aplastic anaemia and leucopenia

Aplastic anaemia is failure of production of all bone marrow cells (pancytopenia), with the result that there is loss of defence against infection, and the systemic and oral effects are not unlike those of acute leukaemia. The management is to stop any drugs that may be responsible and to give antibiotics and transfusions. Oral health care management is as for acute leukaemia (see below).

Leucopenia is a deficiency of white cells, which can be a chance haematological finding and may cause no symptoms until it becomes so severe as to impair defences against infection. Lymphopenia in an apparently healthy person may be a sign of HIV infection.

Agranulocytosis is the term given to the clinical effects of severe neutropenia, namely fever, prostration and ulceration, particularly of the gingivae and pharynx.

Drug-induced leucopenia is the commonest cause (Table 26.4), and stopping the drug is the immediate management.

Certain other factors are important in the oral health care of these patients (Table 26.5).

In cyclic neutropenia there is a fall in the number of circulating neutrophils at regular intervals

---

Table 26.5 Oral health care of leucopenic patients

Attention to oral hygiene
Control oral infections (as for acute leukaemia)
Avoid extractions
Antibiotic cover if surgery is essential and unavoidable

---

of 3–4 weeks. It is therefore necessary to monitor the white cell count daily for several weeks in order to diagnose the condition. It may cause oral ulceration and periodontal breakdown.

Dyshaemopoietic anaemias

These anaemias arise due to deficiencies of iron, folic acid or vitamin B$_{12}$ (see Ch. 7). The oral problems which arise in association with these anaemias are not due to the anaemia per se but to the nutritional deficiencies which caused the anaemia. These tissue signs of deficiency may precede the appearance of changes in the peripheral blood, such as a reduced haemoglobin concentration or an altered mean cell volume, and so when oral symptoms or signs suggest a deficiency, direct assays or ferritin, folate and vitamin B$_{12}$ are mandatory.

The tissue signs of nutritional deficiencies are shown in Table 26.6.

Angular cheilitis. This cracking at the corners of the mouth is usually secondary to candidosis intraorally or due to staphylococcal or streptococcal infection. It is a classic sign, however, of iron deficiency.

Aphthous stomatitis. This is associated with nutritional deficiencies in around 20% of cases (see Ch. 19).

Paterson–Brown–Kelly syndrome (Plummer–Vinson syndrome). This encompasses iron defi-

---

Table 26.4 Important causes of drug-induced leucopenia

Analgesics
Antibacterial agents
Phenothiazines
Antithyroids
Cytotoxics
Carbamazepine

Table 26.6 Tissue signs of nutritional deficiencies

Angular cheilitis
Aphthous stomatitis
Paterson–Brown–Kelly syndrome (iron only)
Glossitis
Infection (especially candidosis)
Koilonychia (iron only)

ciency, dysphagia and postcricoid oesophageal stricture (Fig. 26.1) with ensuing malignant change in the post-cricoid area, oesophagus or stomach in about 4–10% of cases. It is less common nowadays because of the earlier diagnosis of iron deficiency.

Glossitis. Haematinic deficiency is the most important, though not the most common, cause of a sore tongue (Fig. 26.2). Soreness of the tongue can precede any fall in haemoglobin levels, particularly as a result of deficiency of iron, vitamin B_{12} or folate, and can be the first sign of such deficiencies. Later, there may be obvious inflammation and atrophy of the filiform papillae.

Lowered resistance to infection. Oral candidosis is the main example, but, in the past particularly, osteomyelitis could follow extractions in

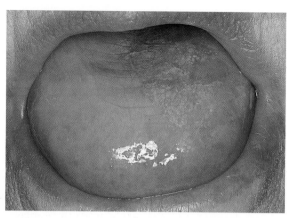

Fig. 26.2 A smooth atrophic glossitis in an elderly female with iron deficiency.

severe anaemia. Currently, sickle cell disease is more important in this context.

Koilonychia. Spooning of the nails is a classic sign of iron deficiency, and was first defined as nails which retained a bead of mercury when placed on them. A drop of water works just as well and is much safer!

Lymphoreticular malignancy

Primary malignant change in the lymphoreticular tissues is of two main types: Hodgkin's disease accounts for about 20% of cases and non-Hodgkin's lymphoma for about 80%. The presentation is usually enlargement of the lymph nodes with a rubbery consistency, as described in Chapter 27 under 'Lymph node swellings'. Oropharyngeal involvement is rare in Hodgkin's disease (less than 1% of cases), but non-Hodgkin's lymphoma more commonly presents in the mouth and can be an oral manifestation of HIV disease (see Ch. 23). The diagnosis and management is discussed fully in Chapter 7.

Myeloproliferative disorders

These may affect the red cells, the white cells or platelets. Myelofibrosis may also occur. The most important condition from an oral view point is leukaemia.

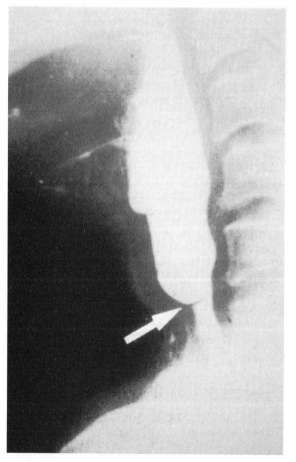

Fig. 26.1 A barium swallow showing an oesophageal web (arrowed) in a patient with the Paterson–Brown–Kelly syndrome (Plummer–Vinson syndrome).

Leukaemia

The effect of malignant overproduction of white cells is the essential feature of leukaemia, and this suppresses other cell lines of the marrow, resulting in anaemia, and thrombocytopenia with a bleeding tendency. The white cells are abnormal, leading to an immune defect. Leukaemia can affect virtually any of the white cell series, but the different types of acute leukaemia cannot be distinguished clinically.

Acute lymphoblastic leukaemia is the most common leukaemia in children (usually aged between 3 and 5 years), while acute myeloblastic leukaemia is the most common type in adults.

The major effects of leukaemia are shown in Table 26.7.

Mucosal pallor or abnormal gingival bleeding, particularly in a child, are strongly suggestive of acute leukaemia. Diagnosis depends on the peripheral blood picture and marrow biopsy.

The main oral problems in acute leukaemia are shown in Table 26.8.

The gingivae become packed and swollen with leukaemic cells particularly in acute myelogenous leukaemias in adults (Fig. 26.3). The gingivae are often purplish, and may become necrotic and ulcerate.

As a result of the immunodeficiency, the first sign of acute leukaemia may occasionally be an infection such as acute osteomyelitis following routine extractions.

Ideally, patients with leukaemia or any others who are to be treated with cytotoxic drugs should have the mouth brought to as healthy a state as possible to control the bacterial population, before complications develop. Mouth care (chlorhexidine mouthwash and an antifungal) will often control severe gingival changes and superficial infections.

Oral ulceration caused by methotrexate, which is a folate antagonist, may be controlled by giving folinic acid mouthwashes.

Extractions should be avoided because of the risks of severe infections, bleeding or anaemia. If unavoidable, blood transfusion and antibiotic cover are required.

Plasma cell tumours (myeloma)

These tumours are derived from B lymphocytes and commonly produce large quantities of immunoglobulin which can be detected in the urine and serum. The commonest oral sign is gingival bleeding, but postextraction haemorrhage and ulceration also occur.

In multiple myeloma the neoplastic proliferation of plasma cells is largely confined to the bone

---

Table 26.7 Major effects of acute leukaemia

Anaemia due to suppression of erythrocyte production
Raised susceptibility to infection due to deficiency or abnormalities of granulocytes
Bleeding tendency (purpura) due to suppression of platelet production

---

Table 26.8 Oral and perioral effects of acute leukaemia

Mucosal ulceration is often a combined effect of immunodeficiency and cytotoxic drugs such as methotrexate
Herpetic infections and candidosis are common, and ulceration may occur
Purpura can appear as excessive gingival bleeding, purplish mucosal patches, blood blisters, or prolonged bleeding after surgery
Anaemic, mucosal pallor may be noticeable, and is an important sign in children among whom anaemia is otherwise uncommon
Cervical lymphadenopathy
Gingival swelling as a result of low-grade infection at the gingival margins but lack of effective white cells

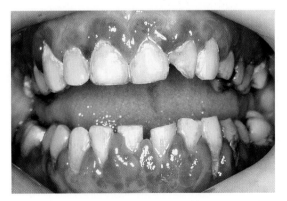

Fig. 26.3 Swollen gingivae in a patient with acute myelogenous leukaemia.

marrow. Proliferating plasma cells form tumours within the bones, leading to bone pain and pathological fractures. The multiple bony lytic lesions classically cause the pepper pot skull, and primary amyloidosis is a fairly common consequence of multiple myeloma which may lead to macroglossia (Fig. 26.4).

Porphyria

This is a rare group of inborn errors of metabolism of pyrrole characterized by the excessive formation of porphyrins (see Ch. 7). The rarest but best known of these is erythropoietic porphyria, and the features, which include skin photosensitivity with bullous lesions and scarring, hirsutism, atrophic cheilitis, advanced periodontitis and erythrodontia (intrinsic staining of the teeth with red-coloured uroporphyrin), are thought to have been the origin of the werewolf legends. Hepatic porphyrias are less rare. The greatest problem with these disorders is impaired liver function and severe neuropathies affecting the limbs and respiratory muscles. Life-threatening exacerbations may be induced by drugs, especially barbiturates or barbiturate-based anaesthetics.

Haemorrhagic diseases

Prolonged bleeding after an extraction for up to 24 h is usually due to local causes or a minor defect of haemostasis, which can be managed by local measures. More prolonged bleeding is significant. Even a mild haemophiliac can bleed for several weeks after a simple extraction. Aspirin and other anti-inflammatory analgesics should be avoided since they impair platelet function. A general consideration of haemorrhagic diseases is found in Chapter 7.

Platelet disorders

These cause purpura (bleeding into the skin or mucous membranes, producing petechiae or ecchymoses) and resulting in prolonged bleeding after injury or surgery. Unlike haemophilia, haemorrhage starts immediately after the injury.

The bleeding time is prolonged, but clotting function is normal. An exception is von Willebrand's disease, where there is an associated factor VIII deficiency.

Deficiency of platelets (fewer than 100×10^9/litre, is termed thrombocytopenia, but spontaneous bleeding is uncommon until the count falls below 50×10^9/litre. The causes of purpura are shown in Table 26.9.

A typical site of oral purpura is the palate where the posterior border of a denture presses into the mucosa (Fig. 26.5). Excessive gingival bleeding or blood blisters are other signs.

Idiopathic thrombocytopenic purpura frequently responds, at least in the short term, to immunoglobulins and corticosteroids, which can be used for urgently needed surgery. For operative treatment, transfusions of platelet concentrates can also be given, but immunosuppressive drugs may also have to be given to prevent platelet destruction by antibodies.

Von Willebrand's disease

Von Willebrand's disease is characterized both by a prolonged bleeding time and a deficiency of von Willebrand's factor and factor VIII. It is inherited as an autosomal dominant trait: both males and females are therefore affected: in contrast, classic haemophilia affects only males.

The deficiency of factor VIII is usually mild in comparison with the platelet defect, so that purpura is the more common manifestation of the disease. The platelet defect is usually correctable

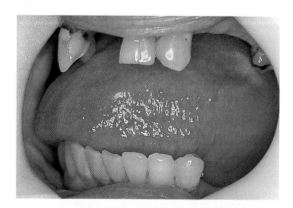

Fig. 26.4 Macroglossia due to primary amyloidosis occurring as the presenting complaint in a patient with multiple myeloma.

Table 26.9 Common causes of purpura

Thrombocytopenia	Idiopathic thrombocytopenic purpura (autoimmune) including HIV infection
	Connective-tissue diseases (especially systemic lupus erythematosus)
	Acute leukaemias and other malignancies
	Drug associated
	Hypersplenism
Vascular disorders	Senile scurvy
	Corticosteroid treatment
	Infective, e.g. meningococcal
	Henoch–Schönlein purpura
Impaired platelet function	von Willebrand's disease
	Aspirin
	Renal failure

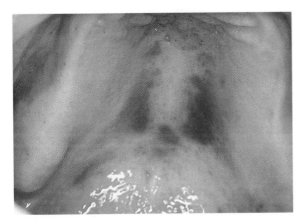

Fig. 26.5 Palatal purpura in a patient with idiopathic thrombocytopenia.

Table 26.10 Important causes of blood coagulation defects

Heritable deficiencies of plasma factors
   Haemophilia A (far the most important cause) and von Willebrand's disease with low factor VIII levels; haemophilia B with low factor IX
Acquired clotting defects
   Anticoagulant treatment, liver disease, Vitamin K deficiency

with desmopressin, which may also be sufficient to correct any significant factor VIII deficiency.

In unusually severe cases the deficiency of factor VIII is such that surgery has to be managed after infusion of von Willebrand's factor concentrates.

Clotting disorders

Important causes are shown in Table 26.10.

Haemophilia A (classic haemophilia)

Haemophilia is the most common and severe clotting disorder. In the past, extractions in haemophiliacs have been fatal, and extractions are still common emergencies on occasions when haemophiliacs need specific treatment. Occasionally the condition is diagnosed because of postextraction bleeding.

Prolonged bleeding deeply into the soft tissues can follow local anaesthetic injections. Inferior dental blocks are most dangerous both because of the rich plexus of veins in this area and because blood can leak down towards the larynx and obstruct the airway.

The characteristic feature is that bleeding starts after surgery after a short delay as a result of normal platelet and vascular responses which provide the initial phase of haemostasis. There is then persistent bleeding, which, if untreated, can continue for weeks or until the patient dies. Pressure packs, suturing, or local application of haemostatics are ineffective.

Inferior dental blocks may cause deep bleeding and airway obstruction in haemophiliacs

Many older haemophiliacs have acquired viral hepatitis or HIV infection as a result of repeated administration of untreated blood products, and are carriers of these viruses.

The principles of management of haemophiliacs is shown in Table 7.15.

It is always wise to plan treatment with the possibility in mind that the next time the patient needs surgery, he or she may have developed antibodies to factor VIII or be in a place where replacement therapy is unobtainable. The number of occasions when replacement therapy has to be given should be kept to a minimum, and as much surgical work as necessary should be done in each session. Radiographs should be taken to forestall any complications as a result of unsuspected disease and to decide whether any other extractions are appropriate at the time. Arrangements must usually be made for admission to hospital.

The risks of bleeding are greatest on the day of operation and again from 4 to 10 days postoperatively. If bleeding starts at any time after the operation, clotting factor replacement or desmopressin must be given or may be given prophylactically on the fourth or fifth day after operation. Administration of tranexamic acid is usually continued for 10 days.

Aspirin and other anti-inflammatory analgesics should be avoided because they impair platelet function.

Christmas disease (haemophilia B)

Christmas disease is inherited in the same way as, and is clinically identical to, haemophilia A. However, factor IX is more stable than factor VIII. Factor IX concentrates are given for replacement. All other aspects of the management of these patients are the same.

Acquired clotting defects

Overall these are more common than the inherited defects. The main causes are summarized in Table 26.11.

Vitamin K deficiency

Extractions or other surgery should preferably be delayed until haemostasis returns to normal. In an

Table 26.11 Important acquired clotting disorders

Vitamin K deficiency
Anticoagulant therapy
Liver disease

emergency, vitamin K can be given, preferably by mouth, and its effectiveness checked by the prothrombin time. If the latter does not return to normal within 48 h there is probably parenchymal liver disease.

Anticoagulant treatment

Coumarin anticoagulants such as warfarin are used for prevention, e.g. of thromboembolic disease, which can complicate atrial fibrillation or insertion of prosthetic heart valves. The underlying condition may therefore influence oral health care management more than the anticoagulant treatment. The latter should be checked regularly to maintain the prothrombin time, which is reported as an international normalized ratio (INR) of 2–3 in most cases but 3–4.5 for those with prosthetic valves.

Short-term anticoagulation with heparin is given before renal dialysis sessions. Heparin is effective only for about 6 h. Extractions or other surgery can therefore be delayed for 12–24 h after the last dose of heparin, when the benefits of dialysis are also maximal.

Liver disease

Obstructive jaundice or extensive liver damage can lead to severe bleeding which is difficult to control. In mild liver disease, vitamin K may be effective. In more severe cases it is valueless, but fresh plasma infusion may control bleeding (see Ch. 7).

Cardiovascular disease

A general consideration of cardiovascular disease is found in Chapter 6.

From the viewpoint of oral health care, cardiac patients fall into two main groups:

- Valvular or related defects (congenital or due to past rheumatic fever) or prosthetic valve replacement. Prophylactic antibiotic cover, particularly before extractions, is mandatory for prevention of infective endocarditis.

• Ischaemic heart disease with or without severe hypertension and cardiac failure. Routine dentistry presents little hazard, but the risk of dangerous arrhythmias must be minimized. Local anaesthetics in normal dosage have only theoretical dangers, but pain and anxiety must, as far as possible, be eliminated. The main risk is from general anaesthesia.

General aspects of management

Patients chiefly at risk are severe hypertensives and those who have angina or have had a myocardial infarct. Anxiety or pain can cause outpouring of adrenaline, which can greatly increase the load on the heart and also precipitate dangerous dysrhythmias. The first essential for these patients is therefore to alleviate anxiety and to ensure painless dentistry. Oral temazepam may be helpful. If sedation is required, relative analgesia is safer because nitrous oxide has no cardiorespiratory depressant effects and is more controllable, but should be administered by an expert. Patients should be asked whether routine oral health care treatment under local anaesthesia is acceptable, and in any session of treatment as little or as much will be done as they feel able to tolerate. For local anaesthesia, an effective surface anaesthetic should be applied, and the injection given as slowly as possible to minimize pain. The most effective agent is 2% lignocaine with adrenaline. The adrenaline content can theoretically cause a hypertensive reaction in patients receiving β-blocker antihypertensives, because of an unopposed α-adrenergic effect. If this is a concern, prilocaine can be used. Doses of local anaesthetics need to be kept to a minimum, and no more than two or three cartridges should be given (or be necessary) for an acceptable session of treatment.

If general anaesthesia is unavoidable, it should be given by an expert anaesthetist in hospital, especially as some of the drugs used for cardiovascular disease increase the risks. Cardiovascular disease is the chief cause of sudden death under anaesthesia.

Cardiac pacemakers

Pacemakers provide a stimulus to cardiac contraction when the normal rhythm is disturbed as a result of, for example, myocardial infarction. Since ultrasonic scalers and electrosurgical equipment may interfere with pacemaker function, they should generally be avoided. Other electromagnetic equipment such as pulp testers do not appear to confer a significant risk.

Infective endocarditis is not a particular risk for wearers of pacemakers, and antibiotic cover is not recommended.

> Antibiotic cover is not needed for those with pacemakers

Oral reactions to drugs used for heart disease

Some drugs used for cardiovascular disease, notably methyldopa, calcium channel blockers such as nifedipine, and captopril can cause oral reactions. Calcium channel blockers often cause gingival hyperplasia.

Other cardiovascular drugs may also complicate oral health care management. Anticoagulants have been discussed earlier. Hypotensive drugs are potentiated by general anaesthetics, and halothane in particular increases the risk of dysrhythmias with digoxin.

Relationship between periodontal disease and cardiovascular disease

Recent evidence links periodontal disease with ischaemic heart disease and myocardial infarction. This relationship persists even when correction is made for associated factors such as smoking. It may be possible that inflammatory mediators and cytokines produced by periodontal inflammation circulate in the bloodstream and increase the atherosclerotic processes in the coronary vasculature. If this were true, improved oral hygiene and oral health care might improve cardiovascular health. Further studies are required to confirm this association. It is important to remember that association does not necessarily mean causation.

Endocrine disorders

Occasionally, oral changes can lead to the diagnosis of unsuspected endocrine disease. Patients with Addison's disease, diabetes mellitus and thyrotoxicosis in particular also need special care when having oral health care operations, and general anaesthetics should be avoided. The endocrine conditions to be considered here are shown in Table 26.12. A general consideration of endocrine disorders is found in Chapter 13.

Acromegaly

Acromegaly is characterized by renewed growth of certain bones, notably the jaws, hands and feet, and overgrowth of some soft tissues. The condylar growth centre becomes active, and the mandible enlarges and protrudes. In radiographs, the whole jaw can be seen to be lengthened, and the obliquity of the angle is increased. Bones become thicker. The teeth become spaced, or, if the patient is edentulous, the dentures cease to fit. Other changes are thickening and enlargement of the facial features, particularly the lips and nose. Headaches and eventual blindness due to the pituitary tumour are common. Mandibular resection may be needed to correct the severe disfigurement, but the pituitary tumour should be treated first.

Adrenocortical insufficiency

Addison's disease can result in brown or almost black pigmentation, which is often an early sign, and, in the mouth, is patchily distributed on gingivae, buccal mucosa and lips.

Addison's disease may sometimes become apparent by development of an Addisonian crisis.

This is characterized by a rapid fall in blood pressure, circulatory collapse (shock) and vomiting. These crises, which may be fatal, are often precipitated by such causes as infections, injuries, surgery or anaesthesia. Immediate treatment with intravenous hydrocortisone and fluid replacement are essential to save life.

Corticosteroid treatment

Corticosteroids when given in sufficiently large doses have important effects, summarized in Table 26.13.

The need to give extra steroids such as intravenous hydrocortisone, in case of circulatory collapse during trauma, surgery, general anaesthesia or infection, must be considered for all patients on systemic steroids or who have used them in the previous 2 years.

Diabetes mellitus

The chief aspects of diabetes mellitus relevant to oral health care management are summarized in Table 26.14. The main problem is hypoglycaemia.

Rapidly destructive periodontal disease can result from severe untreated diabetes mellitus. However, even treated diabetic children have slightly poorer periodontal health than controls. As well as more severe gingivitis, diabetics also have higher caries levels (despite the sugar-controlled diet) and earlier loss of teeth than controls. Infections especially candidosis are more common. Occasionally, in an unrecognized diabetic a dry mouth may be the main symptom of dehydration.

Table 26.12 Endocrine disorders

Acromegaly
Adrenocortical insufficiency
Corticosteroid treatment
Diabetes mellitus
Hyperthyroidism
Hypothyroidism
Hyperparathyroidism
Hypoparathyroidism

Table 26.13 Important side-effects of long-term use of corticosteroids

Depression of adrenocortical function (collapse under stress)
Depression of inflammatory and immune responses
Opportunistic infections
Osteoporosis
Impaired wound healing
Moon face
Raised blood sugar levels
Sodium and water retention (hypertension)
Mood changes

Table 26.14 Complications of diabetes mellitus affecting oral health care
Susceptibility to infection
Hypoglycaemic coma
Diabetic coma
Ischaemic heart disease

Sialosis may be seen. Oral lichenoid reactions may arise as side-effects of chlorpropamide and other hypoglycaemic drugs.

Local anaesthesia should be used for routine dentistry in diabetics. The amount of adrenaline in local anaesthetic solutions is not significant in its effect on the blood sugar. Sedation can be given if required.

Hypoglycaemic coma may be precipitated by dental treatment which delays a normal meal or after a routine dose of insulin. Treatment should therefore be so timed as to avoid these risks. An ideal time for treatment is shortly after the patient's breakfast. Management of surgery in diabetics is detailed in Chapter 13.

Hyperthyroidism – thyrotoxicosis

Oral health care management of thyrotoxic patients may be difficult because of nervousness and excitability. If these and other signs (such as exophthalmos) suggestive of thyrotoxicosis are evident but the patient is not already under treatment, referral to a physician is indicated. Patients with long-standing thyrotoxicosis and older patients with the disease should not be given general anaesthesia, because of the risk of cardiac failure.

Severe thyrotoxicosis with excessive cardiac excitability is a possible contraindication to giving lignocaine with adrenaline. However, the risk appears to be largely theoretical, and no other local anaesthetics can be shown to be safer.

Hypothyroidism

Skeletal development and eruption of the teeth are much delayed in cretinism (congenital hypothyrodism). The face is typically broad and rather flat; this is partly due to defective growth of the skull and facial bones. The tongue is large and usually protrudes.

Ischaemic heart disease or cardiac failure are important complications of adult hypothyroidism. Therefore, it is important to avoid, or use in lower doses, sedatives including diazepam, analgesics such as codeine, and general anaesthetics. Any of these can increase the risk of myxoedema coma. Local anaesthesia is always preferable for these patients.

Hyperparathyroidism

Increased parathyroid activity may cause decalcification of the skeleton and cyst-like areas of bone resorption, and sometimes giant cell lesions.

Hypoparathyroidism

Tetany more often results from overbreathing, commonly neurotic in origin (hyperventilation syndrome), than hypoparathyroidism. In mild cases, tetany is latent, but can be triggered by tapping on the skin over the facial nerve; this causes the facial muscles to contract (Chvostek's sign). An early symptom of tetany is paraesthesia of the lips and extremities.

In the rare early onset type of hypoparathyroidism there may be aplasia or hypoplasia of the developing enamel, which becomes deeply grooved. The main effects are retarded new bone formation and diminished resorption. These changes are the results of ectodermal defects associated with this disease.

Gastrointestinal disorders

Coeliac disease (gluten-sensitive enteropathy)

This is a hypersensitivity to gluten, a constituent of wheat and other cereals not uncommon in some ethnic groups such as Celtic descendants, though not always recognized if not severe.

Coeliac disease is a genetically determined hypersensitivity to gluten that affects the jejunum. Patients may appear otherwise well; a few fail to thrive and/or have other manifestations of malabsorption. A small percentage of patients with aphthae have coeliac disease causing malabsorption and deficiencies of haematinics, resulting in oral ulceration. Oral features of coeliac disease may include ulcers, angular stomatitis, glossitis and dental hypoplasia.

A blood picture and haematinic assay may suggest malabsorption, but transoral small bowel biopsy is required for definitive diagnosis. Deficiencies should be rectified and the patient must thereafter adhere to a gluten-free diet. The oral lesions then invariably resolve or ameliorate.

Crohn's disease

Crohn's disease is a chronic inflammatory bowel disease of unknown aetiology, affecting mainly the ileum.

It presents typically with abdominal pain, persistent diarrhoea with passage of blood and mucus, anaemia, and weight loss. However, any part of the gastrointestinal tract can be involved including the mouth. The clinical oral features are described on page 321.

An oral biopsy may confirm the presence of lymphoedema and granulomas; blood tests, and intestinal radiology, endoscopy and biopsy may be required to exclude gastrointestinal lesions.

Secondary deficiencies should be corrected. Intralesional corticosteroids may help control oral lesions such as swelling, but occasionally systemic sulphasalazine or other agents are required.

Gardner's syndrome

This genetic syndrome characterized by osteomas, fibromas and epidermoid cysts includes colonic polyposis. This is discussed further in Chapters 10, 12 and 27.

Pyostomatitis vegetans

Oral lesions in the mouth, related to inflammatory bowel disease, are termed pyostomatitis vegetans, and include deep fissures, pustules, ulcers and papillary projections (Fig. 26.6).

The course of these lesions tends to follow that of the bowel disease.

Most patients with these lesions have ulcerative colitis or Crohn's disease. Some have liver disease. Oral lesional biopsy and gastrointestinal

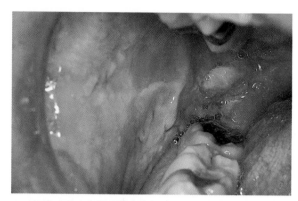

Fig. 26.6 Pustular stomatitis in a patient with pyostomatitis vegetans who also has ulcerative colitis.

investigations are required. Management is with sulphasalazine or systemic corticosteroids.

Granulomatous diseases

Histologically this term refers only to conditions where there is formation of tuberculosis-like follicles, consisting of rounded collections of large, pale histiocytes ('epithelioid cells'), sometimes surrounded by lymphocytes, and often containing giant cells. There are very many causes of this type of reaction, the more important of which are described below (Table 26.15). All of them can affect mouth or cervical lymph nodes.

Foreign body reactions

Granulomas in response to implantation of foreign bodies are usually readily recognizable because of the clinical circumstances, most frequently implantation of amalgam or extrusion of root canal filling material. Such material is usually visible microscopically either directly or by polarized light.

Table 26.15 Important granulomatous diseases

Foreign body reactions
Infections (e.g. tuberculosis).
Midline granuloma syndromes
Orofacial granulomatosis (including Crohn's disease and Melkersson–Rosenthal syndrome)
Sarcoidosis

Infections

Several infections result in granulomatous responses, and these are shown in Table 26.16.

The most important are discussed in Chapter 5.

Midline granuloma syndromes

In these diseases, the main features are variable degrees of destruction of the central facial tissues and a fatal outcome. They are not reliably clinically distinguishable, but are now recognized to result from either Wegener's granulomatosis or a peripheral (nasopharyngeal) T cell lymphoma.

Wegener's granulomatosis is a potentially lethal but uncommon disease whose main features are summarized in Table 26.17 (see also Ch. 14).

Nasal discharge is typically the first sign, and there can be destruction of, for example, the palate (Fig. 26.7) and the nasal septum, and a saddle nose deformity. In a few patients a characteristic proliferative gingivitis is the first sign. The changes initially resemble pregnancy gingivitis, but the gingivae become swollen with a granular surface and dusky or bright red in colour ('strawberry gums') (Fig. 26.8).

Early cytotoxic treatment may be life-saving.

Nasopharyngeal T cell lymphomas can start in the nasal cavity and cause extensive destruction of

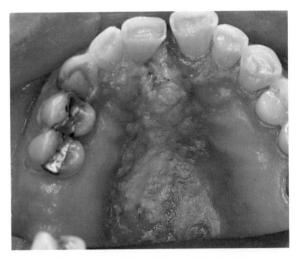

Fig. 26.7 Palatal necrosis in a 58-year-old man with Wegener's granulomatosis.

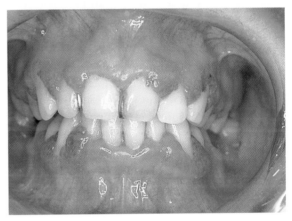

Fig. 26.8 'Strawberry gums' as the presenting symptom in a patient with Wegener's granulomatosis.

the centre of the face. Nasal obstruction, discharge and crusting are typical early signs. Extension through the palate can cause ulceration.

In the past, death could result from infection secondary to facial tissue necrosis. Usually death now results from dissemination of the lymphoma, but this may be delayed by radiotherapy.

Orofacial granulomatosis

Orofacial granulomatosis or lymphoedema is a clinical syndrome of signs which can occur in isolation or may be the oral manifestation of intestinal Crohn's disease. If intestinal symptoms

Table 26.16 Granulomatous infections
Cat scratch fever
Deep mycoses
Leprosy
Syphilis
Toxoplasmosis
Tuberculosis and non-tuberculous mycobacterioses

Table 26.17 Important features of Wegener's granulomatosis
Granulomatous inflammation of nasal tract
Cavitation of the lungs
Renal damage
Proliferative gingivitis occasionally
Oral ulceration occasionally
Antineutrophil cytoplasmic antibodies (ANCAs) typically present
Histologically, granulomatous inflammation with giant cells and vasculitis

occur in these patients, then gastrointestinal investigation is warranted. Patients should be followed to see if intestinal symptoms develop subsequently.

Melkersson–Rosenthal syndrome is an associated disorder where the patient has the features of orofacial granulomatosis but with an associated fissured tongue and recurrent facial palsy, which presumably arises due to pressure from granuloma in the stylomastoid canal.

A full description of the oral lesions, causes and management of orofacial granulomatosis is given later in this chapter.

Sarcoidosis

Sarcoidosis is a chronic disease of unknown cause, in which granulomas form particularly in the lungs, lymph nodes (especially the hilar nodes), salivary glands and other sites such as the mouth.

Oral lesions indistinguishable from orofacial granulomatosis may be seen. Clinical involvement of the major salivary glands is uncommon. In over 50% of patients with bilateral hilar lymphadenopathy, biopsy of a labial salivary gland shows typical granulomas which are non-caseating, contain multinucleated giant cells and are surrounded by lymphocytes.

Immunological disorders

Many of the immunologically mediated diseases have some oral health care relevance, as summarized in Table 26.18.

Immunologically mediated disease will be considered under the headings of allergy, atopic disease and autoimmune disease.

Allergy

Semantically speaking, allergy refers to the clinical manifestations of specific IgE-mediated immediate hypersensitivity responses. In clinical practice, however, allergy encompasses all those conditions where a person is immunologically hypersensitive to an exogenous agent whether it is IgE mediated or not. For example, patch testing measures a delayed immune response, but patients still perceive themselves as 'allergic' to substances to which they are hypersensitive in this way, such as nickel.

This broad interpretation of allergy means that a number of diverse mechanisms may be involved, and this is reflected in the range of oral conditions which may be due to or complicated by allergy. The important oral diseases in which allergy plays a part are shown in Table 26.19, and these will be discussed in turn.

Angioedema

Angiodema may be hereditary, acquired or idiopathic in nature. Clinically there is a recurrent non-itchy oedema commonly affecting the face, tongue, pharynx and larynx. This can lead to respiratory embarassment, and, in severe cases, death. Hereditary angioedema is a rare autosomal dominant genetic disorder due to a C1 esterase inhibitor defect. This leads to an unimpeded complement response in inflammation, causing oedema due to stress, allergy or trauma.

Acquired angioedema can arise due to abnormal antibodies against C1 esterase inhibitor, or more commonly as a reaction to drugs such as angiotensin-converting enzyme inhibitors, nonsteroidal anti-inflammatory drugs, food additives

---

Table 26.18 Aspects of immunologically mediated diseases affecting oral health care

Systemic effects affecting oral health care
    management
Immunologically mediated oral disease
Risks of abnormal reactions to drugs (e.g.
    penicillin anaphylaxis)

Table 26.19 Oral disease in which there may be an allergic component

Angioedema
Aphthae
Contact cheilitis
Erythema multiforme
Lichen planus
Orofacial granulomatosis
Plasma cell gingivitis

or latex rubber. Because of the potential serious- ness of the condition, patients require urgent management with airway maintenance to treat the acute attack. Patients should then be referred to a specialist. Those with hereditary angioedema can be treated prophylactically with stanozol or fresh frozen plasma (containing C1 esterase inhibitor), and those with acquired angioedema require avoidance advice and the availability of self- administered steroids, adrenaline or antihista- mines.

Aphthae

Many patients with recurrent aphthous stomatitis are patch test-positive to some substances, espe- cially foods and food additives, and one-third of all patients can relate the onset of some of their ulcers to the ingestion of foods (see Ch. 19). The commonest foods responsible are cheese, choco- late, nuts, tomatoes and citrus fruits, and the commonest additives are benzoates and cinna- mon aldehyde, which are often found in processed foods and carbonated drinks. It is thought that the acute inflammatory mediators released by the hypersensitivity reactions to the foods spark off the ulcerative process. Patients with troublesome ulceration should be patch tested if this facility is readily available, or asked to look for foods in their diet which they seem to per- sistently ingest prior to getting fresh ulcers. Patients can also be asked to empirically eliminate convenience foods and carbonated drinks for a few weeks to see if this is of clinical benefit.

Contact cheilitis

Patients may present with dry, flaky skin on their lips or lip swelling. This is most likely due to a contact allergy. This may be due to cosmetics, soaps or shampoos, or may be due to foods or even nickel in cutlery. Once *Candida* has been excluded, then referral for patch testing is pre- ferred. Symptomatic improvement can be obtained immediately with the use of a steroid ointment or cream. Hydrocortisone should be used in the first instance, or if this is unhelpful the condition will often respond to beta- methasone.

Erythema multiforme

This immune complex disorder, which may pres- ent as a stomatitis, cheilitis and skin lesions, is dis- cussed fully in Chapter 20. It is one of the vesiculobullous disorders. The immune complex reaction may be the result of a response to her- pesvirus or to drugs such as sulphonamides. It may also arise as a result of food or environmental 'allergy', and if no cause is found the patients should be patch tested.

Lichen planus

Lichen planus, or lichenoid reactions, are fully dis- cussed in Chapter 21. Lichenoid reactions may be the result of drug sensitivity, especially to non- steroidal anti-inflammatory drugs, hypoglycaemics or antihypertensives. They may also be seen in con- tact with amalgam restorations. Up to 40% of patients patch tested show a positive response to mercury or amalgam. Regardless, research studies suggest that some patients with clinical lichen planus will improve if their amalgams are removed even if they are patch test-negative and their lichen planus is not in obvious contact with amalgam restorations (Figs 26.9 and 26.10). Patients with severe symptomatic lichen planus should therefore be considered for removal of their amalgam fillings if this is possible. Patients with troublesome symp- toms should also be patch tested since some will be found to be allergic to foods or food additives, and improve with dietary advice and manipulation.

Orofacial granulomatosis

As described earlier in the chapter, Crohn's dis- ease may present with oral manifestations. These oral signs and symptoms also occur occasionally as mentioned earlier in sarcoidosis, and most commonly such oral problems occur without any concurrent evidence of Crohn's disease or sar- coidosis. For this reason the term 'orofacial gran- ulomatosis' has been coined to cover the clinical symptoms of orofacial lymphoedema with its associated features. Since granulomas are not clinically detectable, orofacial lymphoedema is probably the preferred term. The features of oro- facial granulomatosis, or orofacial lymphoedema, are shown in Table 26.20.

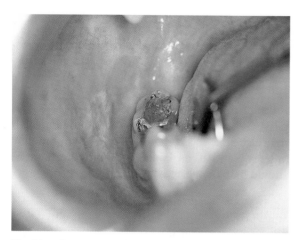

Fig. 26.9 Contact lichen planus adjacent to an amalgam restoration.

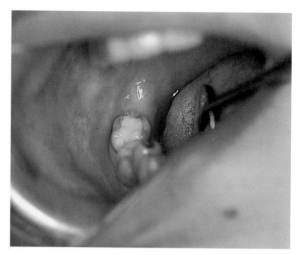

Fig. 26.10 The same patient as in Figure 26.9 after replacement of the amalgam with a composite restoration.

Table 26.20 Signs of orofacial lymphoedema

Lip swelling
Facial swelling
Angular cheilitis
Mucosal tags
Cobblestoning
Ulceration
Aphthae
Full-thickness gingivitis
Palatal (papillary) hyperplasia

The lip and facial swelling is permanent, but may increase or decrease dramatically in response to exposure to allergens as discussed below. When the lip swelling worsens, tissues become more turgid due to oedema in the tissues, and the vertical fissuring seen in association with the lip swelling becomes exaggerated (Fig. 26.11). There is almost always an associated bilateral angular cheilitis (Fig. 26.12), which improves with steroid therapy. The intraoral buccal cobblestoning and mucosal tagging is also the result of intense lymphoedema (Fig. 26.13). The ulceration may be typically aphthous in nature, especially if there is a concurrent nutritional deficiency (which is common, for example, in intestinal Crohn's disease), or there may be deep intransigent ulceration which persists indefinitely without healing (Fig. 26.14). The full-thickness gingivitis (Fig. 26.15), and less commonly hyperplastic palatal inflammation (Fig. 26.16), is due to granulomatous inflam-

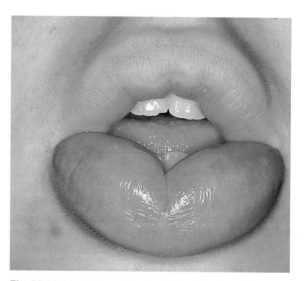

Fig. 26.11 Lower lip swelling due to lymphoedema in a patient with orofacial granulomatosis.

mation, and is particularly severe in the mixed dentition phase. Soft tissue swellings occasionally arise due to areas of non-specific infection, and may cause severe pain. The condition affects individuals of all ages, but is particularly prevalent in children and adolescents, when the emotional sequelae of the facial deformities are particularly severe.

The diagnosis is clinically obvious, but biopsy is confirmatory. Biopsy must be deep (down to

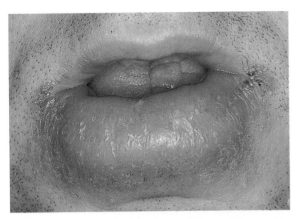

Fig. 26.12 Angular cheilitis and lip swelling in a 63-year-old man with orofacial granulomatosis.

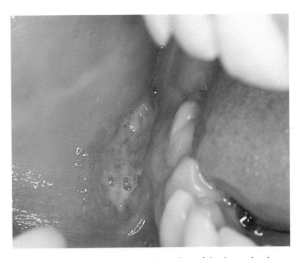

Fig. 26.14 Deep intransigent ulceration of the buccal sulcus in a 13-year-old girl with orofacial granulomatosis.

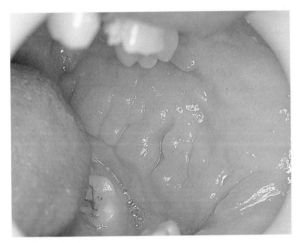

Fig. 26.13 Buccal cobblestoning in orofacial granulomatosis.

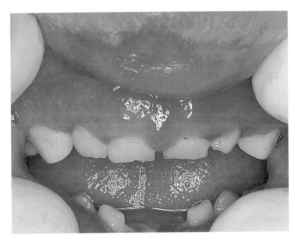

Fig. 26.15 Full-thickness gingivitis in a child with orofacial granulomatosis.

muscle) if the non-caseating granulomas are not to be missed. Other histological features include lymphocytic infiltration and intercellular oedema. Tuberculosis should be excluded. A number of other investigations are needed for successful management of orofacial lymphoedema. These include a careful history of gastrointestinal symptoms, and anyone with intestinal symptoms such as pain, rectal bleeding or diarrhoea should be investigated by a gastroenterologist to exclude intestinal disease. In children, leucocyte labelling is a non-invasive method of assessing gastrointestinal inflammation. Angiotensin-converting enzyme levels are raised in sarcoidosis, and so this

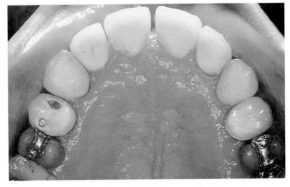

Fig. 26.16 Papillary hyperplasia of the palate in a patient with orofacial granulomatosis.

is also a useful screening test in addition to chest radiography.

As alluded to above, the central abnormality appears to be granuloma formation in the orofacial tissues which interefere with proper lymphatic drainage. When food allergy is superimposed on this problem, the condition becomes clinically obvious. About 85% of patients with orofacial lymphoedema who are patch tested will show a reaction to benzoates (E additives) or cinnamon aldehyde, as compared to 25% of controls without orofacial lymphoedema. Dietary manipulation, if this is successfully implemented, will cause significant improvement in many cases. Strict oral hygiene measures are also important, and empirical therapy with erythromycin for 3 months is occasionally helpful. Steroid therapy, either intralesional or systemic, is sometimes required to control the clinical features. Surgical reduction of the lips provides only temporary benefit in the absence of elimination of the causative factors such as foodstuffs. Antihistamines are unhelpful.

> Patients with orofacial lymphoedema may react to benzoates or cinnamon aldehyde

Plasma cell gingivitis

This condition, which usually arises due to toothpaste allergy, is discussed in Chapter 21.

Atopic disease

Drugs used in the treatment of atopic disease (particularly asthma) may complicate oral health care treatment. Antihistamines can cause drowsiness, potentiation of sedatives and hypnotics, and dry mouth. Corticosteroids are given systemically for severe asthma. They can increase susceptibility to infection, particularly oral candidosis, but more important is the risk of circulatory collapse. Sprays used to deliver corticosteroids directly to the airways can promote oropharyngeal candidosis.

Contact dermatitis to materials used in dentistry is a hazard to dentists and, especially, laboratory technicians. Methyl methacrylate monomer in particular is known to be a sensitizing agent, but contact dermatitis is surprisingly rare. The incidence of latex allergy, however, is increasing (see Ch. 12).

Autoimmune diseases

Autoimmune disease is characterized by autoantibody formation, and may be organ specific in nature or non-organ specific: the so-called connective tissue disorders or collagen diseases. The organ specific diseases with specific autoantibodies are shown in Table 26.21.

The main types of non-organ specific autoimmune disorders are shown in Table 26.22, and these are discussed in turn.

Systemic lupus erythematosus (SLE)

SLE can have effects on almost any of the body systems (Table 26.23), but oral mucosal lesions are seen in only about 20%. The oral lesions somewhat resemble lichen planus (see Chapter 21). Sjögren's syndrome may be seen.

The chief oral health care considerations are summarized in Table 26.24.

Table 26.21 Autoimmune diseases with specific autoantibodies

Pernicious anaemia[a]
Idiopathic and drug-associated thrombocytopenic purpura[a]
Drug-associated leucopenia[a]
Autoimmune haemolytic anaemia
Addison's disease[a]
Hypothyroidism (Hashimoto's thyroiditis)
Hyperthyroidism
Idiopathic hypoparathyroidism
Pemphigus vulgaris[a]
Mucous membrane pemphigoid[a]

[a]Can give rise to characteristic intraoral changes.

Table 26.22 Connective tissue diseases

Lupus erythematosus
Rheumatoid arthritis
Sjögren's syndrome
Systemic sclerosis

Table 26.23 Organs and tissues affected in SLE

Joints	Joints pains and arthritis
Skin	Rashes
Mouth	Stomatitis, Sjögren's syndrome
Serous membranes	Pleurisy, pericarditis
Heart	Endocarditis, myocarditis
Lungs	Pneumonitis
Kidneys	Nephritics
Central nervous system	Neuroses, psychoses, strokes, cranial nerve palsies
Eyes	Conjunctivitis, retinal damage
Gastrointestinal tract	Hepatomegaly, pancreatitis
Blood	Anaemia, purpura

Table 26.24 Features of systemic lupus erythematosus affecting oral health care

Corticosteroid and other immunosuppressive drugs
Painful oral lesions
Sjögren's syndrome
Bleeding tendencies (antiplatelet antibodies or anticoagulants)
Anaemia
Cardiac disease and risk of endocarditis

Discoid lupus erythematosus mainly causes mucocutaneous lesions essentially similar to those of SLE but without the latter's serological changes (see Ch. 21).

Rheumatoid arthritis

Arthritis is the most prominent feature of rheumatoid arthritis. The temporomandibular joints are frequently involved in the more severe cases (see Ch. 14). The chief importance of rheumatoid arthritis, however, is its association with Sjögren's syndrome. Drugs used in the management of rheumatoid arthritis can also affect oral health care or occasionally cause oral reactions. Care should be taken not to forcefully extend the neck, as this may cause atlantoaxial subluxation.

Sjögren's syndrome

This is discussed in Chapter 24.

Systemic sclerosis (scleroderma)

Clinically the most common early sign is Raynaud's phenomenon and joint pains. Later the skin becomes thinned, stiff and pigmented, and the facial features become smoothed out and mask-like. The oral features are summarized in Table 26.25.

Infections

The oral manifestations of infections are considered fully in Chapter 22.

Liver disease

A general consideration of liver diseases is found in Chapter 10. The main effects of liver disease relevant to dentistry are summarized in Table 26.26. Rarely, liver disease has followed oral health care treatment when halothane has been given, or as a result of transmission of viral hepatitis.

A full consideration of viral hepatitis is found in Chapter 5.

Neurological disorders

A general consideration of neurological disorders is found in Chapter 9. The oral manifestations are considered in Chapter 25.

Nutritional deficiencies

Patients with nutritional deficiencies are common in the developing world but are rarely seen

Table 26.25 Possible oral features of systemic sclerosis

Sjögren's syndrome
Limited opening
Telangiectasia
Widened periodontal ligament shadow
Gross resorption of the jaws (rarely)

Table 26.26 Important aspects of liver disease relevant to dentistry

Haemorrhagic tendencies
Impaired drug metabolism
Transmission of hepatitis
Sialosis
Lichen planus
Xerostomia
Halitosis

elsewhere. Those most liable to be affected in the West are the elderly, food cranks and alcoholics living on a grossly unbalanced diet, or patients with malabsorption. The main oral effects of vitamin deficiencies are shown in Table 26.27.

Several oral conditions of doubtful cause, such as periodontal disease, have been ascribed to vitamin deficiencies though the patient is otherwise healthy and well fed. In such cases, giving vitamin preparations brings benefit only to the multimillion pound vitamin industry.

Vitamin A

Successful treatment of keratotic plaques (leukoplakias) with retinoids (vitamin A derivatives) has been claimed but is short lived. The toxic effects of these drugs are severe, and they are teratogenic. Epidemiological studies suggest an association between low vitamin A intake and oral and other cancers.

Riboflavin (Vitamin B₂)

Riboflavin deficiency can occasionally result in angular cheilitis, consisting of red, painful fissures at the angles of the mouth, and shiny redness of the mucous membranes. The tongue is commonly sore and red. A peculiar form of glossitis in which the tongue becomes magenta in colour and granular or pebbly in appearance, due to flattening and mushrooming of the papillae, may be seen but is uncommon. The gingivae are not affected. The disorder clears up within days when riboflavin (5 mg three times a day) is given. Riboflavin is ineffective for the commonly seen cases of glossitis and angular stomatitis, which are rarely due to vitamin deficiency.

Nicotinamide

Pellagra, which affects the skin, gastrointestinal tract and nervous system, is rare but very occasionally may result from malabsorption or alcoholism. The tip and lateral margins of the tongue become red, swollen and, in severe cases, deeply ulcerated. The dorsum of the tongue becomes coated with a thick, greyish fur which is often heavily infected. The gingival margins also become red, swollen and ulcerated, and generalized stomatitis may develop.

Vitamin B_{12} and folic acid

Mouth ulcers, glossitis or angular cheilitis may result from deficiency of these vitamins (see p. 309).

Vitamin C

Scurvy is now exceedingly rare. In advanced cases, swollen bleeding gums may develop. There is no evidence that deficiency of vitamin C plays any part in periodontal disease except in frank scurvy, and there is no reason for giving ascorbic acid to healthy patients with periodontal disease.

Vitamin D

Deficiency of vitamin D during skeletal development causes rickets (see Ch. 14). However, there is no basis for the idea that dental caries is due to poor calcification of the teeth, and the giving of vitamin D and calcium for caries is valueless.

Table 26.27 Oral effects of vitamin deficiencies	
Deficiency	Oral effects
Vitamin A	Unconfirmed contribution to leukoplakia and cancer
Riboflavin (Vitamin B₂)	Angular stomatitis and glossitis
Nicotinamide	Glossitis, stomatitis and gingivitis
Vitamin B₁₂	Glossitis, aphthae
Folic acid	Glossitis, aphthae
Vitamin C	Gingival swelling
Vitamin D	Hypocalcification of teeth (severe rickets only)

Pregnancy

A general consideration of pregnancy is found in Chapter 16.

Oral effects, and oral health care management of pregnant patients are summarized in Table 26.28.

Only a minority of women in late pregnancy become hypotensive when laid supine, as a result of the swollen uterus impeding venous return; they should be treated in a sitting position or lying to one side. Respiratory reserve is decreased, and there is a risk of fetal hypoxia. Neonatal respiration is further depressed by drugs such as general anaesthetics and sedatives, especially barbiturates, diazepam and opioids, all of which cross the placenta. Local anaesthesia is generally safe. The main risks of fetal abnormalities are from drugs and radiation: the hazard is greatest during organogenesis in the first trimester. Aspirin may increase the risk of neonatal haemorrhage. Systemic corticosteroids can cause fetal adrenal suppression. However, the only drugs known to be teratogenic are thalidomide (used experimentally for major aphthae), etretinate (used experimentally for leukoplakia) and possibly azathioprine (used experimentally for Behçet's syndrome and sometimes for connective-tissue diseases). Few drugs are known to be teratogenic for humans, and in many cases the risk is no more than theoretical or results only from prolonged high dosage. For example, any teratogenic risk of metronidazole for humans has never been substantiated. Non-steroidal anti-inflammatory drugs in high dosage may cause premature closure of the ductus arteriosus and fetal pulmonary hypertension. Because of the theoretical risk of toxicity from mercury during insertion or removal of amalgams, it is recommended that these procedures should be avoided during pregnancy.

The risks from oral radiography are small, but only essential radiographs should be taken, the minimal radiation exposure should be given, and a lead apron should be worn by the patient.

Psychiatric disorders

A general discussion of psychiatric disorders can be found in Chapter 15. The oral problems seen in association with psychological problems are described in Chapter 25.

Renal disease

Renal disease has become more important in dentistry because of the increasing number of patients who, as a result of renal dialysis or transplantation, survive renal failure. Aspects of renal disease relevant to dentistry are summarized in Table 26.29.

Patients receiving regular dialysis, remain otherwise in reasonably good general health. However, they are heparinized before dialysis, and haemostasis is impaired for 6–12 h. These patients are also at greater risk of becoming carriers of hepatitis B or C.

Further, the permanent venous fistula for the dialysis lines is susceptible to infection, and antibiotic cover should be given for oral health care surgical procedures.

Renal osteodystrophy and secondary hyperparathyroidism can result from prolonged dialysis

---

Table 26.28 Pregnancy – oral and management considerations

Risks to the mother
Aggravated gingivitis and epulis formation
Variable effect on recurrent aphthae
Risk of hypotension when laid supine
Possible hypertension of pregnancy
Possible iron or folate deficiency
Vomiting, especially with general anaesthesia
Aspirin may cause neonatal haemorrhage

Risks to the fetus
Radiography hazardous, especially in first trimester
Respiratory depression due to sedatives, including
   benzodiazepines
Dental pigmentation due to tetracycline
Theoretical risk of depressed vitamin B_{12} metabolism
   by nitrous oxide
Prilocaine may rarely cause methaemoglobinaemia
Thalidomide, retinoids, azathioprine and possibly other
   drugs are teratogenic
Risk of toxicity from mercury during amalgam removal
   or insertion

Placement of amalgam restorations should be avoided during pregnancy

Table 26.29 Aspects of renal disease affecting oral health care management

Bleeding tendency
Impaired drug excretion
Possible hepatitis B or C carriage
Permanent venous fistulae susceptible to infection
Secondary hyperparathyroidism
Immunosuppressive treatment for nephrotic or transplant
  patients
Oral disease in chronic renal failure

or renal failure, and are now a more common cause than primary hyperparathyroidism of osteolytic giant cell lesions, which may first appear in the jaws.

Normal renal functions and health can be restored to renal transplant patients apart from the possible complications of prolonged immunosuppressive treatment. These patients have often also been on dialysis while awaiting a compatible donor.

Some patients with chronic renal failure are unsuitable for, or unable to obtain, dialysis or a transplant. They can show a variety of oral effects, as summarized in Table 26.30.

The factors affecting the oral health care of patients with renal disease are shown in Table 26.31.

Table 26.30 Oral changes seen in renal failure

Mucosal pallor (anaemia)
Xerostomia
Purpura
Mucosal ulceration
Candidal or bacterial plaques
White epithelial plaques
Giant cell lesions of the jaws (secondary
  hyperparathyroidism)
Drug adverse effects, e.g. gingival hyperplasia

Table 26.31 Possible factors affecting oral health care management of patients with renal disease

Corticosteroid and other immunosuppressive treatment
Bleeding tendencies
Reduced resistance to infection
Anaemia
Impaired drug excretion
Hypertension
Hepatitis B or C carriage
Underlying causes of renal failure (e.g. diabetes mellitus,
  hypertension or connective-tissue disease)

Miscellaneous orofacial lesions

There are a whole range of simple lumps and bumps and other lesions which occur in the mouth which commonly cause diagnostic problems and unnecessary concern to the patient. These may occur in any area of the mouth, including the floor of mouth, the buccal mucosa, tongue, lips and gingivae. Swellings of the floor of mouth are called ranulas (known as ranula because of the resemblance to a frog's belly). The commonest cause of a ranula is a mucocele, but carcinomas and salivary gland tumours also occur in this region.

Other miscellaneous lesions, including bony lesions, halitosis, taste disturbances and extraoral lesions, will also be discussed.

Intraoral

The common lesions occurring on the buccal mucosa include swellings, and these will be discussed below.

Buccal swellings

Differential diagnosis of simple buccal swellings is shown in Table 27.1, and these will be discussed in turn.

Carcinoma

This is discussed fully in Chapter 21.

Table 27.1 Differential diagnosis of mucosal and gingival swellings

Carcinoma
Denture-induced hyperplasia
Fibroepithelial polyp
Fibroma
Fordyce spots
Gingival swellings
Haemangioma
Lipoma
Lymphangioma
Malignancy
Neurofibroma
Papilloma
Pyogenic granuloma
Salivary gland lesions

Denture-induced hyperplasia

Where a denture flange irritates the vestibular mucosa, a linear reparative process may be initiated. In time, an elongated fibroepithelial enlargement may develop (Fig. 27.1). Several leaflets with a fairly firm consistency may develop. Such a lesion is little different in structure from a fibroepithelial polyp. Although rarely symptomatic, a denture-induced hyperplasia should be excised and examined histologically, particularly if modification of the denture does not induce the lesion to regress.

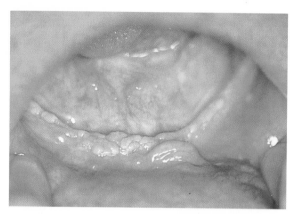

Fig. 27.1 Denture-induced hyperplasia of the lower labial sulcus in a patient with a loose-fitting denture.

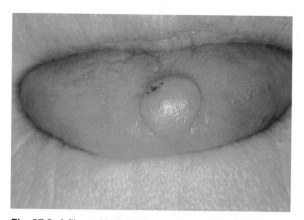

Fig. 27.2 A fibroepithelial polyp on the tip of the tongue.

Fibroepithelial polyp (fibrous lump)

When oral tissues are traumatized, healing is usually rapid and complete, with negligible scar formation. Sometimes a more vigorous and extensive healing process ensues, producing a localized tissue overgrowth which generally takes the form of a smooth, sessile or pedunculated polyp (Fig. 27.2). Such fibrous lumps are common. They may become ulcerated if traumatized but otherwise are usually asymptomatic, and some patients tolerate such polyps for months or years. They tend to be soft, especially if they have been chewed by the patient, and are often misdiagnosed as 'lipomas'. If they are interfering with the patient's chewing or the patient is concerned, the fibrous lump should be excised with its entire base and examined histologically.

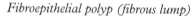

> Most buccal 'lumps' are fibrous polyps

Fibroma

The true fibroma – a benign neoplasm of fibroblastic origin – is rare in the oral cavity. It is probable that many lesions called fibromas in the past were actually fibroepithelial polyps. The true fibroma is a continuously enlarging new growth, not necessarily arising at a site of potential trauma. It is a pedunculated growth with a smooth non-ulcerated pink surface. Removal should be total.

Fordyce spots

These are ectopic sebaceous glands, and look like grains of sand under the mucosa (Fig. 27.3). They occur in about 50% of the population, and can be quite noticeable. They are totally harmless, and require no active treatment other than reassuring the patient of the benign nature of these 'lesions'.

Gingival swellings

Fibrous epulides should be removed down to the periosteum, which should be curetted thoroughly. Such excision will create an open wound which should be dressed. Removal of a large epulis from the labial aspect of the maxillary gingiva may create an unsightly gingival defect, about which patients should be warned in advance.

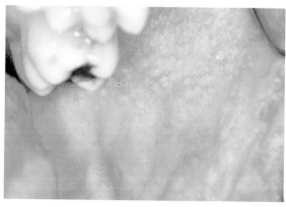

Fig. 27.3 Fordyce spots on the buccal mucosa.

Giant cell epulis. The giant cell epulis characteristically arises interdentally, adjacent to permanent teeth which have had deciduous predecessors (Fig. 27.4). Classically, the most notable feature is the deep-red colour, although older lesions tend to be paler. The resorption of deciduous teeth and remodelling of the alveolus at the mixed dentition stage indicate the osteoclastic potential of the area from which giant cell epulides arise. The lesion probably arises because chronic irritation triggers a reactionary hyperplasia of mucoperiosteum and excessive production of granulation tissue. Giant cell granulomas are also a feature of hyperparathyroidism, and levels of plasma calcium, phosphate and alkaline phosphatase should therefore be assayed and the area examined radiographically.

Pregnancy gingivitis and pregnancy epulis. Pregnancy gingivitis is characterized by soft, reddish enlargements, usually of the gingival papillae. The lumps vary from small smooth enlargements to more extensive, ragged, granular lumps which sometimes resemble the surface of a strawberry. A similar appearance may complicate the use of oral contraceptives. Sometimes there is a localized epulis – a pregnancy epulis. Poor oral hygiene predisposes to these changes. Changes of pregnancy gingivitis usually appear about the second month of pregnancy, and reach a peak at the eighth month. They may revert soon after parturition to the previous level of gingival health. Therefore, conservative treatment is indicated unless an epulis interferes with occlusion or is extremely unsightly – when it can be excised. The patient's chief concern is usually of gingival bleeding, particularly on eating or toothbrushing. This tendency to bleed is an indication of the considerable vascularity of the affected tissues. Histologically, a pregnancy epulis is a pyogenic granuloma.

> Most pregnancy epulides resolve postpartum

Lumps and swellings related to drug therapy. This is a particularly important cause of gingival swelling to consider since it may be possible to change the drug. Improving the oral hygiene is

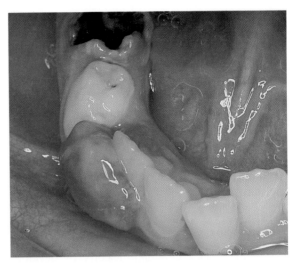

Fig. 27.4 A giant cell epulis affecting the lower arch in a child.

necessary and gingival surgery may also be needed. Enlargements related to oral contraceptives are referred to in the previous section.

The anticonvulsant phenytoin (Epanutin or Dilantin), used mainly for the control of grand mal epilepsy, can produce a variable extent of gingival enlargement, which characteristically affects the interstitial tissues first but which may later involve the marginal and even attached gingiva. The buccal and labial gingiva are mainly involved. The enlargement rarely affects edentulous sites. It is characteristically firm, pale and tough, with course stippling (Fig. 27.5).

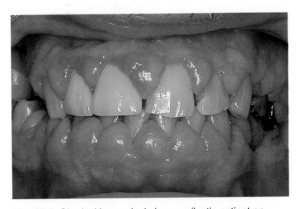

Fig. 27.5 Gingival hyperplasia in an epileptic patient on long-term phenytoin.

Nifedipine (an antihypertensive agent) and other calcium channel blockers may cause gingival hyperplasia typically affecting the papillae, which become red and puffy and tend to bleed.

The immunosuppressive drug cyclosporin is particularly used to suppress the cell-mediated response after organ transplants. One side-effect is gingival hyperplasia, initially of papillae.

Eruption cyst. Occasionally a cyst develops over an erupting tooth. This appears as a bluish swelling over the tooth, and is treated simply by incision.

Haemangioma

Haemangiomas are benign lesions of developmental origin – hamartomas. They may be capillary or cavernous. They are seen most often on the tongue or lip, as bluish or purplish soft lesions (Fig. 27.6). The characteristic feature is that they blanch on pressure, or contain blood on aspiration with a needle and syringe. They may not need treatment, but if they do for aesthetic or functional reasons, they can often be treated with cryosurgery or laser. Very large haemangiomas may need to be treated by the surgeon with embolization. Occasionally, intraoral haemangiomas may be associated with the Sturge–Weber syndrome, a congenital syndrome comprising angiomas of the face, angiomas of the lep-

tomeninges, intracranial calcification, mental retardation, contralateral hemiplegia and epilepsy (Fig. 27.7).

Lipoma

This benign neoplasm presents as a slow-growing, spherical, smooth and soft semifluctuant lump with a characteristic yellowish colour caused by the fat which makes up the bulk of the lesion. It is far less common than a fibroepithelial polyp.

Lymphangioma

Lymphangioma is of similar structure to a haemangioma, but contains lymph rather than blood.

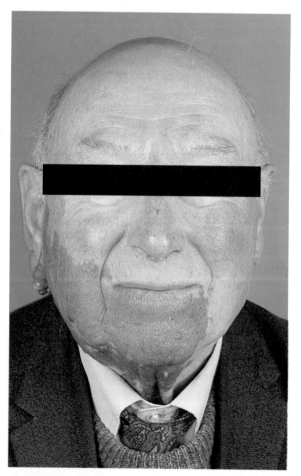

Fig. 27.7 Facial angioma in a patient with Sturge–Weber syndrome.

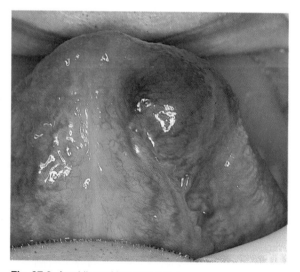

Fig. 27.6 A sublingual haemangioma.

It is uncommon in the mouth, and often has a 'frogspawn' appearance. It is treated in the same way as a haemangioma.

Malignancy

Malignant tumours are discussed elsewhere, but obviously enter the differential diagnosis of a buccal lump. These lesions may be haematogenous (e.g. leukaemia or lymphoma) as well as carcinomas, Kaposi's sarcoma and metastatic tumours.

Neurofibroma

Neurofibroma is an uncommon lesion, and typically affects the tongue. It represents a benign overgrowth of all elements of a peripheral nerve (axon cylinder, Schwann cells, and fibrous connective tissue), arranged in a variety of patterns.

Neurofibromas may occur multiply as a feature of neurofibromatosis (von Recklinghausen's disease) (Fig. 27.8) and rarely may undergo sarcomatous change.

Papilloma

This benign neoplasm of epithelium, caused by papillomaviruses, appears most often at the junction of the hard and soft palates (Fig. 27.9). The papilloma is a cauliflower-like lesion with a whitish colour, and may resemble a wart. Papillomas of normal colour may be confused with the commoner fibroepithelial polyps, although the latter are commonest at sites of potential trauma. Unlike papilloma virus lesions of the uterine cavity, which may undergo malignant transformation, papillomas in the oral cavity appear to remain benign. However, oral papillomas should be removed and examined histologically to establish a correct diagnosis. Excision must be total, deep and wide enough to include any virally infected cells beyond the zone of the pedicle.

Pyogenic granuloma

A pyogenic granuloma appears to represent an excessive reaction to trauma or infection. The lesion usually affects the lip or tongue, and may grow to 1 cm or more in diameter (Fig. 27.10). Basically red in colour, with a thin or ulcerated epithelium, it may bleed readily if traumatized. Clinically, a pyogenic granuloma may occasionally resemble a capillary haemangioma. These lesions should be excised, but will readily recur if excision is not adequate. A major point of difference between the pyogenic granuloma and capillary haemangioma is that the latter usually contains few inflammatory cells. The histological

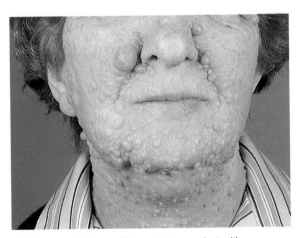

Fig. 27.8 Multiple neurofibromata in a patient with von Recklinghausen's disease.

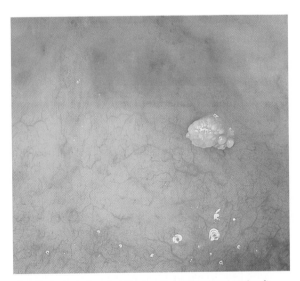

Fig. 27.9 A viral wart at the junction of the hard and soft palate.

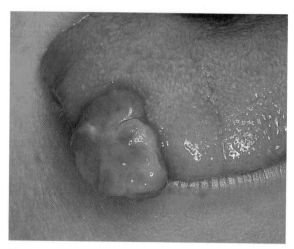

Fig. 27.10 A large pyogenic granuloma on the tongue of a 30-year-old female.

Table 27.2 Brown or black lesions affecting the oral mucosa

Localized	Amalgam tattoo
	Kaposi's sarcoma
	Malignant melanoma
	Naevus
	Peutz–Jeghers syndrome
	Pigmentary incontinence
Generalized	Addison's disease
	Drugs
	Racial and familial
	Smoking

features of the so-called pregnancy epulis are identical to those of pyogenic granuloma (see above).

Salivary gland lesions

These are discussed fully in Chapter 24.

Brown or black lesions

Extrinsic staining

Extrinsic staining is most commonly a problem of the teeth. If the mucosa is affected it is usually the tongue which displays extrinsic staining, and this is discussed under tongue lesions.

Intrinsic staining

The commonest causes of intrinsic brown lesions of the oral mucosa are shown in Table 27.2.

Amalgam tattoo. Amalgam tattoos are common causes of blue-black pigmentation seen in the mandibular gingiva or at least close to the teeth, or in the scar of an apicectomy where there has been a retrograde root filling (Fig. 27.11). Amalgam incorporated into the wound causes a tattoo. Radio-opacities may or may not be seen on radiography. These lesions are innocuous, although biopsy may be indicated to exclude a naevus or melanoma if clinical doubt exists.

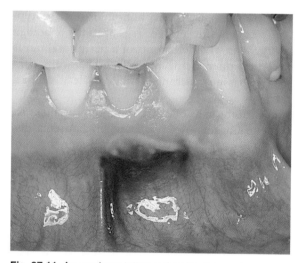

Fig. 27.11 An amalgam tattoo at the site of a previous apicectomy.

Kaposi's sarcoma. This will be discussed under bluish lesions.

Malignant melanoma. Malignant melanoma may arise in apparently normal mucosa or in a pre-existing pigmented naevus, usually in the palate (Fig. 27.12). Features suggestive of malignancy include a rapid increase in size, change in colour, ulceration, pain, the occurrence of satellite pigmented spots or regional lymph node enlargement.

> A change in size or colour, ulceration, pain, satellite lesions or neck nodes suggests a malignant melanoma

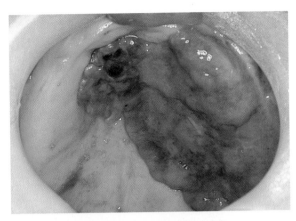

Fig. 27.12 A malignant melanoma of the palate.

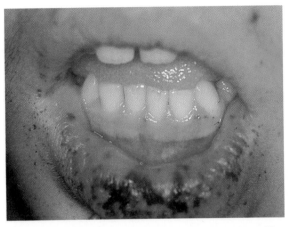

Fig. 27.14 Perioral and labial pigmentation in a patient with Peutz–Jegher syndrome.

Naevus. Pigmented naevi are seen particularly on the vermilion border of the lip and on the palate (Fig. 27.13). These lesions are usually brown, macular, do not change rapidly in size or colour, and are painless. Excision biopsy is recommended for cosmetic reasons, to exclude malignancy, and because of the premalignant potential of some – particularly junctional naevi.

Peutz–Jegher syndrome. The Peutz–Jegher syndrome shows characteristic perioral pigmentation resembling freckles (Fig. 27.14), and is associated with gastroduodenal polyps in about 40% of patients. Endoscopic removal of these polyps is advocated to prevent intussusception. There is also a risk of malignant transformation in these polyps.

Pigmentary incontinence. When there is chronic irritation, for example from occlusal trauma, this is typically associated with a frictional keratosis. Occasionally, however, it may also produce mucosal pigmentation (Fig. 27.15), which histologically is called pigmentary incontinence. This also occurs in smokers (see below).

Addison's disease. Addison's disease (adrenocortical hypofunction) is usually autoimmune (idiopathic). Previously it was commonly due to tuberculosis, and this cause is becoming more common in those with HIV disease. Hyperpigmentation is generalized but most obvious in areas normally pigmented (e.g. the areolae of nipples, genitalia, skin flexures, and sites of trauma). The oral mucosa may show patchy hyperpigmentation (Fig. 27.16). Generally, however, the patient feels unwell and is hypotensive. It is extremely unlikely that Addison's disease would be found to be the cause of intraoral pigmentation in an apparently healthy fit adult patient: most have weight loss, hypotension and weakness. The diagnosis of Addison's disease is discussed in Chapter 13.

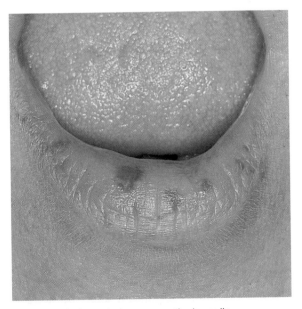

Fig. 27.13 A pigmented naevus on the lower lip.

> Addison's disease is unlikely in an apparently fit patient with pigmentation

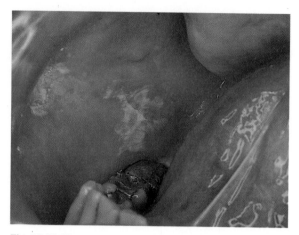

Fig. 27.15 Pigmentation associated with frictional keratosis.

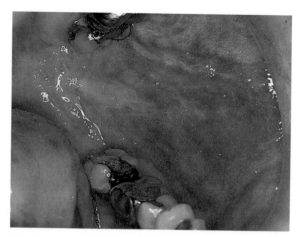

Fig. 27.17 Racial pigmentation of the buccal mucosa in an Asian patient.

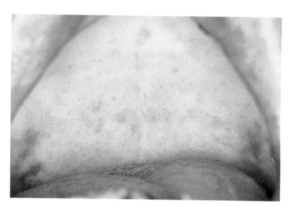

Fig. 27.16 Intraoral pigmentation in a patient with Addison's disease.

Drugs. Intraoral pigmentation is sometimes the result of taking certain drugs, particularly anti-malarials, oral contraceptives and phenothiazines. The recent onset of patchy pigmentation in a patient taking such medication can be presumed due to the drug.

Racial and familial. Probably the commonest cause of generalized patchy pigmentation is racial or familial. Dark-skinned individuals often have patchy pigmentation (Fig. 27.17), especially of their attached gingivae, and these sometimes seem to change over a period of time, causing the patient concern. Reassurance is all that is required.

Smoking. Smoking is a cause of general irritation to the oral mucosa, and sometimes smok-ing-related keratoses are also associated with pigmentation.

Management

Most pigmented lesions are innocent and only require patient reassurance. If an amalgam tattoo is suspected, a radiograph will often show submucosal amalgam. If clinical doubt exists about the diagnosis or the patient is anxious, a biopsy is diagnostic.

Bluish lesions

Haemangiomas, Kaposi's sarcoma, and some cysts may present with a bluish appearance, as may some drug-induced pigmentation. Central cyanosis may also cause a bluish discoloration of the oral mucosa.

Haemangioma

This lesion has been discussed above (see p. 332).

Kaposi's sarcoma

This lesion is discussed fully in Chapters 5 and 23.

Tongue lesions

Various conditions specifically affect the tongue, and it is convenient to discuss these together from a diagnostic and management point of view. The most prevalent lesions affecting the tongue are shown in Table 27.3.

Black or brown hairy tongue

Black hairy tongue (Fig. 27.18) affects the posterior dorsum of the tongue; the filiform papillae are excessively long and stained. Black and brown hairy tongue appears to be caused by the accumulation of epithelial squames and the proliferation of chromogenic microorganisms. Patients with black hairy tongue may find the condition to be improved by increasing their standard of oral hygiene, brushing the tongue with a toothbrush or using sodium perborate or sodium bicarbonate mouthwashes. Occasionally, a black hairy tongue may be caused by antimicrobial therapy, especially with broad-spectrum drugs such as tetracyclines. The latter condition is related to overgrowth of *Candida* species and may respond to withdrawal of the drug.

Table 27.3 Common tongue lesions
Black or brown hairy tongue
Geographic tongue
Glossitis
Fissured tongue
Normal structures

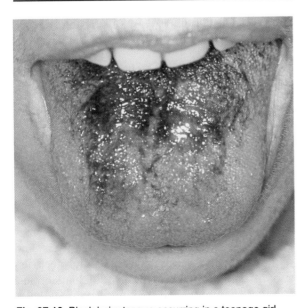

Fig. 27.18 Black hairy tongue occurring in a teenage girl.

A common problem is that of furred tongue. Coating of the tongue is quite commonly seen in healthy adults, particularly in edentulous patients, those who are on a soft, non-abrasive diet, those with poor oral hygiene, or those who are fasting. The coating in these instances appears to be of epithelial, food and microbial debris, which collects since it is not mechanically removed. Indeed, the tongue is the main reservoir of some microorganisms such as *Candida albicans* and some streptococci. The coating appears more obvious in xerostomia and in ill patients, especially those with poor oral hygiene, those who have a febrile illness, or those who are dehydrated.

Superficial brown staining of the teeth and soft tissues, often the dorsum of the tongue, may be caused by cigarette smoking, some drugs (such as iron salts), some foods and beverages (such as coffee and tea), and chlorhexidine. Such discoloration is easily removed, and is of little consequence.

Geographic tongue (erythema migrans or benign migratory glossitis)

Geographic tongue is a peculiar condition which affects all ages, from babies to the elderly. It is also known as migratory glossitis or erythema migrans. It usually affects the tongue, although less commonly it may affect other oral mucosal sites. It is characterized by erythematous patches surrounded by a margin of white pinhead lesions, which start by completely surrounding the erythematous patch but then break up, leaving a 'gap' in the periphery (Fig. 27.19). The patch tends to expand and spread away from the gap, with the small pinhead lesions at the advancing front. These white pinhead lesions are intramucosal microabscesses, and histologically the condition resembles psoriasis, although there is no reliable connection between these two diseases, and psoriasis is seldom seen in the mouth.

Geographic tongue may be quite severe, and in these circumstances tends to cause lobulation and fissuring of the tongue (see later). Because of the atrophic nature of the erythematous patches, patients tend to have tongues which are sensitive to hot or spicy foods, although this is widely variable between patients, and may not be related to

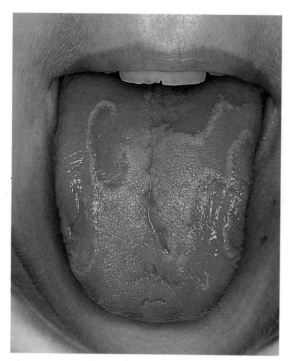

Fig. 27.19 Geographic tongue.

the apparent clinical severity. Patients who complain of a sensitive tongue should be investigated as if they had non-specific glossitis, since the two conditions may coexist (see below).

Geographic tongue is a condition with a genetic predisposition, as demonstrated by HLA associations; there are no known disease associations such as nutritional deficiencies or systemic disease, and so patients should be reassured about the benign nature of the condition. Mouthwashes and topical steroids are unhelpful, although some patients empirically improve with zinc sulphate three times daily for 3 months.

Glossitis

Glossitis is a term used to describe the symptom of tongue discomfort. Glossopyrosis (burning tongue) and glossodynia (painful tongue) are archaic alternative terms. The commonest cause is functional dysaesthesia, but several organic causes exist which must be excluded (Table 27.4).

Atrophic glossitis occurs in deficiencies of iron, folic acid and vitamin B_{12} (Moeller's glossitis).

Table 27.4 Organic causes of glossitis
Atrophic
Frictional
Geographic
Infection

There may be a coexisting anaemia but the atrophy of the lingual epithelium is due to the nutritional deficiency rather than the anaemia, and, indeed, may antedate the appearance of peripheral blood changes. Moreover, the tongue may be symptomatic or frankly painful before epithelial atrophy is clinically evident, and so nutritional deficiencies should be excluded when a patient complains of a painful tongue, even if it looks normal. As a result, it is often difficult to be confident about differentiating a functional dysaesthesia or burning tongue from a nutritional glossitis, and in these circumstances, blood tests are indicated. The factors suggesting a functional component to a patient's glossitis are discussed in Chapter 25.

When atrophy occurs, the filiform papillae are lost, and the dorsum of the tongue becomes smooth, glassy and erythematous (see Fig. 26.2). There may be other associated tissue signs of deficiency, such as aphthae, angular cheilitis or intraoral candidosis. Replacement therapy restores the appearance of the tongue to normal and renders the patient asymptomatic. An underlying systemic cause for a nutritional deficiency should always be pursued.

Geographic tongue has already been discussed above. Infectious causes such as candidosis or staphylococcal mucositis should also be excluded, by microbiological sampling with a swab or saline rinse, if clinical doubt exists. Erythematous candidosis may specifically present as median rhomboid glossitis, and this is discussed fully in Chapter 22.

Fissuring of the tongue may present in a number of ways: the tongue may be regularly fissured as an inherited phenomenon – the so-called scrotal tongue (Fig. 27.20). This is harmless and requires no intervention. Occasionally, deep fissuring is seen with chronic candidal infections, and these fissures may be painful. Antifungal therapy improves the situation. Patients with severe

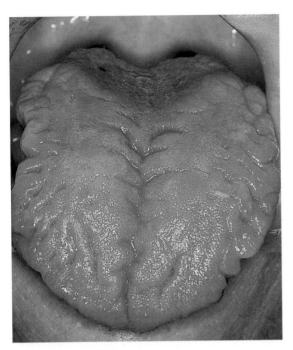

Fig. 27.20 Scrotal (plicated) tongue.

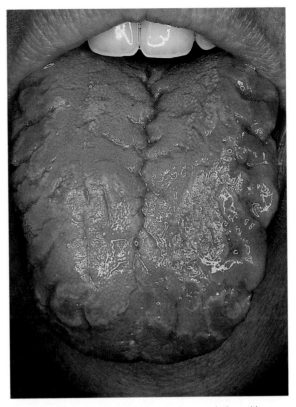

Fig. 27.21 Geographic tongue seen in association with fissuring and lobulation of the tongue.

geographic tongue tend to get lingual swelling, resulting in lobulation of the tongue, which may become quite dramatic (Fig. 27.21). Patients with long-standing xerostomia also display a characteristic cobblestone appearance on the dorsum of their tongues (see Fig. 24.11). Finally, the tongue may become crenated due to either the tongue swelling (rarely amyloid causes macroglossia) (see Ch. 26) or due to the tongue pressing against the teeth. This is usually a sign of stress.

Occasionally, patients present with concern regarding the appearance of their tongue, and examination reveals that they are worried about a normal structure. This is usually the foliate papillae area which has been noticed (Fig. 27.22). Pointing out the bilateral nature of these 'lesions' ('foliate papillitis') helps the reassurance process. The circumvallate papillae also give rise for concern when the patient has protruded his or her tongue far enough to see these structures. This is more easy in patients who have no lower natural dentition. Lastly, patients may become alarmed about the appearance of the sublingual salivary glands and duct orifices, and require firm reassurance about the normality of these structures.

Lip lesions

The most frequently encountered lesions affecting the lip are discussed elsewhere, such as allergic cheilitis, angular cheilitis, carcinoma and mucocele. Angiomas, as discussed previously, may be more noticeable on the lip.

Lip fissures may present as part of the lip swelling seen in patients with orofacial lymphoedema, but may also occur for no apparent reason, and are commoner in winter months. Lip fissures are often very intransigent, and the dryness and fissuring does not significantly improve with hydrocortisone cream. Patients should try a strong steroid cream such as betamethasone prescribed by their doctor, and if this fails to improve the situation the patient may need the fissure stretched under local anaesthetic to encourage healing, or in extreme circumstances surgical excision of the fissure area is indicated.

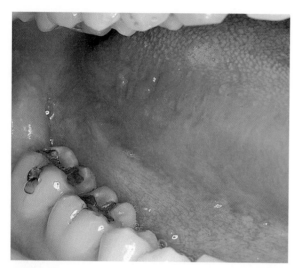

Fig. 27.22 Normal foliate papillae on the lateral margin of the tongue.

Bony lesions

Osteodystrophies fall within the realm of oral surgical practice and are not discussed further here. They are, however, considered in Chapter 14. Benign osteomas, however, commonly present as diagnostic problems. They may occur as mandibular tori or torus palatinus. These are developmental benign exostoses with a smooth or nodular surface. Torus palatinus occurs in the centre of the hard palate (Fig. 27.23); torus

mandibularis is lingual to the lower premolars, and is usually bilateral (Fig. 27.24).

Multiple osteomas may also occur in the alveolar bone (Fig. 27.25), and the tuberosities may also undergo benign enlargement, although this is frequently not osseous but simply fibrous. Reassurance is the treatment of choice unless they are causing mechanical problems, when they should be surgically removed.

Gardner's syndrome, which is characterized by multiple osteomas, is discussed in Chapter 26.

Halitosis

Halitosis or 'bad breath' is a common complaint. It usually arises due to bacterial odour from oral infection (e.g. secondary to a primary herpes infection) or simply poor oral hygiene. Infections of the sinuses or respiratory tract may occasionally cause a similar problem, and there are several other miscellaneous causes to be excluded, especially smoking (Table 27.5).

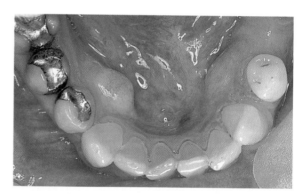

Fig. 27.24 Bilateral torus mandibularis.

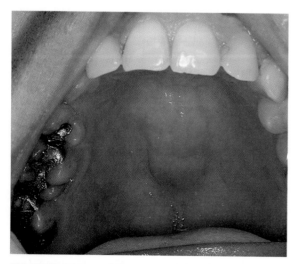

Fig. 27.23 A torus palatinus.

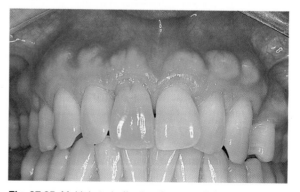

Fig. 27.25 Multiple tori affecting the upper labial alveolus.

Table 27.5 Causes of halitosis

Smoking
Starvation
Xerostomia
Drugs
Foods, e.g. garlic
Gastrointestinal disease
Oral infections
Psychogenic
Renal failure
Respiratory tract infections
Cirrhosis
Diabetic ketosis

Some patients, however, present complaining of halitosis when their mouth is clean and uninfected. In these circumstances the problem is usually psychogenic and a perceived problem either for the patient only or occasionally his or her partner.

Treatment comprises correcting the underlying cause, and when this is psychogenic, reassurance can be reinforced with the use of a hydrogen peroxide or perborate mouthwash, since regular treatment with these will optimize oral hygiene and provide reassurance to the patient.

Disturbance of taste

Disorders affecting taste are shown in Table 27.6.

Taste and olfaction are both susceptible to the general sensory phenomenon known as adapta-tion, i.e. the progressive reduction in the appreciation of a stimulus during the course of continual exposure to that stimulus.

Probably the most common causes of loss of senses of taste and smell are viral upper respiratory tract infections which affect olfaction, but also, thereby, decrease the appreciation of food. Olfaction may also be impaired after head injuries, due to tearing of olfactory fibres, and in ageing.

Dry mouth for any reason can distort taste, as can drugs (particularly penicillamine and captopril), nutritional deficiencies (especially of zinc), ageing, and various disorders.

Lesions in the nose (especially respiratory infections) or in the olfactory pathway may cause anosmia. Other causes of anosmia include some endocrine disorders (especially hypothyroidism), Parkinson's disease, and some other cerebral disorders. Unilateral anosmia is often unnoticed by the patient.

Both olfaction and taste are susceptible to genetic and hormonal factors. For example, sensitivity to the bitter taste of phenylthiourea is genetically determined, and some other patients are genetically unable, for example, to smell fish. There appear to be no significant differences in the senses of olfaction and taste between sexes, but both senses vary through the menstrual cycle and may be distorted during pregnancy, often with the appearance of cravings for unusual foods.

Disorders of these senses can be distressing and sometimes incapacitating, and can cause anorexia and depression. The causes of an unpleasant taste are shown in Table 27.7.

Extraoral

Facial swelling

Swelling of the face is common after trauma, and often associated with infections of dental origin, but may also arise from a number of varying pathologies which should be included in the differential diagnosis (Table 27.8).

Neck lumps

Occasionally the salivary glands, thyroid gland or other structures may cause neck swellings. More

Table 27.6 Disorders affecting taste

Local disorders	Xerostomia
	Sepsis
	Various foods
	Irradiation or burns
	Zinc and other deficiencies
	Cytotoxic drugs
Disorders affecting cranial nerves	Damage to lingual nerve, chorda tympani or facial nerve
	Bell's palsy
Cerebral disorders	Brain tumours
Others	Psychogenic disorders
	Smoking
	Old age
	Cancer
	Cirrhosis
	Drugs

Table 27.7 Causes of unpleasant taste

Dental infections
Nasal sinus or pharyngeal disease
Salivary gland disorders causing xerostomia
Psychogenic causes
Drugs
   Drugs causing dry mouth
   Metronidazole, lithium, gold, etc.
Gastric regurgitation

Table 27.8 Causes of facial swelling

Inflammatory	Infections
	Bites
	Crohn's disease
	(orofacial granulomatosis)
	Sarcoidosis
Traumatic	Injury
	Postoperative
	Surgical emphysema
Immunologically	
mediated	Angioedema
Other	Masseteric hypertrophy

diffuse swelling of the neck may be caused by infection, haematoma, oedema, surgical emphysema or, rarely, a neoplasm. However, by far the most common causes of lumps in the neck are swollen lymph nodes.

The site of the lump in the neck will give a good indication of the tissue of origin, and the age of the patient suggests the most likely diagnosis. The duration of the lesion is clearly relevant: one that has been present since an early age is likely to be of congenital origin, while a lymph node enlargement appearing in later life and persisting may be malignant.

Lymph node swellings

Swollen lymph nodes in the neck are common, and therefore an important part of the examination of every dental patient is inspection and palpation of the cervical lymph nodes. Most frequent is an enlarged jugulodigastric (tonsillar) lymph node, inflamed secondary to a viral upper respiratory tract infection.

Nodes also enlarge in oral infections or local infections in the drainage area (virtually anywhere

The commonest neck lumps are swollen lymph nodes

in the head and neck). Enlarged cervical lymph nodes may also be related to malignant disease in the drainage area (e.g. carcinoma) or may be a manifestation of systemic disease (e.g. HIV, leukaemia or lymphoma).

Lymph nodes that are increasing in size and that are tender may be inflammatory. Those that are hard or rubbery may be malignant. Lymphadenopathy in the anterior triangle of the neck alone is often due to local disease, especially if the nodes are enlarged on only one side, or occasionally glandular fever. Generalized lymphadenopathy with or without enlargement of other lymphoid tissue such as liver and spleen (hepatosplenomegaly), however, suggests a systemic cause.

The local cause of lymph node enlargement may not always be found despite a careful search. For example, children occasionally develop a *Staphylococcus aureus* or mycobacterial lymphadenitis (usually in a submandibular node) in the absence of any obvious portal of infection. More serious is the finding of an enlarged node suspected to be malignant but where the primary neoplasm cannot be found. Nasopharyngeal carcinoma is a classic cause of this, and the opinion of an ear, nose and throat specialist should therefore be sought.

Lymph nodes may also swell when there are disorders involving the immune system more gen-

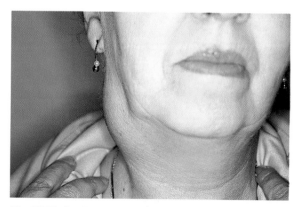

Fig. 27.26 Swollen cervical lymph nodes.

erally, such as the glandular fever syndromes, HIV and various other infections. In the systemic infective disorders such as tuberculosis, the nodes are usually firm, discrete, tender and mobile. Enlarged nodes are also found in neoplasms such as lymphomas and leukaemias (Table 27.9 and Fig. 27.26). In the lymphomas, particularly, the nodes may be rubbery, matted together and fixed to deeper structures, and in these lymphoproliferative states there is usually enlargement of the liver and spleen (hepatosplenomegaly).

> Enlarged, tender neck nodes tend to be inflammatory

Table 27.9 Causes of cervical lymph node enlargement

Inflammatory	Infective	Local	Bacterial, e.g. dental abscess Viral, e.g. herpes simplex
		Systemic	Bacterial, e.g. tuberculosis or syphilis Viral, e.g. glandular fever or HIV
	Non-infective	Sarcoidosis Crohn's disease Connective tissue diseases	
Malignancy	Primary	Leukaemias Lymphomas	
	Secondary	Metastases	

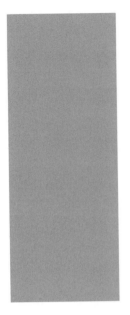

Index

Rosemary

This book is dedicated to all my very good friends.

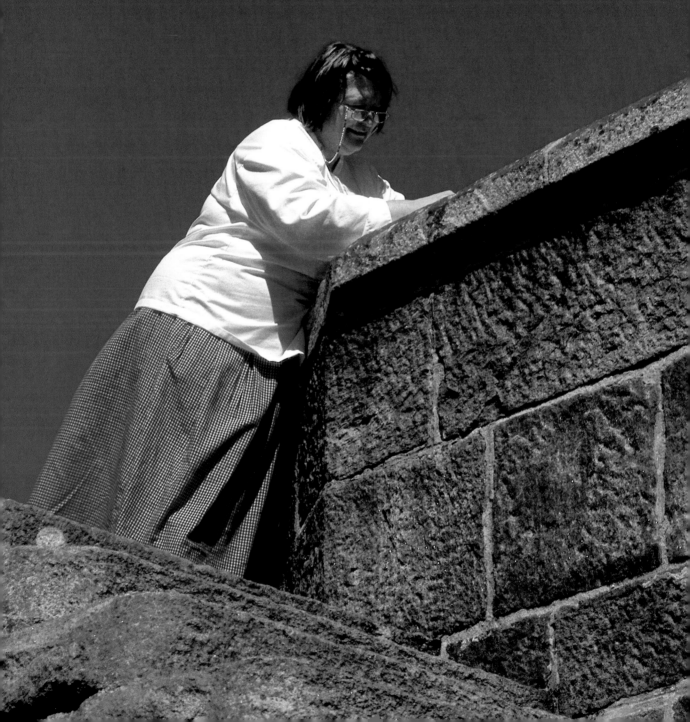

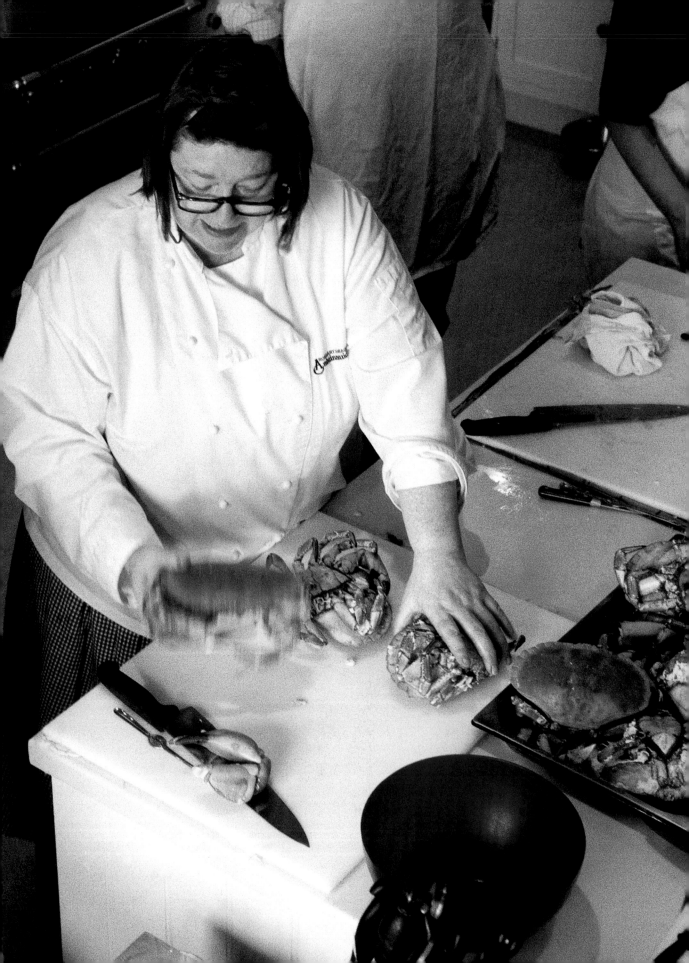

Rosemary

Castle Cook

Recipes from Rosemary Shrager's
Cookery School on the Isle of Harris

Photographs by
Christopher Simon Sykes

Text by Rosemary Shrager
and Sue Gaisford

ADELPHI PUBLISHERS

Rosemary, Castle Cook
Recipes from Rosemary Shrager's Cookery School
on the Isle of Harris

Published by Adelphi Publishers, London

Text by Rosemary Shrager and Sue Gaisford
Photographs by Christopher Simon Sykes

Designed by Broadbase

© 2001 Everyman Publishers Plc
© 2009 Adelphi Publishers
Text copyright © Rosemary Shrager and Sue Gaisford
Photographs © Christopher S. Sykes /
The Interior Archive

Adelphi Publishers
Northburgh House
10 Northburgh St
London EC1V 0AT
books@everyman.uk.com

ISBN 978-0-9562387-1-9

Printed and colour separated in the Far East.

Contents

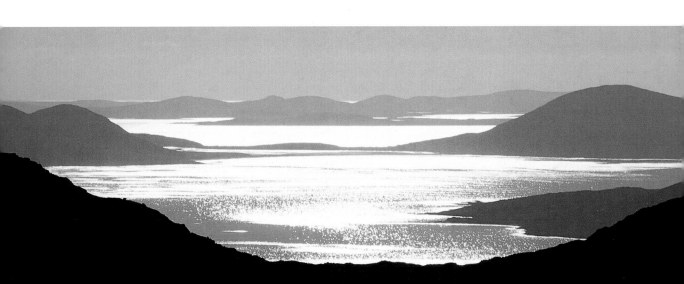

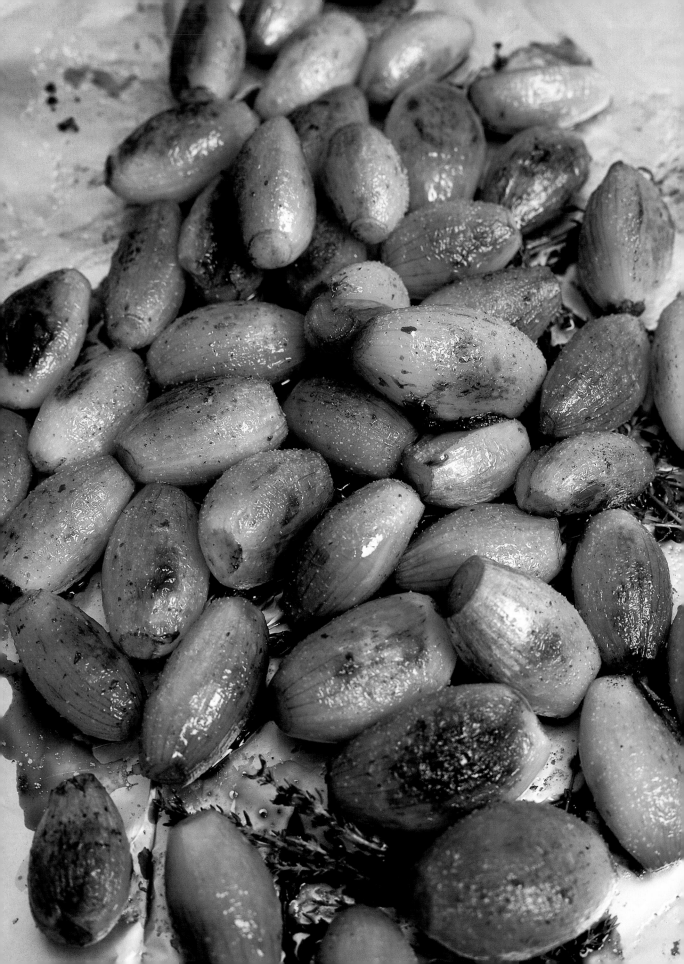

Rosemary is a very courageous woman always striving for perfection. She has an instinctive feel and passion for both finding and respecting the best raw ingredients. I know that Rosemary is one of the very best, and that her natural modesty as well as her relentless search for perfection are a gift of God.

She is also a great teacher with a tremendous ability to communicate her passion. Her chocolates are a must. And her smile is so heartwarming.

Pierre Koffmann

Why buy another cookery book? It's a

hard question to answer. All I can say is that I have hundreds. One of my most treasured possessions, for example, is a little book by Edouard de Pomiane, illustrated by Toulouse-Lautrec and published at the turn of the last century. I can never resist bookshops and I still haunt them, hoping always to come across, say, a Brillat-Savarin, a rare first edition of Hannah Glasse, or a collection of brilliant ideas by a cook I've never come across before.

This book is largely inspired by the magnificent fresh ingredients to be found on the Isle of Harris. I went there to cook for the season and loved it so much that now I seem likely never to leave this enchanted place. The fish, particularly, is the best and freshest I have ever found, and the sweet lamb and lean venison from the hill would make any cook leap at the chance to do her very best with them. But thanks to modern marketing and communication, most of these ingredients can now be found in supermarkets all over the world.

I have worked for some of the best chefs of our time – particularly Pierre Koffmann and Jean-Christophe Novelli, for whose encouragement I am profoundly grateful. My style is based on classic French tradition, with my own personal twist. Sometimes I literally dream up recipes at night, sometimes I am fired by a sudden idea and experiment until I find what I consider the very best way of putting it into practice.

Although I have usually suggested the ideal way of achieving the desired effect, I do hope that you will improvise and experiment with these recipes. Not everyone can have a flourishing herb garden, or several stock-pots on the go at the same time, and occasionally dried herbs, a bought bouillon or a stock-cube will have to be used. Don't worry. Above all, don't forget that good cooking will generate laughter, friendship and camaraderie. It really should be fun!

I hope that you will find plenty to read and enjoy in this book, and that one day I might see you on a cookery course.

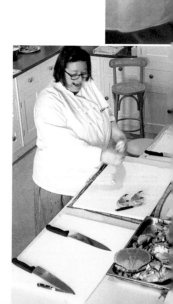

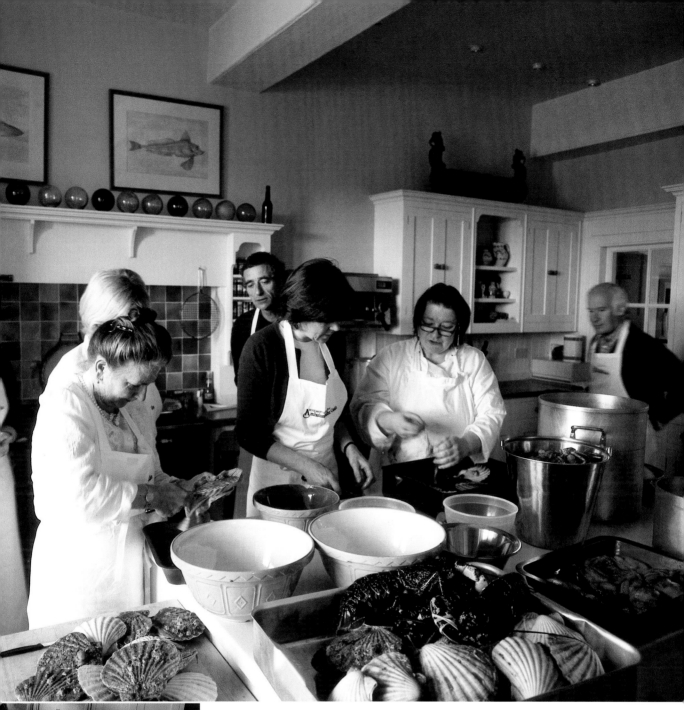

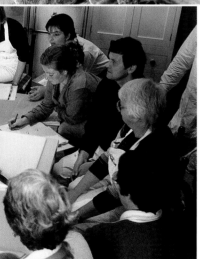

A morning shellfish class at Rosemary's Cookery School.

Shellfish

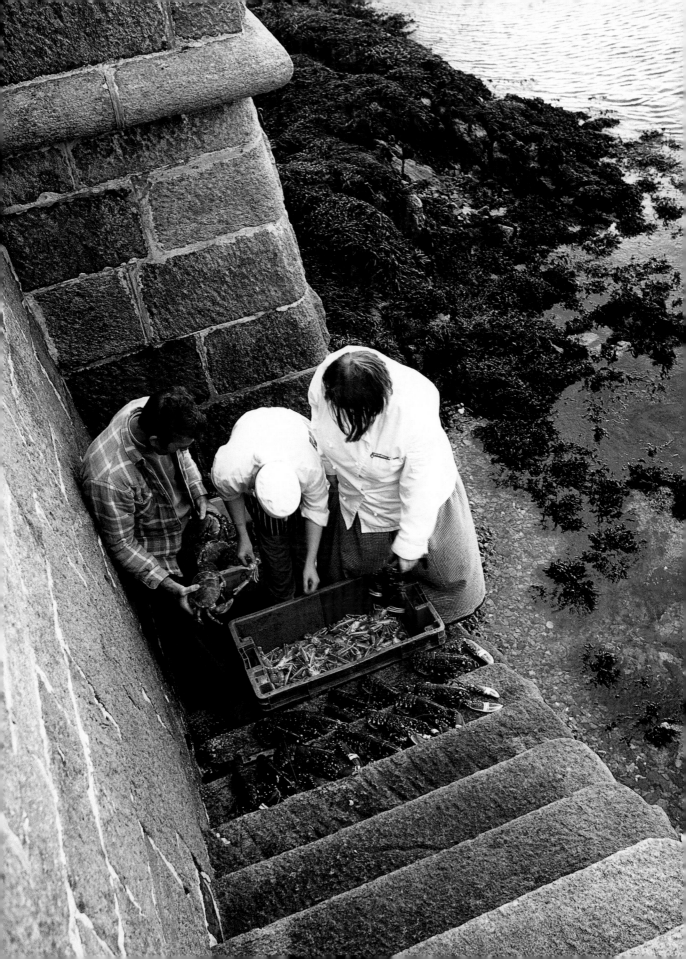

Mussel and Octopus Spaghetti

Some people are rather squeamish about octopus. Give them this: they'll probably not realise what it is, but when you tell them they'll be converted. There is a theory that the way to soften up an octopus – which does tend to be a tough creature – is to add a wine cork to the court-bouillon as it cooks.

Serves 4

1 kg mussels
500 g octopus
350 g spaghetti
2 shallots, finely chopped
4 cloves garlic, finely chopped
8 tomatoes, skinned, deseeded and chopped
2 tablespoons parsley
150 ml white wine
1 litre court-bouillon (see Basics)
olive oil and extra virgin olive oil
seasoning

Simmer the octopus for an hour in the court-bouillon. While it is cooking, clean the mussels, removing the beards and any barnacles, and cook them in the wine, in a large pan, until they have all opened (discard any that remain stubbornly closed after 5 minutes). Strain them, reserving the wine in which they were cooked and remove half of them from their shells.

Drain and skin the octopus and chop it up into small pieces: add it to the shelled mussels. Now soften the shallots and the garlic in olive oil, stir in the tomatoes and add the reserved wine, letting it simmer for a few minutes until it thickens. Then stir in the octopus and shelled mussels and let the whole thing warm gently for a couple of minutes.

Boil the spaghetti until just soft and strain it. Add the mussels still in their shells to the cooked spaghetti, with some extra virgin olive oil, the parsley and seasoning. Finally stir in the octopus and mussel sauce.

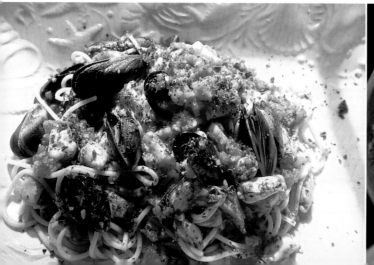
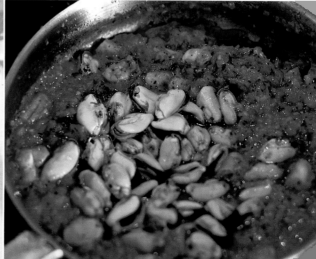

Mussel Soup

Serves 4

2 kg mussels
4 shallots, finely chopped
2 cloves garlic, finely chopped
4 sprigs parsley
zest of one orange
1/2 bottle white wine
60 g butter
1 rounded tablespoon flour
500 ml fish stock (see Basics)
100 ml double cream
1 teaspoon cumin
seasoning
1 tablespoon chopped chives for garnish

Clean the mussels, removing the barnacles and beards. Simmer half the shallots, garlic, parsley and orange zest in the wine for a minute or two then add the mussels and boil them until they are all open. If, after 5 minutes, some of them haven't opened, throw those away. Strain the juice through a fine sieve and reserve it.

Take about 20 of the best looking cooked mussels and reserve them for later. Then shell all the others. Rinse the pan and soften the rest of the shallots in the butter, then add the flour and cumin and cook it gently for a minute before stirring in the vinous mussel-juice and the fish stock. Simmer it gently for about 15 minutes before adding the shelled mussels for the last 5 minutes.

Liquidise the soup and pass it again through a fine sieve, pushing it all through, even if it takes a bit of time. Finally heat it through gently with the rest of the mussels, and serve it sprinkled with chives.

Crab The shores of Great Britain are surrounded by crabs and the Isle of Harris is no exception. The heavier a crab is, the better. Another good sign, besides weight, is a fine encrustation of barnacles and other knobbly bits: this indicates that the crab hasn't recently lost its shell.

A good deal of folklore surrounds the sexing of fish but in this case the general preference for the male is justified, if for nothing else than for the meatiness of its claws. To find out which you have picked up, turn it over and inspect the back – taking great care as the claws can be vicious if they haven't been secured. If it is a male, it will have a long, narrow tail, folded onto the shell; the female has a broader, slightly heart-shaped tail.

As with lobsters, it is a good idea to put them in the fridge for several hours to become soporific before cooking them in a large pan of rapidly boiling salted water. Most crabs weigh about a kilo and will take about 25 minutes to cook – obviously, allow a little more time for the larger ones.

You'll need plenty of time to prepare them: it is a fiddly business, requiring separate bowls for white meat and brown, a bucket for the rubbish and a large glass of white wine to see you through. But it really is worth it, not only for the sense of achievement when you have finished but because the taste is exquisite.

Start by snapping off all the legs and claws and remove all the white meat from them, using skewers or similar implements. Turn the crab on its side, head downwards, and give it a bash (2) with your fist: this should separate the body from the shell. Next, press your thumb down on the mouth and crack it. The head should come away: discard it along with the 'dead man's fingers' and (3) anything that looks greenish or watery.

Now take all the brown meat from the shell, then take the white meat from the centre of the crab (4) and from the claws (5), scraping it out from all the little nooks and crannies: it is worth doing this properly as this is the sweetest meat. Congratulate yourself: you have finished.

It is wonderful just like this, with a little lemony mayonnaise and some fresh bread – or you could try one of the following recipes.

Crab Soup

If you are happy to prepare the crabs yourself, which does take time, take the meat from the shells, separating brown meat from white and keeping both; you will also need to keep the shells. If this doesn't take your fancy, ask your kind fishmonger to do it for you.

Serves 8–10

2 large cooked crabs
500 g prawns, shell-on (optional)
2³/₄ litre fish stock (see Basics)
¹/₂ bottle dry white wine
1 small bulb fennel, chopped
1 large onion, chopped
1 leek, chopped
1 carrot, chopped
4 cloves garlic, chopped
2 sprigs fresh thyme
a pinch of cayenne papper
250 g tomatoes, quartered
2 tablespoons tomato purée
2 potatoes, chopped
4 tablespoons olive oil
1 tablespoon saffron mayonnaise (see Basics)
seasoning

Using a large pan, soften the fennel, onion, leek, carrot and garlic in 3 tablespoons of the olive oil. Add the crab shells and the wine: bring it to the boil and allow it to simmer for a minute or two. Now add the fish stock and simmer for a further 30 minutes. Strain it into a large bowl, pressing the contents thoroughly so as to extract maximum flavour.

Wipe out the pan and heat the remaining tablespoon of olive oil with the tomatoes and thyme, cooking them together for a moment before adding the purée and cooking for another minute. Add the strained stock, the brown crab meat, the potatoes and the prawns and simmer for a further 10 minutes. Finally, liquidise the soup and rub it through a fine sieve.

Mix the white crab meat with the saffron mayonnaise, season and serve the soup with two teaspoonsful of this mixture floating on top of each bowl.

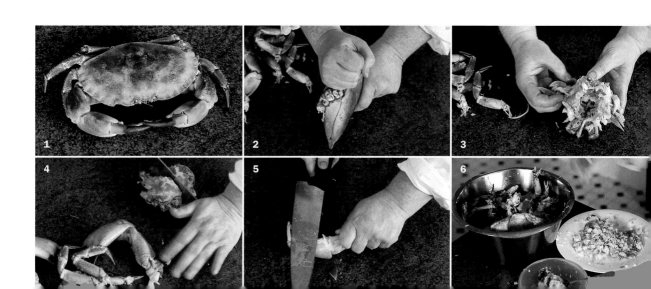

Crab Soufflé

Despite their reputation, soufflés are dead easy to make. The only problem is getting your guests ready to eat them just as soon as you have taken them from the oven. When Lily Macdonald was in charge of the cooking at Morsgail Lodge, Lewis, in the early 1960s, she used her famous cheese soufflé as an extra dinner-bell: 'I'd cook for about 18 in the dining-room and 8 ghillies in the staff-room', she told us 'and they'd stay drinking gin in the hall forever, unless I told them there was a soufflé – then they'd know they had to hurry'. This one makes use of our local crab – but you can flavour the recipe with many other ingredients, exactly as you like, bearing in mind that it is vital that the basic sauce has a strong taste.

Serves 6

60 g butter
60 g plain flour
300 ml milk
300 g prepared white crab meat
1 tablespoon grated Gruyère cheese
3 tablespoons grated Parmesan cheese
10 egg-whites
4 egg-yolks
a good pinch of cayenne pepper
1 teaspoon garam masala
seasoning

You will also need 6 ramekin dishes, well buttered, sprinkled with one tablespoon of the Parmesan and then chilled in the fridge.

Oven 180C/ 350F/ Gas 4

Use the first three ingredients to make a very thick white sauce (see Basics), taking care not to brown the roux. After two minutes of gentle cooking, remove the pan from the heat and stir in both cheeses.

Allow it to cool a little and fold in the crab. Now beat in the egg-yolks, one at a time, and add spices and seasoning. Transfer it to a large bowl.

Whisk the egg-whites until they hold their shape and stir a little into the mixture to slacken it, then fold in the rest. Take care not to be too energetic about this, so as to retain as much air as possible. Spoon the mixture into the cold ramekins and level the surfaces. Run your thumb around the inside edge of each dish to help the souffles rise evenly.

Bake for 10 minutes – check after 8 – and serve instantly.

Crab Risotto

You can vary this dish by adding a few mussels, if you like – in which case, keep them in their shells for maximum dramatic effect – or cooked fresh green peas, in season. Be prepared to be flexible about the liquid: you may need a little more, or a little less. The final result should be creamy.

Serves 6 as a first course, or 4 as a light lunch

400 g white crab meat
250 ml dry white wine
250 g arborio/risotto rice
2 shallots, finely chopped
1 medium leek, finely chopped
1 dessertspoon tarragon
1 dessertspoon chives
115 g butter
600 ml fish stock (see Basics)
150 ml double cream
a good pinch of cayenne pepper
seasoning
1 dessertspoon chervil for garnish

250 g cooked mussels (optional)
150 g fresh peas (optional)

Soften the shallots and the leek in the butter, then turn the rice in the mixture and add the wine. Over a very low heat, allow the rice to absorb the wine, stirring continuously, then gradually add the fish stock, keeping the heat low and waiting until it is nearly dry before each addition.

After about 25 to 30 minutes, when the rice still has a little bite left, fold in the tarragon and chives followed by the crab meat, the cream, cayenne, seasoning and – if you're using them – the cooked mussels and/or peas.

Sprinkle the chervil over the top before serving.

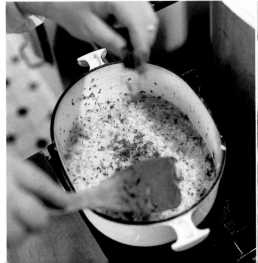
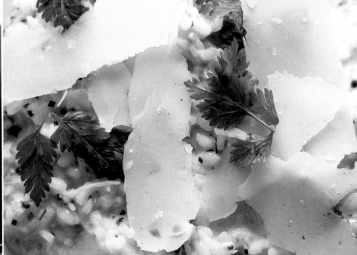

Castellated Crab

Wonderful crabs can be fished from the waters just below the walls of Amhuinnsuidhe Castle. This recipe is one for the cook/architect. It is a bit fiddly to assemble but you can prepare it all up to an hour in advance and it will undoubtedly impress your guests. Of course it is also scrumptious.

Serves 6 as a first course, or 4 as a light lunch

450 g white crab meat
2 ripe avocado pears
6 large ripe tomatoes
1 teaspoon dill
2 tablespoons mayonnaise (see Basics)
seasoning
juice of 2 lemons
1 sprig fresh dill for garnish

You will also need a metal or plastic ring, about 6 cm in diameter (or 8 cm if you think of serving this dish as a light lunch) and 5 cm in height.

Skin the tomatoes and remove the seeds; dice and season them and put them aside. Skin the avocadoes, chop them in horizontal rings and put them into the lemon juice. Mix the crab meat with the dill and mayonnaise and season the mix.

Build each little circular castle from the bottom up, using your ring and compressing the layers as you go. Start with a layer of diced tomato, followed by avocado, followed by one layer of crab. Put more avocado on top of the crab and finish with another layer of tomatoes, topped with a frond of dill. Serve it with some basil oil.

Basil Oil

Basil is particularly good with all tomato dishes. This oil will keep for about three weeks.

Serves 6

150 ml extra virgin olive oil
a good bunch of basil
salt

Liquidise the basil with about one dessertspoon olive oil. Stir in the rest of olive oil and salt and leave it in a bowl for about a day before straining it through muslin (or a tea towel) so that it is clear. Store it in a screw-topped jar.

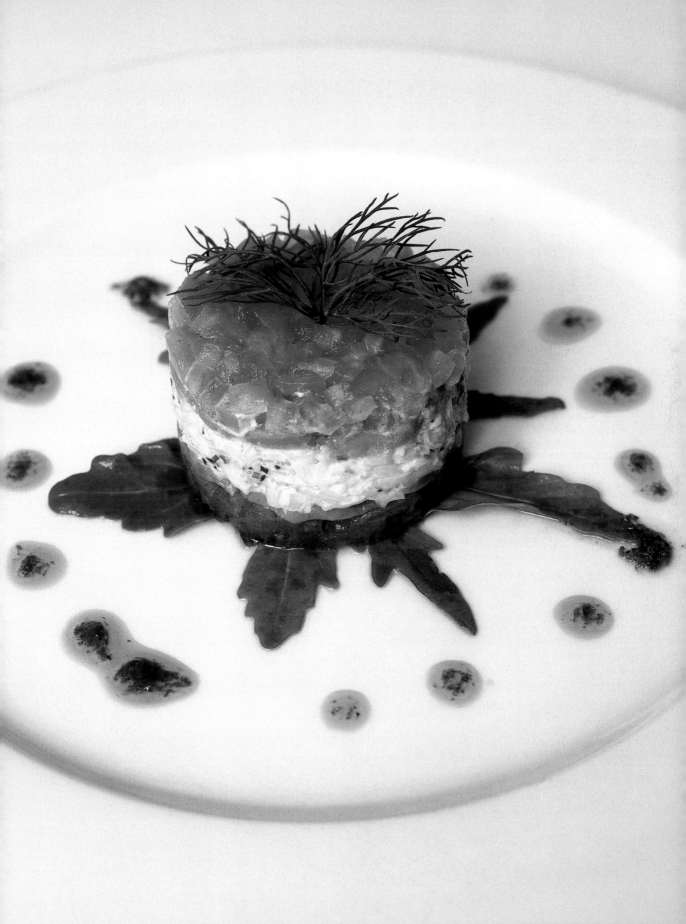

Lobster

Lobster The cold waters of the Sound of Taransay are home to many fine lobsters. Every chef who lives near the sea thinks his or her local lobsters are the best. However they are all wrong. Mine are.

Alive, lobsters are very dark blue-black in colour: when cooked they turn a reddish pink. I tend to prefer the smaller specimens, weighing only about 600 g each, as they are generally the sweetest and most succulent. A local fisherman told me that one of the reasons ours are so sweet is that the rocks in the neighbourhood of the Sound provide plenty of cubby-holes in which they can rest.

The way to sex a lobster is to turn it upside down and check the length of the spikes underneath the tail: the longer ones are male, the shorter female. The only reason for finding out (unless of course you're another lobster) is that some people prefer the taste of the female, though I think there's little to choose between them.

There are many theories about the best way of killing a lobster but at Amhuinnsuidhe, I prefer to send them into a sleepy state first by putting them into the fridge for at least four hours. Then I plunge them into rapidly boiling sea water (or salted water), the lid clapped on again as soon as

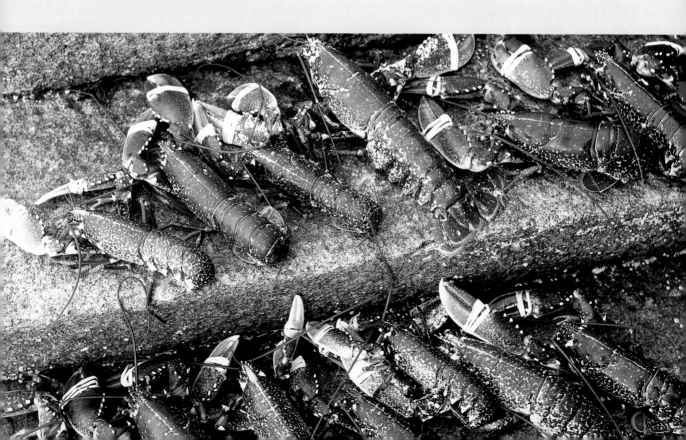

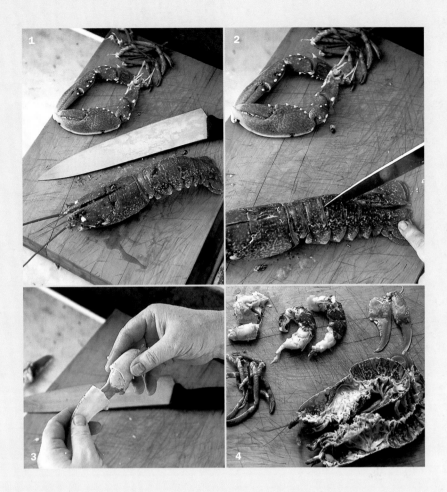

possible to retain the heat (I would never boil more than three at a time, as it's important that the temperature rises again very quickly). An alternative way of killing them is to dispatch them briskly with a large, sharp knife.

To clean them, snap off the two large claws, then the legs (1). Stretch the lobster out and slice it in half lengthwise firmly, with a large knife (2). Remove the meat from the claws (3). Identify, remove and discard the stomach-sack from its head, then the intestine – a thin black line running down towards a smaller bag in the tail. Remove any coral you may find and also any dark greenish meat for possible future use: this latter is the liver, or 'tomalley' and turns bright red when cooked. Everything that remains is delicious (4).

There are several lobster recipes in this section, so the only other thing to add here is that the big mistake some people make is to cook them for too long, turning them rubbery. Seven minutes (from boiling point) per 600 g is the maximum time you should give them .

Lobster Salad
with Lime and Tarragon

'A woman should never be seen eating or drinking, unless it be lobster salad and champagne'.
Lord Byron (1788–1824)

So here is a lovely, fresh summer salad, which you might like to use for a special picnic when you can expect to be publicly observed.

Serves 4

4 live lobsters, each weighing 600 g
4 sprigs dill

For the lime mayonnaise:
1 egg-yolk
150 ml sunflower oil
juice of 1$^1/_2$ limes, strained
zest of 1 lime
1 tablespoon fresh tarragon leaves, finely chopped
seasoning

Make the lobsters sleepy by refrigerating them for a couple of hours – four if you can – while you make the mayonnaise (see Basics). Stir in the lime juice and zest and the herbs. Season to taste.

Cook and clean the lobsters as described on page 20. Arrange the meat on a plate, keeping it whole as far as possible and serve it garnished with dill and accompanied by the lime mayonnaise and the following salad.

New Potato and Broad Bean Salad

Serves 4

750 g new potatoes, scraped
180 g young broad beans
$^1/_2$ bulb fennel, diced
1 tablespoon mint leaves, cut into strips

For the vinaigrette:
150 ml extra virgin olive oil
juice of 1 lemon, strained
1 tablespoon dill, finely chopped
seasoning

Unless the beans are very tiny, slip the skins off them before cooking them briefly in boiling water. Put the new potatoes into boiling water, with a little salt and a sprig of mint and cook them for 10 minutes or until they are tender.

Drain them and cut them into small cubes. As they cool a little, combine all the ingredients for the vinaigrette in a large bowl, add the warm vegetables and mix everything together.

Lobster with Turbot

I admit that this dish is not cheap. But if you want to push the boat out one day, do give it a try. It is sumptuous.

Serves 4

2 live lobsters, each weighing 600 g
500 g turbot, skinned and filleted
750 ml fish stock (see Basics)
a good bunch of tarragon
a good bunch of parsley
a good bunch of dill
300 ml double cream
60 ml dry vermouth
30 g butter, melted
sprigs of chervil to garnish
salt
4 carrots
4 courgettes

Oven 200C/ 400F/ Gas 6

Make the lobsters sleepy for a couple of hours in the fridge and then plunge them into a large pan of boiling water, clapping the lid on tight and boiling them for 7 minutes. Clean them, discarding the stomach, intestine and liver (see page 21) and reserve the meat.

Next, peel the carrots and courgettes and, with a small paring knife, shape them into little barrels, producing 'turned' vegetables. Boil them (separately) in salted water until just tender, then drain and refresh them.

Heat the fish stock with the bunches of herbs and simmer until reduced by a half. Remove from the heat and allow the herbs to infuse for half an hour.

Strain the sauce, return it to the pan with the cream and reduce again for 5 minutes before stirring in the vermouth – the sauce should still be quite thin. Add salt to taste and set it aside.

Cut the turbot into rectangles, roughly 8 cm x 3 cm, salt them and bake them for 5 minutes on a buttered tray.

Heat the sauce, stir the lobster meat and the turned vegetables into it, then simmer the whole pot gently for a couple of minutes to warm it up. Serve it with the turbot, garnished with chervil. Baby new potatoes go well with this dish.

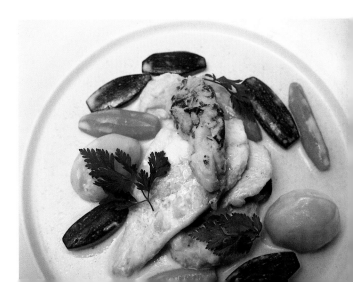

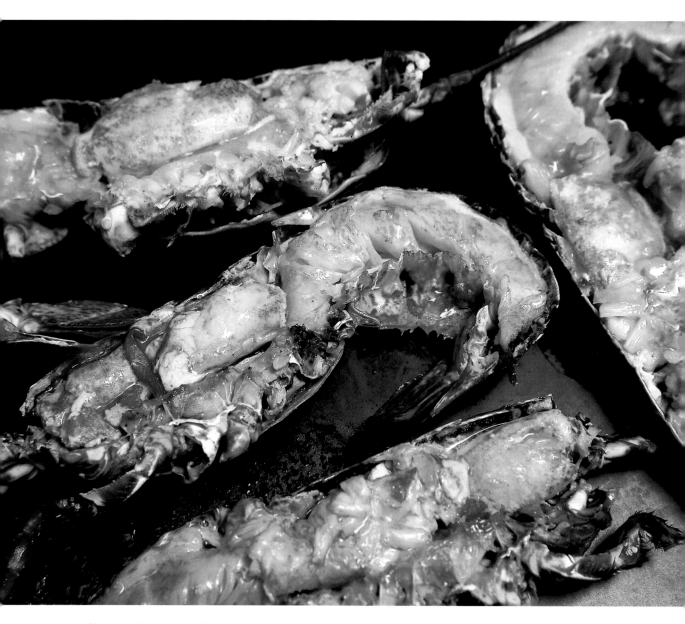

Above, roasting lobsters. *Opposite page*, choosing lobsters with John.

Roast Lobster Sauternes

This is one of the favourites at Amhuinnsuidhe: everybody seems to love it. It is simple to make, once you understand how the anatomy of the fish works. You can make the whole dish in advance, up to ✳.

Serves 4

4 live lobsters, each weighing 600 g
120 g butter, melted
1 tablespoon chives, chopped
1 tablespoon dill, chopped

For the sauce:
1 shallot, finely chopped
170 ml dry white wine
300 ml double cream
170 ml Sauternes
salt

Oven 220C/ 425F/ Gas 7

Cook the lobsters and allow them to cool.

Remove the two large claws, then the legs. Cut the lobsters in half lengthwise, firmly, with a large knife – you want to keep the shell intact (see illustration 4 on page 21). Identify, remove and discard the stomach-sack. Do the same with the tiny, black thread-like intestine and then find the greenish meat (the tomalley) near the head and reserve it for future use in pasta or sauces. Take all the meat out of the claws and pack it into the clean head.

Now make the sauce. Simmer the shallot with the white wine and reduce it to one third. Add the cream and reduce it again, by half, then stir in the Sauternes and some salt. ✳

Brush the surface of the lobsters with the melted butter and sprinkle them with salt. Roast them for 10 minutes. Reheat the sauce and serve with the fish, sprinkled with fresh herbs.

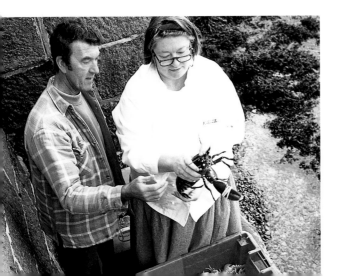

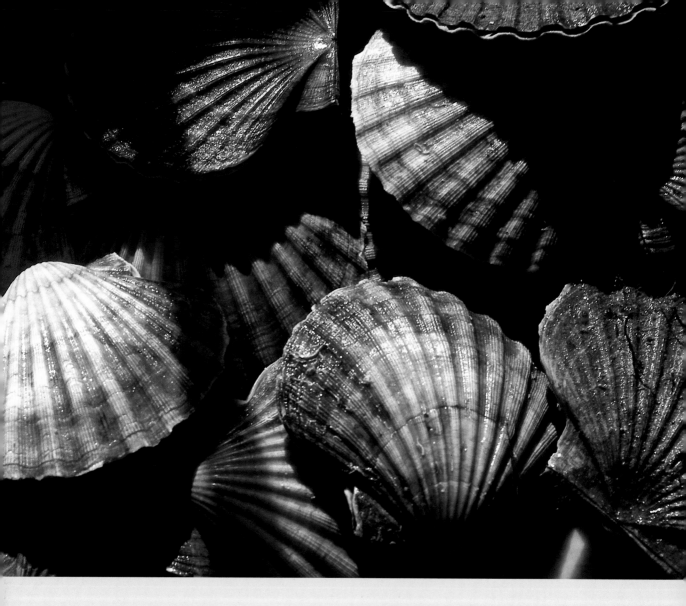

Scallops

These wonderful molluscs are very plentiful in the Western Isles, readily available to us at our beck and call. We buy them alive, for maximum freshness, so that they are often still actually pulsating as they are shelled: this sometimes alarms the guests on our courses. We usually refer to them as scallops but many Hebridean people call them clams, which confused me when I first arrived.

I only buy scallops from divers who have gathered them by hand: this is not merely to do with the quality of the scallops themselves, but because divers can find them in places where dredgers cannot reach. Also, the dredgers do considerable harm to the ecology of the seabed. Ours tend to be larger than those found in shops – I weighed one, out of interest, whose meat alone weighed 150 g.

In the sea, a scallop propels itself about by skilful snapping of the shells: it's very charming to watch. However, the shells are clamped tight shut when you come to try and cook them and have to opened with great care.

Hold the scallop, flat side up – you might like to protect your hands with a thick cloth. Put the point of a small, strong knife into the gap near the hinge and twist it sharply to open it (1). Then take a longer-bladed knife and slide it right across, just inside the flatter shell, severing the connecting muscle: this automatically opens the whole thing up. Scoop it from the other half, with a similar action, keeping the contents intact (2). On a board, cut off the frill (which is really the scallop's 50 eyes) and keep it for sauces. Discard everything else except the pink roe and the white meat. Keep these covered, on a cloth in the fridge for as little time as possible.

As with so many fish, scallops must never be overcooked – they need the briefest time imaginable and are even perfectly delicious eaten raw, finely sliced and dressed with olive oil, pepper and lemon juice.

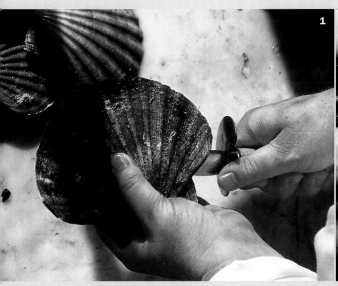
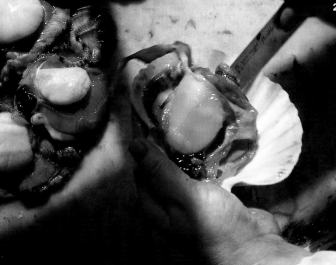

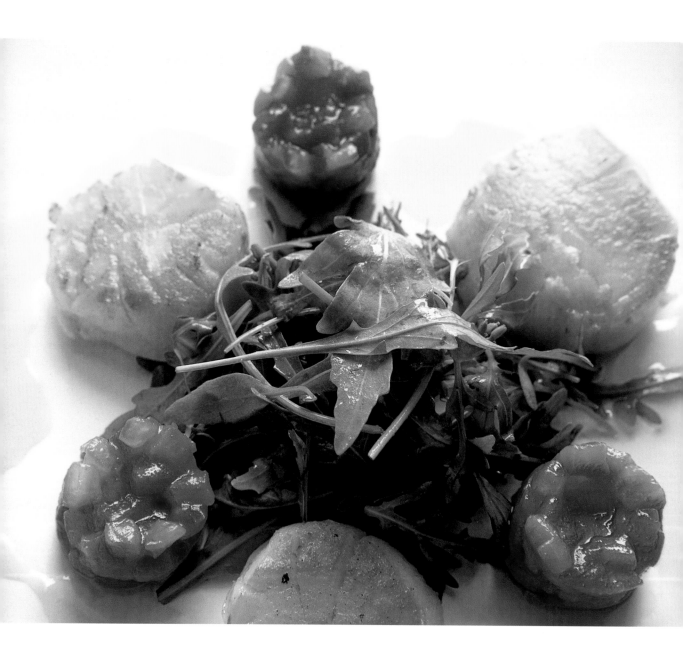

Seared Scallops
with Rocket and Red Pepper Salsa

Really fresh scallops take well to very rapid searing. In this case, the scallops are turned in oil before cooking: it is important not to shift them about in the pan but just to turn them once. If you don't like red peppers, this recipe is just as good if you use a little extra virgin olive oil and balsamic vinegar as a dressing.

Serves 4 as a first course

12 fresh scallops, shelled and cleaned
1 bunch of rocket, prepared

For the red pepper salsa:
2 large red peppers
1 large tomato
$\frac{1}{2}$ small fresh red chilli, deseeded and very
 finely chopped
olive oil
1 teaspoon lemon juice
1 teaspoon white wine vinegar
$\frac{1}{2}$ teaspoon caster sugar
salt

Oven 220C/ 425F/ Gas 7

Roast the peppers with a little olive oil for 25 to 30 minutes, turning them once. Cool them a little, plunge them into cold water, remove the skins and seeds and chop them very finely.

Skin, deseed and chop the tomato, equally small, mixing it with the peppers, sugar, chilli, a good pinch of salt, the vinegar and one tablespoon of olive oil.

Salt the scallops and turn them in cold olive oil. Heat a dry frying pan and sear the scallops rapidly, turning them only once.

Toss the rocket with the lemon juice and a tablespoonful of olive oil. Put a little pile of rocket in the middle of each plate and surround it with scallops and a spoonful of the red pepper salsa.

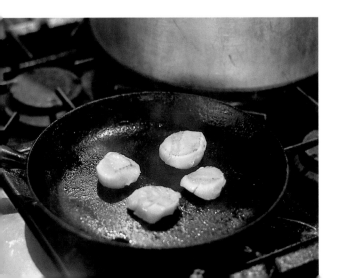

Mousseline of Scallops

This is a pretty first course, light and delicate.

Serves 4

250 g fresh scallops, with no coral
1 egg-white
2 large carrots
275 ml double cream
1 teaspoon salt
a pinch of cayenne pepper
250 g fresh spinach
**50 g butter, and a little more for buttering
  the moulds**

For the sauce:
250 ml fish stock (see Basics)
**a good handful of mixed fresh herbs – dill,
  tarragon, parsley, coriander, in whatever
  combination is available**
4 tablespoons dry white wine
1 shallot, finely chopped
150 ml double cream
240 g cold butter, cut into small cubes

You will also need 4 little moulds – ideally,
90–100 ml dariole moulds, but small ramekins
will do – generously buttered.

Oven 190C/ 375F/ Gas 5

Using a mandolin or a potato-peeler, slice the
carrot lengthwise into very thin, broad strips.
Blanch them for 2 minutes, then refresh and dry
them on kitchen paper. Use them to line the
moulds, leaving enough overlap to fold over
the top.

Put the scallops into a food-processor and
process until smooth. Add the egg-white, cayenne
and salt. Using the 'pulse' button, add the cream,
taking care not to curdle it by over-mixing. Pass
it through a sieve, one spoonful at a time then
spoon the mixture into the moulds, smoothing
the surface. Fold the slices of carrot over the
top. Wrap each in buttered tinfoil and bake in a
bain-marie for 20 minutes.

While it cooks, prepare the sauce: put the stock
with the herbs in a saucepan and bring it to the
boil. Simmer until it is reduced to about a third,
then strain it into a jug. Put the chopped shallot
into the saucepan, add the wine and boil it, until
the liquid has evaporated to about a tablespoonful.
Over a low heat, beat in the butter thoroughly,
little by little, followed by the cream and finally the
reduced stock from the jug. Season to taste.

Wash and drain the spinach; turn it gently in the
melted butter over a low heat until it wilts, then
strain it.

Turn each mousseline onto a bed of spinach and
serve warm, surrounded by the sauce.

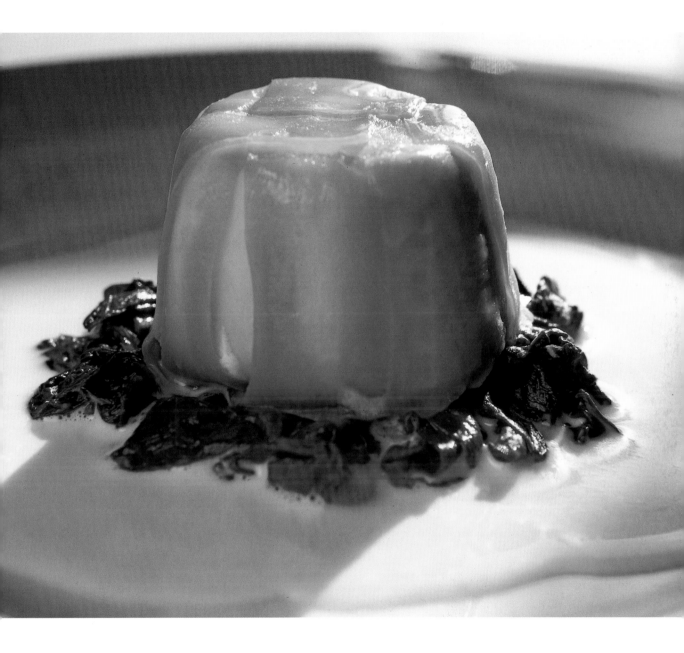

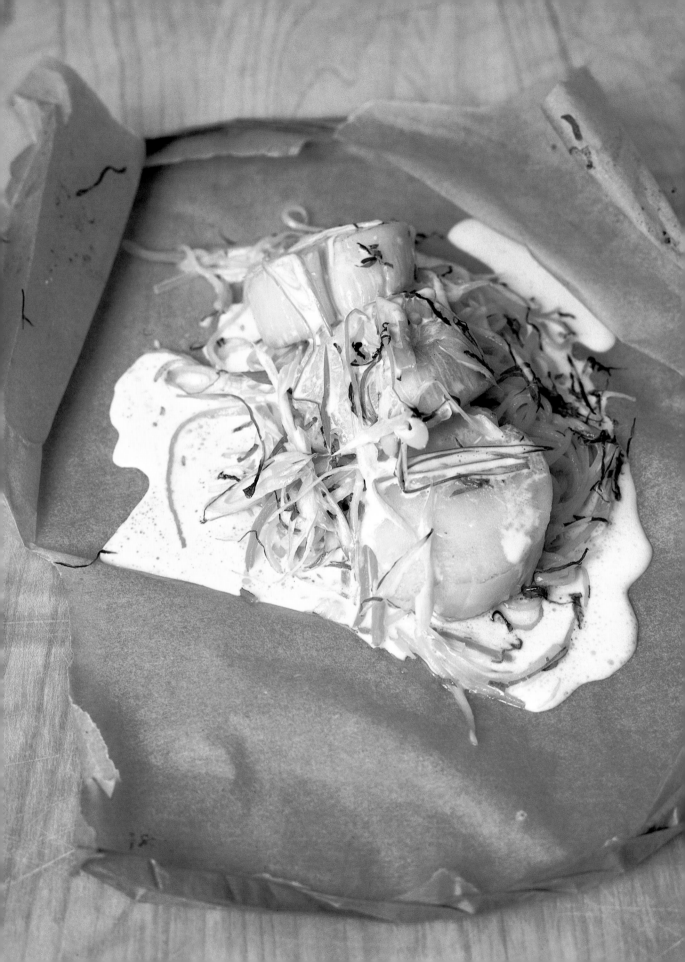

Scallops in a Paper Bag
with Egg Noodle and Ginger

Serves 4 as a first course

8 large scallops
75 g fine egg noodles
2 shallots, finely chopped
100 g carrots, cut into fine julienne strips
3 cm root ginger, cut into fine julienne strips
4 spring onions, cut into fine julienne strips
1 tablespoon chopped basil
100 ml fish stock (see Basics)
140 ml double cream
60 g butter
olive oil
seasoning

You will also need 4 sheets of parchment paper, 25 cm x 38 cm (greaseproof will do, but it is not quite as good).

Oven 220C/ 425F/ Gas 7

Prepare the scallops (see page 27), reserving the juice and frills, then slice them in half horizontally, adding a little olive oil. Boil the noodles until almost cooked.

Soften the shallots in the butter with the carrots, ginger and seasoning and cook them gently for 3 minutes. Take them out and reserve them, leaving any juices in the pan – to which you now add the juice and frills from the scallops, and the fish stock. Bring it to the boil and reduce it for a minute before adding the cream. Strain it and pass it through a fine sieve. Fold the basil into the noodles and season them, adding just a little of the sauce to slacken the texture slightly.

Sear the scallops very rapidly in a dry pan. Make paper parcels: using one sheet per person, fold the papers in half, widthways, to give them a crease, and open them up again. Pile up tiny quantities of noodles, vegetables, and 4 slices of scallop per person on one side of the fold (1). Pour some sauce over the whole (2). Fold the paper over the top and crimp it, as in a Cornish pasty (3). Cook them for 5 minutes. Snip a hole in the top of each bag to let the steam escape.

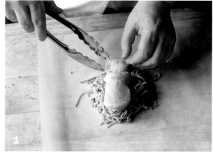
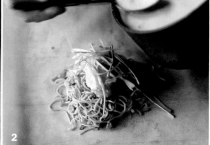
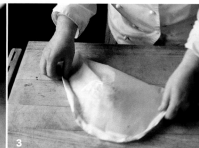

Langoustines are sometimes called Dublin Bay prawns, but neither is an appropriate name for a shellfish so common around the Hebrides. Perhaps it is for this reason that the islanders call them simply prawns.

There is a long-standing prejudice against eating such shellfish in the islands. It is quite possible that it dates from the time of the Clearances, when people who stayed on the island were so destitute that shellfish were their only diet. They have become an atavistic symbol of utter, hopeless destitution. On the other hand, they are still there to be fished, and bringing them ashore provides a welcome and comparatively profitable living for the fishermen.

Most of the langoustines here are caught by the fleet which goes out from Rodel harbour. There are about 20 boats and they travel daily 12 miles to the south, where a hundred pots, or creels, are strung out on a line, each baited with half a herring. There's a buoy at each end, so that the fishermen can lift the whole line at once to empty the pots. They always throw the smallest back, to give them – as one of them, Donald Norman Maclean, says – 'a fighting chance'.

I buy them in 3 sizes, the largest being almost as big as a small lobster. They are fiendish creatures to handle, being all spikes and lashing claws. I always cool them off in the fridge for several hours to lessen the peril to my hands.

It is fine to cook them briefly, whole, in boiling water for 5 minutes and serve them with garlic butter, but several of my recipes require you to take them apart raw. It's not difficult. Take the pincers off first and then the head, scooping out and discarding the inside and reserving the shell for stock. Take the rest of the shell off the tail – take care, it can be quite sharp – and add it to the stock-pot. Use the meat as described in the following recipes.

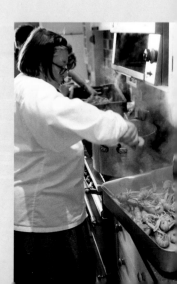

Seafood Feuilletés

This little jewel-box of light, crispy pastry can be filled with any treasures from the sea. Here I use langoustines and scallops. If you use frozen pastry it works but, if you go to the trouble of making your own, it is magnificent. It can be prepared a few hours in advance, up to the ✶.

Serves 4 as a generous first course

500 g puff pastry (see Basics)
8 large langoustines or Dublin Bay prawns, shelled
8 large scallops, shelled, washed and cleaned
450 g fresh spinach, washed and prepared
30 g butter
3 tablespoons extra virgin olive oil
1 egg-yolk, lightly beaten
1 tablespoon chives, chopped
a handful of fresh tarragon leaves

For the sauce:
1 shallot, chopped
230 ml fish stock (see Basics)
115 ml dry vermouth
2 pieces of preserved stem ginger in syrup,
  chopped, syrup reserved
a good pinch of saffron
200 ml double cream
seasoning

Oven 200C/ 400F/ Gas 6

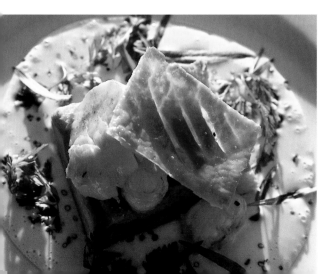

Roll out the pastry to 1 cm thickness then cut it into 4 rectangles. Using a sharp knife, score the pastry 1 cm inside the edge, like a picture frame, taking care not to cut it all the way through. Put the squares onto a baking tray and brush them with egg-yolk, making sure you don't go over the edges or the pastry will not rise evenly. Bake for 15 minutes, until golden brown.

While it is still hot, remove the inner squares (which are going to be the lids) and discard the stodgy insides, so that you have 4 clean boxes. ✶

Blanch and refresh the spinach. Drain it and squeeze all the water from it. Make the sauce by softening the shallot in the vermouth and reducing it, before adding the fish stock and reducing it again, to a third. Add the ginger, the saffron and the cream and simmer for two minutes. Season and add a little ginger syrup, to taste. Keep it warm.

To finish the dish, make sure the scallops are dry, then slice them in half horizontally and turn them, with the langoustines, in the olive oil and a pinch of salt. Sear them quickly on both sides in a very hot, dry frying pan. Pop the pastry cases in the oven for a minute if you need to reheat them.

Turn the spinach in the butter over a gentle heat and assemble the feuilletés by putting a spoonful of spinach in the bottom of each pastry-box and filling it with shellfish and some sauce. Sprinkle with chives and tarragon and put the lid on top.

Langoustine Salad
with Orange and Olive Oil Dressing

Squat lobsters or 'squatties' as we call them, are becoming increasingly available in supermarkets. They are as tasty as their larger cousins and can be used in their place if you like. This simple salad is served with a delicious orange-flavoured cold dressing, and with tossed mixed herbs. It can be prepared up to the ✱ as much as a day before.

Serves 4

**about 20 langoustines or 40 squat lobsters,
    shelled**
mixed herb and salad leaves
2 tomatoes, skinned, deseeded and diced
1 tablespoon chives, chopped
1 tablespoon vinaigrette (see Basics)
olive oil
seasoning

For the dressing:
3 shallots, finely chopped
4 cloves garlic, finely chopped
75 ml white wine vinegar
175 ml olive oil
150 ml water
zest and juice of 2 oranges
1/2 red chilli, finely diced
some sprigs of oregano, parsley, basil
2 bay leaves
1 teaspoon caster sugar

Salt the langoustines and leave them to stand. Make the dressing by combining all the ingredients in a small pan, bringing it to the boil and allowing it to simmer and thicken slightly for 20 minutes before cooling and straining it through a fine sieve.

Heat some olive oil in a frying pan and cook the langoustines gently for 30 seconds on each side turning them only once. Cool them on kitchen paper to remove excess oil, then toss them in the dressing and chill them until required. ✱

Toss the mixed herbs with the vinaigrette and serve the langoustines with the dressing spooned over them, arranged around a little pile of herb salad, the whole garnished with the chives and tomatoes.

Squat lobsters, or 'squatties'.

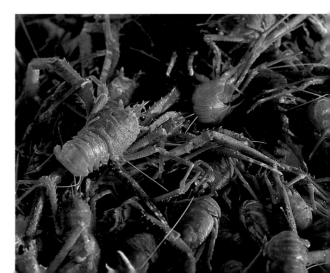

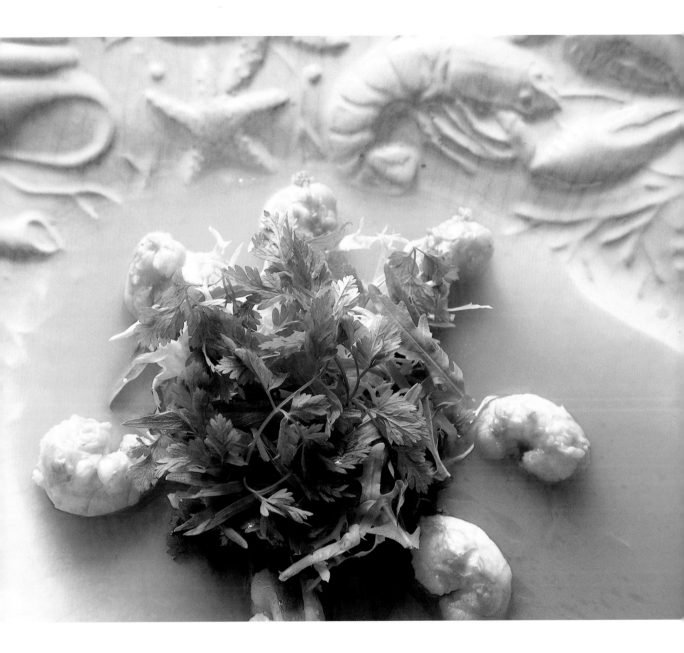

Langoustine Ravioli
with a Red Pepper Sauce

This is one of my very favourite dishes. It really isn't too difficult to make and the wonderful thing about it is that you can prepare it well in advance and leave it sitting in your fridge until you're ready to use it.

Serves 4 as a first course

1 portion pasta (see Basics)
24 langoustines (or Dublin Bay prawns)
2 egg-yolks, lightly beaten
1 tablespoon finely chopped chives for garnish
a bunch of chervil for garnish

For the marinade:
1 rasher bacon, finely diced
2 small shallots, finely diced
1 small clove garlic, finely diced
1 teaspoon fresh root ginger, finely diced
20 g butter

For the sauce:
4 medium red peppers
200 ml double cream
30 g butter
3 tablespoons olive oil

Oven 220C/ 425F/ Gas 7

Remove the heads and shells from the langoustines – take great care as they can be sharp. Combine the marinade ingredients in a small frying pan and allow them to cook very gently, until all the flavours have intermingled. Transfer it to a large bowl and turn the prepared langoustines in it. Allow it to cool.

Put two langoustines together at 8 cm intervals along each ribbon of pasta (1), then brush outside the fish and along the edges with egg-yolk. Cover the whole thing with a second ribbon and press down to make ravioli squares (2), before cutting them apart into individual parcels. Pinch the edges together, using floured fingers. Put the parcels, uncovered, into the fridge while you make the sauce.

Roll the peppers in the olive oil then roast them for 25–30 minutes. Remove them from the oven, plunge them into cold water and slip them out of their skins. Chop them on a board, discarding the seeds and the core, and puree them in a liquidiser. Then bring them to simmering point in a small pan, with the cream. Pass the mixture through a fine sieve and keep it warm.

Cook the ravioli for 4 minutes in plenty of boiling salted water, drain it thoroughly until all the water has run out and finish the sauce, just before serving, by whisking in the butter. Finally, sprinkle the chopped chives and sprigs of chervil on top of the ravioli.

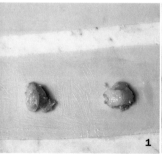 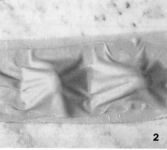

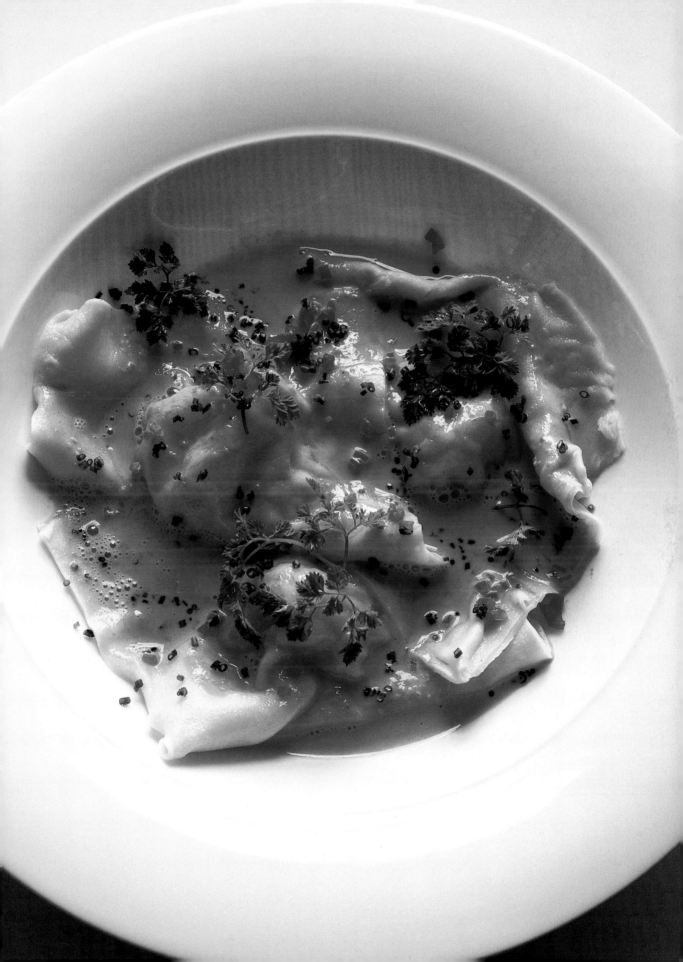

Fish

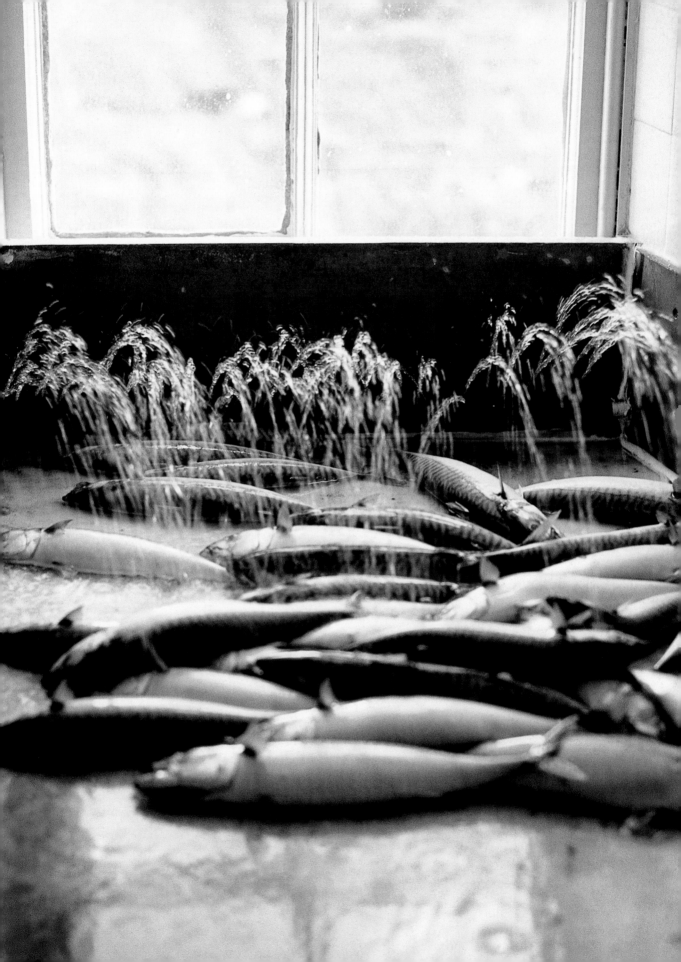

Haddock Tapenade

This is an inexpensive and unusual dish, easy to prepare in advance and very tasty. You can cook the fish as separate fillets or in an open gratin dish, with the cheese-mixture covering the whole surface. I like to use Isle of Mull cheese but a good quality white cheddar will do.

Serves 8 as a first course, or 4 as a main course

4 fresh haddock fillets, each weighing 180–200 g
4 teaspoons tapenade (see Basics)

For the topping:
25 g butter
75 g grated cheddar cheese
50 g full-fat soft cream cheese
1 egg-yolk
2 egg-whites
a pinch of paprika

Oven 200C/ 400F/ Gas 6

Gently melt the butter and cheddar together, stirring very vigorously, then let the mixture cool in the pan. When it is nearly cold, add the cream cheese, stirring it again, thoroughly, followed by the egg-yolk. Add the paprika. Whisk the egg-whites until firm and fold them gently into the cheese-mixture. Put the whole thing into the fridge for a little while, up to half an hour.

Spread a thin layer of tapenade onto each haddock fillet, followed by a layer of the cheese mixture. Bake them, uncovered, in a buttered baking dish for 10 to 12 minutes. Neaten the edges, if you like, and serve it on a bed of ratatouille.

Ratatouille

This wonderfully versatile dish, making use of the abundance of late summer vegetables, is as good cold as hot. You should chop the vegetables very small if you intend to use the ratatouille as part of this haddock recipe, but more coarsely should you want it as an extra vegetable dish with, say, roast lamb.

1 medium onion, chopped
2 cloves garlic, crushed
500 g tomatoes, skinned, deseeded and chopped
1 teaspoon caster sugar
2 courgettes, cubed
1 red pepper, deseeded and cubed
1 aubergine, diced
plenty of extra virgin olive oil
fresh basil

Soften the garlic and onion in the oil, add the tomatoes, sugar, salt and pepper and cook for 5 minutes. Remove them from the pan and set them aside. Wipe the pan with paper, add some more oil and cook the courgettes in the same way, adding them to the tomatoes (they will take a little less time).

Do the same to the other vegetables. Season to taste. Just before serving stir in some basil. It can happily be reheated.

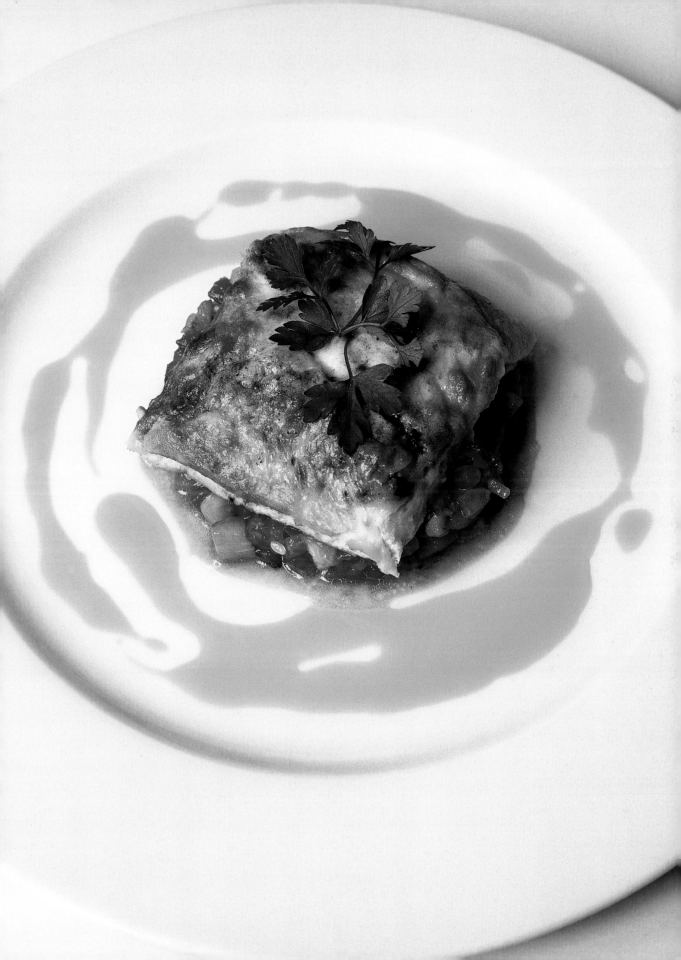

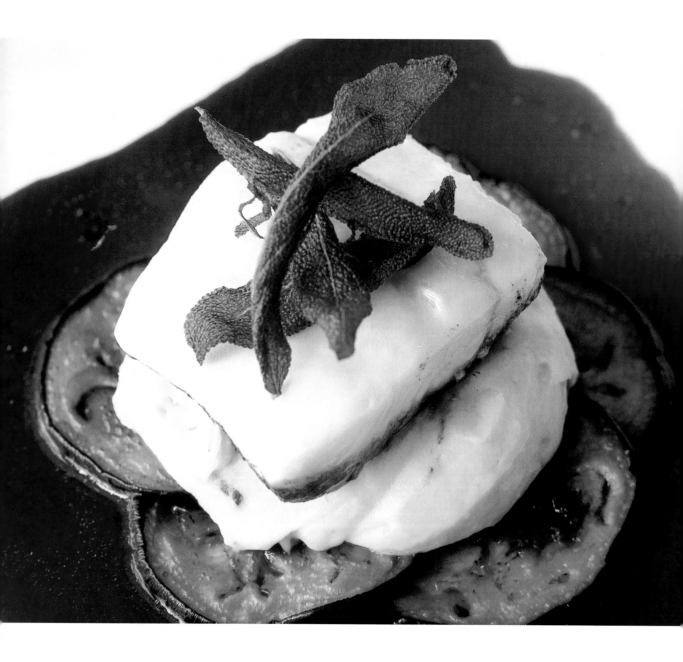

Braised Halibut
with a Rich Red Wine Sauce

I dreamed this up in the early hours of the morning. It may seem controversial to use red wine with fish, but it works like my dream. Halibut is a dry fish which takes well to this kind of treatment, but be sure not to overcook it. You should also take care not to allow the wine to colour the whole fish: it should leave a pink frill around the edge.

Serves 4

4 halibut fillets, skinned, each weighing about 180g
125 ml red wine
2 medium aubergines
olive oil
seasoning
sage leaves for garnish

For the sauce:
280 ml red wine
280 ml fish stock (see Basics)
1 tablespoon redcurrant jelly
60 g butter

For the potatoes:
4 large potatoes
90 g butter
100 ml warm milk
2 sage leaves, chopped
seasoning

Oven 200C/ 400F/ Gas 6

Slice aubergines into 3 mm rounds and bake them in olive oil until soft and golden (not crisp). Drain them on kitchen paper. Prepare the fish by neatening the edges and ensuring that all bones are removed.

Peel and boil the potatoes, then sieve them and beat in the butter and the milk, followed by the sage and seasoning. Keep them warm.

Make the sauce by putting the red wine and jelly in a small pan and reducing it by half. Add the fish stock and leave it simmering until it is again reduced by half.

Cook the fish like this: pour the 125 ml red wine into a shallow ovenproof dish and put the fish fillets on top. Cover the dish with foil and braise it in the oven for 8 minutes, then remove it and leave it to rest, still covered, for 5 minutes.

Deep-fry the remaining sage leaves until crisp (it will take about 30 seconds) and save them for decoration, then finish the sauce by adding the butter to the pan over a low heat, whisking it all the time.

To serve, arrange slices of aubergine in a fan shape. Put a spoonful of potato on top, surmounted by the fish. Decorate it with the crisp sage and surround it with the sauce – the rest of the sauce can be served in a jug.

Halibut with Flageolet Beans

This is a hearty and sustaining dish but it takes time to prepare. You have to start the day before, as the beans need to be soaked in cold water overnight. In some recipes, tinned flageolets can be used instead of the dried variety but in this dish they would not produce quite such a delicious flavour.

Serves 4

**4 halibut fillets, skinned, each weighing
  about 170–180 g**
1 litre fish stock (see Basics)
**200 g dried flageolet beans, soaked overnight
  in cold water**
1 onion, diced
2 cloves garlic, diced
**4 tomatoes, skinned, deseeded and roughly
  chopped**
2 bay leaves
2 medium carrots, sliced into rounds
**2 tablespoons olive oil (and a little more for
  the fish)**
**2 tablespoons fresh coriander, chopped, and
  4 sprigs, for decoration**
4 large sprigs parsley
seasoning

Oven 200C/ 400F/ Gas 6

Using a large pan, soften the onion and garlic in oil, then add the tomatoes, bay leaves, parsley and stir the mixture together for a minute or two, over a low heat. Drain the beans and add them to the pan, then cover them with fish stock.

Allow the pan to simmer gently for about an hour, topping it up with stock from time to time – it should never become dry. Add the carrots and cook for a further half-hour, testing the beans occasionally. When they are tender, fold in the fresh coriander.

During the last half-hour, after you've added the carrots, cook the fish. Sear it on all sides in hot oil, then bake it, uncovered, in an ovenproof dish for 7 minutes.

Serve the fish on a bed of beans, with a sprig of coriander.

Filleting halibut.

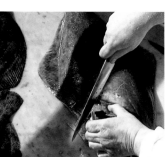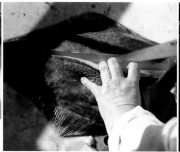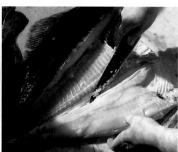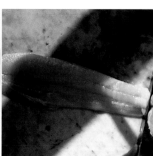

Herrings in Pinhead Oatmeal

Though I had never eaten this dish before
I came to Harris, I now love it – especially for
breakfast. But it makes a good supper, too,
when accompanied by a plain green salad and
new potatoes. Because I am greedy, I have
allowed two herrings per person, but one might
well be enough for a more modest appetite.
If you have trouble finding pinhead oatmeal,
try a good health-food shop.

Serves 4

8 herrings, boned and flattened
250 g pinhead oatmeal
1 tablespoon butter
1 tablespoon olive oil
1 lemon

Spread the oatmeal onto a plate and put the
herrings into it, patting the meal into the surface
of the fish on both sides. Melt the butter and
oil together in a pan and fry the fish on a low
heat for 2 minutes on each side. Serve with a
squeeze of lemon.

Herrings with Couscous

From time immemorial the people of Harris have lived on herrings. Before coming here I had never used them much in cooking, but within weeks of my arrival I was converted. The germ of the idea for this recipe came from a dish I first came across at the Tante Claire restaurant: in that case, the fish was red mullet.

Serves 6 as a first course, or 4 as a light lunch

6 fresh herrings, boned and cut in half
extra virgin olive oil

For the marinade:
6 tablespoons dark soy sauce
1 dessertspoon syrup from a jar of stem ginger
1 dessertspoon sherry

For the couscous:
150 g couscous
200 ml boiling fish stock (see Basics)
100 ml extra virgin olive oil
2 cm grated root ginger
1 red pepper, skinned, deseeded and finely diced
1 tablespoon chives, chopped
1 tablespoon coriander, chopped
seasoning

You will also need a metal or plastic ring, about 6 cm in diameter and 5 cm in height.

Mix the marinade ingredients together and steep the herrings in it for at least an hour. Mix all the couscous ingredients together thoroughly, stirring the mixture frequently.

Take the fish out of the marinade and fry it quickly on both sides in hot oil. Shape the couscous into circles with the ring-mould, and press it down. Run a sharp knife around the inside of the ring to lift it off and arrange the fish on top.

Hamish Taylor's salt herrings.

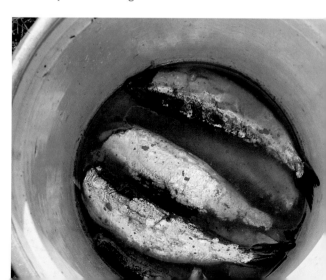

Turbot with Sole Mousse

Turbot is a wonderful, smooth fish which needs very little cooking, but this dish works equally well with other fish, John Dory for example. If you want to push the boat out, garnish it with caviar.

Serves 4

4 turbot fillets, skinned, each weighing about 180 g
170 ml fish stock (see Basics)
60 g butter, melted
half a cucumber
seasoning

For the mousse:
1 sole fillet, skinned weight about 150 g
150 ml double cream
1 egg-white
1 dessertspoon dry vermouth

For the sauce:
100 ml dry white wine
300 ml fish stock (see Basics)
1 shallot, finely chopped
190 ml double cream
75 ml Pernod
salt
a few sprigs parsley, chervil and dill

Oven 200C/ 400F/ Gas 6

Prepare the mousse: puree the sole in a food-processor until smooth. Add the egg-white, vermouth and a little salt and pepper. Switch on again for 5 seconds. Using the 'pulse' button, add the cream slowly, taking care not to overdo it and cause curdling.

Pass the mousse through a sieve, a little at a time, and refrigerate it for at least 2 hours. Put the turbot fillets on a baking tray. Spread the mousse mixture evenly over each of them. Peel the cucumber and slice it paper-thin, then arrange the slices like scales over the fish. Pour the melted butter over the top and bake it for 10 minutes – it may take a little longer.

Meanwhile, make the sauce. Reduce the wine, with the shallot, to about one third. Add the stock and the herbs and reduce, again to about a third. Add the cream and continue reducing for about 5 minutes. Finally, stir in the Pernod and check the seasoning. This is delicious served on a bed of braised fennel.

Braised Fennel

1 large bulb of fennel
60 g butter
salt and pepper

Remove the outer leaves from the fennel and cut it into strips lengthwise, following the grain. Simmer in boiling water for 2 or 3 minutes. Drain and refresh. Turn the fennel in melted butter over a medium heat until warmed through and season it.

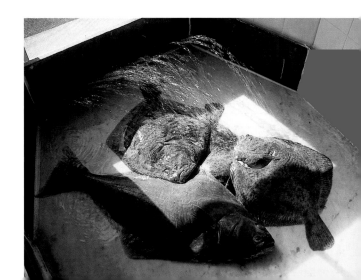

Roast Saffron Monkfish
with Herb Risotto

There is a lot of water in monkfish, so it is better to buy a little more than you think you might need. Saffron is a powerful (and expensive) spice so use it with discretion.

Serves 4

4 monkfish tails, skinned and filletted, each
weighing about 180 g
$1/2$ teaspoon turmeric
350 ml dry white wine
a good pinch of saffron

For the risotto:
250 g arborio/risotto rice
2 shallots, finely chopped
1 medium leek, finely chopped
1 dessertspoon parsley, chopped
1 dessertspoon coriander, chopped
1 tablespoon chives, chopped
115 g butter
500 ml fish stock (see Basics)
55 g grated Parmesan cheese
4 tablespoons double cream
seasoning

Oven 200C/ 400F/ Gas 6

Reduce the wine with the saffron and turmeric over a brisk heat, for 2 minutes, then leave it to cool and infuse for half an hour. Dunk the fish in the saffron-wine, turning it until each whole piece is bright yellow. Leave the fish in the wine for a further half-hour, while you start the risotto.

Melt the butter in a broad, shallow pan (a cast-iron skillet is ideal). Soften the shallots and leek, then add the rice, turning it gently. Drain the fish and add the saffron-wine to the rice-mixture. Cook gently while the rice absorbs the liquid, stirring it all the time. As it begins to dry out, add the stock, little by little, still stirring – you may find that you need a little more than 500 ml. After about half an hour, the rice should be just tender and the liquid absorbed. Finally, fold in the cream, the herbs and the Parmesan, so that it becomes almost like a sauce.

Make sure that the fish is dry, then sear it in hot oil before roasting it in the oven for 7 minutes. Allow it to rest on a grid so that the juices run out. Slice the fish with a sharp knife and serve it over a bed of risotto.

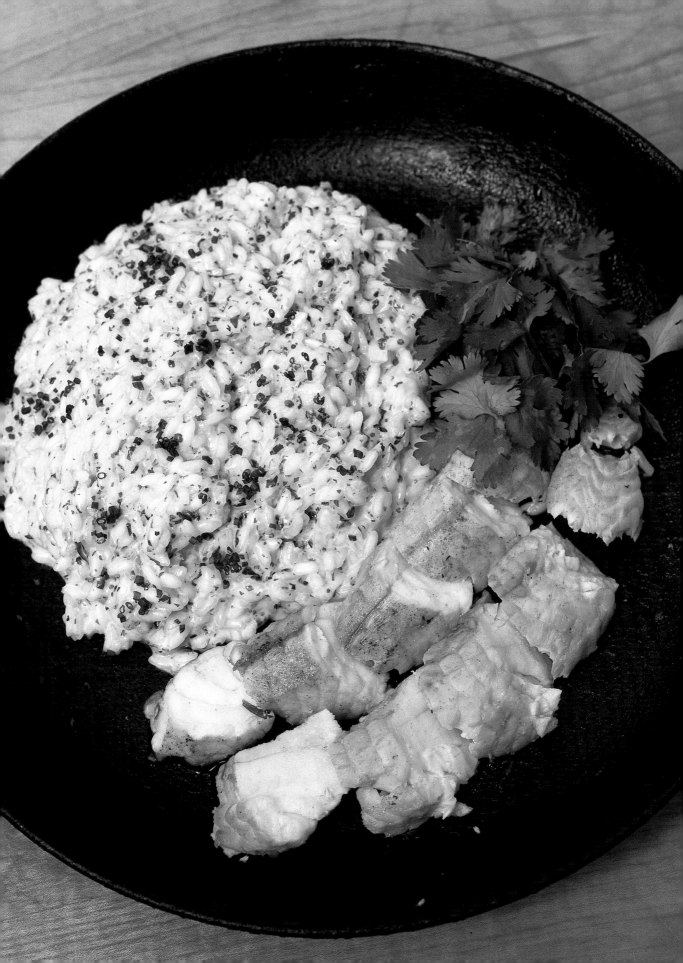

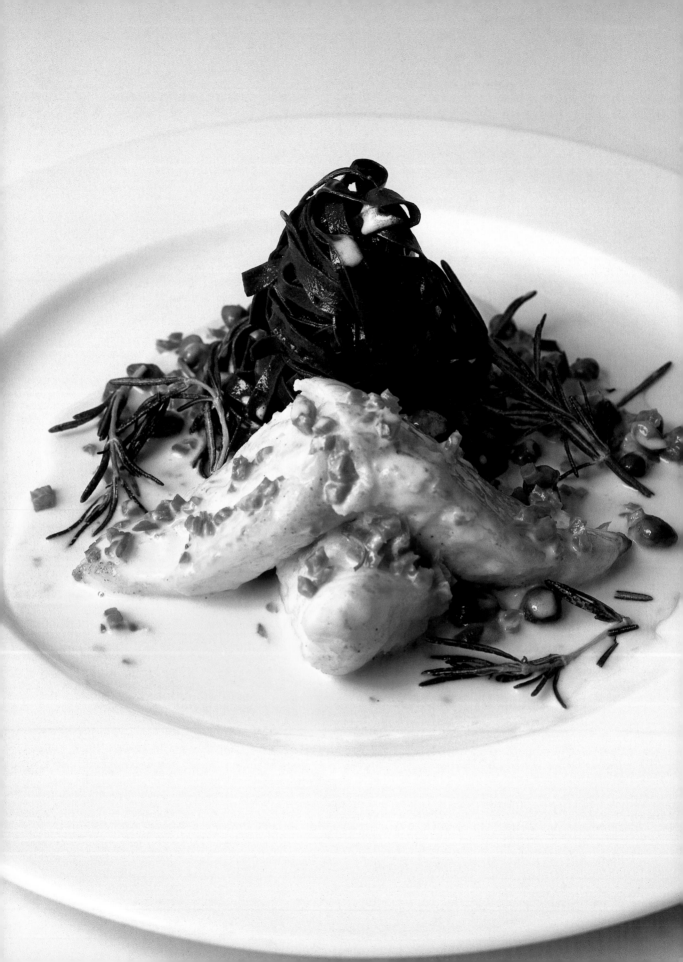

Monkfish with Ink Fettuccine
and a Caper and Rosemary Sauce

The amount of pasta you use depends on how greedy your friends are. The minimum is about 35–40 g per person, but this recipe uses more, and will provide a substantial lunch dish. The sauce is strongly flavoured and very tasty and the colours are pleasingly dramatic.

Serves 4

4 monkfish tails, skinned and filletted, each
**   weighing about 180 g**
250 g ink fettucine
4 slices smoked streaky bacon, chopped small
4 large sprigs rosemary
1 rounded tablespoon capers
100 ml dry white wine
300 ml fish stock (see Basics)
200 ml double cream
2 tomatoes, skinned, deseeded and diced
2 tablespoons butter
3 tablespoons olive oil
60 g clarified butter (see Basics)
seasoning

Oven 200C/ 400F/ Gas 6

Fry the bacon in a tablespoon of olive oil, remove it and keep it for the sauce. Wipe the pan with kitchen paper then pour in the wine and reduce it by half. Add the stock to the reduced wine and reduce the whole again by half. Then add the cream and reduce yet again (yes!), to about one third. Stir in the bacon, rosemary, capers and tomatoes and set it aside.

Cook the pasta in plenty of boiling salted water, drain it and toss it in the butter and the rest of the olive oil. Meanwhile, sear the monkfish in the clarified butter then roast it for 8 minutes. Reheat the sauce and serve.

Sole Amhuinnsuidhe

This is our variant of a classic and spectacular dish, making elegant use of the fine fresh fish we enjoy in the Hebrides. I have used squat lobsters, the delicious little crustaceans that abound here, but prawns are nearly as good. You can also use lemon sole, or plaice, instead of Dover sole. The first part is a little fiddly, but the end result is well worth it. Do be careful when sieving the mousse: if you do too much at a time the cream might curdle. It can be prepared well in advance up to the ∗.

Serves 4

4 small, plump Dover soles
38 prawns or squat lobsters, cooked
220 g salmon fillet, skinned and boned
300 ml double cream
1 egg-white
1 teaspoon salt
60 g butter

For the sauce:
2 tablespoons wine vinegar
2 tablespoons white wine
140 g butter
180 ml double cream
2 tablespoons dry vermouth
1 tablespoon chopped chives for garnish

Remove the head of each fish, and fillet it by cutting through the skin to the spine, then easing the fish off the bone with a very sharp knife either side of the backbone. Turn it over and do the same the other side. With scissors, sever the bone at tail and remove it, making sure that the tail stays attached to the fillets to keep the whole thing together. Trim the smaller bones off the sides of the fish, leaving just a little frill of bone to keep the shape. Arrange the filleted fish, dark side up, on buttered foil on a baking tray, sprinkle it with salt inside and prepare the mousse.

Put the salmon into a food-processor and process it for a minute. Add the egg-white, then, using the 'pulse' button, gently mix in the cream and salt. Sieve it, a little at a time into a clean bowl and chill it thoroughly for an hour in the fridge.

Spoon the mousse (I often use a piping-bag with a broad nozzle for this) into the cavity of each fish (1) and arrange the prawns or squat lobsters along the top (2). Trickle melted butter over the top and cover the whole thing in foil. ∗

Bake for 20 minutes (check after 15 – the mousse should be firm to the touch).

Meanwhile, make the sauce by reducing the wine and vinegar over a brisk heat until only about one tablespoonful is left. Whisk in the butter, little by little, then stir in the cream and the vermouth and check the seasoning. When the fish is ready, allow it to rest for a minute or two and then lift the skin off the top, and discard it, along with the tail.

Pour the sauce over the fish and sprinkle with chives. This is very good served with tagliatelle, sprinkled with fresh tarragon leaves.

1

2

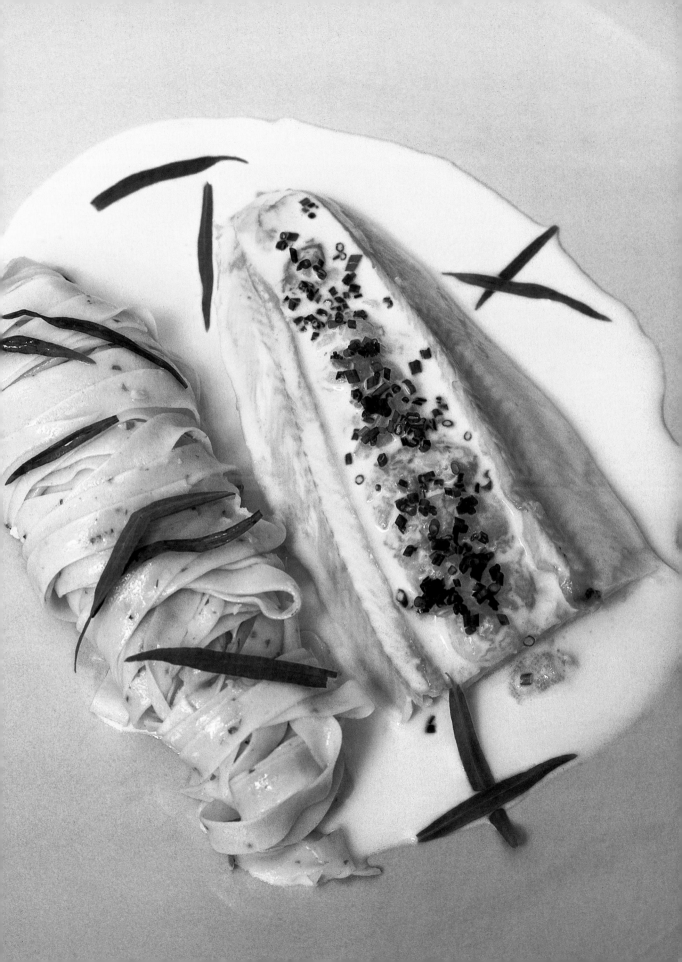

Oriental Sole

This is faintly reminiscent of a classic dish, but where Escoffier might have used cream, these ingredients produce a more aromatic taste. You may think that there will be too much sauce, but Bridget, manager of Amhuinnsuidhe, can never get enough of it! If you only have lemon sole, or plaice, it works just as well.

Serves 4 as a first course

8 fillets of Dover sole, skinned, each weighing 130 g, halved lengthwise
24 large leaves from a Cos lettuce, hard, white central spines removed
1 shallot, finely diced
250 g shitake mushrooms, finely diced
30 g butter
2 medium carrots, cut into fine julienne strips
3 medium leeks, cut into very fine julienne strips
280 ml fish stock (see Basics)
seasoning

For the sauce:
150 ml extra virgin olive oil
150 ml sunflower oil
150 ml dark soy sauce
2 teaspoons chopped root ginger
3 teaspoons runny honey

Oven 200C/ 400F/ Gas 6

Make the sauce by combining all the ingredients in a bowl. Soften the shallot in the butter and add the mushrooms, cooking them together for 2 minutes before straining them. Blanch one leek with the carrots, strain and refresh them and use them to cover the base of a buttered ovenproof dish.

Blanch the lettuce very briefly, 4 leaves at a time, removing it with a slotted spoon to a cake rack to drain thoroughly. Arrange 3 leaves in a star shape, with a spoonful of mushrooms and shallot in the middle. Arrange 2 fillets of fish folded on top of it all (see below) and make a little parcel by bringing the lettuce leaves up from underneath. As you finish each parcel, turn it upside down so that it keeps its shape and arrange them all on top of the vegetables brushing a little melted butter over the top.

Pour the fish stock into the dish and bake, covered with tinfoil, for about 25 minutes – check for firmness after 20. Toss the rest of the leeks in a little plain flour and deep fry them until crisp. Serve a handful of these leeks on top of each fish. Finally pour the sauce around or over.

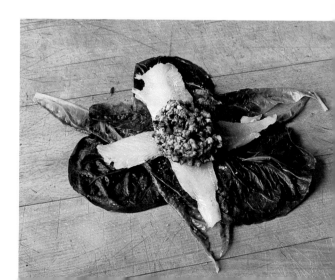

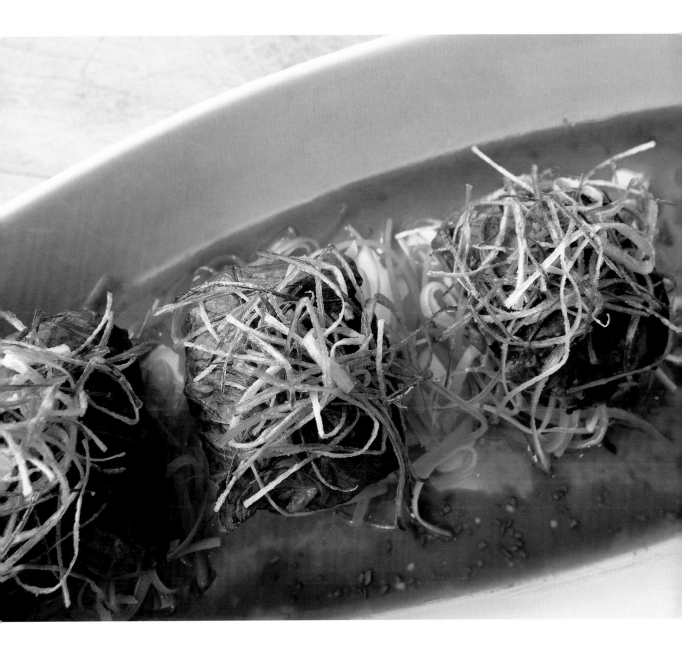

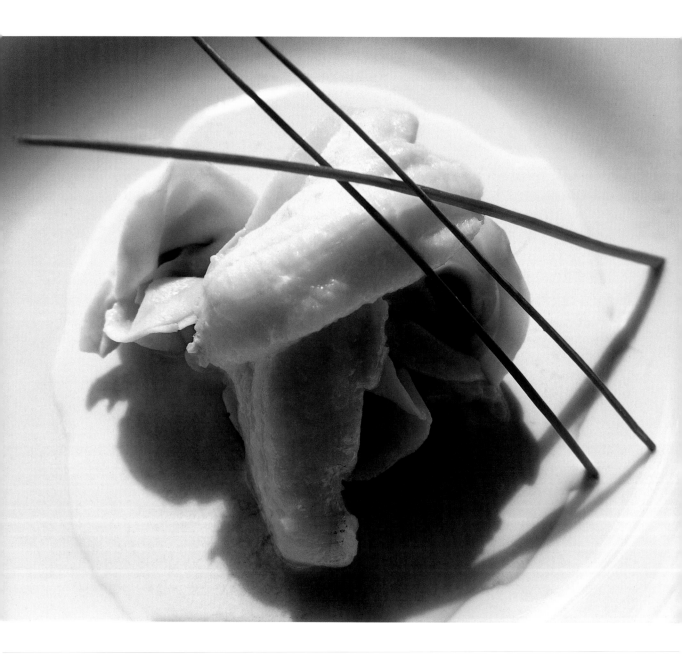

Sole with Spinach Tortellini

This is a light and tasty dish but it does take time to prepare. You'll need a round cutter about 8 cm in diameter. If you like, you can assemble the whole thing a few hours in advance, up to the ✶ and store the tortellini, well spaced, on a floured tray in the fridge.

Serves 4

**4 fillets of sole, skinned, each weighing about
   180 g**
¹/₂ pasta recipe (see Basics)
250 g fresh spinach, washed
4 spring onions, finely chopped
a pinch of chilli powder
1 egg-yolk
1 tablespoon mascarpone cheese
30 g butter

For the sauce:
125 g whole, raw prawns
400 ml fish stock (see Basics)
1 teaspoon tomato purée
2 dessertspoons dry sherry
200 ml double cream
seasoning

Oven 200C/ 400F/ Gas 6

Start with the pasta: prepare it as in Basics up to the ✶, wrap and refrigerate it. Then deal with the spinach: soften the onions in the butter, add the spinach, chilli powder and seasoning to taste, cook for 3 minutes, drain it thoroughly and allow it to cool. Put the mixture into a food-processor, add the cheese and one egg-yolk and process it very briefly. Leave to cool.

Now make the sauce: peel the prawns and reserve them. Put together the heads, shells, tomato purée and the fish stock in a saucepan; bring it to the boil and reduce it by half. Using a potato-masher, smash up all the prawn shells so as to release the maximum flavour, then pass the stock through a sieve. Return the stock to the pan, add the cream and simmer for a couple of minutes. Add the peeled prawns and bring the sauce back to the boil for a minute then liquidise it and sieve it again. Finally return it once more to the pan, add the sherry and warm it through, taking care that it doesn't boil. Set it aside until you are ready to eat.

To make the tortellini, roll out the pasta (again, refer to Basics) and cut it into rounds on a floured surface. Brush the edges with beaten egg-yolk and put half a teaspoon of the spinach mixture in the middle. Fold each into a half moon, bring up the points and twist them together, twice. ✶

Just before you want to eat, bake the fish, covered with foil, on a buttered dish for 3 to 4 minutes. Gently warm the sauce and bring a large pan of salted water to the boil. Cook the pasta for 2 minutes and drain it. To serve this dish, pour some sauce onto each plate then some tortellini, and top it all with the fish.

Graciously acknowledge the applause.

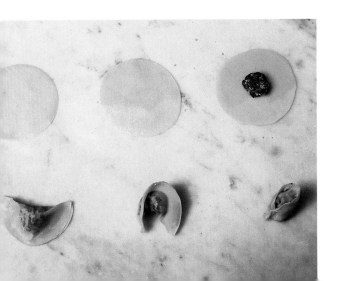

Seafood Tempura
with Pickled Cucumber

This recipe is inspired by Japanese food, which tends to have a wonderful clean taste: this method of cooking makes the most of our super-fresh fish. It has to be deep-fried at the last minute.

Serves 4 as a first course

8 large prawns, shelled
4 large scallops, shelled and dry
12 mussels, cleaned, cooked and shelled
  (see Mussel and Octopus Spaghetti page 12)
sunflower oil
2 courgettes, cut into fine julienne strips
1 aubergine, cut into four fan-shapes
1 piece Nori seaweed
flour for dredging
1 lime

For the batter:
2 egg-yolks
170 ml water
125 g plain flour
1 egg-white
seasoning

For the pickled cucumber:
1 cucumber
1 teaspoon salt
25 ml white wine vinegar
1 tablespoon caster sugar

Start by pickling the cucumber. Peel it and cut it into very, very fine slices. Put it into a colander with the salt, then leave it to drain for about an hour. Finally mix in the vinegar and the sugar.

Now make the batter by beating the egg-yolks and water into the flour, little by little. Then whisk the egg white and fold it into the mixture. Season.

Make 4 bundles of courgette-sticks, wrapped with a strip of piece of Nori. Dredge each bundle in flour and shake off the excess.

Dip the prawns in the batter and deep fry them briskly in hot oil. Do the same with the rest of the fish and the mussels, standing them on kitchen paper afterwards, to absorb any excess oil. Finally, deep fry the aubergine fans and the courgette bundles. Serve the dish garnished with the cucumber and a wedge of fresh lime.

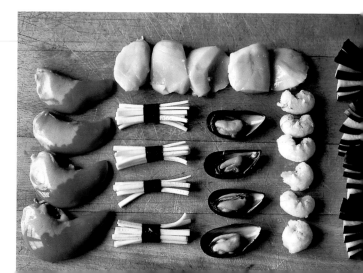

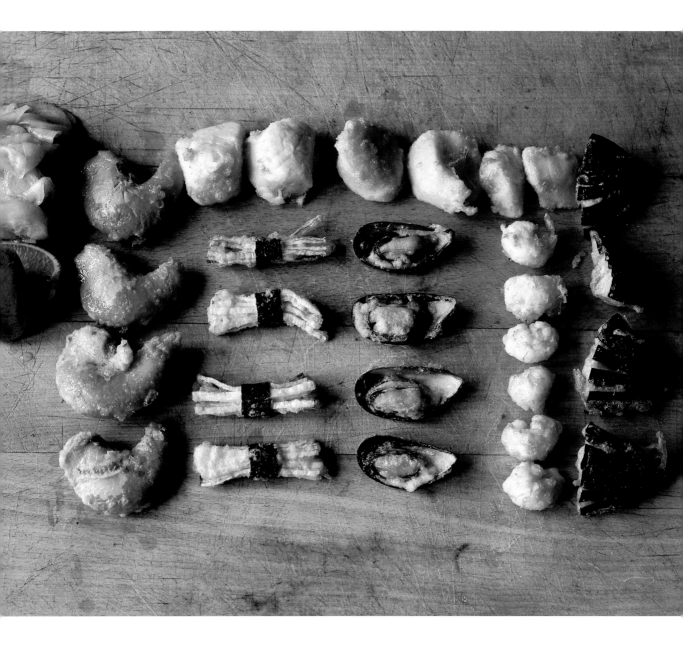

Hebridean Fish Pie

Here is my version of a classic and magnificent dish, warming and comforting, which makes use of the wide variety of fish living in the clear, unpolluted waters around our island. It doesn't really matter which fish you use, but the more variety the better. There is a lot of it: you can use it all at once for a convivial supper party or halve it if there are fewer of you.

Serves 8–10

2^1/$_2$ kg mixed, filleted fish – turbot, haddock, prawns, scallops, salmon, cod, plaice etc.
1 kg mussels
300 ml dry white wine
1 shallot, chopped
1 litre milk
180 g butter
180 g flour
seasoning

For the topping:
1^1/$_2$ kg potatoes, peeled
2 dessertspoons chives, chopped
150 g butter
150 ml milk
1 dessertspoon grated Parmesan cheese
2 beaten eggs

Oven 220C / 425F / Gas 7

Clean the mussels, removing barnacles and beards. Bring the wine and shallot to the boil in a large pan and steam the cleaned mussels in it for 15 minutes, until they are all open – as usual, discard any that fail to open after 5 minutes. Strain them through a fine sieve into a large jug and reserve the liquid.

Put all the rest of the fish (except the prawns) into an ovenproof dish and cover it with the milk. Bake for 15 minutes until just cooked. Allow it to cool, then strain off the milk and reserve it with the wine. Carefully remove the skin and any remaining bones from the fish, keeping it in large chunks.

Make a white sauce (see Basics) with the juices in the jug and any more that may have run from the fish. Use plenty of seasoning.

Arrange the cooked fish, the mussels (in their shells or out of them, as you like) and the prawns in a very large ovenproof dish (or two smaller ones). Pour on the sauce, turning the pieces of fish so that they are all covered and allow it all to cool down while you boil and mash the potatoes in the usual way.

Finally mix the chives and Parmesan into the potatoes and spread them over the top of the fish. Score the top with a fork and pour the eggs over the top. Bake for 30–40 minutes.

Smoked Haddock Lasagne

If you can get hold of some dulse (seaweed) for this, use it instead of the coriander for a real taste of the sea, but remember to soak it first. Either vegetable goes beautifully with the fish – be sure to seek out pale, undyed haddock. If you haven't time to make your own pasta buy it freshly made, or even dried.

Serve it surrounded with a drizzle of extra virgin olive oil and a little reduced balsamic vinegar.

Serves 8 as a first course, or 4 as a main course

**12 sheets lasagne, made from the pasta
  recipe** (see Basics)
1 kg smoked haddock fillets
700 ml milk
120 g butter
100 g flour
2 egg-yolks
150 ml double cream
4 tablespoons fresh coriander
seasoning

You will need a lasagne dish, circa 36 cm x 20 cm, well buttered.

Oven 150C/ 300F/ Gas 2

Cover the fish with the milk and put it into the oven for 15 minutes, then remove it and allow it to cool a little. Strain the fish, retaining the milk, and flake it, making sure there are no skin or bones left.

Make a white sauce (see Basics) with the butter, the flour and the fishy milk, adding the cream at the end and seasoning it to taste. Let it cool a little before beating in the egg-yolks. If using home-made lasagne, remove it from the cold water in which it has been resting and pat it dry with a tea towel.

Build up the dish with layers of pasta, sauce, fish and coriander. Finish with a layer of sauce and sprinkle the last few leaves of coriander on top. Bake for 30 minutes, turning the oven up to 200C/ 400F/ Gas 6 for the last 5 minutes.

Smoked Haddock Tartare

This is a most elegant first course and extremely easy to prepare. Try to find the very best, undyed haddock, which is one of our finest local fish.

Serves 4

500 g smoked haddock, skinned and carefully filleted
4 quail's eggs
rind and juice of 1/2 lemon
1 teaspoon tabasco
1 teaspoon Dijon mustard
1 dessertspoon runny honey
1 shallot, finely chopped
2 gherkins, finely chopped
1 tablespoon chives, chopped
1 dessertspoon tarragon
4 tablespoons extra virgin olive oil
seasoning
6 tablespoons of reduced balsamic vinegar
  (see Basics)
a handful of fresh herbs

For the sauce:
3 tablespoons mayonnaise (see Basics)
1 tablespoon sour cream

You will also need a round cutter, 6 cm in diameter, 5 cm in height.

With a large knife chop the fish into very small pieces – do not be tempted to use a food-processor or it will become mushy. In a large bowl, mix thoroughly the rind and lemon juice, tabasco, mustard, honey, shallot, gherkins, chives, tarragon and olive oil. Add the fish and mix it all together well. Make the sauce by mixing all the ingredients together and put everything into the fridge until you need it.

With the point of a sharp knife cut off the tops of the quail's eggs and tip the raw eggs into simmering water, stirring the water as they go in. It will set very quickly, when you can remove it with a slotted spoon and keep it in cold water until required.

To serve, put the round cutter in the middle of the plate and put a quarter of the fish mixture inside. Pat it down firmly then top it with a dessertspoon of the sauce and carefully remove the cutter. Then put a poached quail's egg on top and finally a little bunch of fresh herbs. Dribble a little of the reduced vinegar around it.

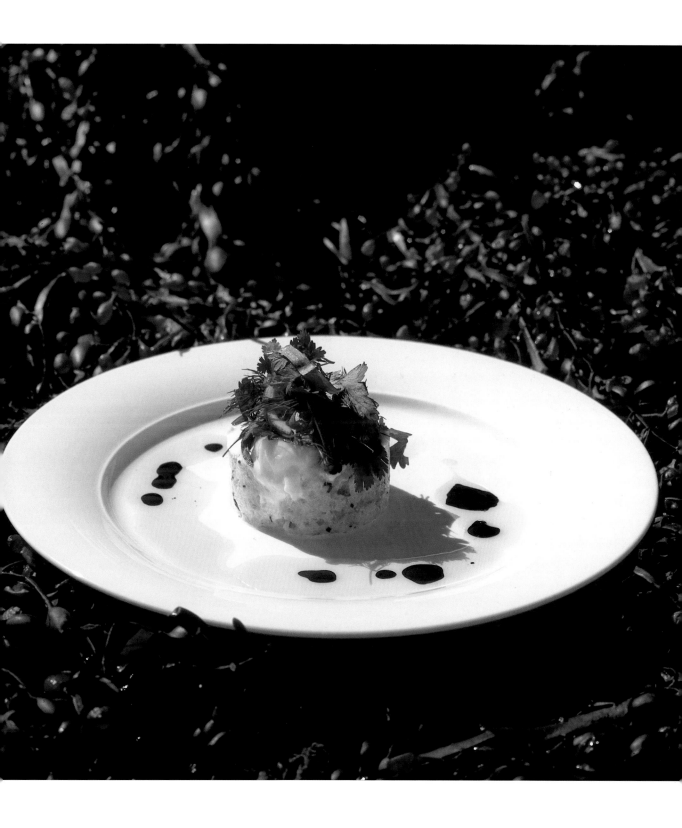

Salmon and Sea-Trout

According to the traveller Martin Martin, tradition has it that if a woman was the first to cross the Barvas River on May 1st, there would be no salmon for a full year thereafter. It would be a brave woman today who would defy such superstition. Martin also maintained that the best time for angling for salmon is 'when a warm southwest wind blows' and that the islanders 'used earth worms for bait, but cockles attract the salmon better than any other'. Today's fishermen often have different ideas.

Below, Alec (left) and Kenny Morrison. *Opposite page,* scaling a salmon.

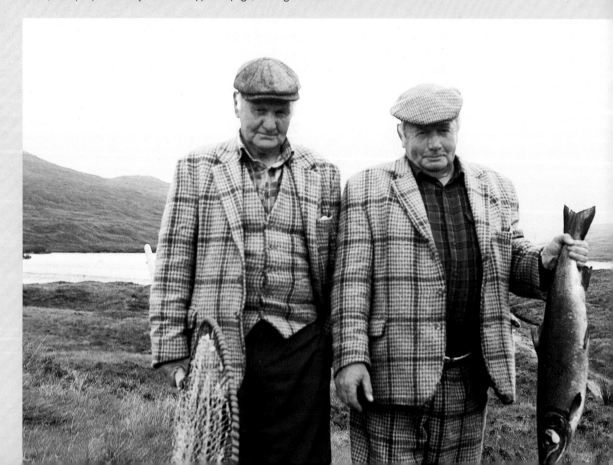

There is a six-loch system at Amhuinnsuidhe, from which we are able to take our own sea-trout. Salmon, of course, is fished throughout the season, from the sweet river which gives the castle its name and from other fine rivers in the surrounding hills. To tell the difference between the two, look at the spots: sea-trout have more of them than salmon and slightly blunter

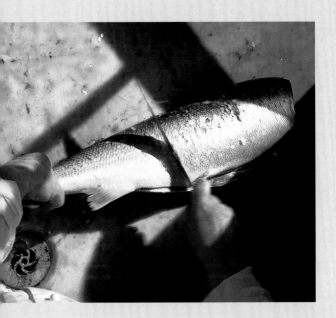

heads. The fish have similar life cycles, both beginning their existence in fresh water, where they stay for between two and three years before heading for the sea. The salmon swim right up to the North Atlantic, to the cold waters around Greenland, the Faroes and Norway but the sea-trout don't travel so far, possibly no further than 30 or 40 miles, feeding on the crustaceans which gives the fish its characteristic pink flesh. Another difference is that the sea-trout return every year to the rivers, while only between five and ten per cent of the salmon come back a second time.

The salmon is widely considered to be the King of Fish and the sea-trout its poor relation. Yet, possibly because it is a more 'local' fish, to a man like Mark Bilberry of the Fishery Trust the sea-trout has a right to the title – and indeed it has a truly wonderful, delicate flavour. It is very seldom farmed, whereas farmed salmon is widely available (though distinctly different from its wild cousin in taste). Finally, a salmon is a slightly larger fish: an 8-lb salmon is a commoner sight than an 8-lb sea-trout, which would be rare indeed. Though I refer to these fish in these recipes as salmon, they would be just as good with sea-trout. For me, the perfect weight is about 5 lbs (2.3 kg).

It is wonderful at Amhuinnsuidhe to see the salmon and sea-trout leaping the rock face up to the river, making their way to the lochs. One tradition at the castle (which I really appreciate) insists that the first of these fish to be caught in the season finds its way to our kitchen – whoever owned the rod that snared it.

We use this fish in so many ways – for gravadlax, for example or in any of the following recipes. However with fish this fresh, little or no cooking is required. You can sear it briefly in a hot pan, or eat it raw, as sushi.

Poached Sea-Trout
with Spring Vegetables

This is one of the simplest and best ways of preparing sea-trout or salmon. If you can't find baby fennel, use ordinary bulbs, cut small – or indeed any young, fresh spring vegetables.

Serves 4

4 sea-trout fillets, each weighing about 200g
1 litre fish stock (see Basics)
200 g butter
1 teaspoon coarse sea salt
20 small new potatoes
120 g sugar-snap peas
12 baby carrots
4 baby fennel, halved lengthwise
100 ml dry vermouth
120 ml double cream
salt and white pepper
sprigs of fennel for garnish

Oven 200C/ 400F/ Gas 6

After making quite certain that no bones have been left in the fish, put them in a large buttered dish, not touching each other. Sprinkle the sea salt over them and pour in the stock. Cover the whole thing in tinfoil and bake it for 8–10 minutes.

Boil the new potatoes and, while they cook, prepare the other vegetables: boil the carrots for a minute, or until just tender, then strain them, saving the water to do the same with the peas and finally the fennel. Mix the potatoes with all the other vegetables and 50 g butter, seasoning with salt and white pepper to taste.

When the fish is ready, measure 300 ml of the stock in which it was poached into a small pan. Reduce it to one third then add the vermouth and reduce it again. Beat in the remainder of the butter and finally stir in the cream and seasoning.

Divide the vegetables into 4 portions and arrange them, prettily, with the fish on top, surrounded by sauce and garnished with sprigs of fennel.

Salmon Fish Cakes

These little things are useful and always popular – perhaps because they remind us of childhood. But the taste is as sophisticated as you want it to be, depending on the flavouring. This recipe uses salmon but you can easily make the cakes with haddock, crab or almost any other fish.

Serves 4, generously

500 g cooked salmon
500 g mashed potato
2 egg-yolks
1 tablespoon parsley, chopped
1 tablespoon coriander, chopped
zest of 1 lemon
a pinch of chilli powder (or more, to taste)

seasoning
60 g flour
3 whole eggs, beaten
100 g white breadcrumbs
90 g butter

Mix the first 8 ingredients together thoroughly in a large bowl, using your hands. Shape them into little patties and, if you have time, leave them in the fridge for an hour to become firm.

Assemble three bowls, the first containing flour, the second the eggs and the third the breadcrumbs. Dip the patties in each bowl, in that order and fry them gently in butter for 3 minutes on each side.

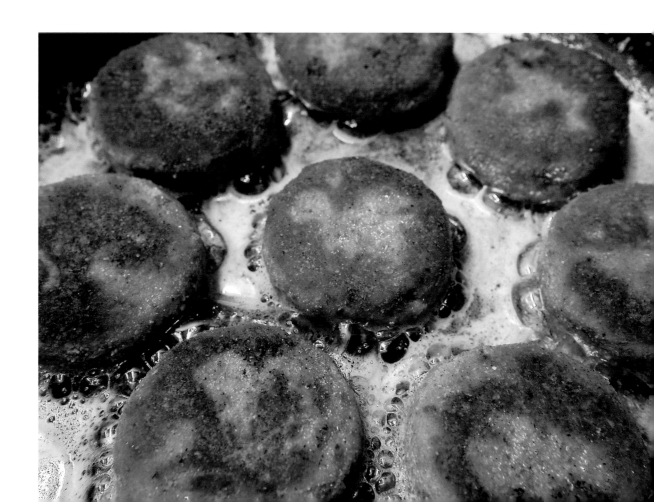

Gravadlax

This means of curing salmon gets its name from the Scandinavian method of burying the fish, with spices, to preserve it. The taste is more delicate than smoked salmon and it really is remarkably easy to make, provided you begin it three days before you'll be needing it. Ask your fishmonger to prepare the fish by descaling and filleting it, removing the head, tail and fins but leaving the skin on. You should be left with two matching fillets.

Serves at least 12

**1 whole salmon, filleted and prepared as above,
   weighing in the end 2–2^1/$_2$ kg**
**1 dessertspoon whole white peppercorns,
   crushed**
150 g coarse sea salt
180 g granulated sugar
4 tablespoons dill, chopped
zest of 2 lemons

For the sauce:
2 egg-yolks
2 tablespoons Dijon mustard
juice of 1 lemon
1 dessertspoon caster sugar
280 ml sunflower oil
1 rounded tablespoon dill, finely chopped

Start with the marinade. Mix the pepper, salt, sugar, lemon zest and half the dill together (1). Make sure that there are no bones remaining in the fish. Put one fillet, skin-side down onto a large doubled sheet of tinfoil. Spread the mixture on top of it (2) and cover it, like a sandwich, with the other fillet, flesh-side down. Wrap it up well and put it on a large dish or tray in the fridge.

Leave it for at least 2 days and nights, turning it every 8 hours and pouring away the liquid.

Open the parcel, separate the fillets and scrape off (3) and discard the marinade-mixture (don't be tempted to wash it off). Sprinkle the remaining dill all over the surface and pat it down (4). Replace the salmon in the fridge, sandwiched in the same way and wrapped in clean foil.

To make the sauce, whisk the yolks and mustard together and add the oil drop by drop, as for mayonnaise, until it thickens. Beat in the lemon juice, sugar, dill and seasoning to taste.

Finally, slice the gravadlax thinly on the slant, starting at the tail-end (5 and 6). Serve with the sauce and toasted brioche (see Basics).

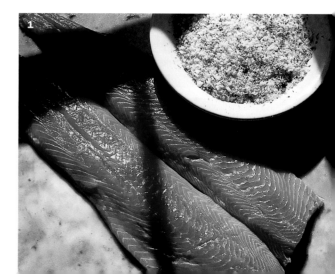

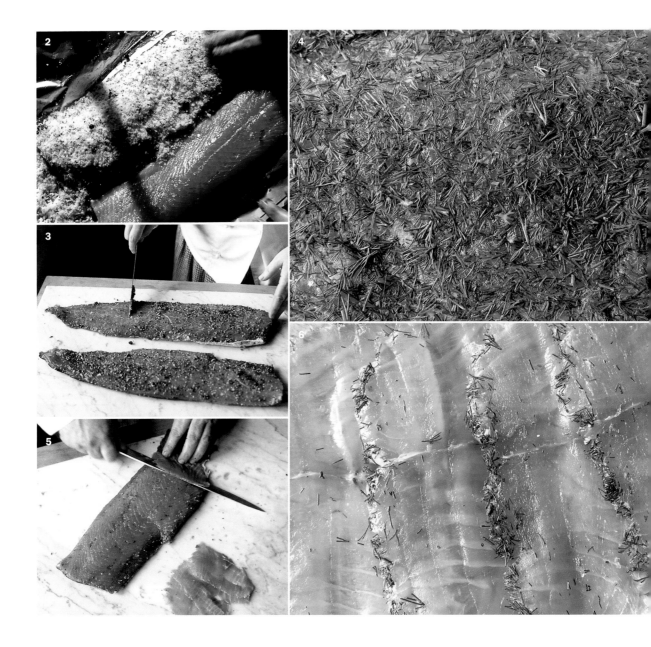

Wild Salmon
with Sorrel and Courgettes

One of the joys of living on Harris is the availability of wild salmon: it is a real treat, particularly when the fish spends practically no time between the rod and the pan! You must be very careful not to overcook it so as not to lose the delicate subtlety of its flavour.

Serves 4

**4 salmon fillets, skinned, each weighing
170–180g**
60g clarified butter (see Basics)
1 teaspoon fine sea salt
Hollandaise sauce (see Basics)
4 medium courgettes
100 g sorrel leaves
4 good sprigs thyme
60 g butter
juice of 1/2 lemon

Check that there are no bones left in the fish and sprinkle each with sea salt. Wash the sorrel and remove the stalks. Cut the courgettes into thin ribbons. Over a high heat cook the vegetables in the butter for no more than a couple of minutes, then stir in the thyme leaves and lemon juice.

Fry the salmon for a minute and a half on each side, over a medium/low heat in clarified butter (I think it is nicer to have them slightly under-done, but if you disagree, cook them for a little longer).

Make a little bed of vegetables in the middle of each plate and rest the salmon on top, surrounded by the sauce.

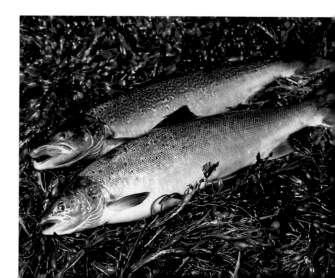

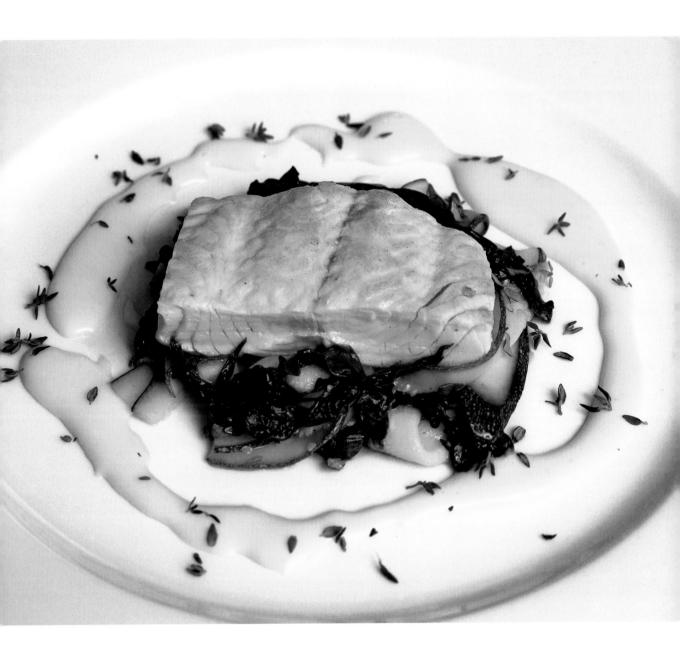

Chicken & Rabbit

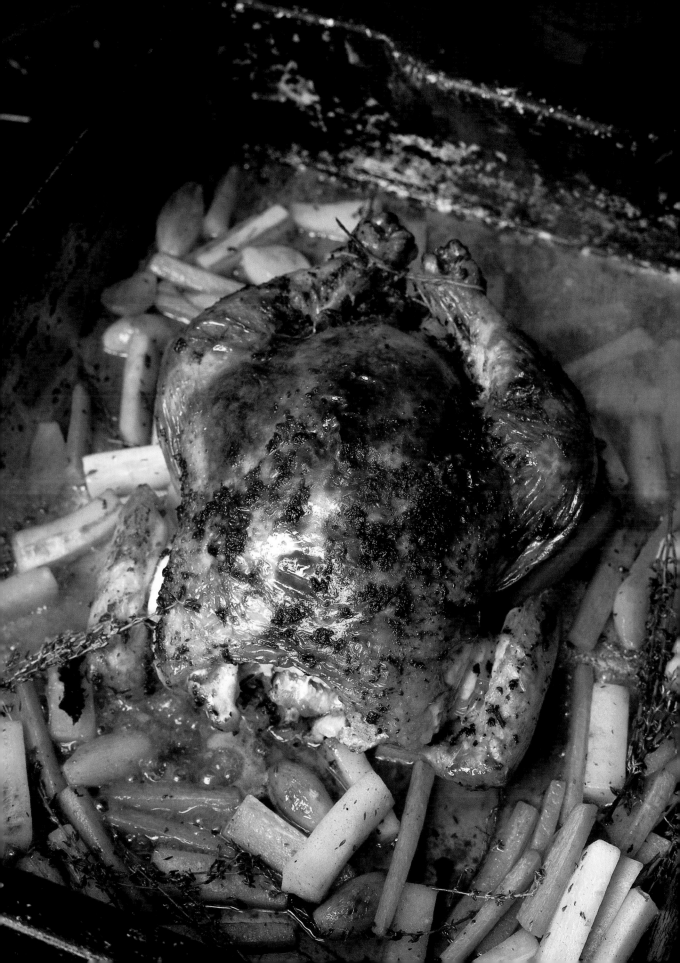

Chicken

'Je veux qu'il n'y ait si pauvre paysan en mon royaume qu'il n'ait tous les dimanches sa poule au pot.'

Henri 1V (1553–1610)

Many an island housewife still keeps a few chickens at home to supplement the family diet. As it is probably the most widely available and versatile meat in the country, I have included several chicken recipes here, as well as one using the baby chicken, or poussin.

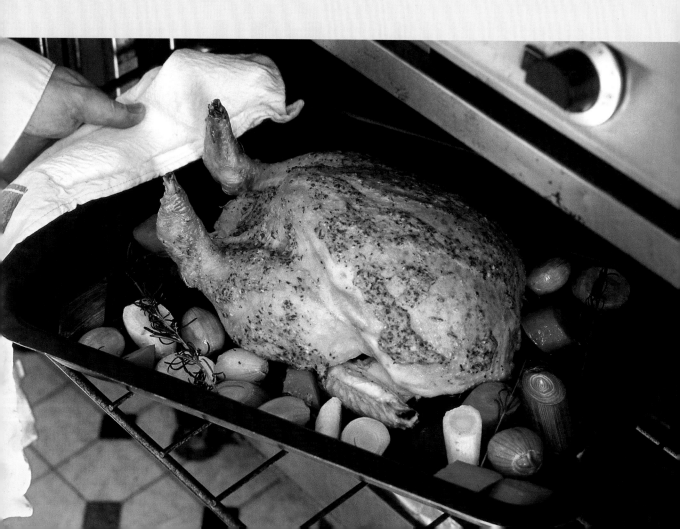

Scalpay Chicken

Serves 6

1 large chicken, weighing about 2 kg
4 rashers smoked bacon, roughly chopped
180 g cold butter
a large bunch of tarragon
a large bunch of parsley
1 small onion
2 cloves garlic
zest of 1 lemon
seasoning

Oven 180C/ 350F/ Gas 4

Put all the ingredients except the chicken into a food-processor and mix them thoroughly. Lift the skin off the breast of the chicken, and around the top of the legs, until it is loose. Smear as much of the mixture as will fit between the skin and the meat and then the rest on top, covering it thoroughly.

Roast, uncovered, for 2 hours, basting it occasionally. Serve it with glazed parsnips and spring greens.

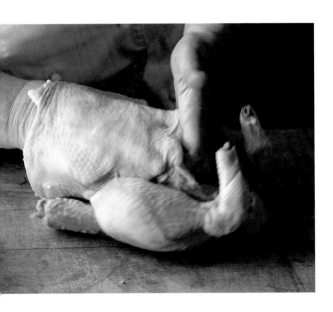

The name of this dish is a shocking pun. The little island of Scalpay lies off the coast, quite close to the castle at Amhuinnsuidhe: the chicken is virtually scalped. It is a mighty tasty variant on plain roast chicken, but you do have to get your hands messy. Should you prefer it, you can cook baby poussins the same way, though they would not take so long to cook.

Glazed Parsnips

Serves 6

4 large parsnips, cut into batons, about 5 cm long
70 g butter
1 dessertspoon caster sugar

Par-boil the parsnips until just soft. Drain them and turn them in melted butter, with the sugar. Fry them for a few minutes until they are golden.

Chicken Mirin

You can steep the chicken in this marinade overnight and then barbecue it, if you like, but I often do it this way instead. The sake and mirin give it an oriental flavour and are readily available in most good supermarkets.

Serves 4

4 chicken legs, boned and flattened
olive oil
seasoning

For the marinade:
125 ml soy sauce
140 ml sake
150 ml mirin
2 cm root ginger, grated
40 g caster sugar

Mix the marinade ingredients together and allow it to infuse for half an hour before straining it. Season the chicken and fry it in olive oil until nicely browned. Pour the marinade over it and let it simmer for 5 minutes, then remove the chicken and reduce the sauce to about a third. Return the meat to the pan and simmer it for a further 5 or 10 minutes, turning it frequently until it has become glossy. Serve it with an oriental salad.

Oriental Salad

The dressing I use for this is magnificent and, what's more, will keep for up to a month in the fridge.

Serves 4

$1/2$ Chinese cabbage, shredded
250 g bean sprouts
1 small tin of water chestnuts, drained and finely sliced
$1/2$ a tin of small tin bamboo shoots, drained and cut into julienne strips
150 g mange-tout, sliced lengthwise

For the dressing:
1 tablespoon olive oil
1 tablespoon sesame seed oil
1 tablespoon soy sauce
1 tablespoon mirin
zest and juice of 2 limes
1 red chilli, deseeded and finely chopped
2 spring onions, finely chopped
1 clove garlic, finely chopped
1 dessertspoon caster sugar
seasoning

Make the dressing first, by combining all the ingredients and leaving it for an hour or two for the flavours to develop. Plunge the mange-tout into boiling water for half a minute, then refresh them. Toss them with all the other ingredients in a large bowl, with the dressing.

Chicken and Potato Pie

This is always a favourite at Amhuinnsuidhe and my 'graduates' report great success with it.
It is easier to slice the potatoes finely if you use a mandolin.

Serves 6–8

500 g puff pastry (see Basics)
4 large chicken breasts, boned and cut into thin strips
720 g peeled potatoes, thinly sliced
130 g butter
3 shallots, finely chopped
2 tablespoons tarragon leaves
2 tablespoons chives, chopped
2 egg-yolks, lightly beaten
240 ml double cream
seasoning

It helps to have a baking-mat, in which case don't bother to butter the tray but put the pastry directly onto the mat.

Oven 180C/ 350F/ Gas 4

Turn the potatoes in half the butter over a gentle heat until they are just tender – don't let them brown. Remove them from the pan and allow them to cool in a large bowl. Meanwhile, soften the shallots in the remaining butter and add the herbs and chicken, turning it over a steady heat for a few minutes until it is partially cooked. Mix it all carefully with the potatoes, season to taste and again, allow it to cool.

Roll half the pastry into a circle about 36 cm in diameter and put it straight onto a lightly buttered baking tray. Brush the edges with egg-yolk then pile the mixture in the middle. Roll the rest of the pastry into a slightly larger circle and cover the pie with it, sealing and crimping the edges. Cut a little circle in the top (about 10 cm diameter) to make a lid, leaving it in place. Brush the whole surface with the rest of the egg-yolk.

Bake the pie for about 50 minutes, checking that it's not too brown – in which case turn the oven down slightly. Heat the cream. Take the pie out of the oven, remove the lid and pour in the boiling cream, lifting the mixture gently to allow it to permeate the pie. Return it to the oven for 10 minutes.

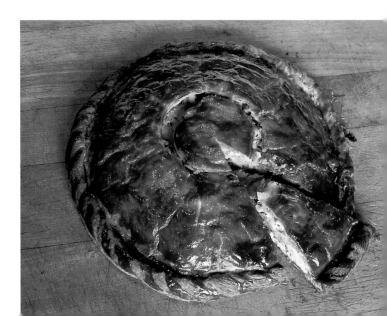

Chicken Taransay

This takes a bit of time to prepare, but it is not expensive and it is unusual – and you can do very nearly all of it in advance (as far as the ✳). It is worth the effort, for the flavour is wonderful. The boning can be a little tricky, so it is as well to stay friendly with your butcher: the skin has to be kept intact, save for one incision underneath, as it is to be used for wrapping.

Serves 4

4 whole chicken legs, boned
8 slices Parma ham
12 chicken livers, sinews removed
1 clove garlic, finely chopped
1 dessertspoon fresh thyme
**1 dessertspoon fresh sage leaves (halve this,
   if using dried herbs)**
seasoning
extra virgin olive oil

You will also need string.

Oven 200C/ 400F/ Gas 6

Dry the livers thoroughly with kitchen paper and toss them in the thyme, sage and garlic. Spread the chicken legs flat, with the skin underneath and season them. Cover each with 2 slices of Parma ham and then 3 chicken livers down the centre (1). Bring the sides in slightly and gently bring the skin up to make a parcel (2). Make a sausage shape, using several pieces of string crosswise and one lengthwise (3). ✳

Brush the little bundles with olive oil and roast them uncovered, for about 40 minutes, then allow them to rest for 5 minutes before removing the string and cutting each into about 6 slices.

Serve them with buttered noodles and a crisp salad.

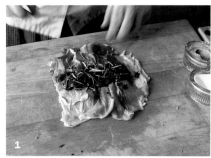
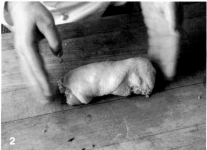
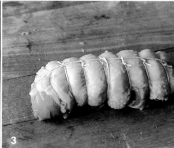

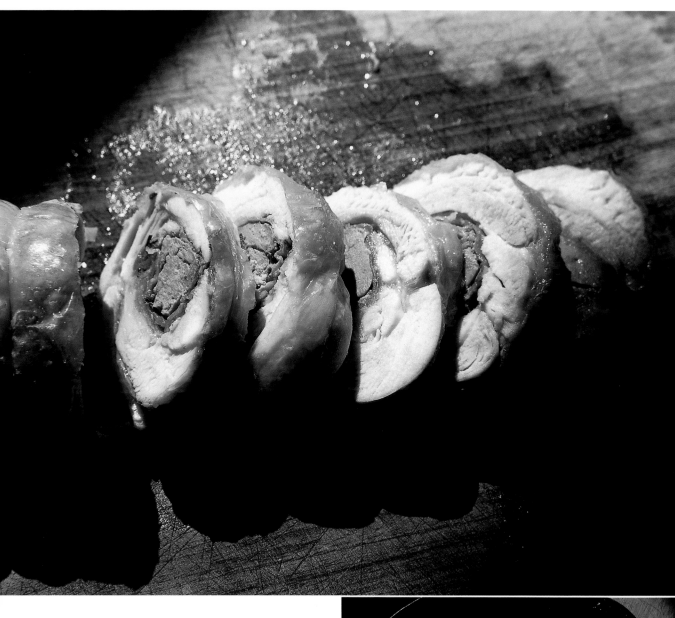

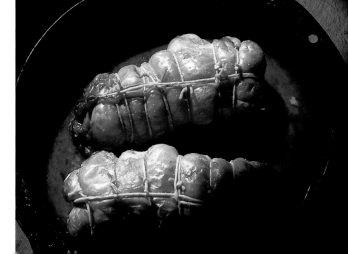

Poussins with Chestnuts

Though the quantities given here will serve four, this is a very well-behaved dish and good for a party, as it can be prepared well in advance and will sit in the oven for ages, coming to no harm. You can adapt it for chicken, pheasant or almost any poultry, but remember that it's a good idea to start it the night before you need it, to give the marinade a chance to do its valuable work.

Serves 4

4 poussins, boned and quartered (you can often buy them ready boned, or you can bone them yourself: if you do, be sure to leave the skin intact and each breast still attached to the wing)
16 very thin slices of streaky bacon
2 tablespoons olive oil
1 dessertspoon flour
2 tablespoons port
2 tablespoons redcurrant jelly
230 ml double cream

For the marinade:
1 stick celery (choose a head of celery with decent leaves, which you can use as decoration)
1 small leek
1 carrot
1 onion
2 cloves garlic
2/3 bottle red wine (sip the rest while cooking; it lubricates the voice and liberates the emotions!)

For the garnish:
12 baby onions
2 sticks of celery, chopped diagonally into lozenge-shaped pieces
1 tin cooked chestnuts (not purée)
30 g butter
1 dessertspoon caster sugar

Oven 200C/ 400F/ Gas 6

Prepare the marinade: chop all the ingredients and mix them with the wine in a large bowl. Wrap each piece of poussin with 4 slices of bacon. Secure each parcel with a cocktail stick and put them into the marinade for several hours (ideally overnight).

Strain the marinade into a jug. Take out the pieces of poussin and dry them. Heat the oil in a heavy casserole and turn the poussin pieces in it until nicely browned. Then remove them with tongs or a slotted spoon and put them aside for a minute. Put the vegetables from the marinade into the casserole, turn them over the heat, then sprinkle them with the flour and add the marinade. Bring the mixture up to boiling point, then return the poussins to the pot. Put the lid on the dish and cook it in the oven for 45 minutes (larger birds need more time).

Meanwhile prepare the garnish: cook the onions and celery in boiling, salted water for 3 minutes. Refresh them in cold water and set them aside.

When the poussins are ready, remove them from the casserole to a serving dish, being sure to remove the cocktail sticks and finish the sauce. Pour the remaining contents of the casserole through a sieve and return it to a clean saucepan over a low heat. Stir in the port, the redcurrant jelly and the cream.

If you want to serve it straight away, finish the garnish now: melt the butter with the sugar in a small frying pan, and add the onions, chestnuts and celery pieces, turning them over the heat for a few minutes, to give them a golden, caramelised character.

If you want to keep it warm, lower the oven heat and put the poussins back into the casserole until you are ready. Then pour the sauce over the poussins and arrange the garnish on each plate.

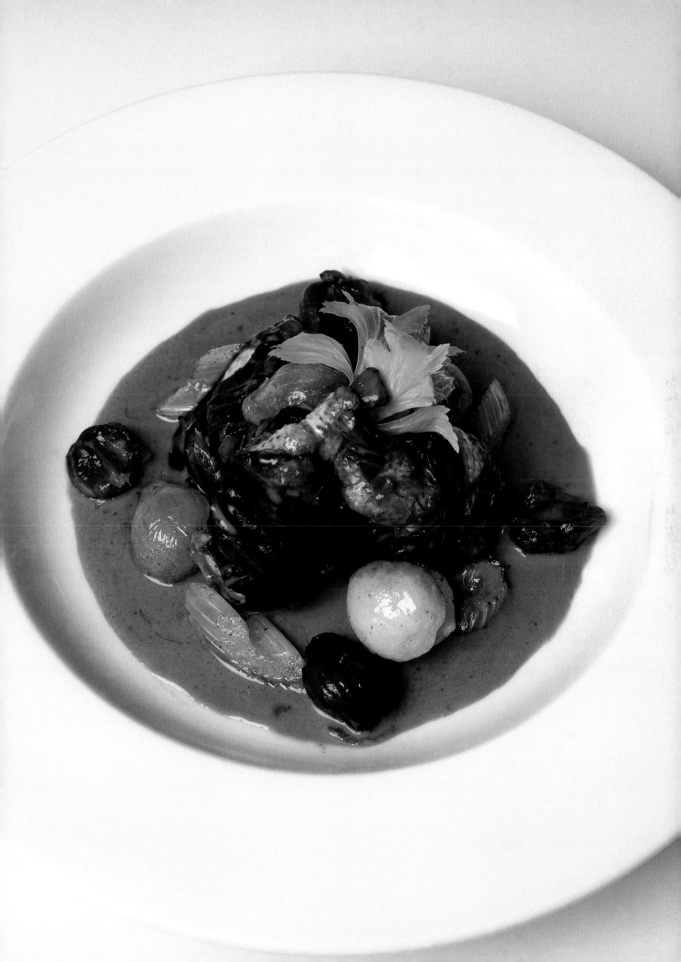

Rabbit

Country people have always known the food value of rabbit, often picking off a couple for the pot at sunset. In recent years, however, it has disappeared from more sophisticated menus. It is time for it to return.

It is available all year round, both wild and from the butcher's, though wild rabbit tends to taste gamier than its tame relations, and can be tougher: it is therefore more suitable for long, slow cooking. As in most parts of Britain, rabbits have long made their homes in the Hebrides and formed a basic element of the diet, though in recent years the proliferation of wild mink has reduced the population. The only kind of rabbit I would not recommend for the pot is a family pet – but then, it is always a nasty thought to eat anything to which you have given a name.

Many people are daunted by the problems of preparing rabbit. If it seems too much for you, your butcher might well help but if you are prepared to give it a try, it's not really very difficult if you follow these instructions.

Start by cutting the skin above the back feet and inside the rabbit's thighs. Then peel it up and pull it rapidly off the body: it should come all in one piece. Remove the head. Slit the carcass up the middle and remove the insides, discarding all of them except the liver and the kidney.

Cut off the legs and the shoulders and you are left with the saddle. If you intend to casserole the rabbit, just chop that into 4 pieces; if you need to use it whole, cut between the 4th and 5th ribs and remove the ribs, carefully sliding your knife underneath so as to keep as much meat as possible. Then remove the backbone, pulling it away so that the saddle remains intact. It is now ready for stuffing.

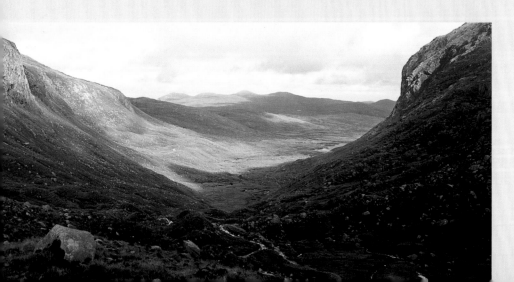

Rabbit with Prunes

This recipe is adapted from one I first came across in the South of France, where prunes are widely used in savoury dishes. It is a rustic, hearty dish, best eaten with plain boiled rice.

Serves 6

2 rabbits, cut into joints
2 onions, finely chopped
450 g Agen prunes, pitted
3 bay leaves
flour for dredging
olive oil
1 litre chicken stock (see Basics)
seasoning
1 dessertspoon fresh thyme

Oven 150C/ 300F/ Gas 2

Soften the onions in one tablespoon of olive oil and remove them, putting them into a large casserole dish. Dredge the rabbit in flour, shaking off the excess and sear it well on all sides before adding the softened onions. Add the bay leaves, seasoning and just enough stock to cover the contents. Cook it for an hour before adding the prunes and cooking for a further hour, or until tender.

Sprinkle the thyme over the top before serving.

Saddle of Rabbit
with Chicken Mousse and Black Pudding

On page 84, you can read of ways of dealing with these animals if you acquire them whole. In this recipe, I assume you have already skinned and prepared them – or asked your famously friendly butcher to do it for you. The joints can be used for rabbit with prunes.

Serves 4

the fillets of 2 saddles of rabbit, all skin and
  bones removed
160 g chicken breast
250 g black pudding, cubed
1 small egg-white
160 ml double cream
¹/₂ red pepper, deseeded, skinned and diced
  (as on page 29)
12 thin slices Parma ham
butter
seasoning

For the sauce:
1 rasher bacon, chopped
1 leek, finely chopped
¹/₂ bottle white wine
170 ml brandy
200 ml chicken stock (see Basics)
60 g butter
1 dessertspoon redcurrant jelly
175 ml double cream
seasoning

Oven 220C/ 425F/ Gas 7

Start by making the mousse. Process the chicken breast, add the egg-white and then carefully 'pulse' in the cream. Pass the mixture through a sieve, a spoonful at a time and chill it for half an hour. Meanwhile, sear the black pudding – very briefly and rapidly – in a little butter; drain and cool it on kitchen paper. When it is cool, fold it into the mousse mixture, with the red pepper and chill it again, for another hour or until really firm.

Spread 3 slices of Parma ham on a sheet of buttered tinfoil, 28 cm square (1), and lay the rabbit fillets, parallel, on top. Season. Spoon the mousse down the centre (2) and fold the ham up around the edges and the ends, making a long sausage of each rabbit. Roll each up in foil, like a cracker (3), and leave them in the fridge to become firm. Roast all 3 sausages in a roasting tin, to which you have added a little water, for about 30 minutes.

To make the sauce, soften the leek and bacon in 20 g butter then add the wine and 120 ml brandy. Bring it to the boil and reduce it to a third, then add the stock and reduce again to a third. Finally add the cream, the redcurrant jelly and the rest of the brandy. Simmer it for a further 5 minutes before passing it through a fine sieve and beating in the last of the butter. Serve the rabbit with buttered tagliatelle and baby leeks.

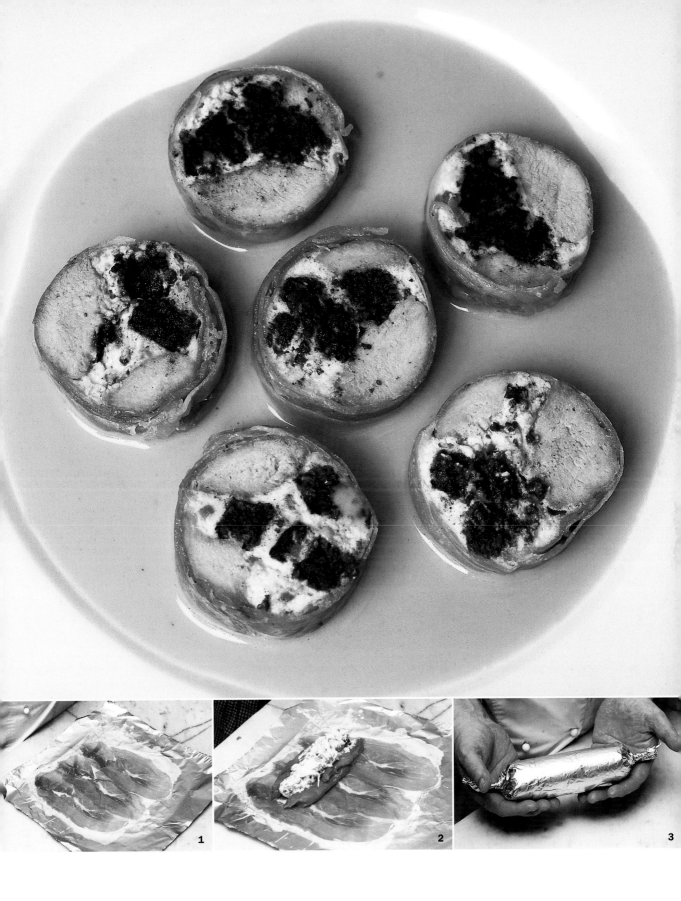

Game

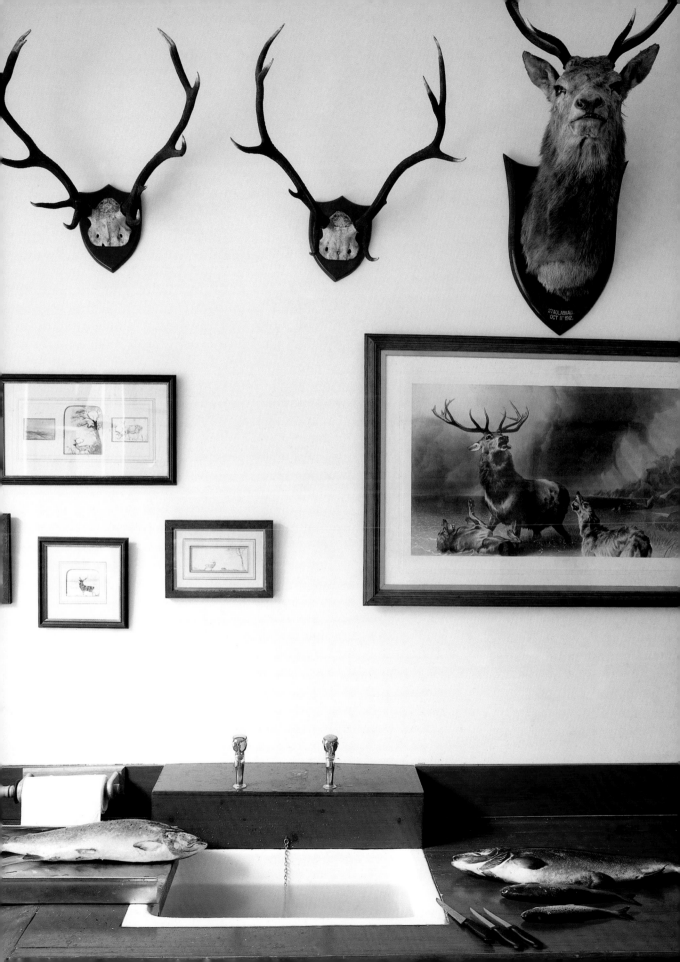

Game Birds

On Harris as everywhere else in Scotland the shooting of game-birds is a seasonal event. On the 'glorious' twelfth of August the shooting of grouse and snipe opens, but in Harris I find that grouse have not yet grown large enough to be really useful until a little later.

Grouse are one of many species of game birds living living on Harris: though they cannot be hand-reared, they need protection from predators and have to be managed. The mistake people often make with grouse is to overcook it, which only makes it tough and dry. I consider that the only way to eat it is the traditional way, for which I have provided a recipe.

Snipe are not resident, but are sometimes intercepted in the course of their migration from Scandinavia to the West Country. Though they are very tiny they are delicious and considered a great delicacy. Again, they take very little time to cook.

Partridge are in season from September 1st until the end of January, along with golden plover, wild geese and wild duck: we seldom use the plover or the wild goose, but we do use a lot of mallard and partridge, always looking for the younger, more tender birds. Partridge are reared on Harris and released at the age of 8 weeks, though a few 'calling-birds' are kept back to ensure that the rest return for food. The meat of a partridge is very pale and distinctive in flavour but it tends to dry out rapidly so that it has to be carefully cooked.

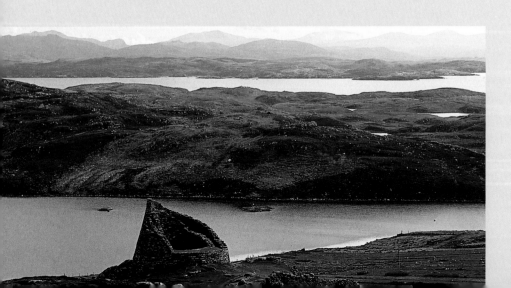

Lily MacDonald's Snipe

Lily MacDonald came to Amhuinnsuidhe as a winner of a cookery competition which appeared in the pages of *The Stornoway Gazette*. She worked for many years as cook on the estate at Morsgail Lodge, in Lewis, where snipe was always a popular dish. This is a variant on her recipe. Snipe are very tiny birds and you really need two each... and finger bowls.

Serves 4 as a main course

8 snipe, plucked and trussed (see Glossary)
8 small potato cakes (see below)
12 small turnips, turned (see Basics)
8 sprigs of thyme
1 tablespoon olive oil
60 g butter

For the sauce:
1 rasher smoked bacon, diced
1 leek, finely chopped
1 clove garlic, chopped
1 shallot, chopped
$1/4$ bottle red wine
250 ml game stock (see Basics)
50 g butter
15 g bitter chocolate
seasoning

Oven 230C/ 450F/ Gas 8

Sear the snipe on all sides in a mixture of oil and 30 g butter and put them, seasoned, into a roasting pan, a sprig of thyme tucked into each. Boil the turned turnips and refresh them.

Make the sauce by softening the bacon, leek, garlic and shallot in 30 g butter, then adding the wine and allowing it to reduce by half. Add the stock and reduce again by half. Just before serving, stir in the chocolate and the remaining 20 g butter.

Roast the snipe for 8 minutes. Meanwhile fry the turnips in 30 g butter, with a little seasoning. Serve each snipe on a potato cake, accompanied by the turnips and the sauce.

Potato Cakes

450 g waxy potatoes, peeled
4 very thin slices bacon, finely chopped
75 g clarified butter (see Basics)
seasoning

Grate the potatoes on a coarse grater. Fry the bacon (not too crisply, as it is to be cooked again) and drain it on some kitchen paper. Mix the bacon, potatoes and clarified butter together in a bowl and sear them in a hot, non-stick pan, in little spoonfuls, patting them into cakes and turning them until they are completely cooked.

Partridge
with Celeriac and Potato Galettes

The smoky flavour of celeriac is a perfect complement to a roast partridge and the dish is elevated to grandeur by its magnificent sauce. The celeriac is an ugly brute but don't be put off.

Serves 4 as a main course

4 young partridges
4 thin rashers bacon
4 sprigs rosemary

For the celeriac and potato galettes:
1/2 large celeriac
1 large potato
60 g clarified butter (see Basics)
celery salt

For the sauce:
1 leek, chopped
1 rasher bacon, chopped
45 g butter
1/4 bottle dry white wine
300 ml game stock (see Basics)
100 ml Armagnac
50 ml fresh orange juice

Oven 230C/ 450F/ Gas 8

Check that the partridges are clean and properly plucked before trussing them with the bacon on top and the rosemary tucked inside, ready to roast.

Make the sauce by softening the leek and bacon in 30 g butter, before adding the wine. Boil briskly to reduce it by half then do the same with the game stock, this time reducing it to a third. Then add the Armagnac and the orange juice and reduce again, finally beating in the remaining 15 g butter.

Peel the celeriac and the potato and coarsely grate them. Mix them together in a bowl with the clarified butter and celery salt and allow the mixture to solidify a little. Make little flattened galettes from the mixture and fry them on a low heat, very gently as they will be quite loose, until they are golden brown.

Roast the partridges for 15–20 minutes. Let them rest for 10 minutes then remove the breasts and legs and put them back for a minute or two before serving them, on top of the celeriac and potato galettes, surrounded by the exquisite sauce.

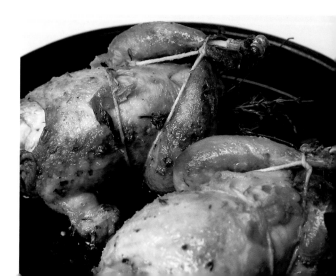

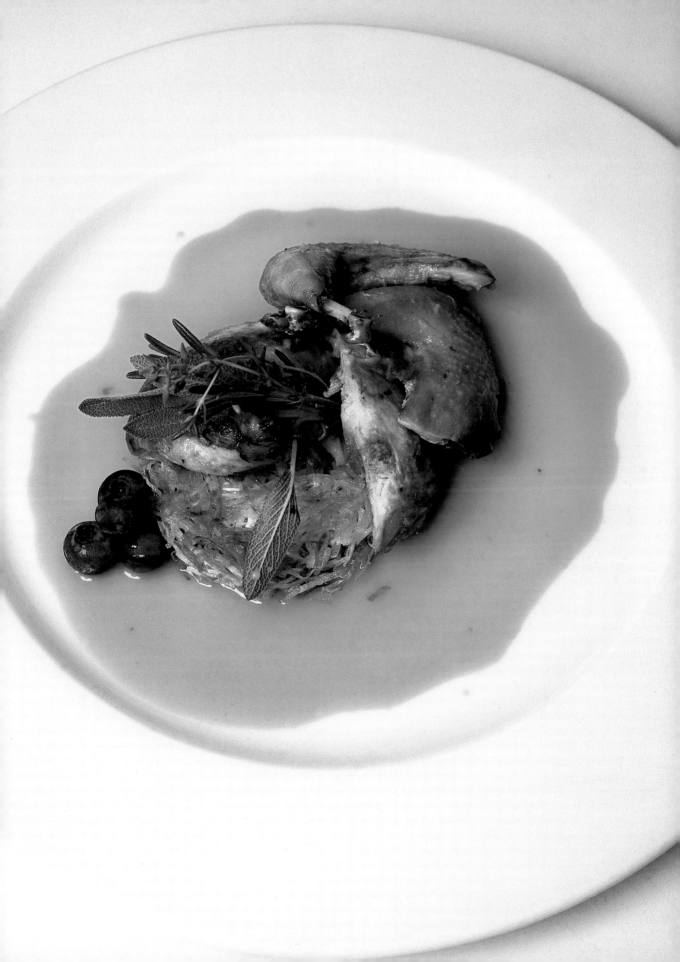

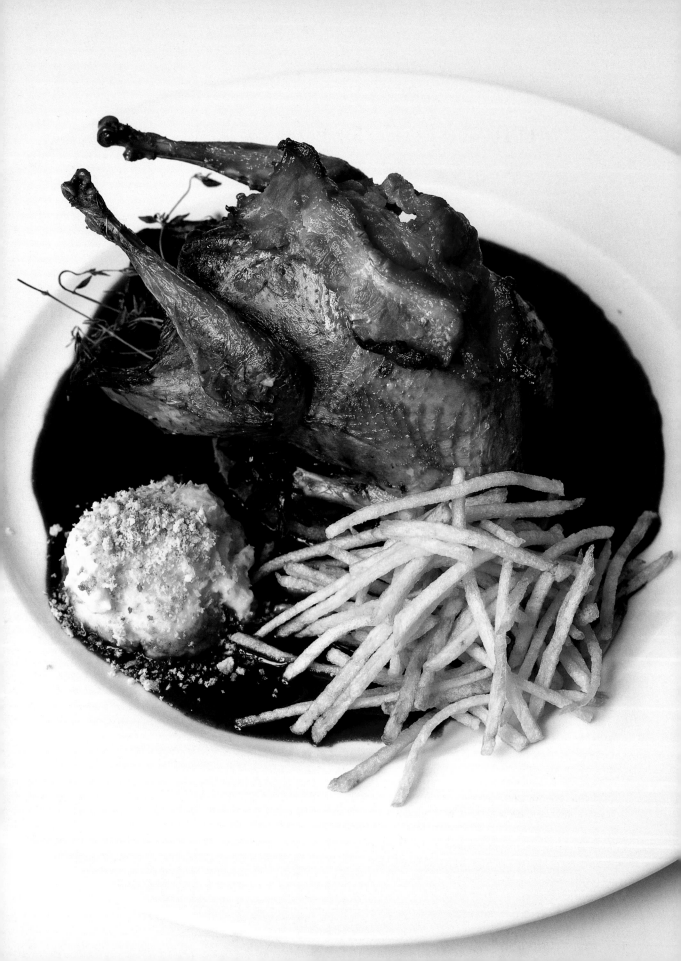

Traditional Roast Grouse

There are no real grouse-moors on Harris, but we 'walk-up' some grouse in the summer, which produces a variable number of birds a year. If you are offered the choice, select young ones, which will be sure to be succulent. For me, there's only one way of eating grouse, which is set out below. You can prepare it all in advance, up to ✳.

Serves 4

4 young grouse, trussed (see Glossary)
4 rashers streaky bacon
4 slices white bread
120 g clarified butter (see Basics)
4 sprigs thyme
olive oil
bread sauce (see Basics)
2 tablespoons toasted breadcrumbs
seasoning

For the sauce:
1 stalk celery, finely chopped
1/2 leek, finely chopped
1 shallot, finely chopped
60 g butter
1/2 bottle red wine
400 ml game/chicken stock (see Basics)
110 ml blackberry purée
1 tablespoon rowan jelly

Oven 220C/ 425F/ Gas 7

Truss each grouse with bacon on the breast and a sprig of thyme in the cavity. Sprinkle salt and pepper on top. Cut the bread into 8 cm circles, brush them on both sides with clarified butter and bake them for 5 minutes until they become large golden brown croutons, turning them if necessary. Remove them and allow them to cool on a rack.

Next prepare the sauce: soften the leek, shallot and celery in 30 g of the butter and add the wine and then the stock, reducing by half after each addition. Stir in the purée and the jelly and reduce again until it reaches a good consistency, then season it to your taste and strain it through a fine sieve. ✳

Sear the grouse on all sides in hot oil and then roast them for 15 minutes, turning them every 5 minutes (if you prefer your grouse less pink, cook them for 5 further minutes but no more). Remove them, cut off the string and allow them to rest for a further 10 minutes. Finish the sauce by whisking the remaining butter into it. Serve each bird on a crouton, with bread sauce, toasted breadcrumbs and game chips, accompanied by the sauce.

Game Chips

A deep fryer is useful for this, but you can use an ordinary pan. Ideally, fry the chips twice – the first time, well in advance, until almost cooked; the second time very rapidly just before you're ready to eat.

6 large potatoes
sunflower oil
salt

Heat the oil to 190C. Cut the potatoes into very small chips and fry them briskly until golden brown. Drain them on folded kitchen paper.

Umbrian Duck

This is a real staple of the Amhuinnsuidhe kitchen. It is both easy and pleasing to make and tremendously impressive to serve. It is also very useful to have in the fridge as it can be produced at a moment's notice. You do, however, have to start some weeks in advance.

Serves 4 as a first course

2 Barbary duck breasts, each weighing about 360 g
40 g coarse sea salt
10 juniper berries, crushed
10 black peppercorns, crushed
10 allspice berries, crushed
1 bay leaf
rind of 1 orange

You will also need some cotton muslin and some string.

Cover the duck breasts, skin-side down, with the remaining ingredients (1). Put them in an oval gratin dish (or a plate), cover and refrigerate for 36 hours (2). Then scrape all the mixture off and discard it. Roll each breast into a sausage shape (3), wrap it in muslin (4) and secure it firmly with string at each end and then at intervals of 2 cm (5).

Hang it in a cool place to dry, by an open window for example (6), for 2 or 3 weeks. Then keep it in the fridge until you need it. Serve it sliced extremely thin, with a lentil salad and a special herb salad.

Lentil Salad

The quantities given are small, just enough for an accompaniment to the duck breasts, but this is so delicious on its own that I usually make three times as much.

120 g Umbrian lentils
3 cloves garlic, finely chopped
1 shallot, finely diced
2 tomatoes, skinned, deseeded and diced
1 dessertspoon fresh thyme
1 bay leaf
120 ml white wine
extra virgin olive oil
chicken stock (See basics)
seasoning

Soften the shallot in olive oil, then add the garlic, lentils, herbs and wine, with just enough stock to cover everything. Cook slowly for 45 minutes, topping up occasionally with stock if necessary. Strain and allow to cool. Then stir in the tomatoes and enough olive oil to make it shiny. Finally, season it according to your taste.

Special Herb Salad with Garlic and Walnut Vinaigrette

1 handful of rocket
1 handful of chervil
1 handful of coriander
1 handful of French parsley
a few tarragon leaves

For the dressing:
4 cloves garlic, crushed
6 tablespoons extra virgin olive oil
3 tablespoons walnut oil
juice of ¹/₂ lemon
seasoning

Mix the dressing ingredients in a bowl and leave to infuse for 4 hours, then strain the mixture into a jug. Carefully rinse the herbs, remove any stalks and toss them together with one tablespoon of dressing and serve the rest separately (or reserve it for another occasion).

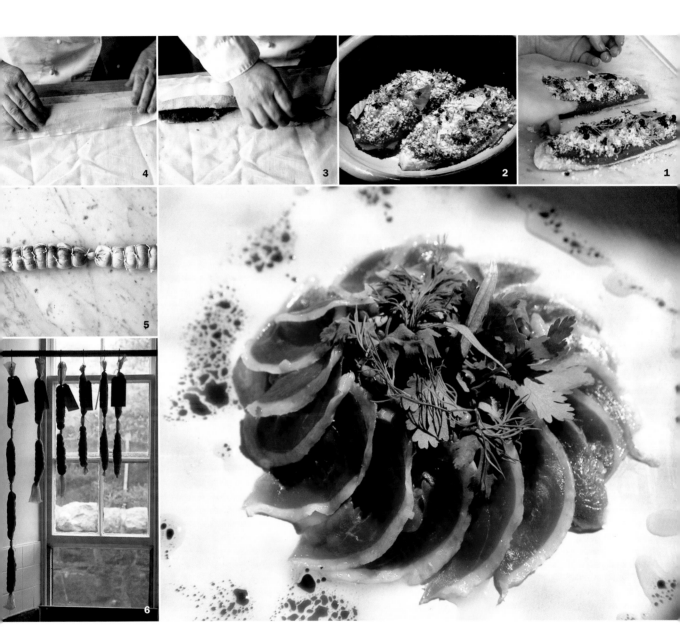

4

3

2

1

5

6

Roast Wild Duck Breasts
with Chanterelles and a Blackcurrant Sauce

It is becoming increasingly easy to buy wild duck breasts in supermarkets without having to have the rest of the bird. You can use Barbary duck if you like. This is a very sophisticated way of preparing them.

Serves 4

2 wild ducks
450 g chanterelles
1 clove garlic, finely chopped
90 g butter
extra virgin olive oil
seasoning

For the sauce:
2 rashers streaky bacon, diced
1 leek, diced
1/2 bottle red wine
1 sprig thyme
1 clove garlic, roughly chopped
300 ml game/chicken stock (see Basics)
120 ml port
2 tablespoon blackcurrant purée
   (or 1 tablespoon Ribena)
90 g butter
seasoning

Oven 220C/ 425F/ Gas 7

Remove the breasts of the ducks and take the skin off (it should come away quite easily). Marinade the breasts in olive oil, garlic and seasoning for 2 hours. Use the rest of the birds to make the game stock (see Basics).

Prepare the mushrooms by chopping off the bottoms of the stalks and wiping the flat caps clean. Make the sauce by softening the bacon, garlic, leek and thyme in 60 g of the butter before adding the wine and then the stock, reducing by half after each addition. Pass it through a fine sieve and then stir in the port and blackcurrant purée (or Ribena) and let it simmer for 5 minutes.

Sear the duck breasts in a dry pan (they will still be coated with the oily marinade) and roast them, uncovered, for 5 to 7 minutes, depending on their size, before letting them rest for a further 10 minutes, on a rack.

Finally fry the mushrooms and season them. Cut each breast into 5 slices and serve the duck on top of a little heap of mushrooms, surrounded by the sauce.

Quail is a comparatively new entry on British menus but it is becoming increasingly popular. Originally a wild bird, it is now farmed all over the British Isles and quail's eggs are nearly as readily available as chickens'.

'We loathe our manna, and we long for quail.'
John Dryden (1631–1700)

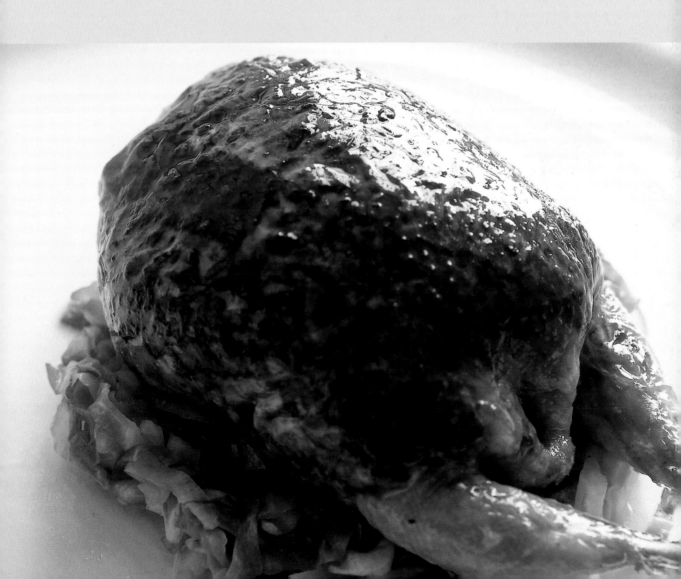

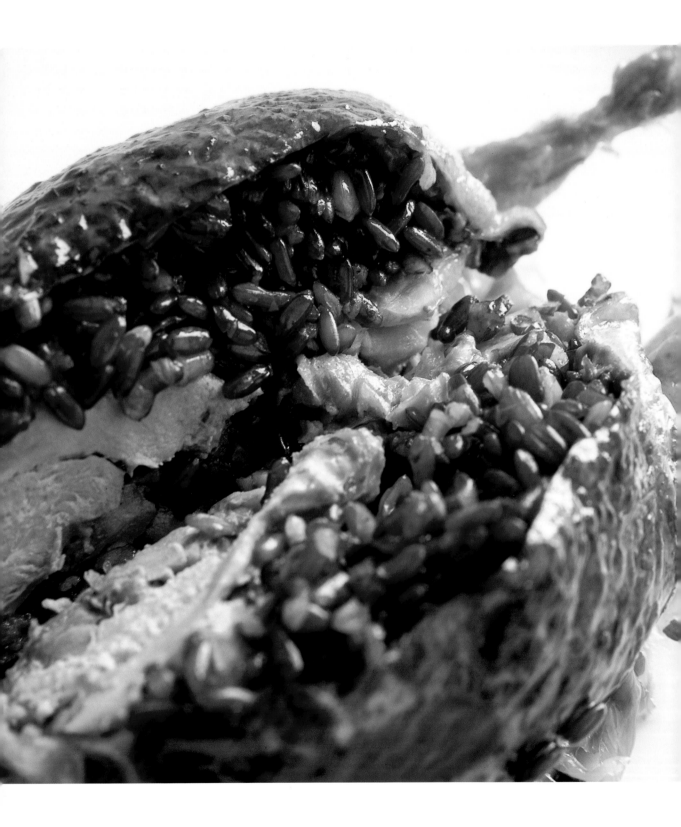

Red Roast Quail
with Honeyed Spring Greens

For this recipe, the little birds are filled with a pilaff of nutty red Camargue rice which has a very distinctive taste. It can be prepared well in advance, up to the ✳ and then quickly cooked. If you are daunted by the thought of boning the quail yourself, look out for ready-boned birds in the better supermarkets.

Serves 8 as a first course, 4 as a main course

8 quail
250 g red Camargue rice
1 medium carrot
1 medium leek
1 stick celery
1 small onion
60 g butter
1 dessertspoon crème de cassis
250 ml hot chicken stock (see Basics)

You will also need a sheet of greaseproof paper, a small, very sharp knife for boning the quail, 8 thin wooden skewers and some string.

Oven 180C/ 350F/ Gas 4

Chop all the vegetables into very tiny dice. Melt the butter in a roasting tin and turn the vegetables in it, warming them through. Add the rice and continue turning everything together over a low heat for a couple of minutes. Pour in the hot stock and cover the tray with the greaseproof paper, letting it rest lightly on the surface of the pilaff. Bake for 45 minutes or a little longer until the rice is tender and still slightly nutty, topping up with stock if it is drying too quickly.

Meanwhile, bone the quail. Turn each bird upside down and make an incision along its length. Cut around the bony central part of the bird and remove it, then carefully remove the longer leg-bones, always taking care not to damage any more of the skin.

When the pilaff is ready, take it out of the oven and allow it to cool. Increase the oven heat to 200C/ 400F/ Gas 6.

Spread the flattened quail skin-down onto the board. Lift the breasts up, spoon the pilaff onto the skin, put the breasts back on the pilaff. Pull the skin up around the sides and secure it by weaving the skewer through. Turn each bird on its side and tie the legs together with string, so that it looks like a minuscule turkey. ✳

Roast them for 10 minutes, then take them out and pour a spoonful of cassis over each bird. Return them to the oven for a further 5 minutes. Serve on a bed of honeyed spring greens.

Honeyed Spring Greens

500 g spring greens
1 tablespoon of runny honey
30 g butter

Shred the spring greens finely. Blanch them for a minute and refresh them. When you're ready to serve warm them in the butter over a low heat then add the honey and seasoning. Cook gently for 2 or 3 minutes.

Aunty's Quail

One day, long before I went to work for him, I was bold enough to ring Pierre Koffmann, just to tell him how much I admired his work. We talked about food for a while and out of that conversation a recipe was born. I have named it in appreciation of his wonderful restaurant Tante Claire and in gratitude for his help.

Serves 4

6 quail
500 g puff pastry (see Basics)
4 large Savoy cabbage leaves, blanched and refreshed
1 large chicken breast, weighing 150 g
1 small egg-white
150 ml double cream
2 egg-yolks
seasoning

For the sauce:
1 rasher bacon, chopped
1 leek, chopped
30 g butter
6 medium mushrooms, quartered
250 ml white wine
300 ml quail/chicken stock (see Basics)
120 ml cream
150 ml Armagnac
a few tarragon leaves
seasoning

Oven 200C/ 400F/ Gas 6

Cut the breasts and the legs off the quail. Make 300 ml stock from the other bones (see Basics). Take the skin off the breasts and season the meat. Take the central cores out of the cabbage leaves and dry them. Set them aside while you prepare a mousse. Process the chicken breast with the egg-white, blending it really thoroughly. Carefully add the cream, using the 'pulse' button so that it doesn't curdle. Season the mixture.

Roll out the pastry thinly. Cut 4 discs, 9 cm in diameter and then another 4, 12 cm in diameter. At the centre of each smaller circle put a small piece of cabbage and 2 quail breasts. Spoon some mousse on top of this, followed by one more quail breast and a little more mousse (1). Cover it all with more cabbage and paint egg-yolk around the rim before putting the larger circle of pastry on top, pressing it gently together to make a small, round parcel and trimming the edges (2).

With a little icing-nozzle – or a very sharp knife – cut a hole from the top to allow steam to escape (3), brush egg-yolk all over the top and bake on a buttered tray for 30 minutes (4).

Make the sauce by softening the bacon and leek in butter. Add the wine and the mushrooms and reduce to a third before adding the quail stock and reducing again. Add the Armagnac, reducing a last time. Finally add the cream and seasoning. Sear the quail's legs on all sides and roast them for 15 minutes. Serve 3 around each little pie, surrounded by the sauce, garnished with a little fresh tarragon.

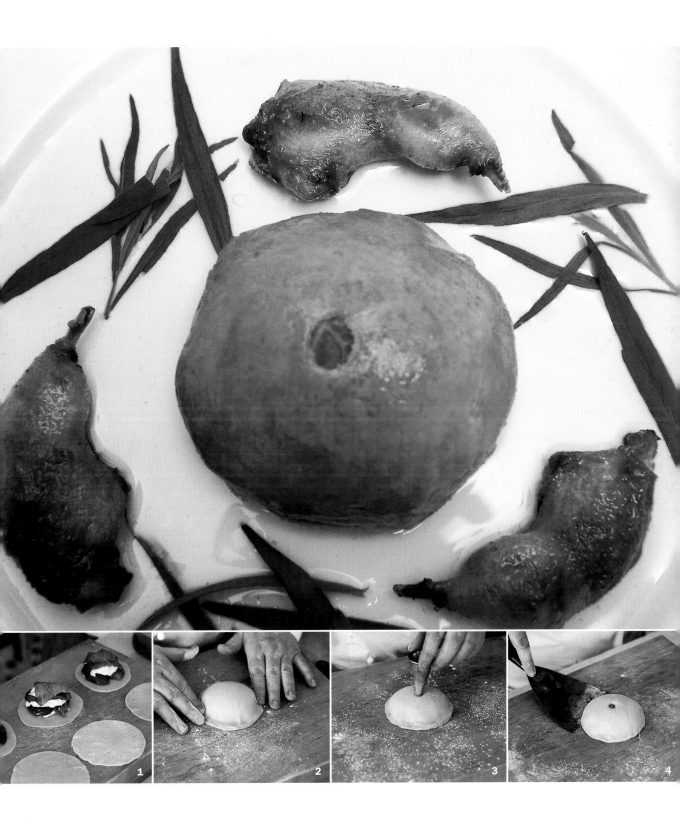

Venison
Red deer roam freely over the high hills of Harris. The herds are carefully tended by Kenny Morrison, his brother Alec and Roddy Macleod, grand stalkers all. The season for stags runs from August to mid-October and the season for hinds follows on over the winter, until February 15th.

The meat is sweet and tender, with very little fat; we hang it for 2 or 3 days and then use it in various ways. I like to cook the saddle, mostly – which comprises the fillet and loins – but the haunch is good for slow roasting and casseroles while meat from the shoulder or the flank makes an unusual terrine.

Although there is not much red deer available outside Scotland, other varieties, such as the fallow and the sika, are becoming more widely farmed elsewhere in the British Isles, and their meat is also delicious.

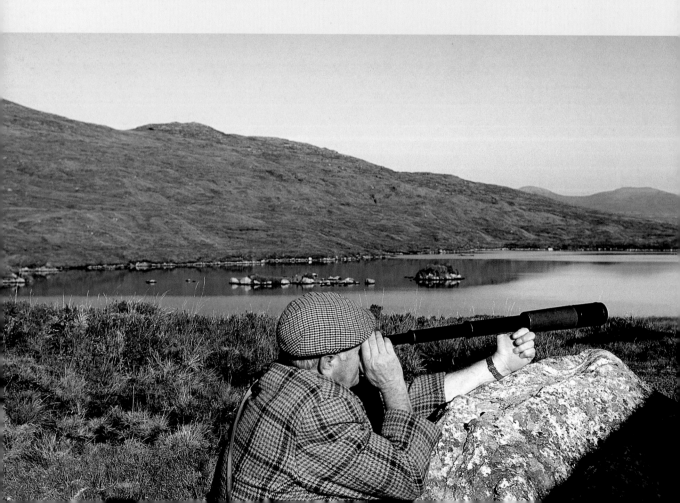

Loin of Venison
with Red Cabbage

Don't waste this scrumptious dish on anyone but your very best friends. This cut of venison comes from a saddle and is tastier than the very best fillet steak. Ask your butcher if you can have the bones for stock.

Serves 4

2 pieces of loin of venison, weighing about 600 g in all
1 medium red cabbage, very finely shredded
90 g butter
1 large onion, chopped very small
4 slices bacon, chopped very small
2 apples, peeled and diced
4 tablespoons red wine vinegar
4 tablespoons clear honey
3 level teaspoons salt
pepper
2 tablespoons olive oil
1 rounded tablespoon marmelade
225 g blueberries (optional)

For the sauce:
1 rasher smoked streaky bacon, chopped
1 leek, finely chopped
1/2 bottle red wine
300 ml venison/game stock (see Basics)
1 dessertspoon rowan jelly
120 ml port
70 g butter
seasoning

Oven 230C/ 450F/ Gas 8

Start with the cabbage. Over a low heat, melt the butter and add the onion. After a minute or two, add the bacon, followed by the cabbage, apples, honey and vinegar. Set it over a very low heat for an hour, stirring occasionally, topping up with a little chicken stock if necessary. Finally add the salt, pepper, marmelade and blueberries.

Next prepare the sauce. Soften the bacon and leek in 40 g of the butter and cook it gently for 15 minutes. Add red wine and reduce to a third then add the stock and the rowan jelly and reduce it again, this time to half, so that the sauce is developing a thicker consistency. Pass it through a fine sieve into a clean pan. Add the port and salt and pepper to taste.

Prepare the venison by removing any trace of fat or sinew, then sear it in hot olive oil. Roast for 8 minutes, until it is just firm to the touch, while you finish off the sauce by beating the remaining 30 g butter into it. Slice the meat and serve it on a bed of red cabbage, ideally with baby onions and potato purée. If you really want to impress, you could scatter a few extra blueberries around the plates.

Medallions of Venison
with Spinach and Morel Sauce

Morels are extremely expensive, but the recipe works quite well with other wild or forest mushrooms.

Serves 4

**2 pieces of loin of venison, weighing about
    600 g in all**
500 g fresh spinach
100 g butter
1 shallot, finely diced
30 g dried morels
1 rasher smoked bacon, chopped
1 leek, chopped
1/4 bottle red wine
2 tablespoons brandy
150 ml double cream
olive oil
seasoning
4 sprigs fresh thyme for garnish

Oven 220C/ 425F/ Gas7

Start by tying the loins neatly with about 8 pieces of string on each, making 2 long sausages and put them into the fridge.

Soak the morels in 200 ml of boiling water for about an hour. Then deal with the spinach: discard all the large stalks, wash the leaves well and melt them gently in 20 g butter; drain them thoroughly and set aside for later.

Start the sauce by straining the morels and reserving the water. Then soften the bacon and leek in 20 g butter, add the wine and reduce it right down to one third. Add the mushroom-water and reduce it again to about a third before stirring in the cream and brandy. Simmer the sauce for a minute, season it and strain it into a clean pan.

Sear the morels briskly for 30 seconds in 30 g butter and keep them warm while you heat the spinach, turning it gently in the rest of the butter. Sear the venison on all sides in a little olive oil and roast it for about 10 minutes. Take it from the oven and let it rest for a minute or two then remove the string and cut the meat into medallions. Serve them on top of the spinach, garnished with thyme and surrounded by the sauce and a scattering of morels.

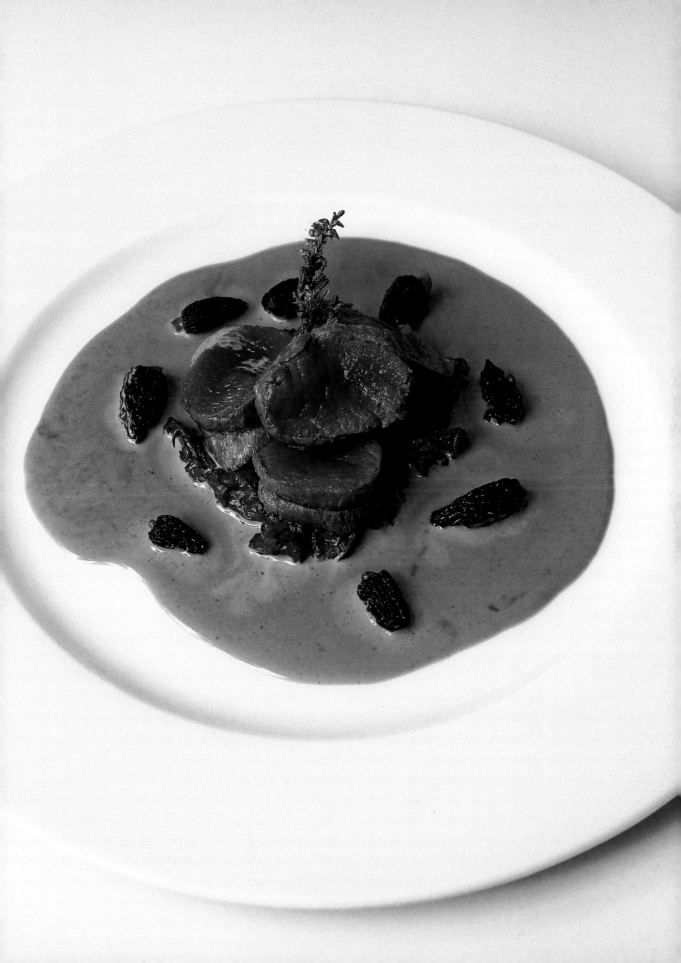

Venison in Red Wine

This is a wonderful, warming winter dish to share with friends old or new. You need to start it the day before your party but, once made, it will wait patiently until you're ready to eat. If you can't get hold of venison, it works nearly as well with beef. I have always used a little chocolate in the sauce: it may seem odd, but it really works.

Serves 12

A haunch of venison, weighing about 7 kg
plain flour, for dredging
6 tablespoons olive oil
50 g butter
3 tablespoons redcurrant jelly
1 tablespoon port
60 g dark chocolate

For the marinade:
2 bottles red wine
2 onions, chopped
1 leek, sliced
2 carrots, chopped
2 cloves garlic, chopped
2 celery stalks, chopped
4 bay leaves
1 teaspoon peppercorns
1 small bunch parsley
4 sprigs thyme

You will also need a very large casserole dish.

Oven 200C/ 400F/ Gas 6

Ask your butcher to take the meat off the bone. Cut it into chunks, about 8 cm square, taking care to remove all sinews (save all the trimmings if you would like to use them for a venison terrine). Combine all the marinade ingredients in a large bowl and turn the meat in it. Leave it overnight.

Strain the marinade, reserving both liquid and vegetables. Remove the pieces of meat, dry them and dredge them well with flour. Heat the oil in a large frying pan and seal them in the oil over a high heat. Put them back into the heavy casserole. Melt the butter in the frying pan and add the vegetables, turning them over a gentle heat for a few minutes, then transfer them to the casserole with the meat. Pour the marinade-liquid in, put the lid on and cook it in the oven for half an hour. Then turn the heat down to 150C/ 300F/ Gas 2 and leave it to cook for a further $3^1/2$ hours.

When the meat is very tender, strain it again, this time discarding the vegetables. Keep the meat warm while you finish making the sauce. Reduce it to half its volume over a fierce heat, then stir in the redcurrant jelly, the port and the chocolate (honestly) and reduce it further, until its consistency is creamy. Check the seasoning, pour the sauce over the meat and keep it warm in the oven until you are ready to eat. Serve with a purée of celeriac and potato and some braised chicory.

Potato and Celeriac Purée

If you've never tried cooking celeriac, do! It's one of my very favourite vegetables. This purée is rather different from ordinary mashed potato – do not be tempted to use a food-processor for the potatoes or they will become gluey.

Serves 12

1.5 kg floury potatoes
1.5 kg celeriac
180 g butter
500 ml hot milk
a pinch of nutmeg
seasoning

Peel the potatoes and boil them until soft, then sieve them and beat in half the butter followed by half the milk. Peel the celeriac, carefully removing all the fibrous matter, and cut it into rough chunks. Boil it until it is really soft then strain it and put it into a food-processor with the rest of the butter. Once it is smooth, sieve it and add it to the potatoes. Mix them well and add nutmeg and seasoning. If you feel you'd prefer it to be a little softer, add more of the milk.

Braised Chicory

Serves 12

6 heads of chicory, halved lengthwise
120 g butter
juice of 1 lemon
12 sprigs thyme
2 dessertspoons sugar
seasoning

Oven 200C/ 400F/ Gas 6

Melt the butter and lemon juice in a shallow dish in the oven. Turn the chicory in the mixture then arrange it, cut side up, with a sprig of thyme on each piece. Sprinkle the sugar over the top, cover with foil and bake for a good half-hour.

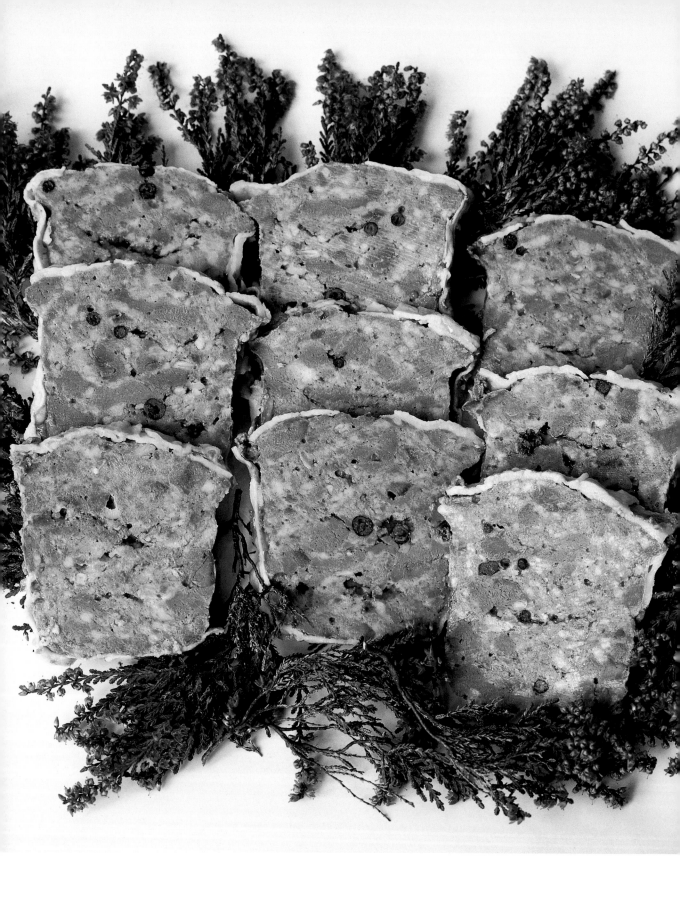

Venison Terrine

Terrines are never difficult to make and this is a very easy one. With a little salad and toast, it makes an unusual first course or light lunch, but you do need to make it the day before you serve it.

**750 g venison shoulder, trimmed of sinews and
  cut into thin strips**
750 g fatty pork, minced
3 tablespoons port
1 egg-yolk
30 juniper berries (approximately)
1 teaspoon salt
2 cloves garlic, pressed or minced
1 dessertspoon redcurrant jelly
20 very thin slices streaky bacon
a good sprinkling of pepper

You will also need some cling-film, some tinfoil and a terrine dish, ideally 26 cm x 10 cm x 7 cm.

Oven 140C/ 275F/ Gas 1

Line the terrine dish with cling-film, then with the bacon, allowing both to hang over the sides, so as to be able to wrap the whole thing up.

Put 250 g of the venison with the pork in a food-processor and process the mixture until it is smooth. Transfer it to a large bowl and add all the other ingredients, mixing it thoroughly with your hands. Transfer the mixture to the terrine dish, fold the bacon and cling-film up over the top, cover it in tinfoil and stand it on top of folded newspaper in a small baking tray.

Half-fill the baking tray with water and put it into the oven for 2 hours. Prod it with a skewer: if it emerges clean and warm the terrine is ready.

Remove the terrine dish from the water and allow it to cool for 12 hours undisturbed. Then take it from the dish, peel off and discard the old cling-film and re-wrap it in a fresh sheet. Refrigerate it until required – it can be kept in the fridge for up to a week.

Venison Carpaccio
with Black Olives and Capers

This exquisite dish works well with our venison, which is seldom hung for more than 3 days. It is absolutely essential that the meat should be trimmed clean of any trace of sinew or fat.

Serves 4 as a first course

500 g loin of venison, prepared as above
1 dessertspoon small capers
12 black olives, stoned and halved
1 small shallot, very finely diced
1 dessertspoon chives, very finely chopped
120 g fresh Parmesan cheese, in the piece
extra virgin olive oil
lots of seasoning

For the marinade:
6 tablespoons extra virgin olive oil
4 dessertspoons balsamic vinegar
salt

Cut the venison into slices about $1/2$ cm thick and put them in between two large pieces of cling-film. Bang them with a rolling-pin (but not too hard) and then roll them out, still between the sheets of film, until they become as thin as Parma ham. Put the venison in the fridge until an hour before you want to serve it.

Put the venison on plates – this is tricky, as the slices are delicate, so peel off one piece of film then invert the meat onto a plate and peel off the top layer. Sprinkle them with salt and pepper and spoon the marinade ingredients, separately, over the slices of venison.

Allow the venison to stand for about an hour at room temperature. Then sprinkle each plate with capers, olives, shallot and chives and shave fine slivers of Parmesan over the top.

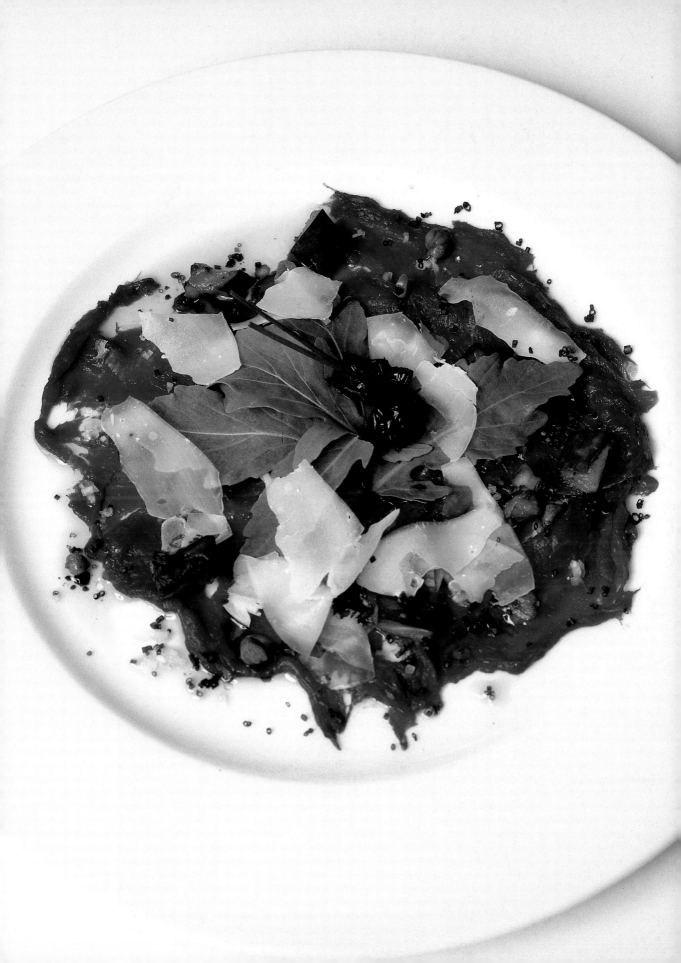

Meat

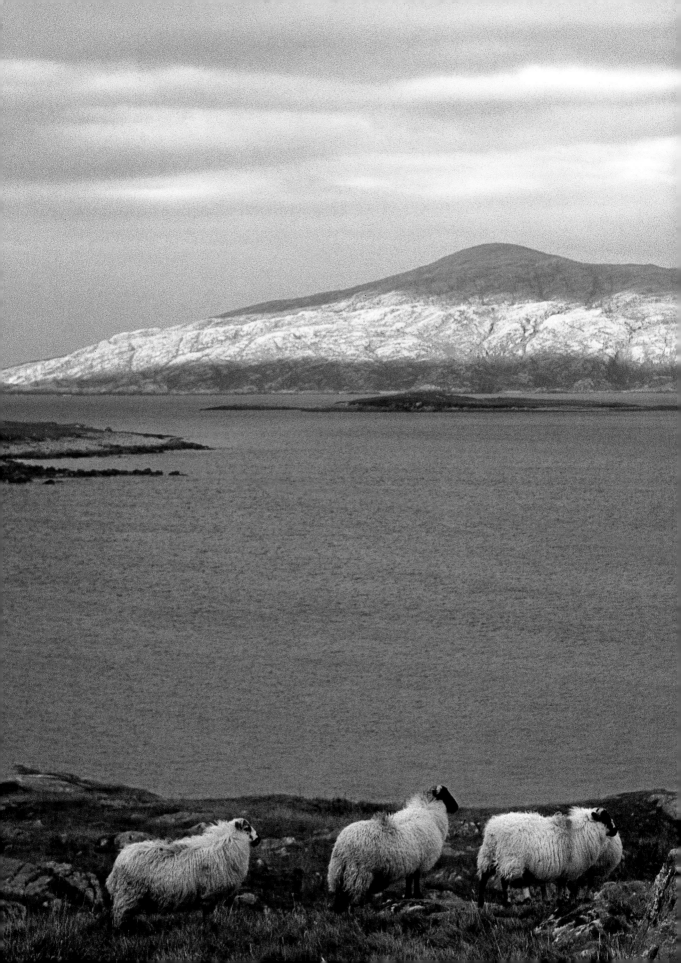

Lamb

Anyone who has ever attempted to negotiate the narrow roads of Harris will know who owns the place: the black-faced sheep. Though they haven't occupied the islands for as long as have cattle, they now roam freely over very nearly every inch, with easy non-chalance. Their wool, as well as their meat, is vital to the economy.

There is a view that a little cross-breeding improves the eating quality of these sheep so that occasionally a Cheviot or a Suffolk ram is brought in for the purpose. At all events, the local custom is to prefer the meat of a wedder, or a two-year-old castrated ram. However, the demands of the mainland mean that these customs are changing a little and a certain number of lambs are now slaughtered every year from late July through to the following February. But at whatever age we eat the meat, it is particularly sweet and good because the animals feed on the wild heather that covers the moors, supplemented by the rich machair grazing on the Atlantic shore. This machair is composed of wind-blown shell sand mingled with the adjacent peat and it produces lush green grass that is used for summer grazing: some of this rich land is also cultivated, producing good crops for winter feed.

Lambs grow on the mountainside for their first summer and those not needed at home are then sold on, generally in October, to the mainland. Many small households and crofters keep a few sheep for home consumption but few would dream of killing them under the age of two. Consequently we use a good deal of mutton at the castle, which takes well to long, slow cooking.

A gigot (spelled as the French do but pronounced 'jiggut') is the cut commonly used for slow roasting while the shoulder is often salted in barrels. The custom is to preserve several pieces together, with layers of salt between them, against the long winter nights.

The mutton is cooked in water for an hour and the fat carefully skimmed off and kept, to be replaced after the salty water has been discarded and fresh water added. This is then cooked with whatever root vegetables are available: it is the basis of a Scotch broth.

Lamb with Fennel, Cardamom
and Button Mushrooms

Serves 4

1 kg lamb, from the leg, cut into 4 cm cubes
1 large onion, sliced
1 bulb fennel, sliced
300 g button mushrooms
60 g butter
zest and juice of 1 lemon
1 tablespoon whole green cardamoms
4 bay leaves
1/2 bottle white wine
150 ml crème fraîche
seasoning

Oven 170C/ 325F/ Gas 3

Sear the lamb briefly in 20 g of butter. Take it out and put the mushrooms, onion and fennel in the same pot, turning them over a gentle heat with the rest of the butter.

Return the lamb to the pot, with the vegetables and add everything else except the crème fraîche. The liquid should nearly cover the meat. If there isn't quite enough, top it up with a little stock. Cover it tightly and put it into the oven for about 1 1/2 hours, giving it a stir now and again.

Take the meat out and boil up the juices in the pan to reduce it a little then add the crème fraîche and seasoning. Serve it with rice and raisins.

Rice and Raisins

250 g Basmati rice
1/2 onion, finely diced
1 good handful raisins
1 tablespoon parsley, finely chopped
1 tablespoon fresh mint, finely chopped
120 ml white wine
chicken stock (see Basics)
olive oil
seasoning

Bring the raisins and wine to the boil together and leave them for 15 minutes to cool before draining the raisins and reserving the liquid.

Soften the onion in a little olive oil, using a large pan. Add the rice, the raisin-wine and just enough chicken stock to cover the rice by about a centimetre. Bring to the boil and simmer gently for about 15 minutes or until the rice is ready and the liquid absorbed. Stir in the raisins, parsley, mint and seasoning.

Braised Knuckle of Lamb

This dish was inspired by a visit to Effie's house where I was very taken by the delicious smell of the Morrisons' Sunday lunch: lamb, covered in sea salt and slow roasting in her Rayburn. You can prepare this well in advance, up to ✳.

Serves 6

6 large knuckles lamb
1 large carrot, roughly chopped
1 large onion, roughly chopped
8 cloves garlic (skins on)
4 sprigs thyme

1 stick celery, chopped
4 bay leaves
1 dessertspoon coarse sea salt
1 dessertspoon black peppercorns
3 dessertspoons heather honey
3/4 bottle red wine
3 level dessertspoons molasses sugar
2 tablespoons soy sauce
olive oil
black pepper

Oven 150C/ 300F/ Gas 2

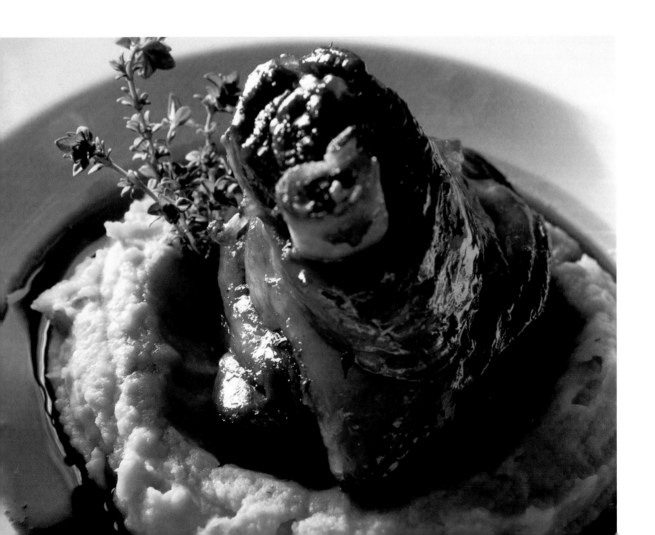

Trim the knuckles so that they will stand on end, exposing the bone. Put all the vegetables and herbs into a large ovenproof dish. Sear the knuckles on all sides in olive oil and add them to the pot, standing up like soldiers in amongst the vegetables. Pour in the honey and wine and sprinkle over the salt and the peppercorns.

Cook the dish, tightly covered, in the oven for 3 hours, until the lamb is coming away from the bone.

Take the knuckles out and put them on a plate while you make the sauce. Strain and discard the vegetables and return the juices to a saucepan, stirring in the sugar and the soy sauce. Reduce the liquid until it is syrupy ✶.

Increase the oven temperature to 200C/ 400F/ Gas 6. Put the knuckles back into the ovenproof dish and pour some of the sauce over them, to coat them. Roast them for a further 20 minutes, basting occasionally and checking that they aren't becoming too dark – in which case cover them loosely with tinfoil.

Serve them with some butter-bean purée and small glazed onions.

Butter-bean Purée

This dish takes time to prepare but it is useful in many ways: it is lovely just eaten as it is, with crusty bread and it is very tasty as a summer salad – in which case end the recipe at ✶✶. As with all pulses, you shouldn't add salt early in the cooking or it hardens the beans.

450 g dried butter-beans, soaked in cold water
 overnight
1 onion, roughly chopped
1 carrot, roughly chopped
2 bay leaves
6 cloves garlic

170 ml extra virgin olive oil
2 tablespoons tomato purée
2 sprigs thyme
1 level tablespoon caster sugar
seasoning

Oven 150C/ 300F/ Gas 2

Drain the beans and cover them with fresh water. Bring them to the boil and cook them for a couple of minutes before draining them again. Return the beans to the pan with the onion and the carrot and again cover them with fresh water; bring them to the boil and simmer them for about an hour – check after 40 minutes: they should be tender. Strain them, reserving the liquid.

Put the beans and other vegetables into an earthenware dish and mix in the olive oil, the garlic, bay leaves, thyme and a little of the reserved liquid, to make a thick sauce. Bake it, covered, for 40 minutes. ✶✶

Puree the mixture in a liquidiser – you may need a little more of the reserved liquid, if it seems too thick. Reheat it gently when you are ready to use it.

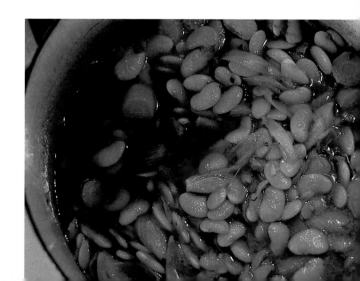

Rack of Lamb
with Ginger and Green Lentils

This is a lovely way to prepare young spring lamb: it is my variation on a classic dish. Trimming the lamb is important: you must be sure that the fat and the skin are removed and the bones are chopped back, to within 5 cm of the eye of the meat.

Serves 4

**4 racks of lamb, each weighing about 200 g
  and trimmed**
4 dessertspoons quince jelly

For the lentils:
150 g Puy lentils
2 cm fresh root ginger, peeled and finely chopped
2 cloves garlic, finely chopped
1 shallot, finely chopped
20 g butter
1 tablespoon mint, finely chopped
100 ml white wine
400 ml lamb/chicken stock (see Basics)
seasoning

For the sauce:
1 rasher bacon, chopped
1/2 onion, chopped
1 tablespoon tomato purée
250 ml red wine
300 ml lamb stock (see Basics)
1 dessertspoon quince jelly
50 g butter

Oven 200C/ 400F/ Gas 6

Sear the lamb on the rack (where the fat is) for a few seconds until it is brown. Melt the quince jelly, slowly, in a saucepan, then cool it a little and, just as it is setting, brush it over the lamb. Sprinkle the mint over the lamb too. Chill it for an hour.

Soften the garlic, ginger and shallot in the butter, then add the lentils and the wine. Bring it to the boil and then add the stock. Simmer it gently for 15 minutes, until the lentils are tender. Strain them and season them to taste.

Roast the lamb – put it in for 15–20 minutes if you like it really rare, longer if you prefer it less pink – and allow it to rest for a further 10 minutes, while you make the sauce.

Soften the onions and bacon in half the butter then add the red wine and tomato purée and reduce it to a third. Then add the stock with the quince jelly and any juices that have run from the meat and reduce the stock again to a third. Pass it through a fine sieve before beating in the remaining butter.

Carve the racks into cutlets and serve them on a bed of lentils, with some braised chicory (see page 109) and dauphinoise potatoes.

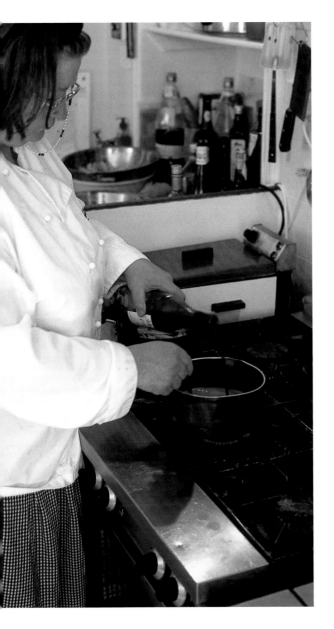

Dauphinoise Potatoes

You can make this dish a few hours in advance and just heat it through at the last minute. If you like, you can cut the finished potatoes into rings, as I do at Amhuinnsuidhe, which looks rather smart. The quantity of cream/milk used will depend a little on the shape of your dish: I use one about 25 cm x 20 cm. A mandolin is useful for slicing the potatoes, or even the fine blade of a food-processor.

Serves 4

1 kg potatoes, peeled and very finely sliced
450 ml double cream
50 ml milk
1 clove garlic, chopped
seasoning
15 g butter

Oven 130C/ 250F/ Gas 1

Stir the seasoning and the garlic into the cream, mixing it well and making sure it is well salted. Butter an ovenproof dish and layer the potatoes into it, pouring over the cream until it just covers them. Bake it for an hour and a half, or until the potatoes are cooked.

Saddle of Lamb
Stuffed with Kidneys and Spinach

'Have you learned to carve? For it is ridiculous not to carve well. A man who tells you gravely that he cannot carve might as well tell you that he cannot blow his nose; it is both as necessary and as easy.'
Lord Chesterfield (1694–1773)

The carving of this dish is not difficult, but the preparation takes time and care – as you might expect from such a seriously impressive party piece. Most of this preparation can be done well in advance (up to ✱). Ask your butcher to fillet and skin the lamb very carefully, keeping the skin intact and giving you the bones for use in stock (see Basics). You should be left with the loins, fillet and flank, which you will be wrapping in the skin.

In fact, there is another way of doing it, if you can get hold of about 500 g caul-fat. If you do, soak it in cold water before squeezing it out, spreading it flat like a cobweb and rolling up the lamb in it; if you do it this way, obviously you won't need the lamb's skin.

Serves 10

1 saddle of lamb, weighing about 4 kg before boning
12 slices Parma ham
2 shallots, finely chopped
800 g fresh spinach
8 lamb's kidneys
60 g butter
seasoning

For the sauce:
1 rasher smoked bacon, diced
1 medium leek, diced
60 g butter
550 ml lamb stock (see Basics)
1 tablespoon tomato purée
280 ml red wine
200 ml Madeira
1 tablespoon redcurrant jelly
seasoning
rosemary as a garnish

You will also need a lot of string, enough to tie up the meat at 2 cm intervals.

Oven 220C/ 425F/ Gas 7

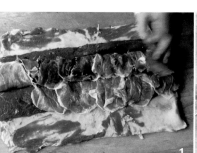 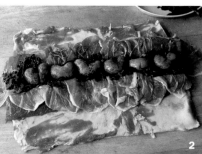 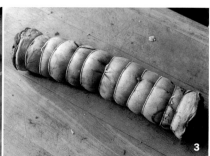

Having asked your butcher to prepare the meat (see above), make sure that all fat and sinews have been removed; season it well and set it aside.

Take the long stalks off the spinach and discard them. Wash the spinach leaves thoroughly and drain them. Soften the shallots in 30 g butter and add the spinach, turning it gently over the heat until it wilts. Drain it thoroughly, pressing all the liquid from it.

Prepare the kidneys by halving them horizontally and removing and discarding the hard sinews. Sear them on all sides in the remaining butter and leave them to cool, allowing all the juices to drain away.

Spread out the skin (or caul-fat), ready for wrapping. Arrange the 2 pieces of loin on it, close to and parallel with the longer side of the skin, with a little trough between them for the stuffing. Put the fillets on top of the smaller ends of the loins, to balance them up.

Line this trough with 8 slices of Parma ham, each crossing the centre and hanging over the side (1) ready to be rolled around the spinach. Line this, again, with half the spinach. Put a row of kidneys along the trough (2) and season them well before covering them with the rest of the spinach.

Now bring up the ends of the ham to make a long sausage. Cover this with the meat from the flank and roll the whole thing up, securing it very tightly with string and using the remaining prosciutto to cover the ends (3). ✶

If you can, leave it for a few hours in the fridge to allow it to settle. Roast it for 35 minutes if you like it rare, longer if not, and allow it to stand, covered in tinfoil, on a rack, for 20 minutes, before carving.

Make the sauce by gently softening the bacon and leek in 30 g butter for 5 minutes. Then add the red wine and Madeira and reduce it to a third of its original volume.

Add the lamb stock, tomato purée and redcurrant jelly and reduce it again to a third until it becomes slightly thicker. Whisk in the remaining 30 g butter at the last minute. Serve with minty new potatoes.

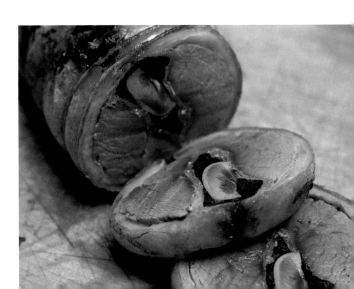

Beef

'Then get me a tender sirloin
From off the bench or hook,
And lend to its sterling goodness
The science of The Cook.

And the night shall be filled with comfort,
And the cares with which it begun
Shall fold up their blankets like Indians
And silently cut and run.'

Phoebe Cary (1824–1871)

Cattle lived in the islands long before the arrival of sheep. The beef industry has, however, changed a good deal since Martin Martin wrote: 'These Cows are very little but very fruitful, and their Beef very sweet and tender'.

At one time, every croft would have had a couple of house cows and they would almost certainly have been shaggy Highlanders: when one was slaughtered, its meat was salted down to see the family through the winter.

Although these lovely creatures do still wander about the roads of Harris, the advent of domestic freezers has caused the gradual disappearance of home salting, until nowadays it is only those who hanker for a nostalgic taste of childhood who even buy salt-beef, let alone produce it at home.

Highland cattle were often crossed with Shorthorn bulls until about 20 years ago. Now, in a constant drive to improve the stock, many more continental strains have been introduced, particularly the Limousin and the Charolais, via the artificial insemination scheme organised on the mainland.

Again, slaughtering habits have changed recently: the custom was always to keep calves until they were nearly 3 years old, but today many of them don't live past 18 months.

If it seems, sentimentally, rather sad to be losing the pure-bred local beef of the islands, there is a very positive side to it. The system of improvement by cross-breeding is working. The beef we buy on Harris today may be descended from an Aberdeen Angus, by way of a Highland, a Shorthorn and a Charolais, but it is still some of the tastiest meat in the world.

Island Meatballs

This is hearty sustaining winter food.

Serves 6

1 kg rump steak, minced twice
1 large onion, finely diced
2 egg-yolks
black pepper
salt
1 teaspoon caster sugar
1 teaspoon ground ginger
1 teaspoon ground cloves
1 teaspoon allspice
olive oil

Soften the onion in a little oil then mix all the ingredients in a large bowl. Roll it into small balls, the size of golf balls, and fry them in oil until brown all over. Serve with a green salad, tomato sauce no. 1 (see Basics) and Rumbledethumps.

Rumbledethumps

If a mixture of potato and cabbage can be known as bubble-and-squeak in England it shouldn't surprise us that the Scottish version makes a heartier noise.

Here is a recipe quoted by Christopher North in his *Noctes Ambrosianae:*
'Take a peck of purtatoes and put them in a boyne – at them with a beetle – a dab of butter – the beetle again – another dab – then cabbage – purtato – beetle and dab – saut meanwhile – and a shake o' common black pepper – feenally, cabbage and purtato throughither – pree, and you'll fin' them decent rumbledethumps'.

Mine is similar.

1 kg potatoes
1 small cabbage
25 g butter
4 tablespoons grated Isle of Mull cheese, or
  any cheddar
1 tablespoon chives, chopped
1 teaspoon ground nutmeg
seasoning

Oven 220C/ 425F/ Gas 7

Boil the potatoes until soft then mash them and allow them to cool. Shred the cabbage and boil it for 3 minutes. Strain and refresh it. Mix the vegetables, chives and seasoning together with 2 tablespoons of cheese.

Melt the butter then shape the mixture into little patties – about 6 cm in diameter – and brush them all over with melted butter. Sprinkle the remaining cheese on top and bake for 20 minutes.

Beef MacLeod

We have named this splendid beef dish after the old Lords of the Isles instead of the hero of Waterloo. Highlander and Aberdeen Angus beef are especially delicious when they have been properly hung: if you can, get a cut called a strip loin instead of sirloin: although it is expensive, it is the best and there is no waste. However, the pudding is good enough to eat on its own, so if a vegetarian should stray into your Sunday lunch party, just increase the quantities.

Serves 8

sirloin of beef, weighing 1.5 kg when trimmed
1 onion, roughly chopped
1 leek, roughly chopped
a good pinch of sea salt
1 tablespoon plain flour
1/2 bottle red wine
250 ml brown stock (see Basics)
olive oil

For the pudding:
230 ml milk
180 ml cold water
2 eggs
200 g plain flour
1 Spanish onion, chopped
1 tablespoon fresh thyme
olive oil
seasoning

You will need 2 muffin trays, bun trays, or similar, for cooking the puddings.

Oven 230C/ 450F/ Gas 8

Start with the pudding. Sear the onion in olive oil until it is brown, sticky and sweet. Add the thyme and season the mixture generously. Leave it to cool. Beat the rest of the ingredients together and chill this batter for an hour, while you start on the meat.

Seal the beef in hot oil until it is browned on all sides. Scatter the onion and leek over the base of your roasting tin and put the beef on top, sprinkling the salt all over it. Roast it for 40 minutes if you like it rare, longer if you prefer it well done. It must stand for 20 minutes, covered in tinfoil, on a grid over a plate to collect the juices, before you carve it.

While it roasts, finish the pudding. Put enough oil into the trays to cover the bottom – probably about a dessertspoonful for each indentation – and heat them in the oven until smoking hot. Take the batter from the fridge and stir in the onion mixture. Remove the trays from the oven and pour the mixture in, enjoying the essential sizzle. Return the trays to the oven for about 15 minutes – check after 12.

Finally, make the gravy: sprinkle the flour over the onion and leek mixture in the base of the roasting tin and stir over the heat before adding the wine. Bring it to the boil and let it simmer for a minute before adding your stock. Simmer it again and finally pour in the juices from the beef, before straining it into a jug. This dish goes very well with rosemary potatoes.

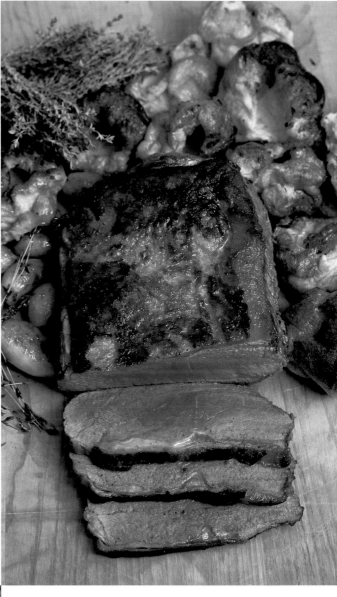

Rosemary Potatoes

Serves 8

The success of this dish depends on your remembering to turn the potatoes several times during cooking, so that they are crisp all over.

1.5 kg small, waxy potatoes
1 rounded tablespoon rosemary leaves
olive oil
coarse sea salt

Oven 230C/ 450F/ Gas 8

Pound the rosemary leaves in a mortar, to release their flavour. Wash the potatoes and cut them into wedges, like large, blunt chips. Combine all the ingredients in a roasting tray using enough olive oil to coat the potatoes and roast them for an hour, turning frequently.

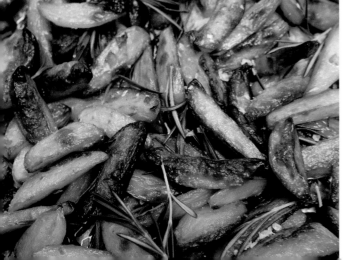

Braised Oxtail

This is one of the classics of British cooking. It is the most wonderfully warming and encouraging dish to serve on a winter's night, with lashing of good red wine and fine company.

Serves 6 to 8

2.5 kg oxtail, trimmed of fat
6 rashers streaky bacon, chopped
100 ml brandy
100 g butter
olive oil
500 ml brown stock (see Basics)
fresh thyme
black peppercorns
4 bay leaves
3 tablespoons parsley
1 tablespoon plain flour
24 shallots, peeled and left whole
8 medium carrots
100 g butter
1 rounded tablespoon caster sugar

For the marinade:
2 bottles of red wine
3 medium onions, roughly chopped
3 large carrots, roughly chopped
2 sticks celery, roughly chopped
8 cloves garlic, chopped

For the garnish:
3 tablespoons lardons – or chopped bacon
2 tablespoons parsley, chopped

Oven 150C/ 300/ Gas 2

Ask your butcher to trim the excess fat off the oxtail and to discard it. Chop the oxtail into pieces and immerse them in the marinade overnight.

Remove the pieces of meat and pat them dry with kitchen paper; strain and reserve the marinade, patting the vegetables dry too, and setting them aside. Seal the meat in a frying pan, in a mixture of oil and some of the butter, browning the pieces on all sides over great heat. Put the meat aside into a very large casserole.

Wipe out the frying pan, melt some more butter and turn the dried vegetables in it until they, too, go brown. Add a tablespoon of flour to the mixture and stir it in. Add the contents of the frying pan to the meat in the casserole.

Deglaze the frying pan with the brandy and add that, too, to the pot. Next, wipe the frying pan again and fry the chopped bacon; add it to the casserole too.

Now boil up the marinade liquid in a clean saucepan and reduce by a third. Add that to the pot, with the thyme, peppercorns and bay leaves and just enough brown stock to cover the contents. Cook it in the oven for 4 hours, or until the meat comes easily away from the bone.

When it is tender, carefully remove the pieces of oxtail from the casserole and pass the sauce through a fine sieve. Stir in the sugar. Allow the fat to rise to the top and skim it off. Return the oxtail to the casserole, with the sauce.

Finally, prepare the remaining vegetables. Slice the carrots into 1 cm rounds and turn them in butter over gentle heat, with the onions, before roasting them for 25 minutes. Stir them all carefully into the casserole and reheat the whole gently.

Garnish the dish with crisply fried bacon pieces and parsley and serve with a parsnip purée.

Parsnip Purée

Serves 8

1.3 kg parsnips
60 g butter
150 ml double cream
nutmeg
seasoning

Peel, roughly chop and boil the parsnips until they are very soft. Strain them and put them into a fodd processor, add the butter and cream, but be careful not to overwork the cream. Heat the purée gently in a saucepan.

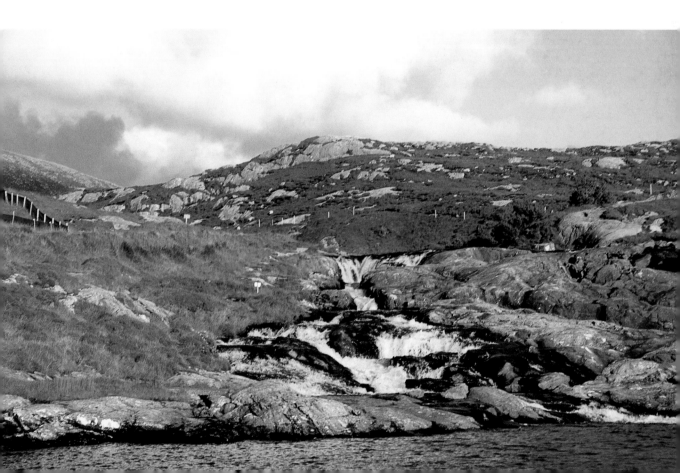

Puddings & Baking

Crème Brûlée

'Health that is purchased by a rigorous watching of the diet is but a tedious disease.'
Baron de Montesquieu (1689–1755)

This is probably the world's most delicious pudding, superb just as it is and also very adaptable. You can put fresh raspberries or strawberries in the bases of the ramekins, or prunes soaked in Armagnac, or virtually anything else you like.

Serves 6

600 ml double cream
200 ml whipping cream
75 g caster sugar
7 egg-yolks
1 vanilla pod
extra caster sugar for the caramel

You will also need 6 ramekin dishes.

Oven 130C/ 250F/ Gas 1

Whisk the egg-yolks with the sugar until the mixture is light. Slit the vanilla pod and add the seeds to the creams, with the pod. Bring it to the boil then strain it and add it to the egg-yolks and sugar, whisking all the time. Then pour it into a jug and fill the ramekins to the top. Bake them in a bain-marie for 2 hours, or until they are set.

Remove the ramekins and allow them to cool. Then sprinkle a thin layer of sugar over the surfaces. Melt the sugar either with a blow-torch or under a fierce grill, just enough for it to caramelise. On no account keep the ramekins in the fridge or the tops will go soggy.

Chocolate Cake

'Love and gluttony justify everything'
Oscar Wilde (1854–1900)

Every cookery book needs at least one good chocolate cake: this is mine. It is deliciously moist and very adaptable: you could layer it with fruit, or dust it with cocoa or icing sugar.

Serves 8

200 g good plain chocolate
2 tablespoons freshly made coffee
1 tablespoon rum
120 g unsalted butter
130 g caster sugar
6 egg-yolks
70 g plain flour
60 g ground almonds
7 egg-whites

You will need a 23 cm cake tin, preferably loose-bottomed.

Oven 180C/ 350F/ Gas 4

Prepare the tin by buttering it thoroughly and dusting it with flour. Melt the chocolate in a bain-marie and stir in the butter, coffee and rum. Allow it to cool a little while you beat the sugar and yolks together, until pale, then beat in the chocolate mixture. Fold in the flour and ground almonds. Beat the egg-whites to soft peak and then fold them, too, into the mixture before transferring it to the tin.

Smooth the surface and bake the cake for about 45 minutes – test it with a skewer: if it comes out of the cake clean, it is ready. Let it settle in the tin for a few minutes then turn it out to cool on a rack.

Raspberries I have used a lot of raspberries in this book, because they are so plentiful on Harris and their season goes from May right through until September.

They are grown in tunnels and their quality is unparalleled. This may be partly because climatic conditions demand that they take a long time to mature and develop their flavour. No chemical sprays are used in their cultivation and they are liberally watered by soft and wonderfully pure rain.

Strawberries are grown in similar conditions, again for a remarkably long season and they too are sweet and good. In many of the following recipes, the two are interchangeable.

Sydney Smith would have been astonished. It was he who wrote that 'no people has so large a stock of benevolence of heart as the Scotch – They would have you even believe they can ripen fruit'. . .

Raspberry soufflés.

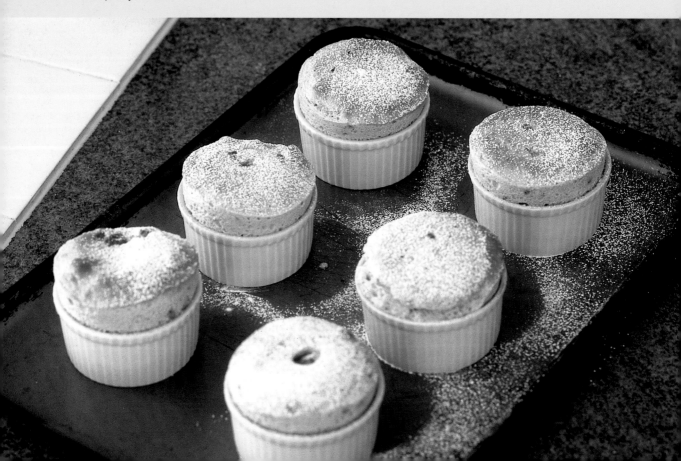

Raspberry Soufflés

Serves 6

200 g raspberries
3 tablespoons crème pâtissière (see Basics)
8 egg-whites
45 g caster sugar
1 egg-yolk
a few drops of good vanilla essence
caster sugar for dredging

You will also need 6 ramekin dishes.

Oven 180C/ 350F/ Gas 4

Butter the ramekins very thoroughly, dredge them with sugar and put them in the fridge. Crush a third of the raspberries with a fork. Mix the crème pâtissière with the vanilla essence, the egg-yolk and the crushed raspberries. Beat the egg-whites until they form soft peaks and then add the sugar and beat again, for a few seconds. Fold one third of this into the raspberry mixture, to slacken it, and then fold in the rest, gently so as not to lose the air. Fold in the rest of the whole raspberries.

Fill the chilled ramekins to the brim. Smooth the tops and run your thumb around each, just inside the rim (this helps rising). Pop the soufflés straight into the oven for 7–8 minutes and serve them immediately, sprinkled with icing sugar.

Raspberry Tart

This simple tart is adaptable for any other fresh fruit.

Serves 6

1 quantity of rich shortcrust pastry (see Basics)
1/2 quantity crème pâtissière (see Basics)
125 ml double cream
450 g fresh raspberries
icing sugar for dusting
fresh mint leaves

Oven 200C/ 400F/ Gas 6

Roll the pastry out into a thin circle. Use it to line a buttered, loose-bottomed 23 cm flan tin. Prick it all over with a fork and bake it 'blind' for 15 minutes – the best way of doing this is to put some tinfoil on top of the pastry and fill it with either ceramic baking-beans, dried peas or rice.

Remove the foil and beans/rice and replace the tart in the oven for a further 5 minutes until it is pale gold in colour (keep an eye on it, that it does not burn).

Remove the pastry again and allow it to cool. Take it out of the tin, with great care, and put it onto a serving dish. Whip the cream lightly and fold half of it into the crème pâtissière, to loosen it. Fold in the rest of the whipped cream and spread it over the base of the tart. Fill it with raspberries. Just before serving dust it with icing sugar and decorate it with mint. Serve it with a raspberry coulis (see next page).

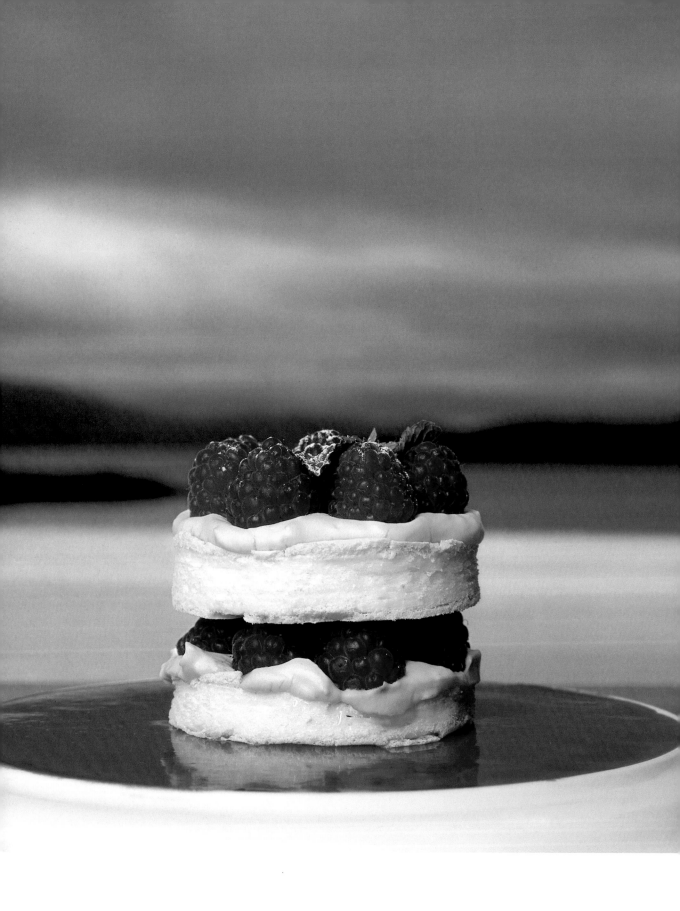

Lady Sophie's Meringue

The benign and gentle spirit of Lady Sophie Scott, who lived at Amhuinnsuidhe long ago, is sometimes thought to drift around the castle. I have named this wonderful pudding after her as it is beautiful, pale, and light as air. It is also remarkably easy to make. Do not be tempted by 'fat-free' crème fraîche, as it hasn't the substance for the job.

Serves 4

6 egg-whites
320 g caster sugar
1 rounded tablespoon cornflour
2 teaspoons lemon juice
240 ml crème fraîche
225 g fresh raspberries

Oven 130C/ 250F/ Gas 1

Line a shallow roasting tin (about 30 cm x 20 cm) with greaseproof paper. Whisk the egg-whites to soft peaks in a clean bowl then add half the sugar and continue whisking. Add the cornflour and the lemon juice, still whisking. Finally whisk in the remaining sugar.

Spread the mixture evenly over the tin and bake it for about 20 minutes, until the surface is beginning to crack. Remove it from the oven and allow it to cool on the tray.

Spread a clean tea towel on the table and invert the meringue onto it, then remove the tin and peel off the paper. Spread the crème fraîche on top and scatter the raspberries over it before rolling it, lengthwise, into a log, using the tea towel to help you handle it. Do not worry that the top appears cracked: it is meant to. Let it settle before putting it onto a serving dish.

An alternative way of serving this, which we prefer at the castle, is to cut circles of the meringue before (and instead of) rolling it, using a round cutter: I also beat some double cream into the crème fraîche if doing it this way and top each circle with prettily arranged raspberries and a mint leaf.

Raspberry Coulis

This can be kept in the fridge for up to 4 days and can be used to accompany sorbets, mousses, ice creams etc. The sweetness of the coulis depends on taste, so you can use more or less syrup, as you like.

Serves 6

250 g fresh raspberries
juice of 1 lemon
about 80 ml of syrup no. 1 (see Basics)

Puree the fruit and the lemon juice in a blender, pass it through a fine sieve it and then add the cold syrup.

Mousse Nouvelle

There are two special things about this glamorous pudding: one is the fact that, though very light in texture, it keeps its shape and can be sliced, almost like a cake: the other is its unusual biscuit base. It is important to use leaf gelatine, which is easier to manage and cleaner in taste than the powdered sort: soak the leaves for at least 15 minutes, in a flat baking tray or loaf-tin, until they are soft enough to squeeze.

I am very grateful to Jean-Christophe Novelli for the original idea, which I have adapted in this recipe. It works equally well with strawberry purée instead of raspberry.

Serves 8

300 g raspberries (fresh, if possible)
75 g unsalted butter
3 gelatine leaves
130 g lightly whipped cream
1 quantity biscuit base (see Basics)

For the Italian meringue:
3 egg-whites
130 g caster sugar

At the castle I use small square moulds, but you can use a 25 cm stainless-steel ring. Failing that, line a loose-bottomed cake tin with cling film (so as to avoid the metal reacting badly with the raspberries). You will also need a sugar thermometer and an electric whisk.

Cut the biscuit base so as to fit snugly inside the ring (or the tin). Soak the gelatine leaves in a bowl of cold water (see above). Rub all but a dozen of the raspberries through a fine sieve into a large bowl and put two tablespoonsful of the pulp into a small pan to warm. Squeeze the water gently from the gelatine leaves and add them to the pan, warming and stirring the mixture until the gelatine has dissolved. Stir in the butter until it too has melted and pour it into the rest of the sieved raspberries. Set it aside, stirring occasionally so that it doesn't start to set.

Make the Italian meringue: put 2 tablespoons of cold water into a small, heavy saucepan and add the sugar. Heat it gently and steadily – have a bowl of cold water and a pastry-brush handy in case crystals begin to form, in which case brush around the inside of the pan to disperse them. When it has reached 120C, set it aside and start whisking the egg-whites. When they have just reached soft peaks, add the syrup slowly and whisk continuously for 5 minutes until it is very smooth. Whisk a third of the meringue mixture into the raspberry mixture then fold in the rest, followed by the cream.

Spoon the mixture into the ring (squares, or tin) and refridgerate the mousse for at least 4 hours. Remove it from the fridge half an hour before serving, surrounded by the remaining raspberries. You could serve this with a raspberry sorbet (see next page) or a raspberry coulis (see previous page).

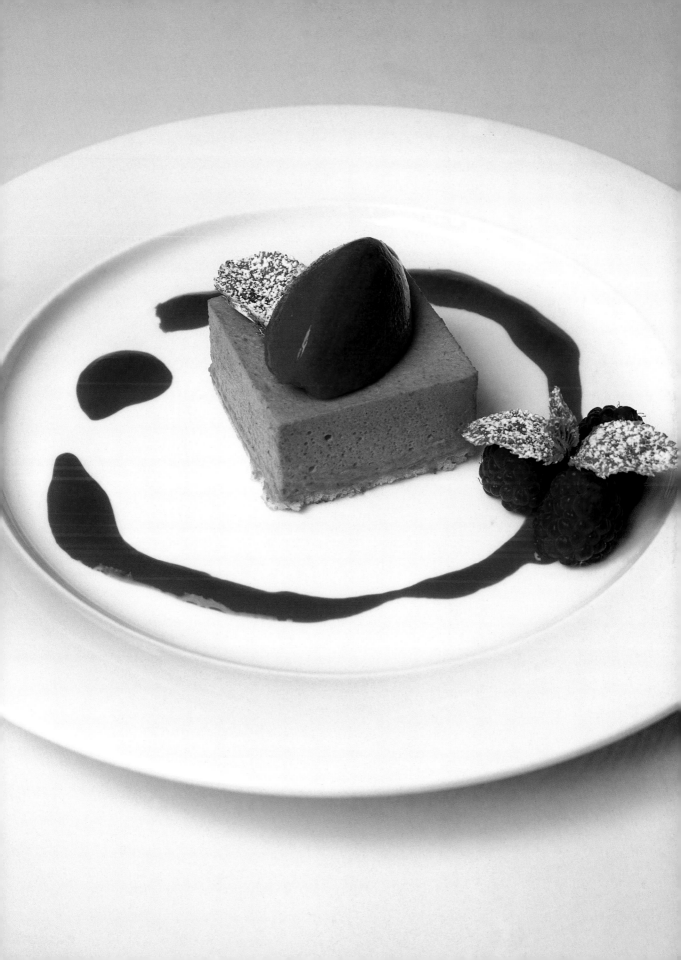

Raspberry Sorbet
with Tuiles

This is another very useful dish to have sitting in your freezer in the event of unexpected guests. It should be removed from the freezer about half an hour before you want to serve it. You really need an ice cream machine, but if you haven't got one, remove the sorbet from the freezer every now and again as it freezes and give it a stir to break down the crystals.

Serves 6

500 g fresh raspberries
juice of 1 lemon
1/2 quantity syrup no. 1 (see Basics)

Pass the raspberries through a fine sieve then stir in the lemon juice and add the syrup. This is a matter of taste: if you think it is sweet enough before you have finished adding it all, just stop. Either put it into an ice cream machine or freeze it, as suggested above. You could serve it with tuiles.

Tuiles

These very fine biscuits are lovely with ice cream and mousse as well as with this sorbet. They are also pretty good just on their own – but they don't keep. Eat them the day you make them. You will need a baking-mat and a sheet of plastic – say the top of an ice cream carton – out of which you have to cut a circle, about 7 cm in diameter.

75 g unsalted butter, room temperature
100 g caster sugar
35 g icing sugar, sieved
4 egg-whites
100 g plain flour

Oven 180C/ 350F/ Gas 4

Beat the butter in a mixer until it is very light. Add the caster sugar and the sieved icing sugar and beat again. Little by little, beat in the egg-whites, followed by the flour. Put the mixture in the fridge – ideally, for 4 hours.

Put your sheet of plastic (out of which you have cut a circle) on top of a baking-mat, on a tray. Spread the mixture thinly over the circle, using a palette knife. As you finish each biscuit, move the template.

When the tray is full, bake the biscuits for about 10 minutes or until golden brown. They harden rapidly as they cool, so if you want to roll them around a rolling-pin, or make baskets of them, do it as quickly as possible.

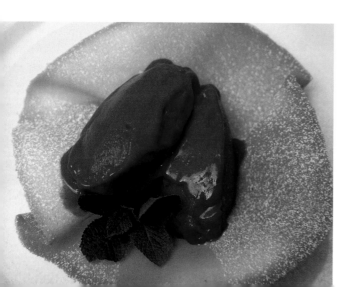

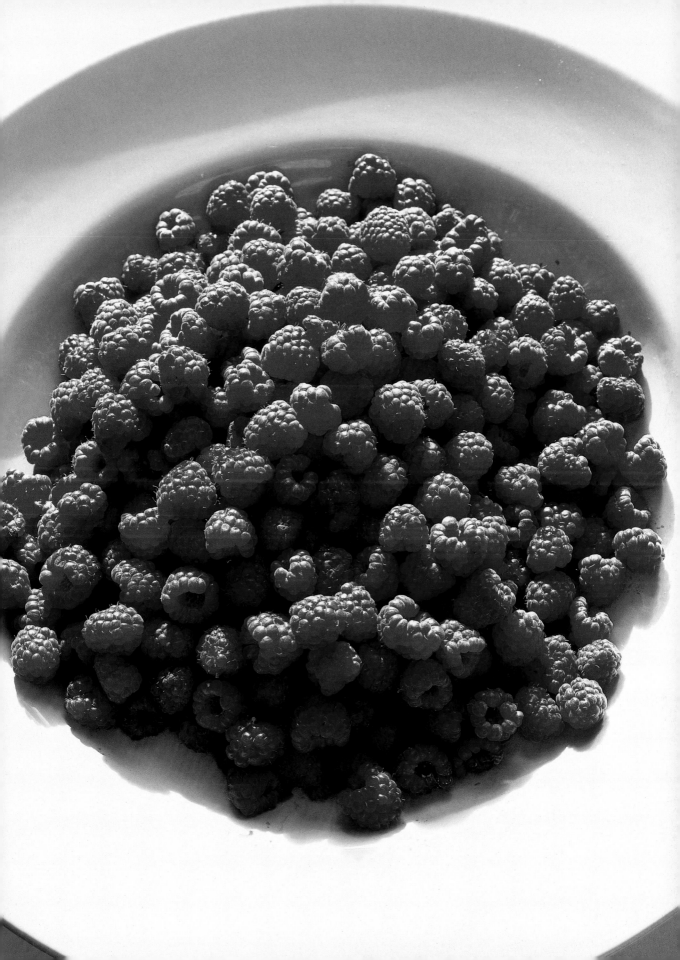

Baking There is a long tradition of home-baking in the islands. It's economical and substantial fare but the skills involved in its production are considerable.

At the castle we are very lucky to be able to learn from Effie Morrison how to turn out some of the finest of such delicacies. In the following section, I am indebted to her for her scones, oatcakes, scotch pancakes and, of course, for her inimitable clootie dumpling.

Oatmeal has always been versatile in this part of the world. In the 17th century it was observed 'When the Cough affects them, they drink Brochan plentifully, which is Oatmeal and Water boil'd together to which they some times add butter'. We tend to use whisky these days, for such purposes.

Another use for oatmeal – which is currently out of fashion – was to use it to make up a cold porridge, which you then put into your sporran and carried into battle. It has also been used for making soap, and there was once a widespread belief that 'there is a notable seasoning of phosphorus in oats which produces the praefervidum in genuine Scotsman'.

It makes very fine oatcakes too.

For oatcakes, scones or Clootie dumpling I happily hand over the apron to Effie.

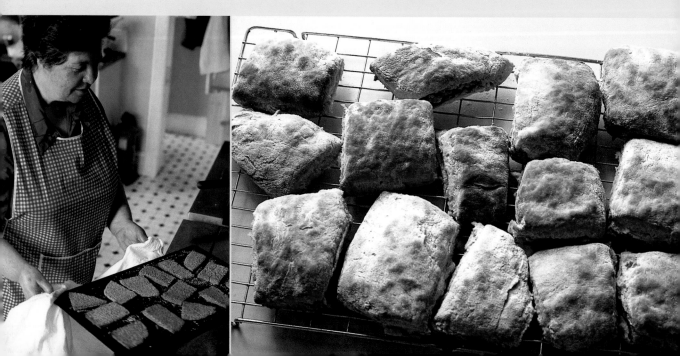

Oatcakes

In the Hebrides, oatcakes are often served with croudie – a soft cream cheese. They break easily, but this crispness is part of their charm.

350 g fine oatmeal
75 g butter
1 pinch baking powder
1 pinch salt

Oven 230C/ 450F/ Gas 8

Mix all the dry ingredients in a bowl. Melt the butter in about 115 ml of water. Add this to the bowl and mix it carefully together with your hands.

Roll out the mixture very gently on a surface which has been lightly sprinkled with oatmeal and cut it into 5 cm squares. Put the squares onto a hot baking tray and bake them for 20 minutes. Turn them over and replace them in the oven for a further 2 or 3 minutes. Leave them to cool.

Shortbread

This is a very useful stand-by for unexpected visitors – or a ceilidh. In the Hebrides, a ceilidh can mean anything from a full-scale dancing-party lasting until dawn to a casual visit.
When scoring the surface, take the knife halfway through the mixture, to make breaking it easier.

200 g unsalted butter
100 g caster sugar
200 g plain flour
100 g rice flour, or fine semolina

Oven 150C/ 300F/ Gas 2

Beat the butter until its pale and creamy then beat in the sugar. Sieve the two flours and beat them in gradually. With floured fingers, press it into a tin – it should be about 1 cm deep. If you decide to use a round tin, score the surface deeply into wedges, if you use a rectangular one, score it into fingers. In either case, prick the top all over with a fork and bake it for about 50 minutes, until it is pale, golden colour.

Allow it to cool a little in the tin, then turn it out onto a wire rack.

Scones

Serves 6

360 g self-raising flour
60 g caster sugar
45 g butter
1 heaped teaspoon cream of tartar
1 level teaspoon baking powder
1 egg
150 ml milk

Oven 200C/ 400F/ Gas 6

Mix the flour and sugar in a large bowl and rub in the butter until the mixture resembles breadcrumbs. Stir in the cream of tartar and baking powder and make a well in the mixture. Pour in the beaten egg and enough milk to produce a very soft consistency and mix it all gently together, drawing in the flour mixture as you go.

Turn the mixture onto a floured surface and roll it lightly until it is about 2 cm thick. Then cut it into triangles, put them onto a buttered tray and bake them for 10 minutes. Remove them and cool them on a rack.

Scotch Pancakes

You can whip up these little pancakes in no time, especially when hungry children are around but beware, you'll never make enough.

Serves 8

250 g self-raising flour
160 g caster sugar
1 heaped teaspoon baking powder
2 eggs
30 g unsalted butter
1 tablespoon golden syrup
200 ml milk

Mix the first three ingredients and stir in the eggs. Beat the milk in gradually, to make a thick batter. Melt the butter and syrup together and add them to the batter. Heat a griddle, or large frying pan, and oil it lightly. Drop spoonfuls of the batter onto it, flipping them over as soon as bubbles appear. Serve them hot, immediately, with butter and jam if you like.

Saint Clement's Cake

I couldn't resist including this light, fresh tasting cake which is made with olive oil instead of butter. I first came across it in Tuscany, when it was made by Conte Contini Bonacossi at La Tenata di Cappezzana: it has no connection at all with the Hebrides!

3 large eggs
300 g caster sugar
300 g plain flour
165 ml milk
165 ml extra virgin olive oil
1 teaspoon grated lemon zest
1 teaspoon grated orange zest
juice of one lemon
1 tablespoon baking powder

Oven 180C/ 350F/ Gas 4

Butter and flour a 25 cm cake tin. Beat the sugar and the eggs until they are pale and creamy. Stir in the remaining ingredients and bake the cake for 30–40 minutes, until it is golden brown. Allow it to cool a little in the tin and then turn it out onto a rack. Serve it with a glass of Drambuie.

Clootie Dumpling

There's a little book of Scottish folklore by Allan Morrison called *Ye Cannae Shove Yer Granny Aff a Bus*. This interesting work of reference contains a vital section on key rules for grannies, including the resounding command 'Make Plenty of Clootie Dumpling'.

This is a substantial and splendid dish. It would make a welcome alternative to Christmas pudding. The quantities are given in cereal-bowlfuls: I could try to translate these into grams, ounces or cups, but hell, it works like this and surely everyone has cereal bowls?

Serves 12 – or more

3 bowls self-raising flour
1 packet Atora suet
1 heaped teaspoon cream of tartar
1 level teaspoon baking powder
1 bowl granulated sugar
1 teaspoon cinnamon
1 teaspoon mixed spice
1 teaspoon ginger
1 bowl sultanas
1 heaped bowl raisins
2 tablespoons golden syrup
2 tablespoons treacle
640 ml hot water (approximately)

1 large piece of cloth, about 80 cm square – cotton sheeting will do.

Set a very large pan of water to simmer on the stove, with a saucer in the bottom to take the pudding. Mix all the dry ingredients together. Add the syrup, treacle and hot water and mix it all

together well. Sprinkle the cloth with water and then lightly dust it with flour. Put the pudding mixture in the middle and bring the sides up, tying it together tightly with string.

Put the pudding in the pan of simmering water: it should come three quarters of the way up the sides. Allow it to simmer gently for 3 hours, topping it up with boiling water as necessary.

Towards the end, set the oven 200C/400F/Gas 6

Take the pudding out and settle it to drain over a large colander or similar. Untie the string and slowly peel away the cloth, leaving a lovely round pudding. Before you take the cloth away completely, you'll have to invert it onto a large plate and pop the whole thing into the oven for 3 minutes to give it a crust.

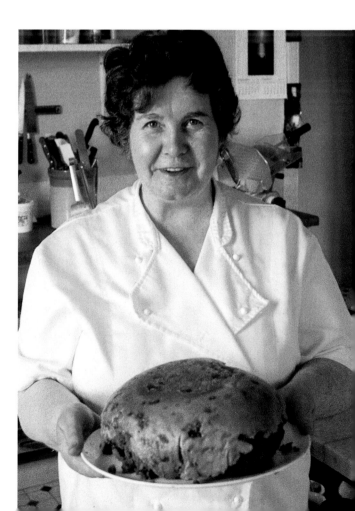

Glossary

Bain-marie
The dish containing the mixture to be cooked is placed in a second larger vessel of barely simmering water. This is a method of gently baking custards, mousselines etc. where direct heat would be too strong.

To blanch
A way of cooking vegetables very briefly, before using them in recipes. Generally, the vegetables are peeled/sliced, then plunged into boiling water for a minute, before being strained and refreshed.

To deglaze
A method of cleaning a pan with another liquid, whilst retaining all the flavours it previously contained. The liquid – often wine or brandy – is poured in, brought to the boil and stirred until everything is incorporated.

Julienne
Vegetables sliced or shredded into slender matchstick shapes.

Marinade
A mixture, usually containing oil, wine, herbs, spices and other flavourings in which meat or fish are immersed before cooking.

To refresh
A way of ensuring that blanched vegetables maintain their colour and/or shape. They are strained, then immersed immediately in very cold water before being strained again and reserved for further use.

To sear
To cook rapidly over a very high heat, in order to seal in the flavour.

To skin tomatoes
Many recipes demand that tomatoes should be prepared in this way. It is quite simple: with a sharp knife, remove the core of each tomato and cut a shallow cross on the round top. Plunge them into boiling water for 20 seconds then into a bowl of cold water: the skins should slip off quite easily. To deseed them, quarter them and scoop out the pips.

To truss
To tie up a bird for roasting. Start by crossing the legs up towards the breast. Then tie the feet together with a long piece of string, which is then passed and crossed underneath the bird and tied in a bow on top of the breast.

To turn vegetables
This is a way of preparing carrots, potatoes courgettes, etc. so that they are of uniform size and shape, for a special garnish. Peel the raw vegetables and cut them into batons, about 5 cm in length. With a sharp knife pare away the corners, producing a barrel shape (see page 23).

Basics

Eggs

When eggs, egg-whites and egg-yolks are used in this book, they are all eggs of 'medium' size (unless I say otherwise).

Ovens

Do remember that all ovens are different so that cooking times may vary. Use your judgement; if it seems to you that something needs a little less or more time than the recipe suggests, you are probably right to follow your instincts. Also, ovens should always be preheated.

Butter

I like unsalted butter, so when butter is mentioned it is always the unsalted kind. Salted butter may very well work with most savoury recipes so it is up to you. Under no circumstances should you use it for pastry!

Olive oil

I use extra virgin olive oil nearly all the time because I, personally, like it enormously. It is usually better to use the extra virgin olive oil for salad dressings but there is no need to use the very best for other purposes such as searing, sealing, frying etc...

Reducing and sieving

I sieve and reduce a lot, and you will, no doubt, be tempted to skip that part: don't, be patient, because it's important. Sieved ingredients have a finer, smoother texture. When reduced they have a much sharper, finer taste, and all this makes for fine cooking, which is what I am striving for.

Quantities

The quantities given in this book are measured in kilograms and litres. If you feel uncomfortable with metric measurements, use the following tables to convert the recipes. Such conversions are always approximate (rounded up or down) so never mix imperial and metric in the same recipe.

Solid measurements

metric	imperial	metric	imperial
25 g	1 oz	350 g	12 oz
50 g	2 oz	370 g	13 oz
85 g	3 oz	400 g	14 oz
100 g	4 oz	425 g	15 oz
140 g	5 oz	450 g	16 oz (1 lb)
170 g	6 oz	675 g	1½ lb
200 g	7 oz	900 g	2 lb
225 g	8 oz (½ lb)	1 kg	2.2 lb
255 g	9 oz	2.3 kg	5 lb
285 g	10 oz	3.2 kg	7 lb
310 g	11 oz	4.5 kg	10 lb

Spoon measurements

1 teaspoon = 5 ml spoon
1 dessertspoon = 10 ml spoon
1 tablespoon = 15 ml spoon

Liquid measurements

ml	fl oz	imperial
15 ml	½ fl oz	
30 ml	1 fl oz	
60 ml	2 fl oz	
150 ml	5 fl oz	¼ pint
190 ml	6.6 fl oz	⅓ pint
300 ml	10 fl oz	½ pint
450 ml	15 fl oz	¾ pint
600 ml	20 fl oz	1 pint
900 ml	30 fl oz	1½ pint
1000 ml (1 litre)	34 fl oz	1¾ pint

Biscuit Base

This quantity is plenty for one mousse.

100 g ground almonds
100 g caster sugar
1 egg
1 egg-yolk
25 g unsalted butter, melted
20 g plain flour
1 dessertspoon Kirsch or similar liqueur (optional)
3 egg-whites
1 dessertspoon caster sugar

You will also need baking parchment, or a 'magic carpet' baking sheet.

Oven 200C/ 400F/ Gas 6

In a large bowl, combine the first 6 ingredients (and the liqueur, if you like). Whisk the egg-whites to soft peaks, then add the spoonful of sugar. Use a little of this to slacken the almond mixture, then fold in the rest gently, so as not to lose too much air.

Spread the mixture on the baking parchment, in a rough circle. Bake on an oven tray for about 10 minutes – check after 5 – until it is pale golden brown. Remove it from the oven and leave it to cool on the parchment until you are ready to use it.

Bread Sauce

Bread sauce is one of those things you either love or hate. If like me you love it, you cannot imagine roast chicken or grouse without it.

Serves 4

1 small whole onion
6 whole cloves
150 g fresh breadcrumbs
500 ml milk

90 ml double cream
seasoning

Stick the cloves into the onion and put it in a small pan with the milk. Bring it to the boil and allow it to cool and infuse. Remove the onion and beat in the breadcrumbs, simmer for about 3 minutes and at the last minute stir in the cream and season to taste.

Brioche

This quantity makes two loaves. If you have a mixer with a dough hook, the process is much easier – but it is quite possible to do it by hand. Prepare it in the evening for the next day's breakfast.

625 g plain flour
45 g fresh yeast
40 g caster sugar
3 level teaspoons salt
6 eggs
225 g unsalted butter, softened
1 egg-yolk for glazing

Butter two loaf tins thoroughly and set them aside while you make the dough. Crumble the yeast and flour together in a bowl. Mix in the sugar and salt and then beat in the eggs, one by one, until they are well incorporated. Add the butter, one tablespoonful at a time. Beat (or knead) it thoroughly for a further 10 minutes.

Turn the dough out onto a lightly floured surface and cut it in two. Shape each half into a ball and tuck it into a tin. Leave it in a warm place for about an hour, to rise, and then put it into the fridge, wrapped in cling-film, overnight.

Oven 200C/ 400F/ Gas 6

Brush the surface of the loaves with egg-yolk, making sure that it doesn't touch the tin – which would inhibit rising – and bake them for 40 to 45 minutes.

Brown Stock

Ask your butcher to let you have some bones for this: it is particularly useful if they contain marrow. Use it for all beef and lamb dishes.

2 kg beef or veal bones
2 large onions, quartered
2 carrots, roughly chopped
2 bay leaves
1 dessertspoon black peppercorns
4 whole cloves
any available herbs

Oven 220C/425F/Gas 7

Roast one of the onions with the bones for about an hour – this length of time gives a good colour and flavour to the stock.

Put the bones and onion with everything else into a large pot and cover it all with water. Bring it to the boil and simmer it for about 4 hours, topping it up when necessary and skimming occasionally. Strain it and allow it to cool. Keep it in the fridge and discard the fat before using the stock.

Chicken Stock

This is the most useful stock of them all. You can make it with the bones of one chicken or of many, depending on circumstance. If you'd like the stock to look darker, roast the bones in a hot oven for an hour before you start.

the bones of one chicken
1 onion, roughly chopped
1 carrot, roughly chopped
1 stick celery, roughly chopped
2 sprigs parsley
2 sprigs thyme
2 bay leaves
1 teaspoon black peppercorns
1/2 bottle white wine

Put everything into a pan and cover it with water. Simmer for 4 hours, skimming occasionally, then strain it through a fine sieve and allow it to cool.

Clarified Butter

This is a very useful commodity. Unlike simple butter, it doesn't burn.

250 g butter

Melt the butter gently in a small pan. Allow it to cool a little until a milky residue has formed at the bottom. Pour off the pure butter into a bowl and store in the fridge until you need it.

Court-bouillon

This stock is sometimes known as a nage and is used to cook fish and in certain sauces.

2 onions
2 leeks
2 carrots
2 sticks celery
2 bay leaves
2 cloves garlic
2 pieces lemongrass
2 sprigs tarragon
2 sprigs parsley
1 dessertspoon black peppercorns
1/2 bottle white wine
1 1/2 litres water

Chop all the vegetables roughly. Put them in a large pan with the wine and bring it to the boil. Allow it to simmer for 5 minutes before adding the water and bringing it back to the boil, simmering it for a further half an hour, skimming occasionally. Leave it to cool before straining it.

Crème Pâtissière

This may be too much for the recipe you have in mind (e.g. Raspberry Soufflé) but it is very useful and keeps well in the fridge.

280 ml milk
25 g plain flour
2 teaspoons cornflour
4 egg-yolks
60 g caster sugar

Whisk the egg-yolks and sugar together and then add the cornflour and flour. Boil the milk and whisk it slowly into the egg mixture. Pour it into a clean pan and bring it slowly to the boil, until it thickens. Simmer it for a minute and then allow it to cool. Cover it with cling-film to prevent a skin from forming.

Fish Stock

The important thing about making stock from fish bones, as opposed to meat, is that it mustn't be cooked too long, or it goes cloudy.

2 kg cleaned bones, skins, heads, tails and fins of white fish
1/2 bulb fennel, roughly chopped
1 leek, roughly chopped
1 onion, roughly chopped
6 sprigs parsley
1 dessertspoon peppercorns
2 bay leaves
1/2 bottle white wine

If you are using fish heads be sure that the blood and liver have been removed before you start. Then cover everything with water and simmer for 20–30 minutes, skimming occasionally. Strain it through a fine sieve and allow it to cool.

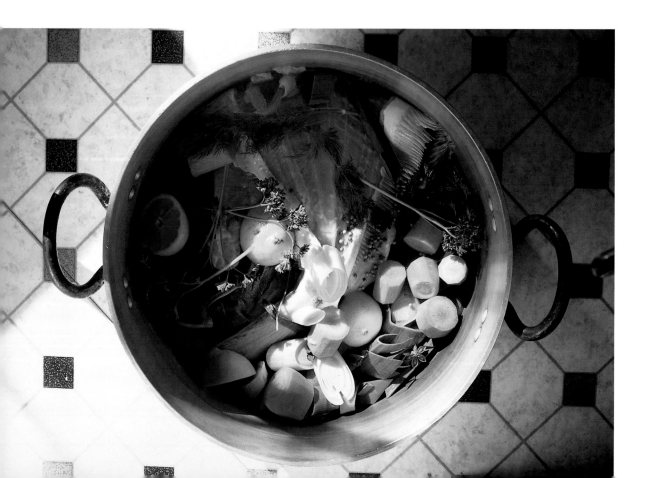

Game Stock

This stock will depend on whatever is available to you. The ingredients suggested below should be seen as a guide – use your discretion, imagination and resourcefulness.

There is no need to peel the vegetables, just wash them.

2 kg carcasses from game birds
venison bones
2 large onions, quartered
2 large carrots, roughly chopped
4 mushrooms
4 cloves garlic
the tops from 2 leeks, chopped
4 stalks celery, chopped
6 sprigs parsley
1 dessertspoon black peppercorns
1 tablespoon juniper berries
4 bay leaves
1 bottle red wine

Oven 230C/ 450F/ Gas 8

Roast the bones for half an hour then put them with everything else into a large pot, cover it all with water, bring it to the boil and simmer it for 4 hours, skimming occasionally. Strain it and allow it to cool. Remove and discard the fat, once it is cold.

Hollandaise Sauce

This is enough to accompany asparagus, salmon etc. for four people. There are many apparently simpler ways to make a similar sauce but this is the very best and not, in fact, very difficult: once you've tried it, you won't want to lower your standards.

240 g unsalted butter, clarified (see page 147)
1 tablespoon white wine vinegar
3 tablespoons water
1 bay leaf
8 peppercorns
4 egg-yolks
juice of 1 lemon
salt

Combine the water and vinegar in a small pan, bring it to the boil and reduce it to one dessertspoonful. Allow it to cool, then put the pan into a barely simmering bain-marie and whisk in the egg yolks, allowing the mixture to thicken slowly while you continue to stir: take care not to turn it into scrambled egg. Remove the pan from the heat and add the clarified butter, little by little, stirring constantly and finally stir in the lemon juice and a good pinch of salt.

If you need to keep the sauce warm before serving leave it over the warm water, off the heat, and stir it occasionally to prevent it from curdling.

Lamb Stock

There are many sheep in the Islands and we find it useful to have this stock ready for casseroles and sauce.

2 kg lamb bones and scrag ends
1 onion, roughly chopped
1 leek, roughly chopped
1 carrot, roughly chopped
4 tomatoes, quartered
6 mushrooms
3 cloves garlic
2 stalks celery, roughly chopped
1 tablespoon tomato purée
1 dessertspoon black peppercorns
6 sprigs parsley
2 sprigs rosemary
4 bay leaves
1/2 bottle red wine

Oven 230C/ 450F/ Gas 8

Brown the lamb for about half an hour in the roasting tin with the onion, leek and carrot. Transfer them to a large pan and add all the other ingredients. Bring to the boil and simmer, to remove the acidity from the wine, then cover everything with water and allow it to simmer again, uncovered, for about 4 hours, skimming occasionally. Pass the stock through a fine sieve and allow it to cool. Remove and discard the layer of fat from the surface when it is cold.

Mayonnaise

This recipe provides the base for a variety of different flavours – herbs, lemon, caper, gherkin, garlic – really anything that takes your fancy. These flavourings should be stirred in, according to taste.

Serves 4

300 ml sunflower oil
2 egg-yolks
3/4 teaspoon salt
1 teaspoon Dijon mustard
juice of 1/2 lemon

Whisk the egg-yolks and mustard together, then add the oil very slowly, drop by drop at first. Add salt to taste and beat in the lemon juice.

To make saffron mayonnaise:
150 ml extra virgin olive oil
1 egg-yolk
1 clove garlic, very finely chopped
a pinch of saffron
salt

Steep the saffron in 1 dessertspoon of boiling water and leave it to stand. Beat the egg-yolk and add the olive oil, drop by drop. When it is all incorporated, add the saffron (with the water), the garlic and salt, to taste.

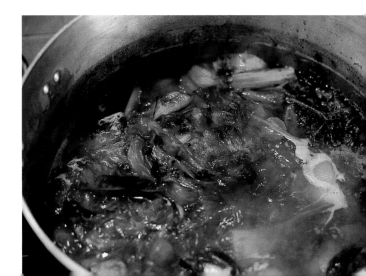

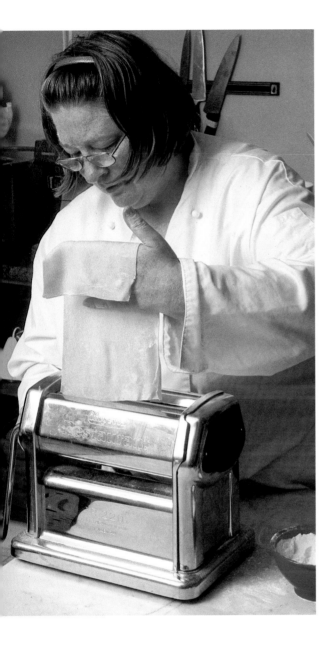

Pasta

This mixture is useful for all the pasta recipes in this book. It is wonderfully versatile: you can even deep-fry it in hot oil and use it for samosas, canapes and garnishes. You really need a pasta machine to make it, but you could use a rolling-pin, if you're blessed with a lot of elbow grease!

Serves 6

300 g white pasta/strong bread flour
3 egg-yolks
2 eggs
2 dessertspoons olive oil
pinch salt

Combine ingredients in a food-processor. Turn the mixture out onto a floured board and knead it lightly ✳, before cutting it into 8 pieces.

Roll each piece through the broadest mangle of a pasta machine 5 times to make sure the texture is smooth, then narrow the aperture until you have made long, broad ribbons and use it immediately.

✳ The mixture dries out quickly, so if you don't intend to use it at once, wrap it in cling-film at this point and keep it in the fridge.

Puff Pastry

The amount given here makes 700 g puff pastry, but I usually make double because, if you don't need to use it all at once, it will freeze very well. Reading this, it may seem to take a very long time to make, but each process only takes a few minutes. The finished product is very useful and much nicer than commercially available pastry.

375 g plain flour
340 g unsalted butter, at room temperature
10 g salt
110 ml water

Mix 250 g of the flour with the salt, 35 g of melted butter and the water in a bowl to make a dough. Shape it into a ball and cut a deep cross into the surface. Cover it with cling-film and put it into the fridge for half an hour. Beat the rest of the butter into the rest of the flour. Wrap this in the same way and put it into the fridge.

Remove the first parcel and put it onto a floured surface. Roll it from the middle into the shape of a four-leaved clover, keeping the centre part slightly thicker than the rest. Take out the other parcel and put it onto the central part, folding the clover leaves over the top. Roll this into a rectangular shape and fold it, from the sides, until it is in three layers.

Put it back into the fridge, on a floured tray, for a further half-hour then repeat the rolling and folding process again, twice. Return it to the fridge for at least two hours before you use it.

If you have any left over, do not scrunch it up into a ball but save it wrapped, in its layers, in the fridge or freezer.

Rich Shortcrust Pastry

It really is worth giving yourself enough time for this pastry to settle in the fridge before using it. It helps considerably to prevent it from shrinking during cooking. Though the quantities are unusual for shortcrust, they produce a marvellously versatile pastry to use with any fruit – or, if you omit the sugar, for savoury flans, pies, tarts etc.

240 g plain flour
170 g unsalted butter
1 dessertspoon icing sugar
1 egg-yolk
2 tablespoons cold water (if using Method 1) or
1 tablespoon cold water (if using Method 2)
a pinch of salt

Method 1:
Chop the cold butter roughly and put it into a food-processor with the flour. Zap it briefly until it looks like breadcrumbs then add the icing sugar and salt and give it another second of whizzing. Finally add the yolk and water, mixed, and continue just until it forms a ball. Take it out of the machine and put it onto a lightly-floured surface, taking care not to handle it too much. ✶

Method 2:
Allow the butter to soften at room temperature. Sift the flour with the icing sugar and salt onto a flat surface and make a well in the centre. Pour in the mixed yolk and water and draw the flour in slowly with your fingertips until it is well incorporated. ✶

✶ Wrap the ball of pastry in cling-film and put it into the fridge for half an hour.

Syrup no. 1

This is a simple syrup to be used for coulis and sorbets.

250 g caster sugar
250 ml water

Bring the ingredients to the boil, stirring throughout. Simmer it for 2 minutes and then allow it to cool. Keep it in the fridge until required.

Syrup no. 2

This syrup is useful for poaching fruit.

500 ml water
250 g caster sugar
1 vanilla pod (optional)

Bring all the ingredients to the boil, stirring throughout. Simmer it for a minute and then allow it to cool. Keep in the fridge.

Tapenade

This tasty and useful paste can be kept in the fridge for months and can be used for many recipes – canapes, sauces (for pasta) and toppings, for instance. It also makes a delicious dip.

200 g olives, pitted
50 g capers, drained
50 g anchovies, with oil
1 clove garlic
a good pinch of cayenne pepper
1 tablespoon good olive oil

Combine the first 5 ingredients in a food-processor, then add the olive oil. Store the paste, covered, in the fridge.

Tomato Sauce no. 1

750 g tomatoes, skinned, deseeded and chopped
1 tablespoon tomato purée
150 g cold unsalted butter
1 dessertspoon caster sugar
seasoning

Liquidise the tomatoes with the tomato purée and sieve the mixture into a saucepan. Heat it gently, without boiling and beat in the remaining ingredients.

Tomato Sauce no. 2

This can be used cold, as a salsa.

**1.5 kg tomatoes, skinned, deseeded and
 chopped
1 shallot, finely chopped
1 clove garlic, finely chopped
basil
extra virgin olive oil
seasoning**

Soften the garlic and shallot in the oil then add
the tomatoes, the basil and the seasoning and
simmer for a further 10 minutes.

Venison Stock

**1¹/₂ kg venison bones
2 onions, roughly chopped
2 carrots, roughly chopped
1 leek, roughly chopped
3 sticks celery, roughly chopped
4 tomatoes, quartered
4 mushrooms
2 cloves garlic
2 sprigs thyme
1 dessertspoon black peppercorns
1 tablespoon tomato purée
1 dessertspoon juniper berries
2 bay leaves
1 bottle red wine**

Oven 230C/ 450F/ Gas 8

Ask your butcher to chop the bones up roughly.
Roast them in a baking tin with the onions,
carrots and leek. When they are well browned,
transfer them to a large pan and add everything
else.

Bring to the boil and simmer for 5 minutes to
reduce the wine a little and add enough water to
cover the bones. Allow it to simmer, uncovered,
for 4 hours, skimming occasionally. Pass through
a fine sieve and allow it to cool. Remove and
discard the layer of fat that will form when it has
been in the fridge.

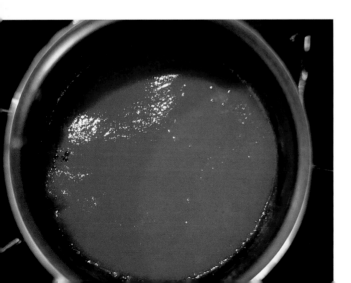

Vinaigrette

I like to keep a large jar of this readily to hand as it is so useful. If, however, this seems too much for you, merely halve the quantities.

250 ml olive oil
250 ml sunflower oil
100 ml white wine vinegar
1 teaspoon Dijon mustard
2 cloves garlic, peeled but not chopped
seasoning

Put the garlic into a screw-top jar. Mix the vinegar and mustard together and then add the two oils and seasoning to taste (a liquidiser is not essential, but it does produce a superb liaison). Pour it on top of the garlic and keep it in a cool place, but not the fridge. Shake it before use.

White Sauce

This simple sauce can be flavoured with anchovies, parsley, cheese, onions – almost anything you like. The important thing is to cook it long enough for it not to taste floury, and to keep stirring it so that it does not burn. Conventionally, equal quantities of flour and butter are used but I find that using a little more butter lessens the risk of lumps and makes a nicer sauce.

40 g unsalted butter
35 g plain flour
350 ml milk, warmed
seasoning

Melt the butter in a saucepan then remove it from the heat and stir in the flour. Return it to the heat and cook it for a minute, stirring it constantly and then add the milk, gradually, until it thickens. Allow it to simmer gently, as you stir, for another few minutes.

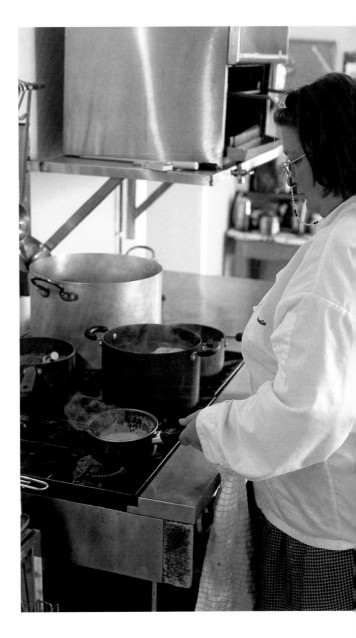

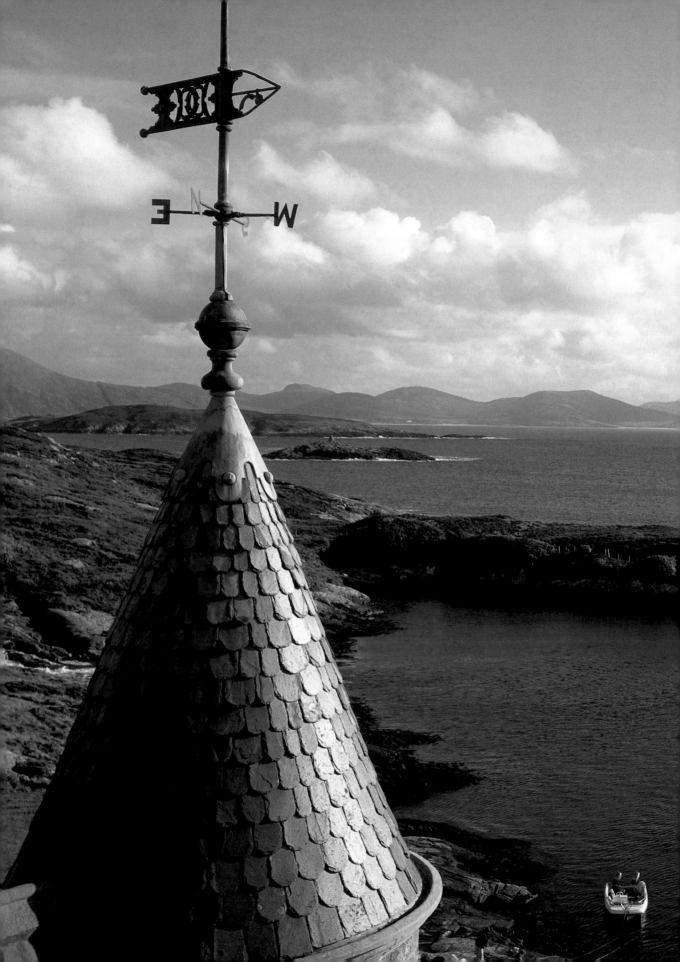

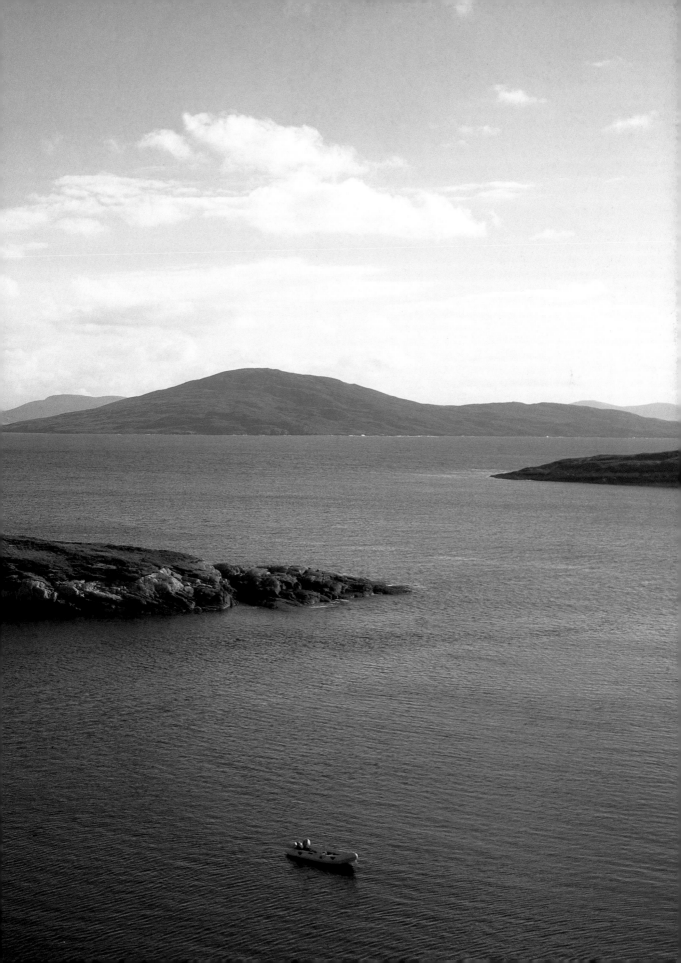

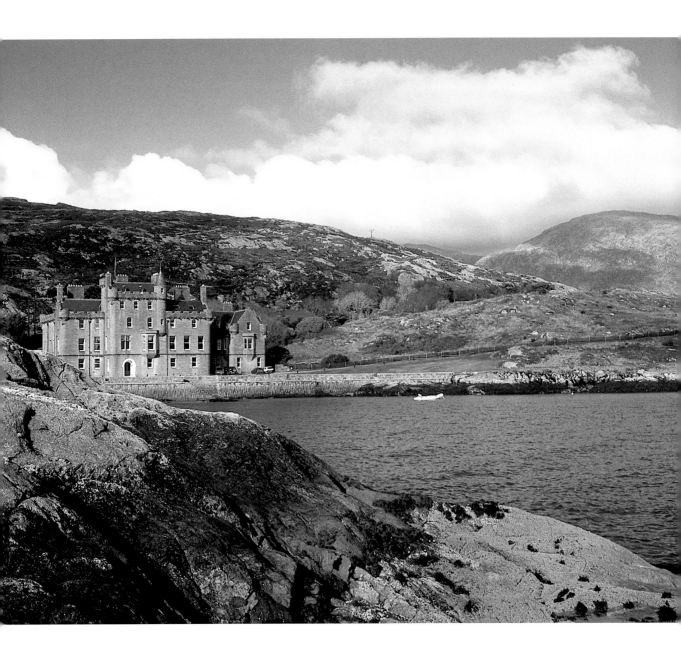

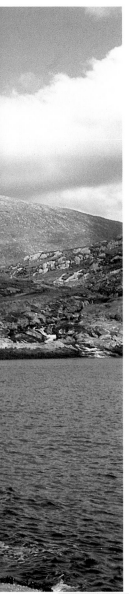

Amhuinnsuidhe Castle, home of Rosemary

Shrager's cookery school, stands sturdy, grey and crenel-
lated, facing the Sound of Taransay on the Isle of Harris. It
is a remote and isolated spot, part of a small Hebridean
community clinging to the furthermost limits of the
inhabited world.

A pleasing Norse legend about these Western Isles suggests an explanation of their shape and position. The story goes that in the time of the
Norsemen they formed one large land-mass known as The Long Island. In
the hope of shifting the whole place nearer to Norway, the Vikings put a
rope through a hole in the cliffs at the Butt of Lewis and began towing it
home. All was going rather well until a mighty storm arose, snapping the
rope and breaking up the land into a scatter of islands. They settled where
they now lie off the north-west coast of Scotland, forming a short, curving
chain and dwindling in size towards the south.

On the map today they look a little like the skeleton of an antediluvian
fish. The largest of them, the head of the fish, is the Isle of Lewis. The Isle of
Harris is at the base of the skull: though connected to Lewis geographically,
its mountains are higher and its character subtly different. But there's one
thing that all these islands have in common: theirs is a largely oral tradition.
Hebridean history is passed down through generations, legend mingling
indissolubly with memory: generally untrammelled by dates, it is often
embroidered by hearsay and imagination. Now and again, however, a fact
or two can be established, particularly when tangible corroboration comes
unexpectedly to light.

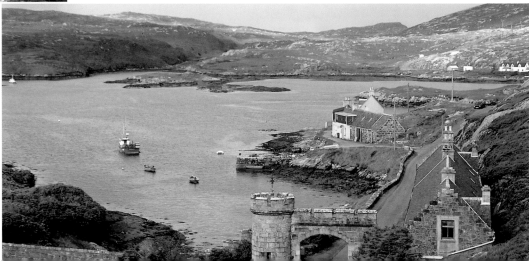

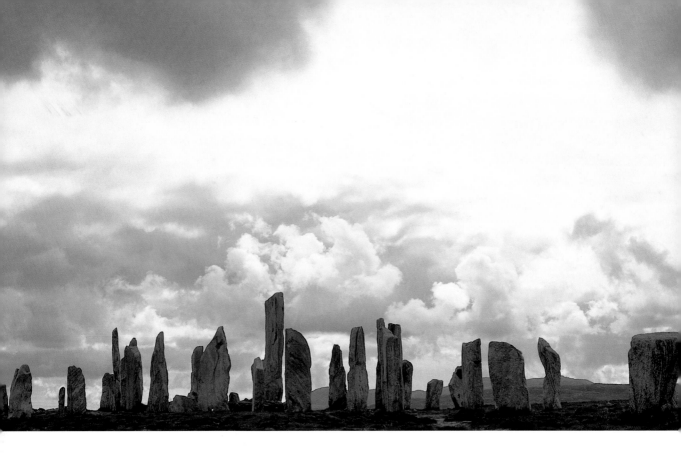

One such piece of evidence surfaced in 1991 when some scallop-fishermen, working the waters off the eastern coast of Harris towards the Shiant islands, dredged up a remarkable catch. It was an exquisite torc dating from about 1000 BC. Made of gold which was probably mined in the Wicklow mountains of Ireland, it offered a tantalising glimpse of an ancient yet sophisticated and mobile society with a long and complex pedigree. Even with modern methods of communication, these islands can still seem wild and desolate from the perspective of cosmopolitan, mainland Britain – yet they have been inhabited for at least five thousand years.

Such history as can confidently be ascertained is long and often turbulent. Standing stones bear mute if enigmatic testimony to the importance of the place in Neolithic times, long before Christianity came to the Hebrides – and

stayed. The Viking empire held sway for four centuries before sovereignty moved to the Lords of the Isles, then away to the mainland and the royal houses of Scotland and, later, of England. Throughout most of this time, however, real power on the Isle of Harris was held by the Macleod family. Their formidable ancestor is thought to have been a Viking called Olvir the Unruly and many of their descendants still inhabit the island.

Amhuinnsuidhe Castle

Alexander, the last of the Macleods to own the island, disliked it. He chose to spend all his life and fortune in Edinburgh and upon his bankruptcy in 1834, the Isle of Harris was sold to the Earl of Dunmore.

Charles Adolphus, the seventh Earl of Dunmore, was a keen fisherman. Using the architect David Bryce he built his castle beside a secluded and beautiful bay, choosing a spot where a river, bursting with salmon, cascaded over rocks to the sea (Amhuinnsuidhe means 'sitting on the river' in Gaelic). Over three years from 1864–7, the Ayrshire stones of which it is constructed were shipped in from Glasgow, already cut and shaped, at enormous expense. Sadly, when the young earl showed it to his English bride, she was disappointed and claimed, they say, that her father's stable-block at Holkham Hall was bigger. To please her an extra wing was added, causing such acute financial embarrassment that, in 1868, the family had to sell the estate.

Of the subsequent owners, the Scotts are the most affectionately remembered, having cared for the estate and its families for many decades. Under their aegis many writers visited Amhuinnsuidhe, including J. M. Barrie who brought the four orphaned Llewellyn Davies boys here for two months during the summer of 1912. Lady Sophie Scott was particularly well-loved. Childless herself, she would send food and blankets to families with new babies and her children's parties are still fondly recalled. A pudding in this book is named after her, as is a pretty bedroom at Amhuinnsuidhe and her ashes, together with those of her husband, are in a cairn on the hill above the castle.

Life on Harris

Today the hills of Harris form one of the last great unspoiled wildernesses of Europe. Along the west coast broad beaches of silver sand sparkle against the clear turquoise waters of the Atlantic, often unmarked even by footprints. Beside these beaches lies the machair, the flat sandy coastal plain of peat onto which lime-rich shell-sand is regularly blown. For a brief spell every summer the machair blooms with a succession of wild flowers: daisies, buttercups, purple orchids and harebells. Strips of machair enriched by seaweed are carefully cultivated; lambing sheep graze it in spring before being herded

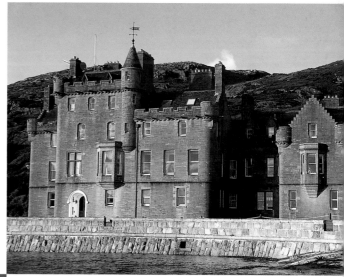

Opposite page, Calandish stone circle on the Isle of Lewis. *Above,* the castle. *Left,* a beach on Harris and undoubtedly one of the most beautiful in Europe.

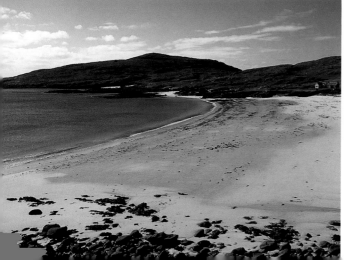

up to the hills, as they have been for centuries; at one time to the sheilings, now to their summer grazing.

The Harrisman

Hamish Taylor was born on Harris in the house next door to where he now lives, on the rocky coast at Flodabay. As is the case with many of today's residents, he makes his living outside the traditional areas of crofting, tweed-weaving and fishing: he is a radio engineer, working with specialist radio navigation equipment for ships... and he is also an expert on seaweed. Occasionally he visits the cookery school to talk about the various types of seaweed to be found on the shores and to discuss their uses – most Harris people no longer use it directly for food, but dig it instead into the otherwise thin and unproductive soil.

Hamish is an Elder of the Church of Scotland. It is a broad church whose practices fluctuate according to local tradition. On Harris, strict Sunday observance is still the norm and many activities are discouraged. Another local custom ensures that Communion is celebrated only twice a year, always on the same Sundays in each village. When Hamish speaks of the traditional crofting year, he uses this as an example:

"Tradition matters a lot here. One family might always cut their seaweed on the first Tuesday after Finsbay Communion (that's near the beginning of March). I used to think such traditions quaint, but I respect them now. Bladder-wrack cut then, from the middle range of the tide, has time to decompose for a couple of weeks by which time you'd be ready to plant potatoes, to give them their best

chance. Crofting families will be turning the ground with the seaweed and planting oats, too, during that time – and cabbages, carrots and turnips. There are fewer cattle to eat them these days, but oats are still grown – some for oatmeal, some for next year's seeds.

In May, the peat-cutting starts. We'll be handling it for the next few weeks. It's cut, then you lay it flat on the heather for three weeks. Then you build a small pyramid of four or five peats, with air-flow between them so that they dry for another month. Then you make bigger piles of them until they are dry and ready to take home in creels for winter fuel. In June, July and August the grass is growing, so we would cut it and make hay. In September and October it would be time to harvest the oats. The potatoes are ready too, but we have little frost here because of the Gulf Stream so they can wait, if they have to.

Sheep and cattle are the only animals we use traditionally: the ground is too steep and hard for horses. All the cultivation had to be done by spade and everything carried in a willow creel on your back. But traditionally every family had two milk cows and a few sheep, marked with colours and ear-tags.

As for fishing, there is a difference between summer and winter. Summer herring are very

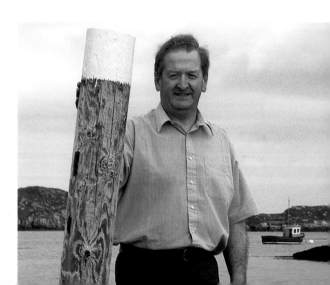

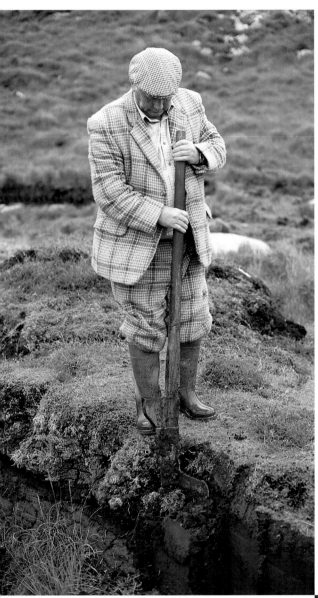

fat and oily. They are excellent eating but no good for salting: they're too oily. In winter the herring come inshore to spawn, after the end of September. They are thinner then, and grand for salting. I've some in barrels now. People have always known easy ways to catch fish. You can see old fish-traps across most of our estuaries - low walls built at the place where the lagoon dries out every day, but where there'd be enough water for the fish to swim in with the tide and shoal. And then, as the tide fell and the fish began to worry, the wall would break the surface and they would be caught. It's using nature and working with it: both clever and passive. There were so many fish then that my mother would speak of not being able to sleep at night for the sound of jumping fish.

This fish-diet was high in calories and salt. People needed that because they were so active, to replace the salt they lost in sweat. So much salt did them less harm when they were doing so much manual work - and fishing still absorbs a fair proportion of men of working age here.

There is little poaching. There is a story of a rainy day when the wife of the then owner of Amhuinnsuidhe took her guests out with umbrellas onto the bridge near the castle, to

Opposite page, Hamish Taylor. *Above,* peat digging. *Right,* Kenny (in front) and Alec Morrison.

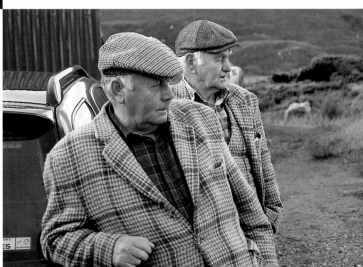

watch the salmon leaping up the falls. They looked downstream and there the fish were, leaping by the dozen. But when they turned to watch their progress upriver, they had disappeared. The answer was that a famous ghillie of the time was under the bridge waiting for the fish, with a gaff and a mail-bag! But there were plenty salmon to go round, anyway.

We say that if there were no watchers, there would be no poaching. Part of the fun when you're young is outwitting the watchers, up on the hills or beside the rivers. Besides, where some speak of poaching, my kind might speak of fishing, or hunting. There's a world of difference between doing it for financial gain and going out to fetch one for the pot – or to bait the ghillie! I remember there was one old ghillie who was also a watcher. He was called Big John Morrison. I went to see him when he was an old man in the hospital and I asked him: 'You know those nights you'd chase me all over the countryside – did you recognise who it was?' And he answered me straight away: 'Every time,' he said, 'and was I glad to see you.'"

Hamish speaks proudly of the islanders' famous reputation for scholarship. There is a higher per capita proportion of university graduates here than anywhere else in Scotland. He wonders whether it is because they have always had to use intelligence and common sense in order to look after themselves, to work alongside nature – or perhaps a diet of oily fish is really good for the brain.

He gives an example of this natural intelligence: in his photograph album is a picture of a man, spruced up in his Sunday best and smiling modestly. It is Murdo Macdonald. He lived right out in the wilderness between Huishnish and Uig. He went to school only one day in his life, in 1938, and that was to take his Highers. He got them all, including exams in Latin, Greek and Hebrew.'

Murdo's sister had taught him the alphabet. After that he learned everything by using the books carried on the Fleetwood trawlers which moored in the deep water at Loch Resort – they were his mobile library. "There is a minister still in Tarbert", says Hamish.

Below, time out on the hills. *Below right,* Murdo Macdonald.
Opposite page, Rosemary and Jonathan Bulmer examining the day's catch.

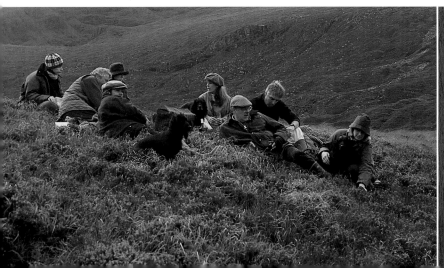
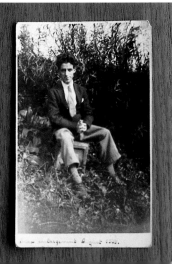

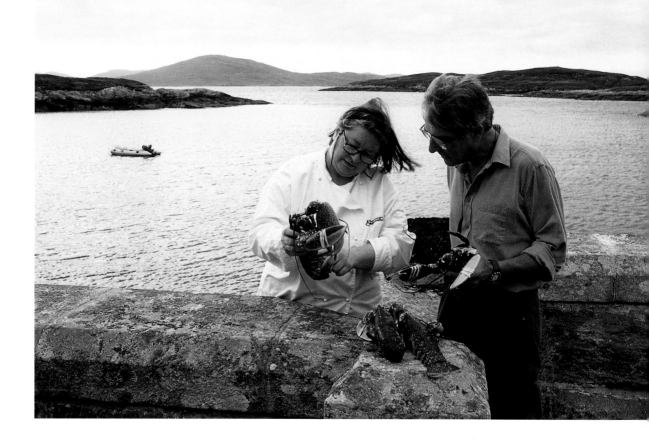

"Mr. Macrae, who's 82 now, and he passed his Highers on the same day. After Murdo passed, he'd intended to study Divinity at Aberdeen University. But he got sick and he was taken to Stornoway Hospital. And there, a doctor – a man who was highly trained – gave him the wrong medicine. And he didn't survive."

There's a lesson in that story and it could be this: given just a whiff of a fair chance, the inhabitants of this remote and physically challenging island easily take their place among the most highly motivated and resourceful people in the world.

The Landowner

Many of the residents of the tiny hamlet of Amhuinnsuidhe earn their living working at the castle or on the estate. The current owner, Jonathan Bulmer, has been in charge since 1995: it is he, in co-operation with Rosemary Shrager, who founded the famous cookery school. There he presides, a warm and generous host. He explains something of his passion for his home:

"The light in the Hebrides is a revelation. The poet Kathleen Raine once described it as 'a quality of the imagination'. There is a limpidity and cleanness in the air which is unique, even when the mist is down and rain sweeps horizontally across the hills. The ocean is never very far away and the great weather fronts drive in from the west. When the clouds lift and the hot sun burns away the mist from the hills and the lochs, the long, white beaches sparkle with the clarity and freshness of creation newly minted.

It is the sea, the endless Atlantic ocean stretching beyond comprehension to the west, that dominates. You see it from the top of every hill whose contours it has formed, you hear it in the dark winter nights and you

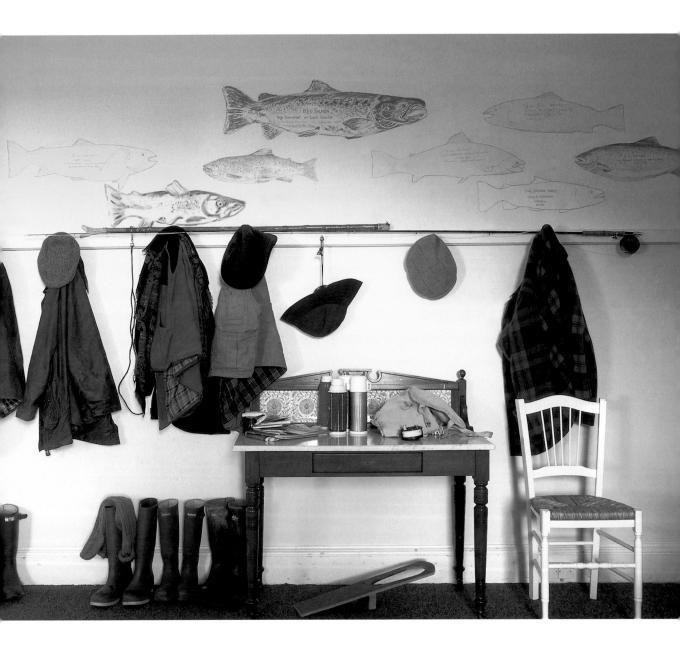

smell it on the warm summer breezes even in the deepest glens. It is the ocean that has shaped these islands and it dominates them still, lulling them summer-long in a sleepy embrace, chiding, chastising and terrifying with its winter storms, providing livelihood and taking life with equal invincible indifference.

For generations the sea, the sheep and cattle on the summer pastures, the potatoes and barley grown on the lazy-beds near the shore and up into the hills, all sustained a way of life that was self-sufficient, proud and civilised. Donald Monro, High Dean of the Isles, writing in 1559 describes a country 'verey fertill and fruitfull for corne, store, and fisching,' and 'many forrests, querin are aboundance deir bot not grate quantitie, verey faire hunting games without any woodes, with infinite slaughter....'

The ancient Forest of Harris had been preserved for deer by the Macleods since time immemorial. Roddy Macleod, our head stalker, was born on the island of Scarp, as was his brother George; the Maclennans at Govig came from Scarp and Peter Dan ran his sheep at Kinloch Resort – it seems only the day before yesterday. The postman, now retired, recalls walking from Morsgail to Kinloch Resort and Hamnavay twice a week – a round trip of thirty miles – barefoot. St Kilda was evacuated in 1930, Scarp in 1971, Taransay in 1974, Deirascleit and Kinloch Resort in the 1950s. Their black- houses are roofless, their schoolhouses in ruins, visited only for the gathering and the dipping of sheep, their communities all finally defeated by the ineluctable demands of an industrialised and uncaring world. The

vast hinterland of moor and rock, hill and loch is now largely trackless, treeless, home only to the red deer, sheep, golden eagle, golden plover, divers, grouse and snipe.

We live by the sea and every year the miraculous run of sea trout and of salmon appears in the sea-lochs and in the bays. They gather, leaping and rolling and splashing in front of the castle. They lie in deep shoals nosing into the fresh water, their fins and tails breaking the surface like plangent kelp. With the first spates of June and then in July they surge up the rivers at Miavaig and Kinloch Resort and into the lochs, driven by the irresistible atavistic urge to regain the burns where they were born. It is primeval, it is awesome – and it is the start of our sporting season.

Every morning the ghillies in their Harris tweeds gather outside the rod-room to greet the guests. There is Roddy Macleod the head stalker, Kenny and Alec Morrison, brothers who have lived here all their lives (Kenny is married to the famous Effie who works with Rosemary in the kitchens), Innes Morrison, Roddy's stepson and Fiona's son and Malcolm Macinnes from Achmore. Tackle is sorted, decisions made and the parties depart for the lochs – by estate road for Scourst

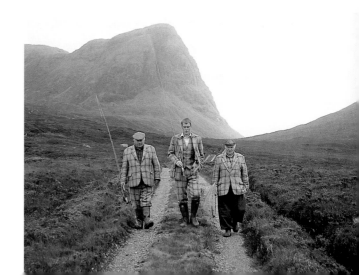

and Vochimid or on foot for the hour's walk to Glinnhe or Ulladale or Mug's.

We fish the lochs from a rowing-boat, traditional, clinker-built, drifting with a rod casting from either end, rowed back at the end of the drift by the ghillie. This can be hard work, for the stiffer the breeze the more likely the salmon are to take. All the lochs are remote and wonderful places but each has its individual magic. Scourst is moody – sometimes dour and sometimes wonderfully productive, Alec's private kingdom; Vochimid the most famous of them all, where J.M. Barrie dreamed up his story of Mary Rose; Ulladale under its huge overhanging cliff where eagles can be seen and heard as they launch their young on their first, terrifying flights; Mug's, a longer walk to what is not much more than a pool in the river, where the running fish can rest.

Amhuinnsuidhe has always been a famous fishery. Its records go back over a century and very little has changed. The fish are still coming and we are still catching them. Although we have not suffered the disastrous declines of some parts of the Western Highlands where the sea trout have all but disappeared we are, these days, a great deal more environmentally conscious and on the whole return the fish we do not want to eat. We also have a Fishery Trust on the islands whose biologists monitor stocks and suggest ways of improving the habitat.

In September the stalking begins in earnest. We aim to cull about forty stags a year and the same number of hinds. This is to maintain the health of the herd and to prevent overgrazing. It is also the most exhilarating of all the days on the hill, a potent cocktail of physical exertion, nervous tension, sublime and ever-changing scenery and the best companionship in the world. The long spy, the slow climb. The inevitable checks and frustrations, the sudden rushes, the hair-raising chances taken and the suppressed excitement of the final approach create a bond between stalker and rifle that is palpable but unstated – at least until the shot is cleanly taken and the tensions dissolved in a dram.

Roddy and Kenny and Alec are intuitive stalkers. They have known every inch of the ground all their lives; they can sense every shift in the wind, every downdraught; how it eddies through a corrie or backs round a cliff and they know by a sixth sense where the deer will be and how they will move, when they will panic and run, when they will feed quietly on, where they will settle. They are patient, calmly reassuring and impressive in their knowledge and skill.

We no longer use ponies to bring back the beasts but drag or 'hump' them to the waiting vehicle. Humping is an old Hebridean tradition: after the gralloch, the stalker ropes the carcass on his shoulders and carries it downhill. The average weight of a stag is 11 stone 6, or 160 lbs. I have only tried this once, with a very small hind, and I managed about two hundred yards and was stiff for a week. There is no more elemental experience than lying up in a remote corrie, pinned down by hinds, while stags roar all around. Or dragging a hind back through the snow, with the full moon rising over Loch Vochimid. These are indeed the days.

There are grouse too at Amhuinnsuidhe, a population which fluctuates wildly according to the success of the breeding season; we

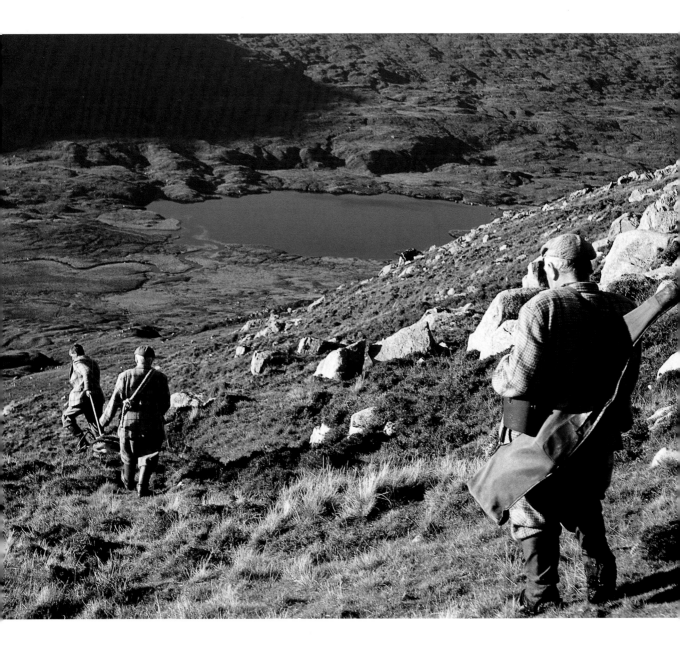

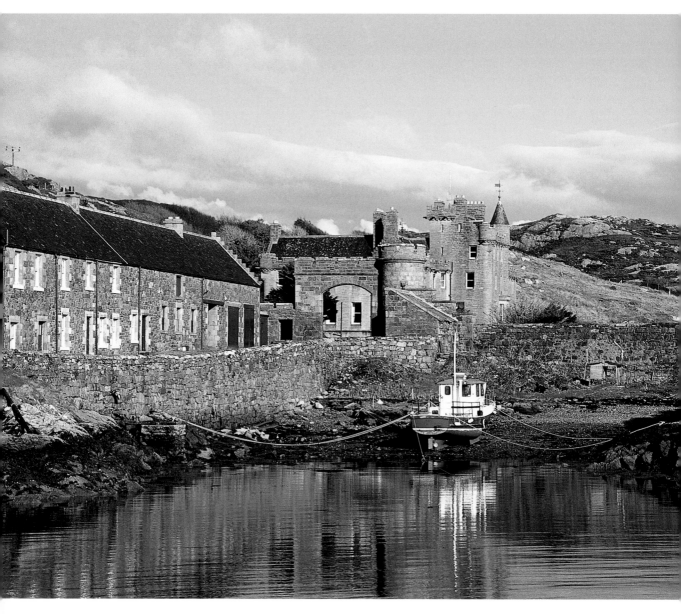

Above, the castle, in the background. *Right*, Sam and Effie peeling prawns outside the kitchens.
Far right, Rosemary with some of her students.

shoot them occasionally over pointing dogs, usually borrowed from Jim McGarrity at Aline. We rarely shoot more than ten or twelve brace in a day but it is always a joy to watch the dogs work and a welcome change from fishing in hot weather. Innes and Malcolm and the river-watchers do their best to control the feral mink who menace all the ground-nesting birds and take a terrible toll of juvenile fish.

The stags and the fishing finish in October. The winter months are spent catching up with the hinds, mending the roads (we have five miles of estate roads which are maintained every winter, literally by hand), repairing and repainting the boats and working on the fabric of the castle and the cottages. We also have a major replanting scheme in the garden and have recently planted 11,000 spring bulbs; thanks to the Gulf Stream there is nothing we could not grow here if we could keep out the salt and the wind, but that may take a long time.

The letting season used to be July, August, September and the first half of October. Now, with the cookery school, the painting and the music we are flat out from April to the end of October and employ up to 25 people, indoors and out, the vast majority of them local.

When I first moved to Amhuinnsuidhe I was asked why. I replied that I thought it was the loveliest place on earth. I still do and I believe, too – thanks to all my friends here who have worked so hard with so much laughter and good grace to make it possible – that we now have a future."

The Cookery School

The school was started in May 1999. Its purpose is to make the best use of both the magnificent raw ingredients provided by the island and waters surrounding it, and to pass on the unique and remarkable skills of the resident chef, teacher and passionate Harris-lover, Rosemary Shrager.

It is also a place of holiday and rest, where the anxieties and cares of bustling urban life can melt away in an atmosphere of timeless harmony – here with the season, the company, the island of Harris, and, of course, The Cook.

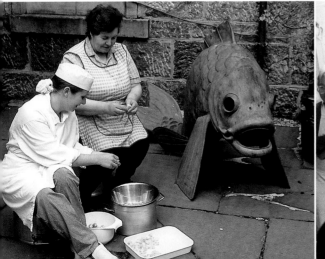

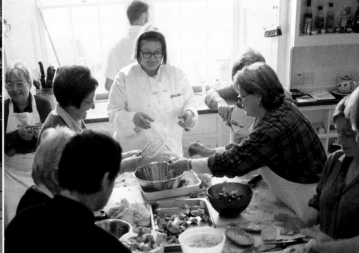

We are very grateful to Jonathan Bulmer, for his patience with this project and for the generous help and support he has given us, to Bridget Miller Mundy whose gentle tact and efficiency have been invaluable and to George Macdonald, Christine MacLeod and the rest of the team at the North Uist Estate office.

We would like to thank Margaret Hewitt and Fiona Macleod who keep the castle clean, comfortable and happy – and indeed all the rest of the staff, particularly Effie and Kenny Morrison and their marvellous family. Sam, a truly superb sous-chef, and her new husband Jonathan have been indispensable in the kitchens, helping us with remarkable, unfailing amiability, efficiency and good grace.

Others who have helped us on Harris are the kindly, invaluable Hamish Taylor; Bill Lawson, the genealogist and historian from Northton and Effie's uncle, Sandy Mackay. He and his charming wife Kirsty have run Amhuinnsuidhe Post Office for 50 years and shared with us their memories of working for the Scott family, long ago.

We are also grateful to Donald Norman Maclean, Ronnie Scott and Charles Macleod for keeping us supplied with fresh fish and meat and to Anderson Road Nurseries and Tony Robson for providing our delicious raspberries. We are grateful, too, to Andrew Farlie for his two excellent sous-chefs, Daren Campbell and Stevie McLaughlin, from *1 Devonshire Place*, Glasgow.

We tested many of these recipes over the millennial winter in East Sussex, where the following people were enormously supportive and produced superlative products for us: Clair Samuells, the splendid and resourceful fishmonger of Wadhurst; Chris Hillary, the magnificent butcher at Mayfield and the staff at Crittle's greengrocers, Wadhurst.

This book owes its very being to the vision, enthusiasm and commitment of David Campbell and the lovely Clémence Jacquinet at Everyman/Adelphi.

Finally, we are very grateful to our friends – especially to Kate and Philip Langford, whose generous hospitality knows no bounds – to our husbands, Michael and Rob, and to all our tolerant, tasting children.

Suppliers

I would like to recommend the following firms who supply their goods by mail order:

For fresh herbs:
Scotherbs,
Kingswell, Longforgan,
Near Dundee DD2 5HJ
Tel. 01382 360642

For fresh shellfish and flatfish
and for smoked salmon:
Ronnie Scott, Unit 2 Rigs Road,
Stornoway, Isle of Lewis HS1 2RF
Tel. 01851 706772

For Hebridean meat and, particularly,
black puddings:
Charles Macleod, Rope Work Park,
Stornoway, Isle of Lewis HS1 2LB
Tel. 01851 702445

For excellent cheeses:
Ian Mellis Cheesemonger,
205 Bruntsfield Place, Edinburgh, EH10 4DH
Tel. 0131 447 8889

For the finest peat-smoked salmon:
Mermaid Fish Supplies, Clachan,
Lochmaddy, North Uist HS6 5HD
Tel. 01876 580209

And finally, for the finest extra virgin olive oil
I am very grateful to my friends Simone and
Robert Benaim and to their olive tree farm,
Podere Sant'Antonio, Monte San Savino,
Arezzo, Tuscany, Italy.

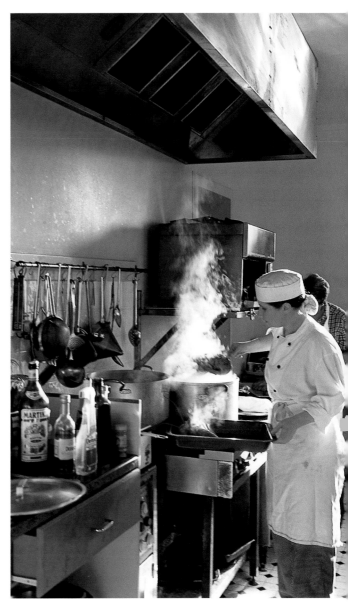

Sam boils lobsters in the castle kitchen.

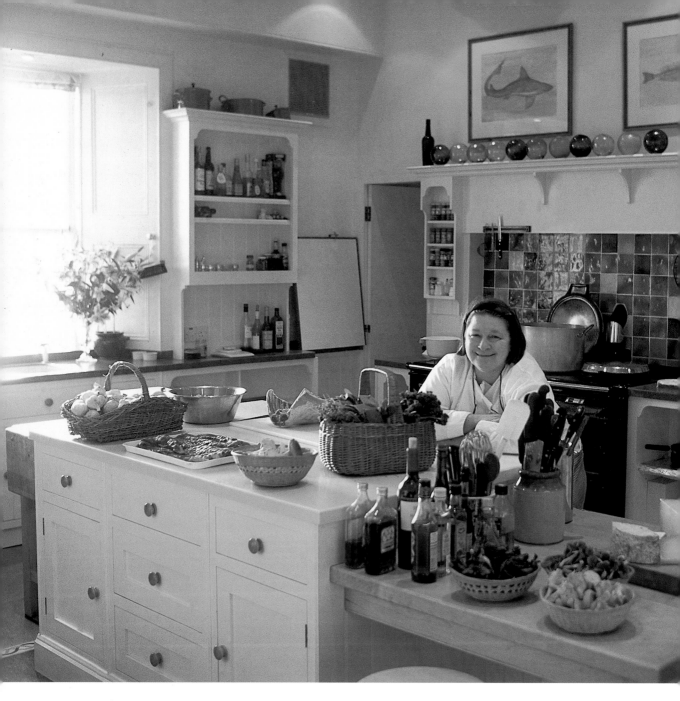

To find out about Rosemary Shrager's
Cookery School at Swinton Park, please
contact Swinton Park, Ripon, North Yorks

Tel. 01765 680900

E-mail: enquiries@swintonpark.com
Website: www.swintonpark.com